PRINCIPLES AND PRACTICE OF PHARMACOLOGY FOR ANAESTHETISTS

Principles and Practice of Pharmacology for Anaesthetists

T.N. CALVEY

BSc MD PhD (Liverpool)
Senior Research Fellow
Department of Anaesthesia
University of Liverpool
Honorary Consultant in
Clinical Pharmacology
St Helens and
Knowsley Health Authority

N.E. WILLIAMS

MB ChB (Liverpool)
FFARCS (England)
Consultant Anaesthetist
St Helens and
Knowsley Health Authority
Part-time Lecturer in
Clinical Pharmacology
University of Liverpool

WITH AN ADDITIONAL
CONTRIBUTION BY

H.L. GORDON

MB ChB (Liverpool)
FFARCS (England)
Consultant Anaesthetist
St Helens and
Knowsley Health Authority

FOREWORD BY

JACKSON REES

MB ChB FFARCS
Honorary Director of Studies
(Paediatric Anaesthesia) and
Clinical Lecturer
Department of Anaesthesia
University of Liverpool

SECOND EDITION

OXFORD

BLACKWELL SCIENTIFIC PUBLICATIONS

LONDON EDINBURGH BOSTON
MELBOURNE PARIS BERLIN VIENNA

© 1982, 1991 by
Blackwell Scientific Publications
Editorial Offices:
Osney Mead, Oxford OX2 0EL
25 John Street, London WC1N 2BL
23 Ainslie Place, Edinburgh EH3 6AJ
3 Cambridge Center, Cambridge
  Massachusetts 02142, USA
54 University Street, Carlton
  Victoria 3053, Australia

Other Editorial Offices:
Arnette SA
2, rue Casimir-Delavigne
75006 Paris
France

Blackwell Wissenschaft
Meinekestrasse 4
D-1000 Berlin 15
Germany

Blackwell MZV
Feldgasse 13
A-1238 Wien
Austria

First published 1982
Second edition 1991

Set by Excel Typesetters Company, Hong Kong
Printed and bound in Great Britain by
Hartnolls Ltd, Bodmin, Cornwall

DISTRIBUTORS
Marston Book Services Ltd
PO Box 87
Oxford OX2 0DT
(*Orders*: Tel: 0865 791155
         Fax: 0865 791927
         Telex: 837515)

USA
  Mosby-Year Book, Inc.
  11830 Westline Industrial Drive
  St Louis, Missouri 63146
  (*Orders*: Tel: 800 633-6699)

Canada
  Mosby-Year Book, Inc.
  5240 Finch Avenue East
  Scarborough, Ontario
  (*Orders*: Tel: 416 298-1588)

Australia
  Blackwell Scientific Publications
  (Australia) Pty Ltd
  54 University Street
  Carlton, Victoria 3053
  (*Orders*: Tel: 03 347-0300)

British Library
Cataloguing in Publication Data

Calvey, T.N. (Thomas Norman)
  Principles and practice of pharmacology for
  anaesthetists — 2nd ed.
  1. Drugs
  I. Title II. Williams, N.E. (Norton E.)
  III. Gordon, H.L.
  615.1024617

  ISBN 0-632-02742-8

This book is dedicated
to our wives

Contents

Foreword to the First Edition

A book with a title such as this might be thought merely to present an account of the drugs used in anaesthesia. In this case, the authors have achieved much more. They have presented their subject in such a way as to give their reader an insight which will make him not only a more competent anaesthetist, but one who will derive more satisfaction from his work by a more acute perception of the nuances of drug administration.

The authors demonstrate their awareness of the unique nature of anaesthesia amongst the disciplines of medicine. This uniqueness arises from the necessity of the anaesthetist to induce in his patient a much more dramatic attenuation of a wide range of physiological mechanisms than colleagues in other disciplines seek to achieve. He must also produce these effects in such a way that their duration can be controlled and their termination may be acute. The anaesthetist may be called upon to do this on subjects already affected by diseases and drugs which may modify the effects of the drugs which he uses. To be well-equipped to meet these challenges he needs a knowledge of the factors influencing the response to and elimination of drugs, and of the mechanisms of drug interaction. Such knowledge is much more relevant to anaesthesia than to most other fields of medicine. The authors of this book have striven successfully to meet the need of anaesthetists for a better understanding of these basic mechanisms of pharmacology. This is illustrated by the fact that one-third of the work is devoted to these principles. This should relieve the teacher of the frustration of having students who seem always to produce answers on the effects of drugs, but respond to the question 'Why?' with a stony silence.

Those sections of the book which deal with specific drugs show the same emphasis on mechanisms of action, thus giving life to a subject whose presentation is so often dull. The trainee who reads this book early in his career will acquire not only a great deal of invaluable information, but also an attitude and approach to the problems of his daily activity which will enhance the well-being of his patients and his own satisfaction in his work.

Jackson Rees

Preface

Since the publication of the first edition of this book in 1982, many new drugs have been introduced into anaesthesia. In a number of instances, accepted explanations for their mode of action have also been modified or altered. The aim of this book, however, is essentially unchanged. It attempts to provide a theoretical background and a general description of drugs that are commonly used by anaesthetists, or which significantly impinge upon anaesthetic practice. All of the original chapters have been extensively revised, and three new topics (variability in drug response, antihypertensive agents, and anticoagulants and related drugs) have been introduced.

This edition is principally intended for candidates preparing for the Part 2 FC Anaes. examination. However, the authors hope that the book may be of interest and value to all those engaged in clinical anaesthesia. For these reasons, an extensive bibliography has been provided for each chapter.

Dr H.L. Gordon has been responsible for the revision of two of the major chapters, and has also provided constructive criticism of other aspects of the book. We are pleased to acknowledge his help, and also that of Dr G. Satchi, Consultant Haematologist, whose advice in the preparation of Chapter 15 is greatly appreciated. The artistic help of Mrs Pamela Williams is also acknowledged. We are grateful to Dr Brenda Phillips for the electromyogram reproduced in Fig. 9.5.

ONE

Drug Absorption, Distribution and Elimination

Drugs can be defined as agents that modify biological systems, and thus produce pharmacological effects. These responses are usually dependent on the transfer of drugs across one or more cellular membranes. The rate and extent of this process is primarily determined by the structure and the physicochemical properties of the cell membrane. In most tissues, the limiting membrane of cells is approximately 10 nm wide, and consists of a bimolecular layer of phospholipids and cholesterol with intercalated molecules of protein (Fig. 1.1); carbohydrate residues may also be present, as glycolipids or glycoproteins. All of these components can migrate within the cell membrane. Some protein molecules are normally incorporated within the phospholipid membrane (intrinsic or integral proteins), while others are situated on the internal or external aspects of the membrane (extrinsic or peripheral proteins). Protein molecules may also be located across the entire width of the membrane; some of them consist of an annulus surrounding small pores or ion channels approximately 0.5 nm in diameter (Fig. 1.1). In capillary endothelial cells, the diameter of these pores is considerably greater (i.e. 4–5 nm), and intercellular spaces may also be present. Integral and peripheral proteins may act as enzymes, receptors, or carrier proteins. Cellular membranes also contain inorganic components (particularly calcium ions, which are associated with negatively charged groups on phospholipids and cholesterol).

TRANSFER OF DRUGS ACROSS CELL MEMBRANES

In general, drugs cross cell membranes by three main methods:
1 Simple diffusion.
2 Non-ionic diffusion.
3 Carrier transport.

Simple diffusion

Simple diffusion is a passive process that depends on differences in the concentration of drugs across cellular membranes. Highly lipid-soluble drugs (e.g.

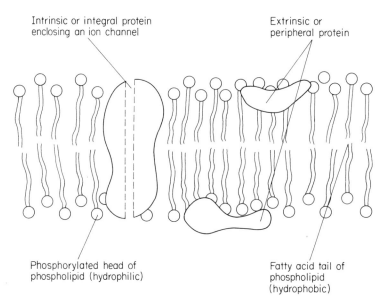

Intrinsic or integral protein
enclosing an ion channel

Extrinsic or
peripheral protein

Phosphorylated head of
phospholipid (hydrophilic)

Fatty acid tail of
phospholipid
(hydrophobic)

Fig. 1.1   Diagrammatic representation of a typical cell membrane.

ethyl alcohol) dissolve in the phospholipid membrane, and easily diffuse across cells. Drugs with a lower lipid solubility (e.g. morphine) diffuse less readily.

The diffusion of poorly lipid-soluble drugs (e.g. quaternary amines) across cells is usually limited by the permeability barrier imposed by the phospholipid membrane. Some polar, small molecular weight drugs may diffuse through the pores in the cell membrane, or penetrate small channels between adjacent cells. The permeability of vascular endothelium is greater than other tissues, and ionized compounds can readily cross capillary membranes.

Non-ionic diffusion

Drugs that are weak acids (e.g. salicylates, probenecid, and barbiturates) or weak bases (e.g. many narcotic analgesics, local anaesthetics, and antihistamines) are present in aqueous solutions (and in physiological conditions) in both an ionized and a non-ionized form. The ionization or dissociation can be expressed as the equations

$$AH \rightleftharpoons A^- + H^+ \text{ (for acids)}$$

and

$$BH^+ \rightleftharpoons B + H^+ \text{ (for bases)},$$

and is obviously influenced by pH; weak acids and bases are predominantly present as the species AH and BH^+ in acidic conditions, but as A^- and B in alkaline conditions. Only the non-ionized forms AH and B are sufficiently lipid-soluble to readily diffuse across cellular membranes. The ionized species A^- and BH^+ cannot readily cross the phospholipid barrier. Since the proportion of the drug that is present in the non-ionized form is dependent on pH, differences in H^+ concentration across cellular membranes can provide a diffusion gradient for the passive transfer of the non-ionic species.

Consider a weakly acidic drug, that dissociates in the manner

$$AH \rightleftharpoons A^- + H^+$$

From the Henderson–Hasselbalch equation, it can be shown that

$$pK_a - pH = \log\frac{[AH]}{[A^-]},$$

where [AH] and $[A^-]$ are the concentrations of the non-ionized and the ionized species, and the constant pK_a (the negative logarithm of the dissociation constant) is the pH value at which $[AH] = [A^-]$. If the pK_a of the drug is 6, at pH 2 (e.g. in gastric secretion), almost 100% is present in the form AH (Fig. 1.2). The non-ionized species will rapidly diffuse into plasma (pH 7.4), where approximately 96% will be converted to A^-, providing a concentration gradient for the continued diffusion of AH. Subsequent transfer of the drug to other sites will also be dependent on the relative pH gradient. At pH 8 (e.g. in interstitial fluid or alkaline urine), the concentration of AH is less than at pH 7.4 (Fig. 1.2). In this manner, a gradient is created for the passive diffusion of AH across renal tubular epithelium, followed by its subsequent ionization to A^- and elimination from the

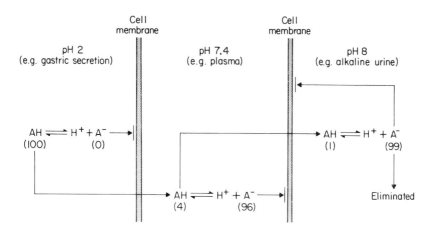

Fig. 1.2 Non-ionic diffusion of the weak acid AH ($pK_a = 6$). Only the non-ionized form AH can diffuse across cell membranes; the diffusion gradient is dependent on pH differences in compartments or tissues. Numbers in parentheses correspond to the percentage of the drug present as AH and A^- at pH 2, pH 7.4, and pH 8.

body (Fig. 1.2). By contrast, at a urine pH of 7 or less, the concentration of AH is greater in urine than in plasma, and the excreted drug will tend to back-diffuse from urine to plasma.

In a similar manner, pH gradients govern the non-ionic diffusion of weak bases which associate with hydrogen ions in the manner

$$B + H^+ \rightleftharpoons BH^+$$

From the Henderson–Hasselbalch equation, it can be shown that

$$pK_a - pH = \log\frac{[BH^+]}{[B]}$$

where $[BH^+]$ and $[B]$ are the concentrations of the ionized and the non-ionized forms, and pK_a is the pH value at which $[BH^+] = [B]$. If the pK_a of the basic drug is 7, at pH 2 (e.g. in the stomach), almost 100% is present as the ionized, poorly lipid-soluble form BH^+ (Fig. 1.3); even at pH 5.5 (e.g. in the small intestine) only 3% is present as the non-ionized species B, and is available to diffuse across the cell membrane. Although the effective pH gradient does not facilitate the non-ionic diffusion of weak bases from the small intestine (pH 5.5) to plasma (pH 7.4), the continuous perfusion of intestinal capillaries provides a small concentration gradient for their absorption.

By contrast, weak bases at pH 7.4 (e.g. in plasma) are mainly present as the non-ionized species B (Fig. 1.3). In these conditions, there is a large concentration gradient that facilitates their diffusion into the stomach (pH 2) and into acid urine (pH 5). After intravenous injection of the narcotic analgesics fentanyl

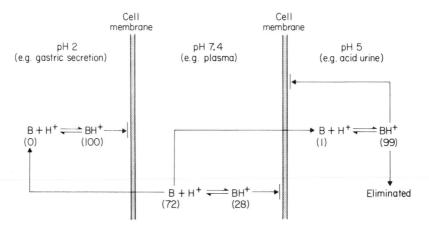

Fig. 1.3 Non-ionic diffusion of the weak base B ($pK_a = 7$). Only the non-ionized form B can diffuse across cell membranes; the diffusion gradient is dependent on pH differences in compartments or tissues. Numbers in parentheses correspond to the percentage of the drug present as B and BH^+ at pH 2, pH 7.4 and pH 5.

and phenoperidine, the initial decline in plasma concentration is followed by a secondary peak 30–40 min later. Both these weak bases are initially eliminated from plasma to the stomach, due to the large concentration gradient in favour of diffusion; their subsequent reabsorption from the small intestine is responsible for the secondary rise in the plasma concentration. Similarly, weak bases rapidly diffuse from plasma (pH 7.4) to urine (pH 5.0) as the non-ionized species B, where they are converted to the ionic form BH^+ and rapidly eliminated (Fig. 1.3).

In theory, modification of urine pH can increase the proportion of weak acids (pK_a = 3.0–7.5) and weak bases (pK_a = 7.5–10.5) that are present in an ionized form in urine, and thus enhance their elimination in drug-induced poisoning. In practice, forced acid or alkaline diuresis has a limited applicability; it is only of value when toxic drugs are (1) non-protein-bound, (2) confined to extracellular fluid, and (3) mainly eliminated unchanged in urine. Unfortunately, many acids and bases are extensively metabolized, and have a large volume of distribution that is consistent with significant sequestration in tissues. In these conditions, only small amounts of the unchanged drug are eliminated in acid or alkaline urine, and the amount of drug available for diffusion from plasma is relatively limited. In addition, forced diuresis is a potentially hazardous procedure, since it requires the infusion of relatively large amounts of fluid and the use of loop diuretics or mannitol to maintain a significant urinary output. Pulmonary and cerebral oedema are possible complications (particularly in elderly subjects). Nevertheless, forced alkaline diuresis is sometimes used in the management of salicylate and phenobarbitone overdosage, and in poisoning with the pesticides 2,4-D (2,4-dichlorophenoxyacetic acid) and mecoprop. Acid diuresis is only rarely of value, but may be used in amphetamine, fenfluramine, and phencyclidine poisoning.

Carrier transport

At some sites (e.g. the small intestine, the proximal renal tubule, the biliary canaliculus, and the choroid plexus), drugs may be transferred across cell membranes by carrier transport systems. The drug initially combines with an extrinsic carrier protein; the drug–protein complex is then transferred across the cell membrane, where the drug is released and the carrier protein returns to the opposite side of the membrane. One type of carrier transport ('facilitated diffusion') is usually responsible for the absorption of some simple sugars, steroids, amino acids and pyrimidines from the small intestine, and for their subsequent transfer across cell membranes (e.g. in red blood cells). Facilitated diffusion is a passive type of carrier transport that does not require energy (either as ATP or an indirect electrochemical gradient).

In contrast, active transport requires cellular or metabolic energy, and can transfer drugs against a concentration gradient. In addition, active transport

Table 1.1 Common acidic and basic drugs eliminated from plasma by active transport in the proximal renal tubule.

Acidic drugs	Basic drugs
Cephalosporins	Choline
Chlorpropamide	Dopamine
Ethacrynic acid	Histamine
Frusemide	Lignocaine
Glucuronide conjugates	Morphine
Indomethacin	Neostigmine
Methotrexate	Pyridostigmine
Oxyphenbutazone	Quinidine
Penicillins	Quinine
Probenecid	Thiamine
Salicylates	
Sulphate conjugates	
Sulphinpyrazone	
Spironolactone	
Sulphonamides	
Thiazide diuretics	

systems are unidirectional, saturable, relatively specific, and can be inhibited (competitively or non-competitively) by other drugs. They are widespread and ubiquitous, and are often concerned with the transport of endogenous substances (e.g. neurotransmitters) across cellular membranes. Active transport plays an important role in the elimination of acids and bases from the body (particularly in the proximal renal tubule and the biliary canaliculus).

In the proximal renal tubule many acidic and basic drugs are eliminated from plasma by active transport (Table 1.1); in consequence, their renal clearance is greater than glomerular filtration rate. Competition between weak acids for proximal tubular secretion may be responsible for drug interactions (e.g. inhibition of urate excretion by diuretic drugs can induce acute gout, and probenecid affects the elimination and the plasma concentration of benzylpenicillin). Basic drugs, including some quaternary amines that are used in anaesthesia (Table 1.1) are eliminated by a separate active transport system in the proximal renal tubule. Both systems can be competitively or non-competitively inhibited by different drugs.

Acidic and basic drugs or conjugates may also be eliminated by active transport from the liver cell to the biliary canaliculus (Table 1.2). In general, drugs or conjugates with a molecular weight of above 400 are eliminated in bile by a process of active secretion that is probably dependent on membrane ATPase. The biliary excretion of some muscle relaxants (i.e. alcuronium, tubocurarine, and vecuronium) probably accounts for their relative safety in patients with poor renal function.

Table 1.2 Common acidic and basic drugs secreted from liver cells into biliary canaliculi.

Acidic drugs	Basic drugs
Amoxycillin	Alcuronium
Ampicillin	Dimethyltubocurarine
Bromosulphonphthalein	Glycopyrrolate
Cephaloridine	Mepenzolate
Glucuronide conjugates of many drugs	Pancuronium
Phenol red	Pipenzolate
Probenecid	Tubocurarine
Radiographic contrast media	Vecuronium
Rifampicin	
Sulphate conjugates of many drugs	

PLASMA CONCENTRATION OF DRUGS AND ITS RELATION TO THEIR PHARMACOLOGICAL EFFECTS

When distribution equilibrium has been established, there is usually a close relationship between the plasma or tissue concentrations of drugs and the intensity of their pharmacological effects. In man, it is usually impossible to determine the effective tissue levels of drugs, although their plasma concentration can often be measured. Factors that modify these concentrations (e.g. absorption, distribution, metabolism and excretion) usually govern the concentration of drugs at their site of action, and thus affect the magnitude and duration of their pharmacological effects. A diagrammatic representation of the relation between drug absorption, distribution, metabolism, and excretion, and the effect of these processes on the tissue concentration of drugs, is shown in Fig. 1.4.

DRUG ADMINISTRATION

In general, drugs may be administered orally, by subcutaneous, intramuscular, or intravenous injection, by local infiltration or topical application, or by inhalation.

Oral administration

Oral administration is obviously most convenient and acceptable for the patient. Nevertheless, non-compliance with prescribed drug therapy is relatively common. Some drugs are unstable in the presence of gastric acid (e.g. benzylpenicillin and erythromycin); others may irritate the stomach and cause nausea, vomiting, or gastrointestinal haemorrhage (e.g. salicylates, phenylbutazone, and concentrated solutions of most salts). These problems can sometimes be circumvented by the

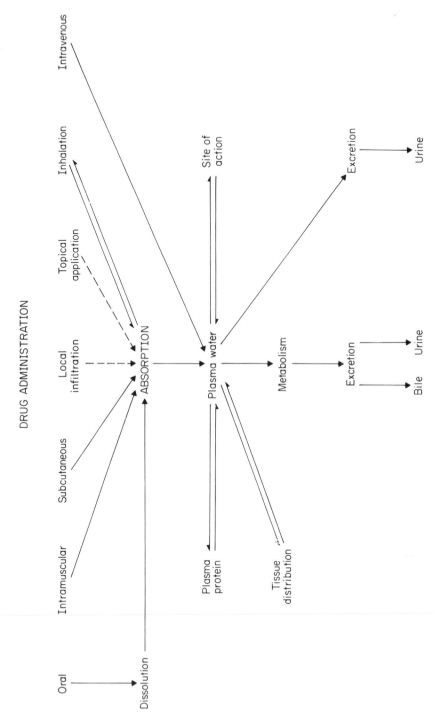

Fig. 1.4 The relation between drug absorption, distribution, metabolism, and excretion, and the concentration of drugs at their site of action.

use of enteric-coated tablets or slow-release preparations, which only dissolve in the small intestine.

When drugs are taken orally, there is usually a latent period of 30–120 min before they reach their maximum concentration in plasma or produce pharmacological effects. The presence of adequate drug concentrations in plasma after oral administration is dependent on:

1 Drug dissolution.
2 Drug absorption.
3 The absence of significant first pass effects in the gut wall or the liver.

Drug dissolution

Since drugs are only absorbed in solution, the dissolution of agents administered as tablets or capsules is essential before drug absorption can take place. Drug dissolution usually occurs in the stomach, and may be dependent on gastric acidity. Variations in the dissolution of tablets and capsules, and the rate and extent of gastric emptying, can thus affect the amount of drug in solution in the upper part of the small intestine (where absorption mainly occurs).

Many pharmaceutical factors may influence the dissolution of tablets and capsules (for instance, particle size, chemical formulation, the presence of inert fillers, and the outer coating applied to the tablet core). In these circumstances, proprietary or generic preparations of the same drug may have different dissolution characteristics and thus produce a range of plasma concentrations after oral administration. Variations in drug dissolution mainly occur with relatively insoluble drugs that are administered orally. The subsequent differences in the proportion of the dose present in the systemic circulation (bioavailability) may be clinically significant. For instance, differences in the potency of digoxin tablets suspected from clinical observations were eventually traced to variations in the dissolution of different preparations of the drug. Similarly, toxic effects were produced by tablets of diphenylhydantoin (phenytoin) when an excipient (calcium sulphate) was replaced by lactose. In these conditions, dissolution was more rapid, resulting in faster and more extensive absorption, and higher blood levels of the drug. Although other examples of differences in dissolution rate resulting in altered bioavailability are common, their clinical significance is a matter of conjecture.

Drug absorption

The absorption of drugs in the stomach and the small intestine is usually dependent on their ability to penetrate lipid cell membranes. Consequently, physicochemical properties of drugs (particularly lipid solubility, ionization, and molecular weight) mainly determine the rate and the extent of drug absorption.

Non-ionized compounds (e.g. ethyl alcohol), and low molecular weight drugs (e.g. urea) readily cross cell membranes by passive diffusion, and are easily and rapidly absorbed from the gut. Drugs that are weak acids (e.g. aspirin and warfarin) are predominantly non-ionized and lipid-soluble in acidic conditions, and therefore should diffuse into plasma more readily from the stomach than from the small intestine. By contrast, basic drugs (e.g. propranolol, amitriptyline and most benzodiazepines) are less ionized and more lipid-soluble in alkaline conditions, and should be preferentially absorbed from the duodenum (pH 5–6). Strong bases (e.g. quaternary amines) are always ionized in solution and are not readily absorbed from the gut.

In practice, other factors influence the site of drug absorption. Mucosal surface area is more extensive in the upper small intestine than in the stomach, and most drugs, whether acids or bases, are predominantly absorbed from the duodenum. Nevertheless, significant amounts of non-ionized compounds and acidic drugs may be absorbed from the stomach, and can produce a relatively rapid increase in plasma concentration after oral administration.

Compounds that affect gastric motility can modify drug dissolution, and influence the rate (but not the extent) of drug absorption. In particular, drugs that slow gastric emptying (e.g. anticholinergic drugs, antihistamines, tricyclic antidepressants and narcotic analgesics) decrease the rate of drug absorption. Other drug interactions (e.g. between tetracyclines and iron preparations, and cholestyramine and digoxin) may affect the extent of drug absorption and thus modify systemic bioavailability. Drug absorption may be reduced in pathological conditions affecting the gastrointestinal tract (e.g. coeliac disease, Crohn's disease, obstructive jaundice, or after extensive resection of the small intestine).

Although most drugs are absorbed from the stomach and small intestine by passive transport (i.e. simple diffusion or non-ionic diffusion), occasionally their absorption is dependent on carrier-mediated processes. Thus, levodopa is absorbed by a carrier that normally transports amino acids; and fluorouracil is absorbed by the carrier that transports pyrimidine bases.

First pass effects

After oral administration and absorption, drugs must pass through the intestinal mucosa and the liver in order to produce their pharmacological effects. Some drugs are absorbed from the small intestine but metabolized by the gut wall (e.g. chlorpromazine, dopamine, and isoprenaline) or by the liver (e.g. lignocaine, pethidine, and propranolol) before they gain access to the systemic circulation ('first pass metabolism'). In these conditions, oral administration may not produce adequate plasma concentrations or reproducible pharmacological effects. First pass metabolism by the liver is relatively common with drugs that have a high hepatic extraction ratio (i.e. when the concentration in the hepatic vein is less than 50% of the concentration in the portal vein). In these conditions, the hepatic clearance of drugs is primarily limited by liver blood flow rather than the activity of drug-metabolizing enzymes. Thus, drugs that modify hepatic blood flow (e.g. propranolol) may affect drug clearance, and influence the magnitude and extent of the first pass effect after oral administration. Most drugs that are given orally have a low hepatic extraction ratio and a limited first pass effect, and their clearance by the liver is dependent on intrinsic enzyme activity rather than hepatic blood flow. Drugs are sometimes given by sublingual or rectal administration in order to evade first pass effects in the liver.

Subcutaneous and intramuscular administration

Some drugs do not produce adequate plasma concentrations or pharmacological effects after oral administration and are usually given subcutaneously or intramuscularly. In particular, drugs that are broken down in the gut (e.g. benzylpenicillin and polypeptide hormones), are poorly or unpredictably absorbed (e.g. aminoglycoside antibiotics and many quaternary amines), or that have significant first pass effects (e.g. narcotic analgesics), are often given by these routes. Drugs are sometimes given intramuscularly when patients are intolerant of oral preparations (e.g. iron salts) or when patient compliance is known to be poor (e.g. in schizophrenia).

The absorption of drugs after subcutaneous or intramuscular administration is not usually dependent on the dissociation constant of the drug or its pH, but is often determined by regional blood flow. Thus, after intramuscular administration, the onset of drug action is usually more rapid (i.e. as fast or faster than after oral administration), and the duration of action is usually shorter, due to differences in the perfusion of muscle and subcutaneous tissues. The subcutaneous administration of relatively insoluble drugs or drug complexes is sometimes used to slow the rate of drug absorption and prolong the duration of action (e.g. with preparations of insulin or penicillin). In these conditions, the dissolution of the drug from the complex and its subsequent absorption governs the duration of drug action.

Intravenous administration

Drugs are usually given intravenously when a rapid or an immediate onset of action is necessary. When given by this route, their effects are usually dependable and reproducible. Intravenous administration often permits the dose of a drug to be accurately related to its effects, and thus eliminates some of the problems associated with inter-individual variability in drug response. Most drugs can be safely given as a rapid intravenous bolus; in some instances (e.g. aminophylline) drugs must be given slowly to avoid the cardiac complications associated with the extremely high plasma concentrations. Irritant drugs (e.g. thiopentone sodium) must be given intravenously in order to avoid local tissue or vascular complications. Some drugs (e.g. diazepam) can cause local complications (e.g. superficial thrombophlebitis) after intravascular administration; it is uncertain if this is due to the pH of the injected solution or to other factors. When drugs that release histamine from mast cells are given intravenously (e.g. tubocurarine and pethidine), local vasodilation and oedema (flare and weal) in the surrounding tissues may be observed.

Topical application and local infiltration

Most drugs are poorly absorbed through intact skin, due to their low lipid solubility. Nevertheless, some extremely potent lipid-soluble drugs (e.g. glyceryl trinitrate, hyoscine, and fentanyl) are absorbed transcutaneously and can produce systemic effects when applied to the skin. In practice, drugs are usually given locally or topically when it is necessary or essential to restrict their action to a region or an area of the body. Local anaesthetics are most commonly given by this method; they are often combined with vasoconstrictors in order to restrict their absorption and prolong the duration of drug action. Local anaesthetics, and other drugs that are used to relieve pain (e.g. narcotic analgesics) are sometimes given by intrathecal and extradural routes (Chapters 8 and 11).

Inhalation

Drugs given by inhalation usually have a rapid onset of action, since there is an extremely extensive epithelial surface available for absorption. In addition to general anaesthetics, other drugs (e.g. corticosteroids and bronchodilators) may be given by this method. The factors that govern the absorption of general anaesthetics from pulmonary epithelium into capillary blood are considered in detail in Chapter 7.

Other methods of drug administration

During the past decade, there has been considerable progress in the development of other methods of drug delivery. Some of these methods may have significant therapeutic advantages. In some instances, the development of sustained and programmed-release preparations allows the use of novel methods of administration. This results in greater convenience and safety, improved bioavailability, and less variability in plasma concentrations. Other advantages include a reduction in side-effects, drug dosage, frequency of administration, and cost.

Timed-release oral preparations usually consist of multi-lamellated erodible polymers, and allow fixed doses of a drug to be released at regular intervals. Some formulations are designed for the slow continuous release of drugs; they may be osmotically active, or incorporate an ion-exchange resin (so that the drug is released in an aqueous medium at an appropriate ionic concentration and pH). A number of therapeutic agents may be administered in this manner (e.g. some opioid analgesics, NSAIDs, bronchodilators, antihypertensive drugs, antiarrhythmic agents, and potassium salts).

Several drugs have been administered by non-invasive routes that avoid presystemic metabolism. The buccal route (i.e. the positioning of tablets between the cheek and the gum) may be used for the administration of glyceryl trinitrate, and tablets of morphine have also been given by this route. Similarly, oral transmucosal administration of opioid analgesics using drug impregnated 'lollipops' have been employed in the management of postoperative pain.

Certain hypothalamic and pituitary polypeptides that are destroyed in the gut are given by nasal administration. This method of drug delivery has also been used for other drugs (e.g. opioid analgesics, histamine antagonists, propranolol, and vitamin B_{12}).

Several drugs are also given by transdermal administration (p. 12). In general, only extremely potent drugs with a high lipid solubility can be successfully given by this route. Glyceryl trinitrate was the first drug given by transdermal administration; the development of rate-controlled release devices with self-adhesive layers has greatly enhanced its applicability and use. Similar transdermal systems are available for the administration of oestradiol, fentanyl, and hyoscine.

In recent years, there have also been advances in the delivery of drugs by parenteral administration. Implantable subcutaneous 'pellets' are frequently used in hormone replacement therapy, and further improvements in this method of drug administration are anticipated (e.g. with insulin and similar polypeptides). Regulated controlled release systems capable of providing increased release rates on demand (e.g. by the external application of magnetic or ultrasonic fields, or the use of enzymes) have also been investigated. The development of mini-infusion pumps for intermittent intravenous drug delivery is particularly valuable in pain relief; some of these devices incorporate electronic pumps to provide 'on-demand' bolus release of the drug according to the patient's needs. Alternatively, the use of gravity methods and balloon reservoir devices provides accurate mechanical control of drug administration. Battery operated syringe drivers for the continuous administration of opioid analgesics are particularly valuable in the domiciliary management of patients with intractable pain associated with malignant disease.

Delivery systems have also been designed to selectively target drugs to their desired site of action, thus avoiding regions where their effects are too toxic or where rapid inactivation may occur. In the future, microparticulate carriers (e.g. liposomes, red cells and microspherical beads) may be widely used in infectious and neoplastic diseases. Similarly, the conjugation of drugs with antibodies may be useful in the treatment of metastatic disease. The more extensive use of 'pro-drugs' may also lead to greater target specificity.

DRUG DISTRIBUTION

After administration and absorption, drugs are initially present in plasma and may be partly bound to plasma proteins. They subsequently gain access to other tissues and organs, and when distribution is complete their concentration in plasma water and extracellular fluid is equal.

The distribution of drugs in the body is extremely variable; it may be assessed by distribution studies in animals, or by pharmacokinetic methods in man (i.e. measurement of the total apparent volume of distribution). Some drugs (e.g. warfarin and tolbutamide) are extensively bound to plasma proteins, and are predominantly distributed in blood. Similarly, ionized compounds (for instance lithium and most quaternary amines) cannot readily penetrate most cell membranes, and are largely confined to extracellular fluid. Since these drugs are poorly distributed in tissues, they characteristically have a low apparent volume of distribution (usually 9–20 litre $70\,kg^{-1}$). By contrast, lipid-soluble drugs with a relatively low molecular weight are widely distributed in tissues. For instance, ethyl alcohol, urea, and some sulphonamides are evenly distributed throughout body water. These drugs usually have a volume of distribution similar to total body water (40–60 litres $70\,kg^{-1}$). Other drugs penetrate cells and are extensively bound to tissue proteins, or are sequestered in fat (e.g. morphine, thiopentone, and digoxin). In these conditions, the volume of distribution is characteristically greater than total body water (i.e. more than 40–60 litres $70\,kg^{-1}$).

Blood–brain barrier

Other drugs are widely distributed in most tissues, but do not readily enter the central nervous system (CNS). In cerebral capillaries, endothelial cells have tight, overlapping junctions which restrict passive diffusion, and pinocytotic vesicles are usually absent. The surrounding capillary basement membrane is closely applied to the peripheral processes of astrocytes (neuroglial cells that play an important part in neuronal nutrition). In order to pass from capillary blood to the brain, most drugs have to cross the endothelium, the basement membrane, and the peripheral processes of astrocytes by simple diffusion or filtration. Some drugs cannot easily penetrate this structural barrier, which is referred to as the 'blood–brain barrier'. In addition, there is a metabolic or enzymatic blood–brain barrier, mainly associated with the peripheral processes of astrocytes. Many potentially neurotoxic agents (e.g. free fatty acids and ammonia) can readily cross the capillary endothelium, but are metabolized before they reach the CNS. Monoamine oxidase and cholinesterases are also present in capillary endothelium, and some drugs (e.g. noradrenaline, dopamine, 5-hydroxytryptamine, and local anaesthetics) may be metabolized as they cross the blood–brain barrier.

In general, low molecular weight, lipid-soluble drugs (e.g. general anaesthetics, local anaesthetics, and opioid analgesics) easily cross the barrier and enter the CNS. When drugs are highly protein-bound (e.g. warfarin and tolbutamide), only the unbound fraction can diffuse from blood to the CNS, so that the concentration of these drugs in the brain may be 1–2% of the total plasma level. Drugs that are highly ionized (e.g. quaternary amines) cannot cross the blood–brain barrier; consequently, muscle relaxants do not enter or affect the brain. Similarly, dyes that are protein-bound (e.g. trypan blue and Evans blue), and drugs with a large molecular weight, do not readily cross the blood–brain barrier. Some drugs (e.g. benzylpenicillin) do not penetrate the barrier or enter the brain unless its permeability is increased by inflammation (e.g. in bacterial meningitis).

In some parts of the brain (i.e. the area postrema, the median eminence, the pineal gland, and the choroid plexus) the blood–brain barrier is deficient or absent. The diffusion of drugs and the exchange of endogenous substrates is not restricted at these sites. For example, in the choroid plexus drugs may freely diffuse from capillary blood to cerebrospinal fluid (CSF) across the relatively permeable choroidal epithelium. Similarly, the ependyma lining the cerebral ventricles does not appear to restrict the diffusion of most drugs. Certain metabolic substrates and hormones cross the blood–brain barrier by facilitated transport; neuropeptides and certain ionized compounds (e.g. benzylpenicillin and probenecid) may be actively secreted from the cerebral ventricles into capillary blood.

The normal impermeability of the blood–brain barrier can be modified by the arterial infusion of hypertonic solutions or by pathological changes (e.g. inflammation, oedema, and acute and chronic hypertension).

Placental transfer

During late pregnancy, structural changes occur in the placenta, involving the gradual disappearance of the cytotrophoblast and the loss of chorionic connective tissue from placental villi. At term, maternal and fetal blood are separated by a single layer of chorion (the syncytiotrophoblast) in continuous contact with the endothelial cells of fetal capillaries. Consequently, the placental barrier consists of a vasculosyncytial membrane, and from a functional point of view behaves like a typical lipid membrane. Most low molecular weight, lipid-soluble drugs are readily transferred across the placenta: their rate of removal from maternal blood is dependent on placental blood flow, the area available for diffusion, and the magnitude of the effective diffusion gradient. In contrast, large molecular weight or polar molecules cannot readily cross the vasculo-syncytial membrane. Almost all drugs that cross the blood–brain barrier and affect the CNS can also cross the placenta, and their elimination by fetal tissues may be difficult and prolonged.

Some drugs that readily cross the placenta are known to produce fetal abnormalities if taken in pregnancy (e.g. cytotoxic agents, folate antagonists, phenytoin, oestrogens, progestogens, aminoglycoside antibiotics, tetracyclines, and antithyroid drugs). Inhalational anaesthetics, intravenous barbiturates, local anaesthetics, and many analgesics (including morphine and pethidine) may diffuse from maternal plasma to the fetus, and when used in labour can cause complications. Similarly, some β-adrenoceptor antagonists (e.g. propranolol) can cross the placenta and may cause fetal bradycardia and hypoglycaemia. When diazepam is used in late pregnancy (e.g. in the treatment of pre-eclampsia and eclampsia), it readily crosses the placenta, but is not effectively metabolized by the fetus. Several of its active metabolites (including both desmethyldiazepam and oxazepam) accumulate in fetal tissues, and can cause neonatal hypotonia and hypothermia. By contrast, ionized compounds (e.g. all muscle relaxants) cannot readily cross the placenta, and their use during late pregnancy or lactation only rarely produces complications.

Local concentration

Some drugs tend to be localized in certain tissues or organs; for example, bromo-sulphonphthalein is concentrated in the liver, guanethidine by postganglionic sympathetic nerve endings, iodine in the thyroid gland, and tetracyclines in developing teeth and bone. The concentration of drugs in these tissues may be much greater than in plasma. Drugs that are widely distributed in tissues and concentrated in cells have an extremely large volume of distribution, which is usually greater than total body water (e.g. the phenothiazines and the tricyclic antidepressants).

After intravenous administration, some drugs are initially sequestered by well-perfused tissues, but are subsequently redistributed to other organs as the plasma concentration declines. Approximately 25% of intravenous thiopentone and methohexitone is initially taken up by the brain, due to its extensive blood supply and the high lipid solubility of the barbiturates. As the plasma concentration falls, the drugs are progressively taken up by less well-perfused tissues with a higher affinity for these compounds (e.g. muscle and adipose tissue). In consequence, intravenous barbiturates are rapidly redistributed from brain to muscle, and finally to subcutaneous fat. Redistribution is mainly responsible for the short duration of action of these drugs; their final elimination from the body may be delayed for 24 h.

Protein binding

Drug distribution may be affected by reversible binding to plasma proteins. When drugs are partially bound by albumin or globulins, only the unbound fraction is immediately available for diffusion into tissues. The concentration of drugs in salivary secretions and CSF may reflect the level of the free or unbound drug in plasma. Alternatively, this may be determined by *in vitro* techniques (e.g. equilibrium dialysis, ultracentrifugation, or ultrafiltration).

Many drugs are partially bound to albumin or globulins (or sometimes to both proteins). Albumin usually plays the most important role in the binding of drugs. It has a number of distinct binding sites with a variable affinity for drugs, and mainly binds neutral or acidic compounds (e.g. salicylates, phenylbutazone, indomethacin, tolbutamide, carbenoxolone, and oral anticoagulants). Some basic drugs and physiological substrates (bilirubin, fatty acids, and tryptophan) are also bound by albumin. Globulins bind many basic drugs (e.g. chlorpromazine, imipramine, lignocaine, bupivacaine, propranolol, alprenolol and opioid analgesics). These drugs are mainly bound by α_1-acid glycoprotein (one of the plasma globulins that play an important part in binding many basic compounds). The plasma concentration of α_1-acid glycoprotein is increased by surgery and by certain pathological conditions (e.g. myocardial infarction, malignant disease and ulcerative colitis). Plasma globulins also play an important part in the binding of elements, vitamins, and hormones. Hydrocortisone (cortisol) is mainly transported in plasma by a specific globulin (transcortin) which has a high affinity for the steroid hormone. Thyroxine, oestrogens, and hydroxocobalamin are also bound to globulins. Some drugs (e.g. tubocurarine and pancuronium) are bound to both albumin and an immunoglobulin (IgG). Indeed, the resistance to muscle relaxants that is sometimes seen in patients with liver disease is usually attributed to the increased binding of these drugs by plasma globulins.

There is considerable variation in the degree of protein binding, even among closely related drugs. Thus, the binding of the semi-synthetic penicillins to plasma albumin at therapeutic concentrations varies from 25% (ampicillin) to 90% (cloxacillin). Protein binding is primarily a method for the rapid distribution of drugs from their site of absorption to their site of action. The binding of extremely lipid-soluble compounds may be essential for their transport in plasma, due to their low inherent solubility in plasma water. During tissue perfusion, the concentration of the unbound drug in plasma falls, and the protein-bound drug dissociates. A continual concentration gradient is therefore provided for the diffusion of drugs from plasma to tissues.

Most of the available evidence suggests that plasma protein binding is only of practical significance when drugs are extensively (i.e. more than 80%) bound at therapeutic plasma concentrations. Drugs that are extensively bound to plasma proteins may interact with each other, since they may compete for and be displaced from related sites on plasma albumin. If two drugs are normally bound at identical or closely related sites on albumin, and both drugs are given to patients simultaneously, increased amounts of either drug may be displaced into plasma and tissue water, thus increasing their effects. Enhancement of the pharmacological response is mainly dependent on the extent of displacement of protein-bound drug, and the subsequent effects on drug elimination. In practice, displacement of drugs from plasma protein tends to cause a temporary rise in the concentration of unbound drug in plasma. Clearance of the unbound drug by renal and hepatic elimination is increased, and the total plasma level falls to a new steady-state, with little or no permanent change in the concentration of the free drug. For this reason, protein-displacement reactions alone are of little or no practical significance. Since all enzymes are also proteins, drugs that displace each other from plasma proteins may interact because they interfere with drug metabolism; in these circumstances, clinically significant interactions can occur.

Some protein-bound drugs have a long duration of action, and are only slowly eliminated from the body. Nevertheless, their prolonged action may not be related to their binding to plasma proteins. The hepatic clearance of many drugs is limited by liver blood flow, and is not restricted by plasma protein binding (which is a rapidly reversible process). Drug dissociation from binding to plasma proteins probably occurs within microseconds or milliseconds; by contrast, the hepatic perfusion time may be several seconds or more. Thus, binding to plasma proteins is not usually the limiting factor governing the uptake of drugs by the liver. Nevertheless, the elimination of extensively bound drugs with a low hepatic extraction ratio may be sensitive to changes in plasma protein binding, which can increase the amount of drug available for clearance by the liver. Similar principles can be applied to the elimination of drugs by the kidney. Protein binding is unlikely to restrict the renal elimination of drugs, either by the glomerulus or the renal tubule. Although only the unbound drug is secreted by the proximal tubule, the resultant decrease in its plasma concentration leads to the immediate dissociation of protein-bound drug in order to maintain equilibrium. Indeed, a number of protein-bound drugs are completely cleared in a single passage through the kidney (e.g. benzylpenicillin).

Binding to plasma proteins is modified in pathological conditions associated with hypoalbuminaemia (e.g. hepatic cirrhosis, nephrosis, trauma or burns). In these conditions, the concentration of the unbound drug tends to increase, and may result in toxic effects (e.g. with phenytoin and prednisolone). Significant changes are particularly likely when high doses of drugs are used, or when drugs are given intravenously. In these conditions, binding to albumin and other plasma proteins may be saturated, causing a disproportionate increase in the unbound drug. Tissues and organs that are well-perfused (e.g. brain, heart and abdominal viscera) may receive a higher proportion of the dose, predisposing them to potential toxic effects. Similar effects may occur in elderly patients and in subjects with renal impairment or uraemia, possibly due to alterations in the affinity of drugs for albumin. In contrast, many basic drugs are bound by the plasma globulin α_1-acid glycoprotein. The plasma concentration of α_1-acid glycoprotein can be modified by a number of pathological conditions (e.g. myocardial infarction, rheumatoid arthritis, Crohn's disease, renal failure and malignant disease), as well as operative surgery. In these conditions, the binding of basic drugs (e.g. propranolol and chlorpromazine) is increased, and the concentration of the free, unbound drug is reduced.

DRUG METABOLISM

Hepatic metabolism is usually responsible for the termination of drug action. It decreases the concentration of active drugs in plasma, and thus encourages their back-diffusion from other tissues and from their site of action. The main purpose of drug metabolism is the conversion of lipid-soluble drugs into water-soluble (polar) compounds, which can be readily filtered by the renal glomerulus or secreted into urine or bile.

Although most agents are primarily metabolized by the liver, a number of drugs used in anaesthesia (e.g. suxamethonium and amethocaine) are hydrolysed in plasma by cholinesterase. Alternatively, drugs may be partly or completely metabolized by other tissues, e.g. the gut (chlorpromazine and isoprenaline), the kidney (ethacrynic acid and dopamine), or the lung (angiotensin I and prilocaine). Nevertheless, the liver plays the major role in drug metabolism.

After oral administration, drugs are absorbed into portal venous blood and may be extensively removed from hepatic sinusoids and metabolized by the liver before they reach the systemic circulation. As mentioned previously, this phenomenon (the first pass effect) is an important cause of the failure to respond to drugs after their oral administration. When lignocaine, propranolol, and most narcotic analgesics are taken orally, significant amounts are extracted from portal blood by the hepatic sinusoids; all of these drugs have a marked first pass effect, and their clearance is predominantly dependent on liver blood flow. By contrast, the elimination of other drugs (e.g. warfarin and tolbutamide) is not determined by hepatic blood flow, but is governed by the intrinsic drug-metabolizing capacity of the liver.

Drug metabolism usually reduces biological activity. Most metabolites have less inherent activity than their parent compounds; in addition, their ability to penetrate to receptor sites is limited, due to their enhanced polarity and poor lipid solubility. Nevertheless, some drugs are relatively inactive in the form in which they are administered, and require metabolism to produce or enhance their pharmacological effects (Table 1.3). Other drugs are metabolized to compounds with a different spectrum of pharmacological activity (e.g. pethidine and atracurium). Certain antibiotics (e.g. ampicillin and chloramphenicol) may be

Table 1.3 Drugs that require metabolism to produce their pharmacological effects.

Drug	Active metabolite
Prontosil red	Sulphanilamide
Chloral hydrate	Trichlorethanol
Cyclophosphamide	Phosphoramide mustard
Cortisone	Hydrocortisone
Prednisone	Prednisolone
Methyldopa	Methylnoradrenaline
Proguanil	Cycloguanil

administered orally as esters; in this form, they are better absorbed than the parent drugs, and are subsequently hydrolysed to active derivatives. Occasionally, drug metabolism results in the formation of compounds with toxic effects. Paracetamol, for example, is partially converted to a highly reactive electrophilic metabolite (*N*-acetyl-*p*-benzoquinoneimine). Unless this metabolite is rapidly conjugated, it alkylates macromolecules in the hepatocyte, causing cell necrosis. Similarly, reductive metabolites of halothane may be bound covalently by tissue macromolecules, resulting in hepatocellular damage. The breakdown of halothane to reactive intermediate metabolites may play an important role in the phenomenon of 'halothane hepatitis'.

The changes carried out by liver cells during the metabolism of drugs are usually divided into two types. Phase 1 reactions (also known as non-synthetic or functionalization reactions) usually result in drug oxidation, reduction or hydrolysis (Table 1.4). Phase 2 reactions (synthetic or conjugation reactions) subsequently occur, involving the combination of unchanged drugs or the products of phase 1 reactions with other chemical groups (e.g. glucuronide, sulphate, acetate, or glycine radicals). Phase 2 reactions enhance the water solubility of drugs or drug metabolites, and thus promote their elimination from the body. Some drugs (e.g. sodium salicylate) are almost entirely metabolized by phase 2 reactions.

Phase 1 reactions

Most phase 1 reactions and glucuronide conjugation are carried out in a specific part of the liver cell (the smooth endoplasmic reticulum or the microsomes; Fig. 1.5). This can be separated from other subcellular particles by ultracentrifugation. Most drug oxidations and reductions, and some hydrolytic reactions, are carried out by a non-specific enzyme system in the hepatic endoplasmic reticulum known as the mixed function oxidase system (Fig. 1.6). An important component of this system is the enzyme cytochrome P-450.

Table 1.4 Typical phase 1 reactions resulting in drug oxidation, reduction, and hydrolysis.

Reaction	Site	Enzyme	Example
Oxidation	Hepatic endoplasmic reticulum	Cytochrome P-450	Halothane → trifluoracetic acid
			Thiopentone → pentobarbitone
	Mitochondria	Monoamine oxidase	Dopamine → dihydroxyphenyl-acetaldehyde
	Hepatic cell cytoplasm	Alcohol dehydrogenase	Alcohol → acetaldehyde
Reduction	Hepatic endoplasmic reticulum	Cytochrome P-450	Prontosil → sulphanilamide
	Hepatic cell cytoplasm	Alcohol dehydrogenase	Chloral hydrate → trichlorethanol
Hydrolysis	Hepatic endoplasmic reticulum	Esterase	Pethidine → pethidinic acid
	Plasma	Cholinesterase	Suxamethonium → succinate + choline
	Neuromuscular junction	Acetylcholinesterase	Acetylcholine → acetate + choline
	Hepatic cell cytoplasm	Amidase	Lignocaine → 2,6-xylidine + diethylglycine

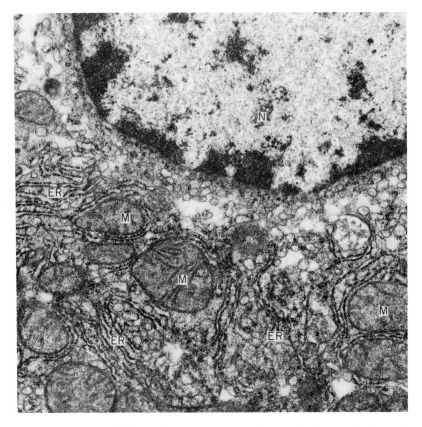

Fig. 1.5 Electron micrograph of part of a mouse liver cell, showing mitochondria (M), endoplasmic reticulum (ER), and the nuclear membrane enclosing the nucleus (N), ($\times 30\,000$). (Courtesy of Mr. Gordon Ross.)

Cytochrome P-450 is a haemoprotein containing iron; in the reduced state, it combines with carbon monoxide, forming a complex which maximally absorbs light at a wavelength of 450 nm. During drug oxidation, the oxidized form of cytochrome P-450 combines with the substrate or drug; the complex is subsequently reduced, combines with oxygen, and accepts an electron to form an 'active oxygen complex'. The active oxygen then combines with and oxidizes the drug, regenerating cytochrome P-450 in the oxidized form (Fig. 1.6). Cytochrome P-450 may also mediate the reduction of certain drugs (e.g. the reductive metabolism of halothane, prontosil, and chloramphenicol; Table 1.4). The reduction of drugs by cytochrome P-450 is dependent on their ability to directly accept electrons from the reduced cytochrome P-450–drug complex (Fig. 1.6), and is enhanced by hypoxia.

Although most oxidations and reductions are dependent on cytochrome P-450,

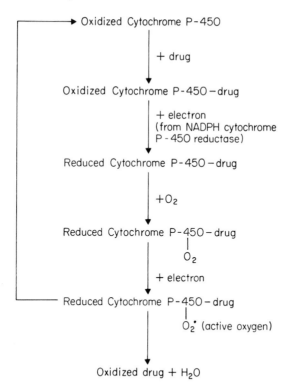

Fig. 1.6   Diagrammatic representation of the mixed function oxidase system (cytochrome P-450).

some drugs (e.g. dopamine and tyramine) are oxidized by monoamine oxidase, which is a mitochondrial enzyme. Ethyl alcohol is oxidized and chloral hydrate is reduced by alcohol dehydrogenase, which is present in the cytoplasm of liver cells (Table 1.4).

The hydrolysis of drugs is a phase 1 reaction that is responsible for the metabolism of esters and amides. Drug hydrolysis may occur in the endoplasmic reticulum and be dependent on microsomal enzyme systems (e.g. the hydrolysis of pethidine to pethidinic acid). Alternatively, it may occur in plasma (e.g. the hydrolysis of suxamethonium and procaine by cholinesterase), at the neuromuscular junction (e.g. the hydrolysis of acetylcholine by acetylcholinesterase), or in the cytoplasm of liver cells (e.g. the hydrolysis of lignocaine and prilocaine by amidases).

Phase 2 reactions

Phase 2 reactions (synthetic reactions) involve the conjugation of other chemical groups with the oxidized, reduced or hydrolysed products of phase 1 reactions. Relatively polar drugs may only be metabolized by phase 2 reactions. These metabolic changes usually involve the addition of glucuronide, sulphate, acetate, glycine or methyl groups. The most important of these reactions is glucuronide conjugation.

The conjugation of drugs to glucuronides is mainly dependent on enzyme systems in the hepatic endoplasmic reticulum. The microsomal enzyme glucuronyl transferase catalyses the transference of glucuronide residues from UDP-glucuronide to unconjugated compounds. This process is responsible for the conjugation of endogenous compounds (e.g. bilirubin and thyroxine) as well as many drugs (e.g. chloramphenicol, morphine, salicylic acid, steroid hormones, sulphonamides and trichlorethanol). Glucuronide conjugation usually results in the formation of acidic drug metabolites with a low pK_a (i.e. relatively strong acids), and consequently increases their water solubility.

Sulphate conjugation may occur in the gut wall or in the cytoplasm of the liver cell. The enzymes involved are normally concerned with the synthesis of sulphated polysaccharides (e.g. heparin). Sulphate conjugation may be the final step in the metabolism of chloramphenicol, isoprenaline, noradrenaline, paracetamol, and certain steroids.

Drug acetylation may take place in several tissues (e.g. spleen, lung and liver). In the liver, Kupffer cells rather than hepatocytes may be responsible for conjugation, which involves the transfer of acetyl groups from co-enzyme A to the unconjugated drug. The rate and extent of acetylation in man are under genetic control. Isoniazid, many sulphonamides, hydralazine, and phenelzine are partly metabolized by acetylation.

Conjugation with glycine may occur in the cytoplasm of the liver cell; bromosulphonphthalein is one of several drugs that are partly eliminated in bile as glycine conjugates.

Enzymes that mediate methylation are present in the cytoplasm of many tissues. Methylation plays an important part in the metabolism of catecholamines (e.g. adrenaline and noradrenaline) by the enzyme catechol-O-methyltransferase.

Enzyme induction

The activity of microsomal enzymes may be enhanced by certain drugs, both *in vivo* and *in vitro*. In these conditions, the rate and extent of drug metabolism is increased. These compounds are known as enzyme inducing agents (Table 1.5); many of them cause an increase in liver weight, microsomal protein content, and the rate of biliary secretion. Characteristically, enzyme induction increases the activity of oxidative enzymes in the endoplasmic reticulum (i.e. cytochrome P-450) and enhances glucuronide conjugation by glucuronyl transferase. The activity of other enzymes (e.g. NADPH cytochrome P-450 reductase; Fig. 1.6) may also be increased, although some hepatic enzymes concerned with drug metabolism are unaffected. Enzyme induction usually takes place over several

Table 1.5 Drugs that induce hepatic microsomal enzymes in man.

Analgesic and anti-inflammatory drugs
  (amidopyrine, phenazone, phenylbutazone)
Anticonvulsants
  (carbamazepine, phenytoin, primidone)
Antibacterial and antifungal agents
  (rifampicin and griseofulvin)
Barbiturates
  (amylobarbitone, barbitone, cyclobarbitone, phenobarbitone)
Inhalational anaesthetics
  (enflurane, halothane, methoxyflurane)
Insecticides
  (aldrin, chlordane, dicophane)
Steroid hormones
  (glucocorticoids, androgens)
Alcohol
  (chronic consumption)
Tobacco
  (cigarette smoking)

days; the rate of metabolism of the inducing agent and of other drugs may be increased, possibly resulting in drug interactions. Barbiturates have a notorious reputation as enzyme inducing agents. Nevertheless, there is little or no evidence that the routine use of thiopentone or methohexitone results in similar effects, or causes drug interactions in man. Many inhalational anaesthetics produce complex effects on microsomal enzymes and the mixed function oxidase system; enzyme induction, enzyme inhibition, or a biphasic response may occur. In addition, the metabolic response to surgery may affect hepatic enzyme systems.

Table 1.6 Drugs that inhibit hepatic microsomal enzymes in man.

Analgesic and anti-inflammatory drugs
  (phenylbutazone, oxyphenbutazone)
Antibacterial drugs
  (chloramphenicol, isoniazid, metronidazole)
Cytotoxic drugs
  (cyclophosphamide)
Monoamine oxidase inhibitors
  (phenelzine, tranylcypromine)
Other enzyme inhibitors
  (allopurinol, disulfiram, metyrapone)
Alcohol
  (acute intoxication)
Other drugs
  (etomidate, amiodarone, cimetidine)

Enzyme inhibition

Conversely, some drugs may inhibit hepatic microsomal enzymes, and may prevent or retard the metabolism of other drugs. Cytochrome P-450 and other hepatic enzymes concerned with drug metabolism may be inhibited in a competitive or a non-competitive manner by many drugs (Table 1.6). Some of these drugs are imidazoles or substituted imidazoles (e.g. etomidate, metronidazole, cimetidine and omeprazole); the imidazole ring may act as a ligand for the haem in the haemoprotein cytochrome P-450, causing inhibition of oxygenation reactions. Etomidate may also suppress steroid synthesis by the adrenal cortex (Chapter 6).

Individual differences in drug metabolism

When some drugs are administered in the same dose to different patients, plasma concentrations may vary over a 10-fold range. This phenomenon is partly due to inter-individual differences in drug metabolism, which are an important cause of the variability in response to drugs (Chapter 5). Most of the available evidence suggests that the rate and the pattern of drug metabolism are mainly controlled by genetic factors. In man, some metabolic pathways are subject to polymorphism (e.g. drug acetylation, ester hydrolysis, and some hydroxylation and dealkylation reactions). Environmental factors (including diet, cigarette smoking, alcohol consumption, exposure to insecticides, and the effects of other inducers and inhibitors on drug metabolism) appear to be of lesser importance.

Drug metabolism may be related to age. Thus, at the extremes of life, the hepatic metabolism of many drugs is modified. Newborn children have impaired drug metabolizing systems (in particular, cytochrome P-450 and glucuronyl transferase may be relatively immature). In the elderly, drug metabolism is also modified; altered environmental influences may be of more importance.

Pathological changes may affect the metabolism and clearance of drugs in an unpredictable manner. In severe hepatic disease (e.g. cirrhosis or hepatitis), the elimination of drugs that are primarily metabolized may be impaired. The reduction in their clearance may result in drug cumulation, and the urinary elimination of their metabolites may be decreased. Liver disease may also enhance and prolong the effects of drugs that are metabolized by plasma cholinesterase. Any decrease in cardiac output (e.g. due to heart block, myocardial infarction or hypertension) may reduce the elimination of drugs whose clearance is dependent on hepatic blood flow. Renal disease usually has little or no effect on drug metabolism, although polar metabolites may accumulate in plasma and produce toxic effects. Thus, norpethidine (a demethylated metabolite of pethidine) is normally rapidly eliminated in urine; in renal failure, its excretion is impaired, sometimes causing cerebral excitation and convulsions.

Hepatic, renal, and cardiac disease are important factors affecting the variable response to drugs (Chapter 5).

DRUG EXCRETION

Almost all drugs and their metabolites (with the notable exception of the inhalational anaesthetics) are eventually eliminated from the body in urine or in bile. Small amounts of some drugs are excreted in saliva and in milk.

The molecular weight of drugs and their metabolites plays an important part in determining their route of elimination (i.e. in urine or in bile). Most low molecular weight compounds and their metabolites are excreted in urine. By contrast, drugs with a higher molecular weight (above approximately 400–500 in man) are preferentially eliminated in bile. Thus biliary secretion plays an

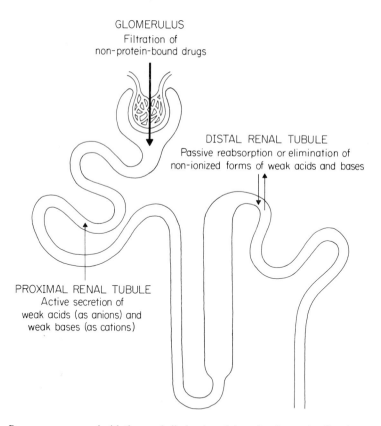

Fig. 1.7 Processes concerned with the renal elimination of drugs by glomerular filtration, proximal tubular secretion, and distal tubular reabsorption or excretion. In the distal renal tubule, weak acids and weak bases may be reabsorbed or excreted into urine, depending on their pK_a values and the pH gradient between plasma and urine.

important part in the elimination of tubocurarine, alcuronium, glycopyrrolate, many steroid conjugates, and some antibacterial drugs (Table 1.2).

The renal elimination of drugs is dependent on three separate processes that take place at different sites in the nephron. These are:

1 Glomerular filtration.
2 Proximal tubular secretion.
3 Distal tubular diffusion (Fig. 1.7).

Glomerular filtration

Glomerular filtration is partly responsible for the elimination of poorly lipid-soluble drugs and drug metabolites in urine. Only the free or unbound fraction in plasma water is available for filtration by the renal glomerulus. Nevertheless, since glomerular perfusion time is probably much longer than the dissociation time from the rapidly reversible binding to plasma proteins, significant amounts of protein-bound drugs may be filtered by the glomerulus.

Proximal tubular secretion

The active secretion of drugs by the proximal renal tubule may lead to their rapid elimination from the body. Proximal tubular secretion is an example of carrier transport, requires the expenditure of cellular energy, and may take place against a considerable concentration gradient. A wide number of drugs and drug metabolites are known to be partly eliminated by this process (Table 1.1). Acidic drugs and basic drugs are secreted by two separate and distinct transport systems. These are located in related sites in renal tubular cells, and both have a requirement for cellular energy. Acidic drugs may compete with each other for tubular secretion; conversely, basic drugs may interfere with the elimination of other bases or cations. Acids do not usually compete with or affect the secretion of bases. Occasionally, the competitive inhibition of the tubular transport of acids or bases is of practical significance (e.g. the inhibition of penicillin secretion by probenecid, or the reduction of urate transport by thiazide diuretics).

During tubular secretion, only the unbound drug is transferred from plasma to tubular cells. Nevertheless, protein or red cell binding does not apparently restrict tubular secretion, and some drugs that are significantly bound to plasma proteins (e.g. phenol red and some penicillins) are completely cleared by the kidney in a single circulation. As discussed above, this probably reflects the rapid dissociation from plasma protein in relation to the time required for renal tubular perfusion.

Distal tubular diffusion

In the distal renal tubule, non-ionic diffusion is partly responsible for the reabsorption and elimination of acids and bases. In this region of the nephron, there is a considerable hydrogen ion gradient between plasma and the normally acid urine. Most acidic drugs are preferentially excreted in alkaline urine, where they are present as non-diffusible anions; in acid urine, they are usually present as non-ionized molecules that can readily back-diffuse into plasma (see p. 4). In these conditions, they are slowly eliminated from the body, and their half-lives may be prolonged. For instance, the weak acid probenecid is actively secreted in the proximal renal tubule as an anion, i.e. $R.COO^-$; in acidic conditions (e.g. in the distal renal tubule) it is partially present in the non-ionized form $R.COOH$, and is extensively reabsorbed. In consequence, its elimination from the body is relatively slow, and its half-life is approximately 6–12 h.

By contrast, basic drugs (e.g. secondary and tertiary amines) are preferentially excreted in acid urine (Fig. 1.3); in these conditions they can readily diffuse from plasma to urine where they are trapped as cations. This provides a gradient for the diffusion of the non-ionized drug from plasma to urine. Many basic drugs are highly lipid-soluble and extensively bound to plasma proteins and may not be significantly eliminated by glomerular filtration or by tubular secretion. Diffusion of the non-ionized species from the relatively alkaline plasma to acidic urine (Fig. 1.3) may be the only method responsible for the elimination of these drugs.

As discussed earlier (p. 5), the effects of changes in urine pH on the elimination of weak acids and weak bases is sometimes used to increase their elimination from the body after drug overdosage.

Biliary excretion

The biliary excretion of drugs and drug metabolites is usually less important than their renal elimination. Nevertheless almost all drugs or their metabolites can be identified in bile after oral or parenteral administration (although only trace amounts of many compounds may be detected). Biliary excretion is usually the major route of elimination of compounds with a molecular weight of more than 400–500.

Ionized or partly ionized drugs (and drug metabolites) are usually eliminated from liver cells by active transport. High molecular weight anions (including glucuronide and sulphate conjugates) and cations (including quaternary amines) are actively transferred from hepatocytes to bile by separate transport systems, which are located in the canalicular membrane. Anions compete with each other for canalicular transport, while basic drugs interfere with the elimination of other bases or cations. Biliary secretion is dependent on the enzyme ATPase; in addition, it is relatively non-specific, saturable, and can be competitively or non-competitively inhibited by other drugs. In many respects, the biliary secretion of anions and cations is similar to their active transport in the proximal renal tubule, and accounts for the high concentrations of certain drugs in bile (in some instances, more than 100 times their plasma level).

The phenomenon is sometimes of practical significance. The visualization of

Chapter One

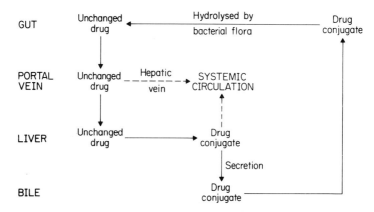

Fig. 1.8 Diagrammatic representation of the enterohepatic circulation of drugs. Only small amounts of the absorbed drug and its metabolites (represented by broken arrows – –►) escape recirculation and enter the systemic circulation.

contrast media during radiological examination of the biliary tract is dependent on their active secretion and concentration in bile. Similarly, the high concentrations of ampicillin and similar antibacterial drugs that are eliminated in bile may account for their effectiveness in the treatment of carriers of enteric fever. Many muscle relaxants are partly eliminated by biliary secretion, and are present in high concentrations in bile. In general, monoquaternary compounds (e.g. vecuronium and tubocurarine) are more extensively eliminated than their bisquaternary analogues (e.g. pancuronium and dimethyltubocurarine), and this may partly account for the differences in their duration of action.

Many compounds that are eliminated in bile as glucuronide conjugates are hydrolysed in the small intestine by bacterial flora which secrete the enzyme glucuronidase. After hydrolysis, the unchanged drug is reabsorbed, metabolized by the liver, and excreted again as a glucuronide conjugate (Fig. 1.8). This 'enterohepatic circulation' of drugs may occur many times before compounds are finally eliminated from the body, and is often associated with a substantial first pass effect and a prolonged plasma half-life. Many steroid drugs (e.g. oral contraceptives and oestrogens) have an extensive enterohepatic circulation. During broad-spectrum antibiotic therapy, bacterial flora are inhibited or destroyed, and glucuronide conjugates are no longer extensively hydrolysed in the small intestine; in these circumstances, drug elimination may be enhanced. It has been suggested that this phenomenon is occasionally responsible for the failure of oral contraception in patients taking broad-spectrum antibacterial agents.

The trace amounts of many drugs that are eliminated unchanged in bile are probably directly transferred from hepatic arterial blood to intrahepatic bile ducts via the peribiliary plexus. The transference of drugs may be modified by the hormone secretin, which also increases bile flow by its action at this site.

Small amounts of most drugs are excreted unchanged in saliva and in milk. The elimination of drugs by these routes is usually dependent on simple physical principles. Non-protein bound, lipid-soluble, small molecular weight drugs can readily diffuse into saliva and milk, where their levels may be similar to the plasma concentration. Since the pH of saliva and milk is slightly acid compared with plasma, the concentration of weak acids will be reduced (although weak bases may be slightly concentrated). Some ions (e.g. chloride and iodide) may be actively secreted into saliva and milk. Nevertheless, drug excretion by these routes is usually of little quantitative significance. Occasionally the elimination of trace amounts of certain drugs in milk (e.g. many opioid analgesics and most hypnotic and tranquillizing drugs) may make breast-feeding inadvisable in patients who are on continual therapy. Muscle relaxants and their antagonists are not significantly eliminated in saliva or in milk.

After intravenous administration, many basic drugs are eliminated into the stomach, where the large pH gradient (approximately $1:10\,000$) favours their non-ionic diffusion from plasma (see p. 4).

DRUG ISOMERISM

Isomers are drugs with the same molecular weight and chemical composition, but which differ in the precise arrangement of their individual atoms or groups. In general, three types of isomerism may occur with drugs:
1 Structural isomerism.
2 Dynamic isomerism (tautomerism).
3 Stereo-isomerism.

Structural isomerism

Structural isomers have an identical empirical formula and basic chemical skeleton, but differ in the positions that are occupied by substituent groups. The inhalational anaesthetics enflurane and isoflurane have the same empirical formula (i.e. $C_3H_2F_5OCl$), but a different chemical structure (enflurane, $CHF_2.O.CF_2.CHFCl$; isoflurane, $CHF_2.O.CHCl.CF_3$), due to the different rearrangement of their substituent groups.

Dynamic isomerism

Dynamic isomers (tautomers) are rapidly interchangeable forms of the same drug. Changes in chemical structure occur when the equilibrium between the two forms is disturbed (e.g. by alterations in pH). Keto–enol isomerism, which occurs with barbiturates and their derivatives, is an example of tautomerism. In neutral solutions, thiopentone and other barbiturates are mainly present in the relatively insoluble keto form ($=C=O$ or $=C=S$). In alkaline solutions, the equilibrium is disturbed in favour of the enol form ($\equiv C\text{-}OH$ or $\equiv C\text{-}SH$). In the enol form, barbiturates are readily ionized and are highly water-soluble (see p. 157).

(see p. 157)

Stereo-isomerism

Stereo-isomers can be defined as drugs with the same chemical structure but a different molecular form ('configuration'). Stereo-isomerism can be divided into two types: (a) optical isomerism; and (b) geometric isomerism.

Optical isomerism

Many naturally occurring and synthetic drugs show the phenomenon of chirality (handedness), i.e. they can exist in right-handed and left-handed forms which may have different effects on enzymes and receptors. These two forms of drugs are non-superimposable mirror-images of each other, and are usually referred to as mirror-image isomers or enantiomers (i.e. substances of opposite shape). Although enantiomers have identical physical and chemical properties, they rotate polarized light in opposite directions due to their molecular asymmetry; for this reason, they are frequently referred to as optical isomers. The symbols (+) and (−), or the letters (*d*) and (*l*) are commonly used to specify the direction of optical rotation (to the right (dextro) and to the left (laevo), respectively).

Alternatively, enantiomers can be defined by their structure or spatial orientation. Thus, amino acids can be defined, on the basis of their structure, as D or L amino acids; drugs are usually specified by the letters R (for rectus or right-handed) and s (for sinister or left-handed). Mixtures of enantiomers in equal proportions have no optical activity; they are usually referred to as racemic (or chiral) mixtures.

Chirality is usually due to the existence of a centre of molecular asymmetry (e.g. the presence of four different chemical groups attached to a single carbon atom). All compounds with this structure may be present as non-superimposable mirror-images, and are usually synthesized as a mixture of R and s enantiomers. In addition, receptors and enzymes are chiral, and possess a centre of molecular asymmetry; they are usually composed of L amino acids.

Approximately 70% of drugs used in anaesthetic practice are chiral compounds; about 20% are given as a single enantiomer, while the remaining 50% are given as a chiral mixture. Normally, organic synthesis results in the preparation of drugs containing 50% of each enantiomer. However, in recent years the rationale of administering drugs as chiral mixtures has been questioned. Chemical methods have been developed for the synthesis and separation of the individual enantiomers of many drugs, so that their individual properties can be investigated; in many instances, methods of measuring their plasma concentration are also available. Recent studies have shown that although the physical and chemical properties of R and S enantiomers are identical, their biological properties may differ significantly. In many instances, their pharmacodynamic effects are unequal; in addition, processes such as drug distribution, protein binding, metabolism and elimination may be stereoselective, and differ with the R and S enantiomers. For example, one chiral form may be more extensively metabolized, undergo chiral inversion, or inhibit the metabolism of its enantiomer. These differences are not surprising, since the individual enantiomers react with receptors or enzymes that are themselves composed of chiral amino acids with stereoselective properties.

Both naturally occurring drugs (e.g. atropine and morphine) and synthetic agents (e.g. most intravenous anaesthetics, inhalational agents, local anaesthetics and inotropic agents) are chiral compounds. Atropine (*dl*-hyoscyamine) is one of the best known examples of a chiral drug. It is present in solanaceous plants as an *l*-isomer; it is converted to a racemic compound during extraction. The *l*-isomer (*l*-hyoscyamine) is about 50 times more active than *d*-hyoscyamine. Morphine is a complex example of chirality; its molecule has five asymmetric carbon atoms, and there are at least 16 possible stereoisomers with the same chemical structure. However, only the naturally occurring *l*-isomer has analgesic activity. All currently used intravenous anaesthetics, with the single exception of propofol, are chiral drugs. Thiopentone and methohexitone are administered as chiral mixtures; experimental studies suggest that the S(−) enantiomers are more potent and more rapidly eliminated. On the other hand, etomidate is used as a single isomer (R(+)-etomidate); its corresponding enantiomer (S(−)-etomidate) has only slight hypnotic activity. Although ketamine is given as a chiral mixture, there is considerable evidence that psychotomimetic emergence phenomena may only be associated with one enantiomer.

In addition, many inhalational anaesthetics (e.g. halothane, enflurane, and isoflurane) and some local anaesthetics (mepivacaine, bupivacaine and prilocaine) are chiral compounds, and are usually administered as chiral mixtures. In the case of these local anaesthetics, the S isomers have a longer duration of action than their R enantiomers, since they produce vasoconstriction. Differences in the rate of metabolism may also be present; thus, S(+)-prilocaine is more slowly metabolized than R(−)-prilocaine; it has been suggested that only the R(−) isomer is metabolized to toluidine and may cause methaemoglobinaemia. Some inotropic agents are also administered as chiral mixtures; in the case of dobutamine, its α-effects and β-effects are associated with different enantiomers.

In the future, it seems likely that most new drugs will be introduced as the single, most active enantiomer rather than as chiral mixtures. When new drugs are developed as racemic mixtures, pharmaceutical manufacturers may be required to show that there are valid pharmacological or medical reasons for their use, and to show that the less active isomer is not associated with adverse effects.

Geometric isomerism

Geometric isomerism usually occurs in drugs containing a carbon–carbon double bond (i.e. C=C). When both carbon atoms have the same dissimilar substituent groups (i.e. compounds of the type abC=Cba, where a and b are dissimilar), geometrical isomerism can occur. In the *cis*-isomer, the two identical groups (a and a, or b and b) are on the same side of the C=C plane; in the *trans*-isomer, the groups a and b are on opposite sides of the C=C plane. Geometrical isomers are not usually optically active, and have different physical and chemical properties. Some anaesthetic agents show *cis–trans* isomerism; for instance, the new muscle relaxant mivacurium is a mixture of three geometric isomers (the *cis–cis*, the *trans–trans*, and the *cis–trans* isomers).

FURTHER READING

Acocella A. Clinical pharmacokinetics of rifampicin. *Clinical Pharmacokinetics* 1978; **3**: 108–127.

Alvares AP. Interactions between environmental chemicals and drug biotransformation in man. *Clinical Pharmacokinetics* 1978; **3**: 462–477.

Asling J, Way EL. Placental transfer of drugs. In: La Du BN, Mandel HG, Way EL (eds). *Fundamentals of Drug Metabolism and Drug Disposition*. Baltimore: Williams and Wilkins, 1971; 88–105.

Axelrod J. The metabolism of catecholamines *in vivo* and *in vitro*. *Pharmacological Reviews* 1959; **11**: 402–408.

Bates IP. Permeability of the blood–brain barrier. *Trends in Pharmacological Sciences* 1985; **6**: 447–450.

Berliner RW. Outline of renal physiology. In: Strauss MB, Welt LG (eds). *Diseases of the Kidney*. London: Churchill, 1963; 30–79.

Blaschke TF. Protein binding and kinetics of drugs in liver diseases. *Clinical Pharmacokinetics* 1977; **2**: 32–44.

Borzelleca JF, Cherrick HM. The excretion of drugs in saliva; antibiotics. *Journal of Oral Therapeutics and Pharmacology* 1965; **2**: 180–187.

Boström H. Sulfate conjugation and conjugated sulfates. *Scandinavian Journal of Clinical and Laboratory Investigation* 1965; **86** (Suppl. 17): 33–52.

Boyd MR. Evidence for the Clara cell as a site of cytochrome P-450 dependent mixed-function oxidase activity in the lung. *Nature* 1977; **269**: 713–715.

Brodie BB, Gillette JR, La Du BN. Enzymatic metabolism of drugs and other foreign compounds. *Annual Review of Biochemistry* 1958; **27**: 427–454.

Calvey TN, Milne LA, Williams NE, Chan K, Murray GR. Effect of antacids on the plasma concentration of phenoperidine. *British Journal of Anaesthesia* 1983; **55**: 535–539.

Clark AG, Fischer LJ, Millburn P, Smith RL, Williams RT. The role of gut flora in the enterohepatic circulation of stilboestrol in the rat. *Biochemical Journal* 1969; **112**: 17P.

Clarke CA, Price-Evans DA, Harris R, McConnell RB, Woodrow JC. Genetics in medicine: a review. Part II: Pharmacogenetics. *Quarterly Journal of Medicine* (New Series) 1968; **37**: 183–219.

Conney AH. Pharmacological implications of microsomal enzyme induction. *Pharmacological Reviews* 1967; **19**: 317–366.

Conney AH, Davidson C, Gastel R, Burns JJ. Adaptive increases in drug-metabolizing enzymes induced by phenobarbital and other drugs. *Journal of Pharmacology and Experimental Therapeutics* 1960; **130**: 1–8.

Crooks J, O'Malley K, Stevenson IH. Pharmacokinetics in the elderly. *Clinical Pharmacokinetics* 1967; **1**: 280–296.

Csáky TZ. Transport through biological membranes. *Annual Review of Physiology* 1965; **27**: 415–450.

Davson H, Danielli JF. *The Permeability of Natural Membranes*, 2nd edn. London: Cambridge University Press, 1952.

Dundee JW, Gray TC. Resistance to *d*-tubocurarine chloride in the presence of liver damage. *Lancet* 1953; **2**: 16–17.

Dutton GJ. Glucuronic acid, free and combined. In: *Chemistry, Biochemistry, Pharmacology and Medicine*. New York: Academic Press, 1966.

Eichelbaum M. Defective oxidation of drugs: pharmacokinetic and therapeutic implications. *Clinical Pharmacokinetics* 1982; **7**: 1–22.

Fehrenbach A. Drugs in breast milk. *British Journal of Pharmaceutical Practice* 1987; **9**: 288–290.

Friedman PJ, Cooper JR. The role of alcohol dehydrogenase in the metabolism of chloral hydrate. *Journal of Pharmacology and Experimental Therapeutics* 1960; **129**: 373–376.

George CF. Drug metabolism by the gastrointestinal mucosa. *Clinical Pharmacokinetics* 1981; **6**: 259–274.

George CF, Shand DG. *Presystemic Drug Elimination*. London: Butterworths, 1982.

Gibaldi M. Drug distribution in renal failure. *American Journal of Medicine* 1977; **62**: 471–474.

Gibaldi M, McNamara PJ. Apparent volumes of distribution and drug binding to plasma proteins. *European Journal of Clinical Pharmacology* 1978; **13**: 373–378.

Gillette JR. Factors affecting drug metabolism. *Annals of the New York Academy of Sciences* 1971; **179**: 43–66.

Gillette JR, Davis DC, Sasame HA. Cytochrome P-450 and its role in drug metabolism. *Annual Review of Pharmacology* 1972; **12**: 57–84.

Goldstein A. The interactions of drugs and plasma proteins. *Pharmacological Reviews* 1949; **1**: 102–165.

Govier WC. Reticuloendothelial cells as the site of sulfanilamide acetylation in the rabbit. *Journal of Pharmacology and Experimental Therapeutics* 1965; **150**: 305–308.

Hasselbalch KA. Die Berechnung der Wasserstoffzahl des Blutes aus der freien und gebundenen Kohlensäure desselben, und die Sauerstoffbindung des Blutes als Funktion der Wasserstoffzahl. *Biochemische Zeitschrift* 1916; **78**: 112–144.

Henderson LJ. Das Gleichgewicht zwischen Basen und Säuren im tierischen Organismus. *Ergebnisse der Physiologie* 1909; **8**: 254–325.

Henry JA. Specific problems of drug intoxication. *British Journal of Anaesthesia* 1986; **58**: 223–233.

Hogben CAM, Tocco DJ, Brodie BB, Schanker LS. On the mechanism of intestinal absorption of drugs. *Journal of Pharmacology and Experimental Therapeutics* 1959; **125**: 275–282.

Inturissi CE, Umans JG. Pethidine and its active metabolite, norpethidine. *Clinics in Anesthesiology* 1983; **1**: 123–138.

Isherwood CN, Calvey TN, Williams NE, Chan K, Murray GR. Elimination of phenoperidine in liver disease. *British Journal of Anaesthesia* 1984; **56**: 843–847.

Kanto J, Erkkola R, Sellman R. Perinatal metabolism of diazepam. *British Medical Journal* 1974; **1**: 641–642.

Kennaghan JB, Boyes RN. The tissue distribution, metabolism and excretion of lidocaine in rats, guinea pigs, dogs and man. *Journal of Pharmacology and Experimental Therapeutics* 1972; **180**: 454–463.

Krakoff IH. Clinical pharmacology of drugs which influence uric acid production and excretion. *Clinical Pharmacology and Therapeutics* 1967; **8**: 124–138.

Milne MD, Scribner BH, Crawford MA. Non-ionic diffusion and the excretion of weak acids and bases. *American Journal of Medicine* 1958; **24**: 709–729.

Nimmo J, Heading RC, Tothill P, Prescott LF. Pharmacological modification of gastric emptying: effects of propantheline and metoclopramide on paracetamol absorption. *British Medical Journal* 1973; **1**: 587–589.

Omura T, Sato R. The carbon monoxide binding pigment of liver microsomes: I. Evidence for its hemoprotein nature. *Journal of Biological Chemistry* 1964: **239**: 2370–2378.

Orloff J, Berliner RW. Renal pharmacology. *Annual Review of Pharmacology* 1961; **1**: 287–314.

Pappenheimer JR. Passage of molecules through capillary walls. *Physiological Reviews* 1953; **33**: 387–423.

Park BK, Breckenridge AM. Clinical implications of enzyme induction and inhibition. *Clinical Pharmacokinetics* 1981; **6**: 1–24.

Peters L. Renal tubular excretion of organic bases. *Pharmacological Reviews* 1960; **12**: 1–35.

Piafsky KM. Disease-induced changes in the plasma binding of basic drugs. *Clinical Pharmacokinetics* 1980; **5**: 246–262.

Prescott LF. Drug conjugation in clinical toxicology. *Biochemical Society Transactions* 1984; **12**: 96–99.

Prescott LF, Nimmo W. *Rate Control in Drug Therapy.* Edinburgh: Churchill Livingstone, 1985.

Price HL, Kovnat PJ, Safer JN, Conner EH, Price ML. The uptake of thiopental by body tissues and its relation to the duration of narcosis. *Clinical Pharmacology and Therapeutics* 1960; **1**: 16–22.

Rane A, Wilson JT. Clinical pharmacokinetics in infants and children. *Clinical Pharmacokinetics* 1976; **1**: 2–24.

Rasmussen F. *Studies on the Mammary Excretion and Absorption of Drugs.* Copenhagen: Carl F. Mortensen, 1966.

Reynolds F. Drug transfer across the placenta. In: Chamberlain G, Wilkinson A (eds). *Placental Transfer.* Tunbridge Wells: Pitman Medical, 1979; 166–181.

Routledge PA. The plasma protein binding of basic drugs. *British Journal of Clinical Pharmacology* 1986; **22**: 499–506.

Runciman WB, Mather LE. Effects of anaesthesia on drug disposition. In: Feldman SA, Scurr CF, Paton WM (eds). *Drugs in Anaesthesia: Mechanisms of Action.* London: Edward Arnold, 1987; 87–122.

Schanker LS. Mechanisms of drug absorption and distribution. *Annual Review of Pharmacology* 1961; **1**: 29–44.

Schanker LS. Passage of drugs across body membranes. *Pharmacological Reviews* 1962; **14**: 501–530.

Scheline RR. Drug metabolism by intestinal microorganisms. *Journal of Pharmaceutical Sciences* 1968; **57**: 2021–2037.

Schou J. Absorption of drugs from subcutaneous connective tissue. *Pharmacological Reviews* 1961; **13**: 441–464.

Singer SJ, Nicolson GL. The fluid mosaic model of the structure of cell membranes. *Science* 1972; **175**: 720–731.

Sjöqvist F, Von Bahr C. Interindividual differences in drug oxidation: clinical importance. *Drug Metabolism and Disposition* 1973; **1**: 469–474.

Smith RL. The biliary excretion and enterohepatic circulation of drugs and other organic compounds. *Progress in Drug Research* 1966; **9**: 299–360.

Somogyi A. New insights into the renal secretion of drugs. *Trends in Pharmacological Sciences* 1987; **8**: 354–357.

Sperber I. Secretion of organic anions in the formation of urine and bile. *Pharmacological Reviews* 1959; **11**: 109–134.

Stoeckel M, Hengstmann JH, Schüttler J. Pharmacokinetics of fentanyl as a possible explanation for recurrence of respiratory depression. *British Journal of Anaesthesia* 1979; **51**: 741–745.

Tillement JP, Lhoste F, Giudicelli JF. Diseases and drug protein binding. *Clinical Pharmacokinetics* 1978; **3**: 144–154.

Tomson G, Lunell N-O, Sundwall A, Rane A. Placental passage of oxazepam and its metabolism in mother and newborn. *Clinical Pharmacology and Therapeutics* 1979; **25**: 74–81.

Tucker GT. Drug metabolism. *British Journal of Anaesthesia* 1979; **51**: 603–618.

Vale JA, Goulding R. Methods to increase drug elimination. *Prescribers Journal* 1979; **19**: 163–168.

Warburg E. Carbonic acid compounds and hydrogen ion activities in blood and salt solutions. A contribution to the theory of LJ. Henderson and KA. Hasselbalch. *Biochemical Journal* 1922; **16**: 153–340.

Weiner IM, Washington JA II, Mudge GH. On the mechanism of action of probenecid on renal tubular secretion. *Bulletin of Johns Hopkins Hospital* 1960; **106**: 333–346.

Wilkinson GR, Shand DG. A physiological approach to hepatic drug clearance. *Clinical Pharmacology and Therapeutics* 1975; **18**: 377–390.

Williams RL, Mamelok RD. Hepatic disease and drug pharmacokinetics. *Clinical Pharmacokinetics* 1980: **5**: 528–547.

TWO

Pharmacokinetics

During the past 20 years, a number of sensitive analytical techniques (e.g. gas–liquid chromatography, high performance liquid chromatography, mass spectrometry, and radioimmunoassay) have been used to measure the concentration of many drugs and their metabolites in plasma and urine. Pharmacokinetics is the quantitative study and mathematical analysis of drug and drug metabolite levels in the body. Changes in drug concentration in relation to time can be used to derive pharmacokinetic constants that adequately account for the behaviour of drugs in the body. These constants can be used to determine the optimum dosage and frequency of administration (or the loading dose and the rate of infusion) required to maintain a steady-state concentration, and to predict the rate and extent of drug cumulation. They can also be used to provide an accurate guide to the modification of drug dosage required in renal and hepatic disease, and to determine the possible effects of other agents and pathological conditions on drug disposition.

The two most important pharmacokinetic constants are the volume of distribution (V) and the clearance (CL). The volume of distribution represents the apparent volume available in the body for the distribution of the drug; the clearance reflects the ability of the body to eliminate the drug. These constants are related to the terminal half-life of the drug ($t_{\frac{1}{2}}$; i.e, the time required for the plasma concentration to decrease by 50% during the terminal phase of decline) by the equation:

$$t_{\frac{1}{2}} = \ln 2 \times \frac{V}{CL}$$

$$= 0.693 \times \frac{V}{CL}.$$

Consequently, the terminal half-life is a hybrid constant, since it is dependent on the primary pharmacokinetic constants V and CL. A prolongation of the terminal half-life may reflect an increase in the volume of distribution, a reduction in the clearance, or both these changes; similarly, a shorter terminal half-life may represent a decreased volume of distribution, an increased clearance, or both phenomena. When the terminal half-lives of drugs are compared, differences between them do not necessarily reflect changes in drug elimination.

VOLUME OF DISTRIBUTION

The volume of distribution represents the relation between the total amount of a drug in the body and its plasma concentration, and thus reflects the process of drug distribution. It is dependent on the partition coefficient of the drug, regional blood flow to tissues, and the degree of plasma protein and tissue binding.

Although the volume of distribution is an apparent volume, and does not correspond to anatomical or physiological tissue compartments, it may be of considerable practical significance. When measured by pharmacokinetic analysis, its value for various drugs in adult man may range from 5 to 700 litres. Drugs with a volume of distribution of 5 to 20 litres 70 kg^{-1} are predominantly localized in plasma or extracellular fluid (e.g. muscle relaxants and other quaternary amines), or are extensively bound by plasma proteins (e.g. warfarin, tolbutamide, chlorpropamide, ibuprofen, probenecid, and aminoglycoside antibiotics). Conversely, when the volume of distribution is greater than the presumed values for total body water (i.e. 50 litres 70 kg^{-1}), there is extensive tissue distribution of drugs (although the specific sites of drug distribution cannot be determined or inferred). In these circumstances, the concentration in tissues is higher than in plasma. The binding of drugs to tissues and tissue proteins is common; drugs with high apparent volumes of distribution include digoxin, fentanyl, pethidine, lignocaine, most phenothiazines, and most antidepressant drugs. The volume of distribution of drugs may be modified by age and physiological factors, since extracellular fluid volume is greater in infants and during pregnancy than in adults; it may also be affected by disease (e.g. renal and cardiac failure).

An appreciation of the total apparent volume of distribution of potentially toxic drugs may significantly affect the management of drug poisoning. Thus, drugs with a large volume of distribution may take many hours or days to be entirely removed from the body, and cannot be reliably eliminated by forced acid or alkaline diuresis. By contrast, drugs with a relatively small volume of distribution may be eliminated by this method (as long as they are not significantly metabolized or extensively bound by plasma proteins). Theoretical considerations suggest that displacement of drugs from plasma protein binding may produce disproportionate changes in the volume of distribution and the concentration of the unbound drug in tissues (depending on the initial value of the volume of distribution).

CLEARANCE

Clearance represents the volume of blood or plasma from which the drug is completely eliminated in unit time; it is usually measured in ml min^{-1}. It can be considered to represent the sum of the different ways of drug elimination that are carried out by various organs in the body; thus,

$$CL = CL_R + CL_H + CL_X$$

where CL_R is renal clearance, CL_H is hepatic clearance, and CL_X is clearance by other routes. Alternatively, clearance can be defined as the rate of drug elimination (in mg min^{-1}) per unit of blood or plasma concentration (in mg ml^{-1}).

In many instances, the renal clearance of drugs can be directly measured by classical methods (or by dividing the total drug eliminated in urine by the area under the plasma concentration–time curve during drug elimination). Consequently, separate estimates may be obtained for renal clearance (CL_R) and extrarenal clearance (CL_{ER}), where $CL_{ER} = CL_t - CL_R$. These values may be useful in assessing the relative importance of renal and hepatic function in drug elimination. When the total body clearance of drugs is predominantly due to renal excretion (i.e. when $CL_R > 0.7 CL$), drug cumulation may occur in renal failure or during renal transplantation. By contrast, when $CL_R < 0.3 CL$, renal disease has little effect on drug elimination. In these circumstances, drug clearance is predominantly dependent on metabolism or biliary excretion. Although these processes may be affected by liver disease, the effects of hepatic dysfunction on the clearance of drugs is usually less predictable.

Nevertheless, the clearance of most drugs from the body is dependent on the liver (either by hepatic metabolism and/or biliary excretion). In steady-state conditions, the removal of drugs by the liver can be expressed by the extraction ratio (ER). This can be defined as:

$$ER = \frac{C_a - C_v}{C_a} = 1 - \frac{C_v}{C_a}$$

where C_a is the drug concentration in mixed portal venous and hepatic arterial blood, and C_v is the drug concentration in hepatic venous blood. The extraction ratio is an overall measure of the ability of the liver to remove drugs from the hepatic capillaries, and reflects drug metabolism, biliary secretion, and other rate limiting processes. It is also one of the main factors that governs the hepatic clearance of drugs.

The most generally accepted model of hepatic clearance assumes that the unbound concentration of drugs in hepatic venous blood and in liver cell water is equal. In these conditions, the elimination of drugs by the liver is dependent on (1) hepatic blood flow, (2) the proportion of unbound drug in blood, and (3) the activity of drug metabolizing enzymes. Hepatic clearance represents the product of hepatic blood flow (Q) and the extraction ratio (ER), i.e.

$$CL_H = Q \times ER.$$

Hepatic clearance can also be expressed in terms of blood flow and 'intrinsic clearance' ($CL_{intrinsic}$), i.e.

$$CL_H = Q \times \frac{CL_{intrinsic} \times f}{Q + (CL_{intrinsic} \times f)}$$

$CL_{intrinsic}$ represents the rate at which liver water is cleared of drug (measured in ml min^{-1}) and f is the fraction of the drug unbound in blood. Intrinsic clearance is independent of blood flow, and represents the maximum ability of the liver to irreversibly eliminate drugs by metabolism or biliary excretion. It has a unique value for different drugs, and can be interpreted in terms of enzyme kinetics as the ratio V_{max}/K_m (p. 62).

When intrinsic clearance ($CL_{intrinsic}$) is relatively low compared to blood flow (Q), then

$$Q + (CL_{intrinsic} \times f) \approx Q$$

and

$$CL_H \approx CL_{intrinsic} \times f.$$

In these circumstances, hepatic clearance is only dependent on intrinsic clearance (i.e. enzyme activity) and the fraction of the drug that is unbound in blood. This type of drug elimination ('capacity-limited' or 'restrictive elimination') is characteristic of the hepatic elimination of phenytoin, tolbutamide, theophylline, warfarin, and most barbiturates and benzodiazepines. These drugs have a limited first pass effect after oral administration and a low hepatic extraction ratio (i.e. less than 0.3). Their clearance is relatively low and is unaffected by alterations in liver blood flow, but is profoundly influenced by changes in hepatic enzyme activity. These changes may be induced by other drugs or environmental agents, as well as age, malnutrition, or disease, which characteristically affect both the total body clearance and the half-life of these compounds. Since $CL_H \approx$ ($CL_{intrinsic} \times$ f), hepatic clearance is also dependent on the fraction of the unbound drug in blood, and may be modified by plasma protein binding. Drugs that are only slightly bound (i.e. 20–30% or less) may be unaffected by changes in protein binding ('capacity-limited, binding-insensitive drugs'). On the other hand, the clearance and terminal half-life of extensively bound drugs will be modified by changes in protein binding ('capacity-limited, binding-sensitive drugs').

When intrinsic clearance ($CL_{intrinsic}$) is relatively large compared to blood flow, then $Q + (CL_{intrinsic} \times f) \approx CL_{intrinsic} \times f$, and the expression

$$CL_H = Q \times \frac{CL_{intrinsic} \times f}{Q + (CL_{intrinsic} \times f)}$$

can be reduced to

$$\mathrm{CL_H} \approx Q.$$

In these conditions, hepatic clearance is primarily determined by liver blood flow ('flow-limited' or 'non-restrictive' elimination). The hepatic clearances of some β-adrenoceptor antagonists, tricyclic antidepressants, opioid analgesics, and lignocaine are dependent on this type of elimination. The hepatic extraction ratio is usually high (i.e. 0.7 or more) and there is usually a substantial first pass effect after oral administration. Characteristically, the clearance of these drugs is relatively high, and is dependent on and determined by liver blood flow (in adult man $21 \, \mathrm{ml \, kg^{-1} \, min^{-1}}$). The half-life may be modified by changes in liver blood flow, but is relatively insensitive to alterations in hepatic enzyme activity or plasma protein binding.

The hepatic elimination of many drugs cannot be readily classified as 'capacity-limited' or 'flow-limited'. Their removal may be partly governed by intrinsic clearance (i.e. enzyme activity and/or biliary secretion) and partly by hepatic blood flow, depending on the conditions in which elimination is assessed. Nevertheless, these concepts provide a physiological approach to the hepatic clearance of drugs, and illustrate the unpredictable relationship between plasma protein binding and drug elimination. When the hepatic clearance of drugs is dependent or partly dependent on intrinsic clearance, significant protein binding may reduce the concentration of the free drug and restrict its elimination. By contrast, when clearance is dependent on hepatic blood flow, protein binding has little or no effect.

TERMINAL HALF-LIFE

Although the terminal half-life of a drug is a hybrid value (i.e. it depends on the primary constants V and CL), it provides a useful guide to the optimum frequency of drug administration. In general, drugs are usually best given (either orally, intramuscularly, or intravenously) at intervals that are approximately equal to their terminal half-lives. In these conditions, there is often an acceptable compromise between the decline in drug concentrations after successive doses, and the necessity for frequent drug administration in order to maintain an adequate plasma level. The terminal half-lives of drugs that are commonly used in anaesthetic practice are shown in Table 2.1. When drugs are administered at intervals that are equal to their half-lives, they cumulate (i.e. there is a progressive rise in plasma concentration) for 4 to 5 half-lives until steady-state concentrations are reached (Fig. 2.1). The latent period before the presence of steady-state concentrations can be avoided by the initial administration of a loading dose equal to twice the normal dose. Similarly, when drugs are given by continuous intravenous infusion, steady-state concentrations are reached (to within 5%) after 4 to

Table 2.1 Plasma half-lives ('elimination half-lives') of drugs commonly used in anaesthetic practice. Values were obtained in patients with normal renal and hepatic function.

Drug	Plasma half-life (min)
Analgesics	
Alfentanil	73–110
Fentanyl	87–346
Morphine	120–180
Pethidine	160–300
Phenoperidine	15–30
Intravenous anaesthetics	
Etomidate	186–282
Methohexitone	60–134
Propofol	184–382
Thiopentone	360–440
Local anaesthetics	
Bupivacaine	180–240
Lignocaine	100–120
Prilocaine	180–300
Muscle relaxants and their antagonists	
Alcuronium	180–220
Atracurium	18–22
Gallamine	80–220
Pancuronium	110–150
Suxamethonium	3–5
Tubocurarine	150–230
Vecuronium	36–72
Atropine	90–200
Neostigmine	15–90
Pyridostigmine	15–130
Other drugs	
Adrenaline	5–10
Diazepam	1200–5400
Hydrocortisone	90–120
Midazolam	120–250
Nitrazepam	1100–1800
Prednisolone	200–300
Sodium nitroprusside	5–10

5 terminal half-lives (Fig. 2.2). If the desired plasma concentration (or the level required to produce a given effect) is known, the dose required after oral or intramuscular administration can be calculated from the clearance, using the expression:

$$\text{required dose (mg)} = \frac{C_p \times I \times CL}{f}$$

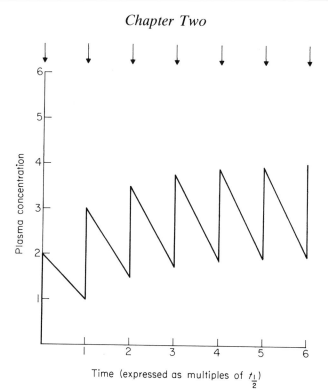

Fig. 2.1 Diagrammatic representation of the cumulation of drugs when they are administered (↓) at intervals that are equal to their half-lives.

when C_p is the desired plasma concentration (mg ml^{-1}), I is the dosage interval (min), CL is the clearance (ml min^{-1}), and f is the fraction of the dose that enters the systemic circulation (i.e. the proportion that is absorbed and is not subject to first pass effects).

Unfortunately, after oral or intramuscular administration of many drugs, precise values for f are not available, and calculation of the required dose may be relatively inaccurate. By contrast, when drugs are given intravenously, the loading dose (mg) is given by $C_p \times V$, and the rate of infusion (mg min^{-1}) by $C_p \times$ CL, where C_p is the desired steady-state plasma concentration (mg ml^{-1}), V is the volume of distribution at steady-state (ml), and CL is the clearance (ml min^{-1}). When drugs are given intravenously over prolonged periods (e.g. opioid analgesics, non-depolarizing muscle relaxants, and antibiotics), this method can be used to produce accurate, constant plasma concentrations (Fig. 2.3). Unfortunately, it depends on the determination of the volume of distribution and the clearance, which may be subject to considerable inter-individual variability. In addition, the loading dose may result in transiently high plasma concentrations above the acceptable range, and may therefore require modification (e.g. by the use of an initial rapid rate of infusion).

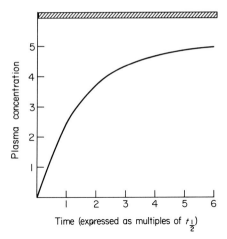

Fig. 2.2 Diagrammatic representation of drug cumulation during continuous intravenous infusion (◫◫◫).

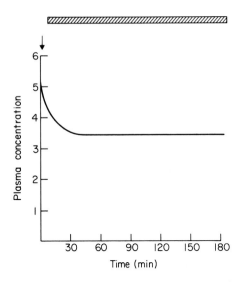

Fig. 2.3 Diagrammatic representation of the maintenance of a constant plasma concentration C_p based on the equations: loading dose (↓) = volume of distribution $\times$ C_p and infusion rate (◫◫◫) = clearance $\times$ C_p.

Pharmacokinetic constants can also be used to predict the effects of altered hepatic and renal function on the plasma concentration of drugs. Chronic renal disease causes a reduction in creatinine clearance and the renal elimination of many drugs. In particular, the clearance of drugs that are almost entirely elim-

Table 2.2 Terminal half-lives and total body clearance of non-depolarizing muscle relaxants in patients with normal and impaired renal function.

Muscle relaxant	$t_{\frac{1}{2}}$ (min)		Clearance (ml min^{-1})	
	Normal patients	Renal failure	Normal patients	Renal failure
Atracurium	18–22	18–22	360–400	340–470
Gallamine	80–220	400–1300	50–100	5–25
Pancuronium	110–150	280–490	75–125	20–50
Tubocurarine	150–230	250–330	80–120	50–70
Vecuronium	36–72	42–94	150–350	130–500

inated unchanged by the kidney (e.g. aminoglycoside antibiotics, some thiazide diuretics, and digoxin) is reduced. In these conditions, the dosage required to produce a given plasma level in patients with reduced renal clearance can be calculated from the equation:

$$\text{required dose} = \frac{C_p \times I \times CL}{f} \quad \text{(see p. 43).}$$

Chronic renal failure reduces the clearance and increases the half-life of most non-depolarizing muscle relaxants (Table 2.2). Although the modification in drug dosage required to produce the plasma concentration associated with neuro-muscular blockade can be calculated, in practice this is rarely carried out. Most of the clinical evidence suggests that the action of large single doses or multiple doses of alcuronium, gallamine, pancuronium, and tubocurarine is prolonged in renal failure, since the plasma concentration of the drug mainly determines the extent and the duration of neuromuscular blockade. In contrast, the effects of atracurium and vecuronium are not prolonged, and these drugs do not cumulate in patients with renal failure.

The terminal half-lives of many drugs may be a guide to their duration of action. For instance, when muscle relaxants are ranked by their terminal half-lives, alcuronium = tubocurarine > pancuronium > gallamine > vecuronium > atracurium > suxamethonium (Table 2.1), and in general this order corresponds to their relative duration of action. Nevertheless, there are many exceptions to this rule; for instance, when drugs act irreversibly (e.g. many cholinesterase inhibitors, monoamine oxidase inhibitors, and some α-adrenoceptor antagonists), their duration of action is unrelated to their clearance or their terminal half-lives. Similarly, the duration of action of intravenous benzodiazepines is not related to these pharmacokinetic constants. Thus, the duration of sedation and anterograde amnesia produced by diazepam and midazolam are similar, despite the wide disparity in their terminal half-lives (Table 2.1). This phenomenon may reflect the rapid fall in their plasma concentration after intravenous administration, due to their relatively high lipid solubility and rapid distribution in tissues. If their plasma concentration falls below the threshold required to produce amnesia during their distribution to tissues, the duration of action will not be dependent on or related to the terminal half-life. Similarly, recovery from the analgesic and respiratory depressant effects of small doses of fentanyl is normally dependent on the rapid decrease in concentration during drug distribution. As the dose of fentanyl is increased, the duration of action rises disproportionately, as recovery is associated with plasma concentrations present during the terminal half-life of the drug. In addition, the duration of action of small doses of fentanyl may be dependent on its method of administration; the slower decline in plasma concentration after intravenous infusion (as compared to bolus administration) can prolong the action of drugs whose effects are terminated by drug distribution.

EXPONENTIAL CHANGES

Changes in the plasma concentration of drugs in relation to time can usually be expressed as mathematical equations containing one or more exponential terms. Similarly, many processes concerned with absorption, distribution, and elimination result in exponential changes in drug concentrations as a function of time. In an exponential change, the rate of increase or decrease of a variable is directly proportional to its magnitude; in mathematical terms,

$$\pm \frac{dX}{dt} \propto X$$

$$\text{or} \quad \pm \frac{dX}{dt} = kX$$

where dX/dt is the rate of increase or decrease of the variable X during an infinitesimal moment of time t, k is a constant, and X is the value of the variable at time t.

On integration of this expression between $t = 0$ and $t = \infty$,

$$X = X_0 . e^{kt} \quad \text{(for exponential growth)}$$
$$\text{or} \quad X = X_0 . e^{-kt} \quad \text{(for exponential disappearance)}$$

where X is the value of X at any time t; X_0 is the initial value of X at zero time; e is the base of natural logarithms (2.718); and k is a constant.

In these conditions, X can be described as an exponential function of time. Consider the equation for exponential disappearance

$$X = X_0 . e^{-kt}.$$

On taking natural logarithms,

$$\ln X = \ln X_0 - kt$$

and
$$\ln \left(\frac{X}{X_0}\right) = -kt.$$

Consequently $k = -\ln(X/X_0)/t$; in this equation k can be considered as a rate constant, and represents the proportional change in X in unit time. Alternatively the rate of exponential change can be represented as the half-time (half-life) or as a time constant.

Since

$$k = \frac{-\ln(X/X_0)}{t}$$

$$t = \frac{\ln(X/X_0)}{-k}.$$

If $(X/X_0) = \frac{1}{2}$, t represents the time for X to decline to half its original value; consequently,

$$t = \frac{\ln\left(\frac{1}{2}\right)}{-k}$$

$$= \frac{\ln 2}{k}$$

$$= \frac{0.693}{k}$$

In these conditions, t represents the half-time (half-life) of the exponential change.

Alternatively, if

$$\frac{X}{X_0} = \frac{1}{2.718} = \frac{1}{e}$$

t represents the time required for X to decline to $1/e$ (37%) of its original value; thus,

$$t = \frac{\ln\left(\frac{1}{e}\right)}{-k}$$

$$= \frac{\ln(e^{-1})}{-k}$$

$$= \frac{-\ln e}{-k}$$

$$= \frac{1}{k}.$$

In these conditions t represents the time constant of the exponential change; it is the reciprocal of the rate constant k.

DETERMINATION OF VOLUME OF DISTRIBUTION AND CLEARANCE

Compartmental models have been widely used to determine the volume of distribution and the clearance of drugs. Nevertheless, the choice of a suitable pharmacokinetic model may be difficult, and can depend on technical, analytical, and sampling factors. The behaviour of some drugs (e.g. tubocurarine) has been described by different pharmacokinetic models, and in these conditions the interpretation of the results may be complex. The calculation of the volume of distribution and the clearance is critically dependent on the choice of model (and on the accuracy with which plasma concentration–time data can be represented by it).

Consequently, in recent years non-compartmental methods have been widely used to determine the volume of distribution and the clearance of drugs. Nevertheless, the distribution and elimination of many drugs in the body can be adequately characterized by simple pharmacokinetic models.

One-compartment model

The decline in the plasma concentration of many drugs after intramuscular administration is consistent with a simple one-compartment pharmacokinetic model. For example, in one study neostigmine (2 mg) was given by intramuscular injection to five patients with myasthenia gravis, and blood samples were removed at 30, 60, 90, 120, 150 and 180 min. The concentration of neostigmine in plasma was then measured. The following table shows the results obtained in one patient.

Time after intramuscular injection (min)	Concentration of neostigmine ($ng\ ml^{-1}$)
30	19
60	14
90	11
120	9
150	7
180	6

When the logarithm or the natural logarithm ($\log_e$ or ln) of the plasma concentration of neostigmine is plotted against time (Fig. 2.4), a straight line is obtained, indicating that the decline in the plasma concentration of the drug is an exponential function of time (p. 47). The decrease in the plasma concentration of

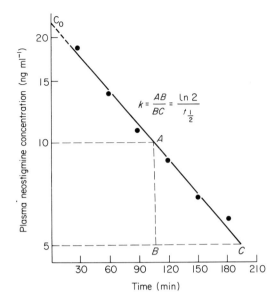

Fig. 2.4 Monoexponential decline in the plasma concentration of neostigmine after intramuscular injection. Data points (•) correspond to the concentration of neostigmine at different times after administration, expressed on a logarithmic (ln) scale. *BC* corresponds to the half-life of neostigmine; the slope of the regression line relating the data points = k = *AB/BC* = ln 2/$t_{\frac{1}{2}}$. C_0 is the extrapolated concentration of neostigmine at the time $t = 0$.

neostigmine is greatest initially (i.e. between 30 and 60 min), and then gradually declines, although a constant proportion of the drug is removed during each time interval.

The slope of the monoexponential decline in the plasma concentration of neostigmine reflects the half-life of the drug. The plasma half-life is defined as the time required for the concentration of a drug in plasma to decline by 50% (i.e. to one-half of its initial value). Since there is a linear relationship between the logarithm of plasma concentration and time (Fig. 2.4), the plasma half-life can be measured from any point on the line. In Fig. 2.4, the plasma half-life is given by

$$t_{\frac{1}{2}} = BC = 93 \, \text{min}$$

as measured by graphical estimation. This corresponds to the time required for the plasma concentration to fall from 10 ng ml^{-1} to 5 ng ml^{-1}. Since the natural logarithm of the plasma concentration of neostigmine was plotted against time, the slope of the monoexponential decline in plasma concentration is equal to

$$\frac{AB}{BC} = \frac{\ln 10 - \ln 5}{t_{\frac{1}{2}}} = \frac{\ln 2}{t_{\frac{1}{2}}} = \frac{0.693}{t_{\frac{1}{2}}}.$$

Drug
administration

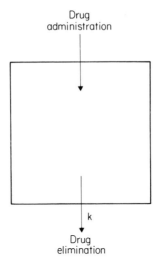

k

Drug
elimination

Fig. 2.5 Diagrammatic representation of a one-compartment, open, pharmacokinetic model. The constant k corresponds to the elimination rate constant, and is measured in units of reciprocal time (e.g. min^{-1}).

The gradient of the line can be used to predict or determine the plasma concentration of neostigmine (C_p) at any time (t) after administration of the drug. It can be shown that the equation relating the decline in plasma concentration to time is

$$C_p = C_0 . e^{-kt}$$

where C_p is the plasma concentration at time t; C_0 is the extrapolated concentration of the drug at $t = 0$; $e = 2.718$ (the base of natural logarithms); and k is the gradient of the decline in plasma concentration.

$$\frac{\ln 2}{t_{\frac{1}{2}}}$$

In this instance, the decline in the plasma concentration of neostigmine after intramuscular injection is consistent with a one-compartment, pharmacokinetic model. According to this model, the body is considered in a highly simplified manner as a single homogeneous entity or compartment (Fig. 2.5). Drugs are administered into, and eliminated from, this compartment (either by metabolism or renal and biliary excretion). The rate of drug elimination is assumed to be proportional to the amount of drug in the body (X) at any time (t), i.e. it decreases exponentially with time and is consistent with first-order kinetics. When expressed as a differential equation,

$$\frac{dX}{dt} \propto X$$

and

$$\frac{dX}{dt} = -kX$$

where X is the amount of drug in the body at time t; and k is the elimination rate constant measured in units of reciprocal time (i.e. per min). The negative sign reflects the removal of the drug from the body. Integration of this expression with respect to time gives the expression

$$X = X_0 \cdot e^{-kt}$$

where X_0 is the amount of drug initially present in the body (i.e. the intravenous dose or the fraction of the dose that is absorbed); and e = 2.718.

The division of this equation by the volume of the compartment (the volume of distribution or V) gives the expression

$$C = C_0 \cdot e^{-kt}$$

which is identical to the equation that describes the plasma concentration of the drug at different times after its administration. The constant k defines the slope of the drug concentration–time relationship obtained from plasma levels (Fig. 2.4); it also represents the elimination rate constant when the data are interpreted by a one-compartment open model. The elimination rate constant k is estimated from the equation

$$k = \frac{\ln 2}{t_{\frac{1}{2}}} = \frac{0.693}{t_{\frac{1}{2}}}.$$

The volume of distribution can be calculated from the expression

$$V = \frac{X_0}{C_0}$$

It corresponds to the volume of the compartment, and represents the relationship between the total amount of drug in the body and the plasma concentration.

The clearance of the drug is given by

$$CL = V \cdot k$$

Thus, clearance corresponds to the volume of the compartment multiplied by the rate of drug elimination (i.e. the volume that is cleared of the drug in unit time). It represents the sum of all the processes of drug clearance that occur in different organs of the body (p. 39). The estimation of renal clearance is simplified by the measurement or calculation of the total area subtended by the plasma concentration–time curve between $t = 0$ and $t = \infty$ (infinity). The area under the curve (AUC) is given by

$$\text{AUC} = \frac{C_0}{k}$$

and the renal clearance (CL_R) by the expression

$$CL_R = \frac{\text{total drug eliminated in urine}}{\text{AUC}}$$

When the pharmacokinetics of intramuscular neostigmine was studied, the plasma concentration data did not exactly correspond to a monoexponential decline (Fig. 2.4). Differences between the data points and the plasma concentration–time regression line were probably due to unavoidable analytical and sampling errors. Although estimates of some pharmacokinetic values (e.g. $t_{\frac{1}{2}}$, k, and C_0) can be made by graphical methods, and other parameters (e.g. V, CL, and AUC) derived from them, this method is time-consuming and relatively inaccurate.

More commonly, plasma concentrations are converted to logarithms, and the linear relation between these values and time (see Fig. 2.4) is derived by least squares regression analysis. The other constants are usually generated by computer programmes. In the example given, when the decline in the plasma concentration of neostigmine after intramuscular injection was interpreted in terms of a one-compartment, open model, the following results were obtained, using a computer programme:

$$t_{\frac{1}{2}} = 91\,\text{min}$$
$$k = 0.0077\,\text{min}^{-1}$$
$$C_0 = 23\,\text{ng ml}^{-1}$$
$$V = 58\,700\,\text{ml}$$
$$CL = 450\,\text{ml min}^{-1}$$
$$\text{AUC} = 2967\,\text{ng ml}^{-1}.\,\text{min}$$

After oral or intramuscular administration, drugs are usually absorbed by first-order processes, and their absorption can be defined and expressed as an absorption rate constant. In the postabsorptive phase, the decline in their plasma concentration can usually be interpreted by a one-compartment open model (as in the example of intramuscular neostigmine). The behaviour of a minority of drugs after intravenous administration (e.g. bromosulphonphthalein, suxamethonium and possibly inulin) can also be described by this simple model, since their plasma concentration usually declines in a monoexponential manner.

It should be emphasized that compartments in kinetic models do not necessarily have any physiological meaning. A one-compartment model is primarily defined by the behaviour of the drug in the body, and not by anatomical or physiological considerations; the model merely implies that the drug does not pass from one part of the body (e.g. plasma) to another at a measurable rate. Although drug concentrations in plasma are probably different from levels in other tissues, a one-compartment model implies that differences in concentration within the body bear a constant relationship to each other. By contrast, the behaviour of many other drugs after intravenous injection cannot be realistically interpreted in terms of a one-compartment open model. In these conditions, paradigms of greater complexity provide a more accurate description of the decline in plasma concentration. In particular, the two-compartment open model has been widely used to account for the behaviour of many drugs that are used in anaesthetic practice and administered by intravenous injection.

Two-compartment model

After intravenous injection, most drugs are initially present in a restricted volume, and are then rapidly distributed throughout the body. During the phase of distribution, there is a rapid decline in plasma concentration; its rate and extent are primarily dependent on the physicochemical characteristics of the drug (e.g. its molecular weight and lipid solubility). When distribution is complete and a state of equilibrium has been established, the subsequent decline in plasma concentration reflects the elimination of the drug.

The decrease in the plasma concentration of many drugs after intravenous injection is consistent with this concept. Thus, after the intravenous injection of phenoperidine, there is a biexponential decline in the plasma level of the drug (Fig. 2.6). An initial rapid fall in concentration (due to drug distribution) is followed by a slower phase of exponential decline (due to drug elimination). The decrease in the plasma concentration of phenoperidine can be resolved into two exponential components by extrapolation. The terminal phase of the decline in plasma concentration (β, slow disposition, or elimination phase) is extended to the ordinate (y axis), which it intersects at point B. Subtraction of the extrapolated values from the initial data points gives a series of residual values, which represent the initial phase of exponential decline. This initial phase (α, rapid disposition or distribution phase) is defined by a regression line that intercepts the ordinate at A. Both the α and the β phases have characteristic slopes α and β) and half-lives ($t_{\frac{1}{2}\alpha}$ and $t_{\frac{1}{2}\beta}$). Numerical values for the slopes α and β can be estimated from the equations

$$\alpha = \frac{\ln 2}{t_{\frac{1}{2}\alpha}}$$

and

$$\beta = \frac{\ln 2}{t_{\frac{1}{2}\beta}}$$

and the concentration C_p at time t is given by the expression

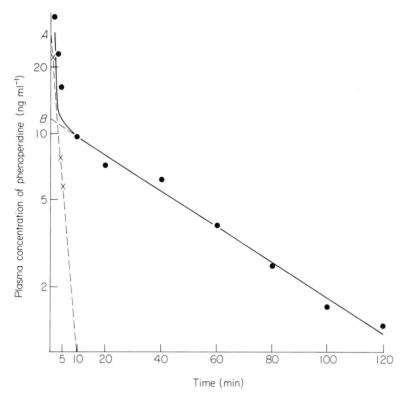

Fig. 2.6 Biexponential decline in the plasma concentration of phenoperidine after intravenous injection. The abscissa (*x* axis) shows the time in minutes; the ordinate (*y* axis) represents the logarithm of the plasma concentration of phenoperidine; data points (●) correspond to the plasma concentration of the drug at different times. *B* represents the initial concentration of the slower phase of exponential decline, extrapolated to zero time. Extrapolated values on this line were subtracted from the data points to give a series of residual values (*x*); the least squares regression line through these points corresponds to the rapid disposition phase.

$$C_p = A \cdot e^{-\alpha t} + B \cdot e^{-\beta t}$$

where *A* and *B* are intercepts on the ordinate (Fig. 2.6) and e = 2.718. The constants α and β are hybrid constants, since they are determined by, and are dependent on, other constants. Values for *A*, *B*, α and β can be derived by graphical methods, or more accurately determined by digital computer pro-grammes. Analysis of the decline in the plasma concentration of phenoperidine (Fig. 2.6) gave the following expression:

$$C_p = 30e^{-0.276t} + 12e^{-0.019t}$$

where C_p is measured in ng ml^{-1} and *t* in minutes.

The biexponential decline in the plasma concentration of phenoperidine was

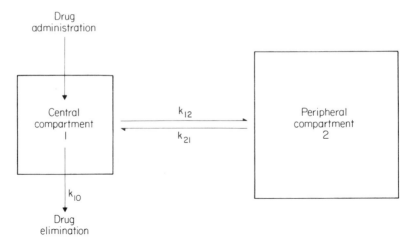

Fig. 2.7 Diagrammatic representation of a two-compartment, open, model, consisting of a central compartment 1 and a peripheral compartment 2. The constants k_{12} and k_{21} govern drug transfer between the central and peripheral compartments; k_{10} is the elimination rate constant.

interpreted in terms of a two-compartment, open pharmacokinetic model (Fig. 2.7). This model consists of a relatively small central compartment, into which the drug is administered and from which it is eliminated, and a peripheral compartment. The rate of drug elimination is governed by the rate constant k_{10}. The peripheral compartment usually has a larger apparent volume than the central compartment; bidirectional (reversible) drug transfer between the two compartments is governed by the rate constants k_{12} and k_{21} (Fig. 2.7). As in the one-compartment model (p. 49), the central and the peripheral compartments have no direct physiological meaning, and their parameters and constants are solely determined by the behaviour of the drug in the body.

The two-compartment model is essentially a theoretical concept which accounts for the observed biexponential decline in plasma concentration (Fig. 2.6). In the case of phenoperidine (and many other drugs), the central compartment probably consists of the blood, interstitial fluid, and some of the intracellular water of highly perfused organs (e.g. the heart, lungs, liver, and kidneys). The peripheral compartment consists of the brain and less well perfused tissues (e.g. most skeletal muscle, fat, skin, and connective tissue). During the distribution phase, the plasma concentration of phenoperidine falls rapidly as the drug is distributed from the central compartment to the peripheral compartment (Fig. 2.7). After the occurrence of distribution equilibrium between the two compartments, removal of the drug is solely dependent on elimination, which is governed by the rate constant k_{10}.

As in the one-compartment model, resolution is dependent on the assumption that both distribution and elimination are exponential, first-order processes (i.e. that the rate at which they occur is proportional to the amount of drug in each compartment). Differential equations can then be derived that express the rate of change of drug in each compartment (i.e. dX_1/dt and dX_2/dt, where X_1 and X_2 are the amounts of drug in each compartment at time t). The solution of these first-order differential equations for dX_1/dt and dX_2/dt, and the conversion of X_1 and X_2 to concentrations, gives expressions that relate the concentration of the drug in the central compartment (C_1) and the peripheral compartment (C_2) to time.

In the case of the central compartment,

$$C_1 = A.e^{-\alpha t} + B.e^{-\beta t}$$

where A, α, B, β are constants, and e $= 2.718$. This is identical to the equation that describes the biexponential decline in the plasma concentration of drugs after their intravenous injection. Consequently values for A, α, B, β can be derived from the measured plasma concentrations. These constants can then be used to derive other parameters of the two compartment open model (e.g. the area under the plasma concentration–time curve (AUC), the clearance (CL), the volume of distribution (V), as well as the rate constants k_{21}, k_{10}, and k_{12}), using the following formulae:

$$\text{AUC} = \frac{A}{\alpha} + \frac{B}{\beta}$$

$$\text{CL} = \frac{\text{dose}}{\text{AUC}} = \frac{\text{dose}}{\dfrac{A}{\alpha} + \dfrac{B}{\beta}}$$

$$k_{21} = \frac{A\beta + B\alpha}{A + B}$$

$$k_{10} = \frac{\alpha\beta}{k_{21}}$$

$$k_{12} = \alpha + \beta - (k_{21} + k_{10})$$

$$V_{\text{area}} = \frac{\text{dose}}{\beta(\text{AUC})} = \frac{\text{dose}}{\beta\left(\dfrac{A}{\alpha} + \dfrac{B}{\beta}\right)}$$

$$V_{\text{ss}} = \frac{\text{dose}}{A + B} \times \frac{k_{12} + k_{21}}{k_{21}}.$$

Analysis of the plasma concentration of phenoperidine after intravenous injection gave the following values, using a digital computer programme:

$$A \quad = 30\,\text{ng ml}^{-1}$$
$$\alpha \quad = 0.276\,\text{min}^{-1}$$
$$t_{\frac{1}{2}\alpha} \quad = 2.5\,\text{min}$$
$$B \quad = 12\,\text{ng ml}^{-1}$$
$$\beta \quad = 0.019\,\text{min}^{-1}$$
$$t_{\frac{1}{2}\beta} \quad = 37.0\,\text{min}$$
$$\text{AUC} = 725\,\text{ng ml}^{-1}.\,\text{min}$$
$$\text{CL} \quad = 2511\,\text{ml min}^{-1}$$
$$k_{21} \quad = 0.090\,\text{min}^{-1}$$
$$k_{10} \quad = 0.057\,\text{min}^{-1}$$
$$k_{12} \quad = 0.147\,\text{min}^{-1}$$
$$V_{\text{area}} = 134\,\text{litre}$$
$$V_{\text{ss}} \quad = 117\,\text{litre}.$$

As shown above, two expressions for the volume of distribution can be derived, V_{area} and V_{ss}. V_{area} expresses the relation between the total amount of phenoperidine in the body and its concentration in the central compartment during the terminal or slow disposition phase (i.e. when distribution equilibrium has been established). V_{area} may overestimate the true volume of distribution when rapid drug elimination occurs and clearance is high. V_{ss} is not dependent on the rate of drug elimination, and therefore provides a more objective and accurate estimate of the volume of distribution.

The pharmacokinetics of drugs whose distribution and elimination are consistent with a two-compartment open model are often determined after rapid intravenous injection, using a bolus dose. In these conditions, the accurate measurement of some kinetic parameters may be relatively difficult. For instance, the estimation of both the clearance (CL) and the volume of distribution (V) are critically dependent on the area under the plasma concentration–time curve between $t = 0$ and $t = \infty$ (AUC). The AUC is determined from the relationship $A/\alpha + B/\beta$; since A is usually large and α is relatively small, any errors or inaccuracy in the determination of these constants may significantly affect the estimation of the AUC. Unfortunately, after the bolus injection of drugs, measurement of A and α may be extremely inaccurate since (1) they are dependent on derived rather than measured concentration, (2) they are usually determined from a relatively small number of points, and (3) the plasma concentration of drugs is rapidly decreasing during the distribution phase, so that minor difficulties in the timing or removal of blood samples may lead to considerable errors.

In consequence, pharmacokinetic parameters that are based on measurements of plasma concentrations after the bolus injection of drugs should be interpreted with circumspection. These values can usually be measured more accurately when drugs are administered by intravenous infusion. In these conditions, pharmacokinetic parameters are best assessed after the administration of

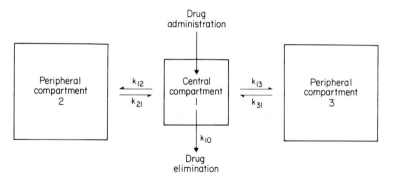

Fig. 2.8 Diagrammatic representation of a three-compartment, open, model, consisting of a central compartment 1 and two peripheral compartments, 2 and 3. Drug administration occurs into, and elimination occurs from, the central compartment. The constants k_{12}, k_{21}, k_{13} and k_{31} govern drug transfer between the central and peripheral compartments; k_{10} is the elimination rate constant.

drugs for several half-lives. Unfortunately, this is rarely possible, and shorter periods of infusion are usually employed. Pharmacokinetic constants applicable to a two-compartment open model can be derived from the postinfusion plasma concentration data by appropriate mathematical techniques. It should be recognized that when drugs are given by continuous intravenous infusion, the subsequent decline in their plasma concentration (and the α or fast disposition phase) is attenuated, since rapid distribution or redistribution no longer occurs. The slower decline in the plasma concentration after intravenous infusion may be clinically significant, and can prolong the effects of short-acting drugs (particularly when their effects are usually terminated by distribution).

Three-compartment models

The kinetics of most drugs after intravenous injection are consistent with a two compartment open model. Nevertheless, in some circumstances models of greater complexity provide a better interpretation of the results. Thus, the decline in the plasma concentration of drugs after intravenous injection can sometimes be resolved into three exponential components, and the plasma concentration C_p after time t is defined by the expression

$$C_p = Pe^{-\pi t} + Ae^{-\alpha t} + Be^{-\beta t}.$$

Values for the intercepts (P, A and B) and the slopes (π, α and β) of the three components can then be obtained, either graphically or by the use of a digital computer programme. The decline in the plasma concentration of the drug can be interpreted in terms of a three-compartment open model, with drug administration into and elimination from the central compartment (Fig. 2.8). Alternatively, the decrease in plasma concentration can be interpreted by a three-

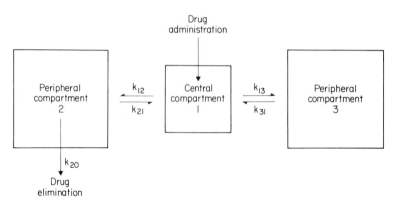

Fig. 2.9 Diagrammatic representation of a three-compartment, open, model, consisting of a central compartment 1 and two peripheral compartments, 2 and 3. Drug administration occurs into the central compartment; drug elimination occurs from peripheral compartment 2. The constants k_{12}, k_{21}, k_{13} and k_{31} govern drug transfer between the central and the peripheral compartments; k_{20} is the elimination rate constant.

compartment model in which elimination occurs from one of the peripheral compartments (Fig. 2.9). The parameters of these models (i.e. clearance, volume of distribution, individual compartmental volumes, and the rate constants governing transfer between compartments) can then be determined.

In some instances, the decline in the plasma concentration of drugs is apparently consistent with both a two-compartment and a three-compartment model. The most appropriate pharmacokinetic model can be selected in the following manner. A semi-logarithmic curve relating plasma concentration to time is resolved into both two and three exponential components, using a digital computer programme. In each case, the residual variation between the experimental points and the computer-derived curves is calculated. If there is no significant reduction in variation when the results are analysed as a triexponential equation, then the biexponential solution (consistent with a two-compartment open model) is assumed to be correct. Although this does not prove that the two-compartment model is correct, it does suggest that the model provides a better interpretation of the results. In practice, the distinction between two-compartment and three-compartment models is small and of little importance. The difference between the experimental points and the computer-derived values may well be less than the accuracy of the analytical method used to measure drug concentrations. Similarly, the timing of the removal of blood samples may influence the choice of a pharmacokinetic model; inappropriate sampling times may fail to identify the initial phase or the terminal phase of exponential decline. In consequence, technical, analytical, and sampling factors may play a disproportionate role in determining the type of pharmacokinetic model that is chosen. For instance, the decline in the plasma concentration of most non-depolarizing relaxants has been analysed by different authors using both two- and three-compartment models; these differences probably reflect the variability in the analytical measurement of plasma concentrations, different sampling times, and possibly other technical factors.

Non-compartmental methods of pharmacokinetic analysis

The various problems associated with resolution of plasma concentration data into specific compartmental models have led to the use of non-compartmental methods of pharmacokinetic analysis. These methods do not depend on the assumption of a specific pharmacokinetic model, although they can be used to estimate drug clearance (CL) and the volume of distribution at steady state (V_{ss}). The terminal half-life can also be derived by non-linear least squares regression analysis, using a digital computer programme; if necessary, the data can be weighted (usually by the reciprocal of the squares of the individual plasma concentrations).

Clearance can be derived from the relationship

$$CL = \frac{dose}{AUC}$$

where AUC is the area under the plasma concentration–time curve between $t = 0$ and $t = \infty$. The AUC can be estimated by the 'trapezoidal rule', which depends on the measurement and summation of the area of each trapezoid between successive sampling times and the corresponding plasma concentrations. The area between the plasma concentration and time of the final sample and $t = \infty$ is estimated from the expression: final plasma concentration × terminal half-life/0.693.

Volume of distribution at steady-state is given by the equation

$$V_{ss} = dose \times \frac{AUMC}{(AUC)^2}$$

where AUMC is the total area under the first moment of the plasma concentration–time curve (i.e. the area under the plasma concentration × time versus time curve, extrapolated to infinity).

Non-linear pharmacokinetics

When drug behaviour is analysed by pharmacokinetic models, it is usually assumed that distribution and elimination are first-order processes. In these conditions, the rate of drug transfer from compartment to compartment is always proportional to drug concentration. This presumption is not necessarily correct. Many physiological processes concerned with drug distribution and elimination are dependent on carrier transport, and are potentially saturable (i.e. they have a maximum, finite, transport capacity). Similarly, many reactions concerned with drug metabolism are saturable, and proceed at a maximal rate in the presence of high substrate concentrations. In these circumstances, drug transport and metabolism occur at a high but constant rate that is not dependent on drug concentration; in mathematical terms, $dX/dt = -k$, where X is the amount of drug in the body or compartment at time t, and k is a constant. This type of kinetics is called non-linear or saturation kinetics, and occurs with the capacity limited elimination of drugs. Metabolic reactions that are subject to saturation kinetics are consistent with Michaelis–Menten kinetics; when saturation occurs, metabolism changes from a first-order process ($dX/dt = -kX^1 = -kX$) to a zero-order process ($dX/dt = -kX^0 = -k$), and is constant and independent of drug concentration.

These relationships can be derived from the Michaelis–Menten equation for enzyme kinetics as expressed in the form

$$v = \frac{V_{max} \cdot C_p}{K_m + C_p}$$

where v is the rate of drug elimination; V_{max} is the maximum rate of drug elimination; K_m is an affinity constant (the Michaelis constant); and C_p is the plasma concentration. When the plasma concentration C_p is much less than K_m, then $v \approx (V_{max}/K_m) \times C_p$; since V_{max} and K_m are both constants, $v \propto C_p$, so that the rate of drug elimination is consistent with first-order kinetics. On the other hand, at higher plasma concentrations C_p may be greater than K_m, so that $v \approx (V_{max} \times C_p)/C_p$ and $v \approx V_{max}$. Thus the rate of drug elimination becomes constant at high concentrations, and is consistent with zero-order kinetics. The affinity constant K_m represents the affinity of the drug for the enzyme, carrier, or transport system; it corresponds to the plasma concentration at which drug elimination is half its maximal rate (i.e. $v/V_{max} = 0.5$).

In practice, the phenomenon of non-linear or saturation kinetics is relatively uncommon, since the capacity of carrier transport systems and metabolic reactions is normally much greater than effective drug concentrations. Nevertheless, in some instances (particularly with drugs that are primarily or predominantly eliminated by hepatic metabolism), non-linear or zero-order kinetics occurs *in vivo*. In these conditions, increases in drug dosage and plasma concentration may cause prolongation in the half-life of drugs, and the area under the plasma concentration–time curve is disproportionately raised. (By contrast, when drugs are distributed and eliminated by first-order processes, all kinetic parameters are by definition independent of the dose.) Non-linear pharmacokinetics may occur during the metabolism of ethanol, salicylates, and phenytoin, due to saturation of hepatic metabolic pathways. In the case of phenytoin, saturation may occur at subtherapeutic or therapeutic concentrations (40–80 μmol litre^{-1}), so that subsequent increments in dosage cause a disproportionate increase in plasma concentration. Saturation kinetics may also occur during the elimination of large or repeated doses of thiopentone; in these circumstances, the terminal half-life of the drug is increased and its pharmacological effects are prolonged, possibly due to zero-order hepatic metabolism. Non-linear pharmacokinetics also occurs in many patients during drug overdosage. It is uncertain whether this reflects saturation of hepatic metabolism, the toxic effects of drugs, or both phenomena. When drugs are eliminated by saturable processes (e.g. after the administration of phenytoin or during drug overdosage), the subsequent decrease in plasma concentration is associated with reversion from zero-order to first-order kinetics. Consequently, the plasma half-life becomes progressively shorter during drug elimination, and the logarithm of the plasma concentration versus time curve is bell-shaped, rather than monoexponential or biexponential.

Compartmental analysis and pharmacological effects

When drugs produce reversible effects at their site of action, there is usually a close correlation between their concentration and their pharmacological effects. When the site of action is in the central compartment, there may be a close correlation between the amount of drug in the compartment and the intensity or magnitude of its effects. Thus, in some studies the serum concentration of tubocurarine (and the amount of the drug in the central compartment) is closely correlated with its effects on neuromuscular transmission, suggesting that the action of the drug is in this compartment. More recent evidence suggests that a better interpretation of the pharmacokinetics and pharmacodynamics of muscle relaxants is obtained when a separate 'effect compartment' is added to a pharmacokinetic model. Thus, when tubocurarine (and other non-depolarizing muscle relaxants) are infused intravenously, there is a short latent period between the rise in plasma concentration and the onset of neuromuscular blockade; when the infusion is stopped the fall in the plasma level occurs slightly earlier than the recovery in neuromuscular transmission. This phenomenon of hysteresis or temporal disequilibrium can be rationalised by the addition of a separate effect compartment (with distinct rate constants) to the central compartment of a pharmacokinetic model.

Hysteresis or temporal disequilibrium occurs with other drugs, and can be interpreted and analysed by statistical techniques. When plasma concentration (abscissa) is plotted against the pharmacological effect (ordinate), a hysteresis loop is obtained by sequentially joining the points relating concentration to effect at different times. When the area enclosed by the hysteresis loop is small and does not differ significantly from zero, the drug probably acts in the same compartment as plasma. By contrast, there may be a considerable latent period between the rise in plasma concentration and the onset of a pharmacological response. Similarly, drug action may persist for some time after the decline in plasma concentration.

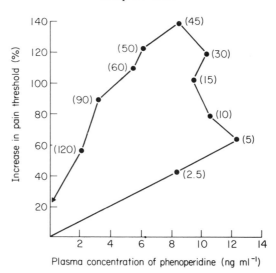

Fig. 2.10   Relation between the plasma concentration of phenoperidine and its analgesic effects. Values in parentheses represent the time in minutes after intravenous injection of phenoperidine. The area enclosed by the hysteresis loop is significantly greater than zero.

In consequence, the area enclosed by the hysteresis loop relating concentration to effect is significantly greater than zero (Fig. 2.10). This suggests that the drug is acting in a compartment that is deeper than plasma, or that its effects on drug receptors are not readily reversible.

BIOAVAILABILITY

When drugs are administered orally, the concept of bioavailability is frequently used to indicate the proportion of the dose that is present in the systemic circulation. It may or may not be the same as bioequivalence. Bioavailability (or biological availability) has been defined as the rate and extent to which a drug is absorbed and becomes available at the site of drug action. Nevertheless, the total amount of drug that is present in the systemic circulation is usually more important than its rate of absorption, and bioavailability is usually defined by reference to the area under the plasma concentration–time curve (AUC). After intravenous administration, drugs can be presumed to have a bioavailability of 100%; consequently, the absolute bioavailability (%) of drugs can be defined as:

$$\frac{(AUC_{0-\infty} \text{ after oral administration})}{(AUC_{0-\infty} \text{ after intravenous administration})} \times 100.$$

Alternatively, the absolute bioavailability of drugs can be measured from the total excretion of unchanged drug in urine after oral and intravenous administration.

Occasionally, absolute bioavailability can be determined without intravenous administration, for example, with drugs that show pH-dependent renal clearance. When intravenous administration is not possible, the relative bioavailability can be measured by reference to a different standard (e.g. an alternative dosage form). Sometimes relative bioavailability is defined by reference to a different route of administration (e.g. subcutaneous or intramuscular injection); in these conditions, it may not be identical with the absolute bioavailability.

Some drugs have a high oral bioavailability (e.g. diazepam, digoxin, phenytoin and warfarin). These compounds are stable in gastrointestinal secretions, are well-absorbed from the small intestine, and are not significantly metabolized by the gut wall or the liver before they gain access to the systemic circulation. In contrast, other drugs have a low oral bioavailability, which may be due to several factors. In the first place, some drugs are unstable or are broken down in the gastrointestinal tract (i.e. benzylpenicillin, heparin, and many polypeptide hormones). Secondly, drugs may be absorbed to a limited extent, due to physicochemical factors (e.g. relatively poor lipid solubility and a high molecular weight). Drugs that are poorly absorbed from the small intestine include neostigmine, glycopyrrolate and aminoglycoside antibiotics. Finally, drugs with a high first pass effect have a low systemic bioavailability, due to their extensive metabolism by the gut and the liver (e.g. morphine, pethidine, propranolol, and lignocaine). This reduces the amount of unchanged drug which gains access to the systemic circulation.

The cause of the reduced oral bioavailability of drugs can often be determined by the isolation and identification of drug metabolites in plasma or urine. When high concentrations of drug metabolites are present, poor systemic bioavailability is usually due to an extensive first pass effect and 'flow-limited' hepatic clearance. On the other hand, if significant amounts of drug metabolites are not identified in plasma or urine, poor absorption (or gastrointestinal breakdown) is probably responsible.

Differences in the oral bioavailability of drugs may be due to several causes. Numerous pharmaceutical factors can influence the dissolution of tablets and capsules. In these conditions, proprietary or generic preparations of the same drug may have different dissolution characteristics and thus produce a range of plasma concentrations after oral administration. These variations in drug dissolution mainly occur with relatively insoluble drugs that are administered orally, and the subsequent differences in bioavailability may be clinically significant (p. 9). Inter-individual differences in hepatic blood flow and first pass metabolism can also lead to variations in bioavailability. With 'flow-limited' hepatic clearance, any reduction in hepatic blood flow may lead to an increase in bioavailability. Drugs that induce or inhibit hepatic microsomal enzymes may also affect systemic bioavailability; for instance, cimetidine can increase the bioavailability of propranolol. Similarly, physiological changes (old age) and pathological factors (hepatic cirrhosis) can impair drug metabolism and increase bioavailability.

Physiological perfusion models

The distribution and elimination of a small number of drugs (e.g. thiopentone, digoxin, lignocaine, methotrexate and inhalational anaesthetics) have been described in terms of physiological perfusion models. These depend on the interpretation of drug distribution in terms of anatomical or physiological spaces, which have defined volumes, perfusion characteristics, and partition coefficients that are specific for each drug. Models, or individual compartments, may either have 'flow-limited' or 'membrane-limited' characteristics (depending on whether blood flow or transmembrane transport is the limiting factor governing drug uptake).

One of the best-known examples of a physiological perfusion model is concerned with the distribution and disposition of thiopentone. The concentration of the drug in blood, skeletal muscle, and subcutaneous fat at various times after its administration was shown to be consistent with a relatively simple model (consisting of a central blood pool and six tissue compartments). This suggested that thiopentone was primarily removed from the brain by lean body tissues (e.g. muscle) and that subcutaneous fat only played a subsidiary role. The model was subsequently refined by the inclusion of compartments representing drug metabolism, plasma protein binding, and tissue binding.

Physiological perfusion models have a number of distinct advantages. They can be used to predict drug concentrations at the site of action in tissues. Distribution and elimination can be precisely described, and they can also take account of local or general physiological changes during anaesthesia (e.g. alterations in cardiac output, regional blood flow and renal function). In some instances, they recognize intra-subject variability in drug disposition. Unfortunately, a number of problems may be associated with their use. They depend on the detailed measurement and analysis of a large number of physiological and pharmacological data, and the collection of appropriate tissue samples from anaesthetized patients is often difficult or impossible. In addition, the models may be described by complex differential equations, and their solution may require access to a digital computer.

FURTHER READING

Allott PR, Steward A, Mapleson WW. Pharmacokinetics of halothane in the dog. *British Journal of Anaesthesia* 1976; **48**: 279–295.

Aziz NS, Gambertoglio JG, Lin ET, Grausz H, Benet LZ. Pharmacokinetics of cephamandole using a HPLC assay. *Journal of Pharmacokinetics and Biopharmaceutics* 1978; **6**: 153–164.

Benet LZ, Galeazzi RL. Noncompartmental determination of the steady-state volume of distribution. *Journal of Pharmaceutical Sciences* 1979; **68**: 1071–1074.

Benet LZ, Massoud N, Gambertoglio JG. *Pharmacokinetic Basis for Drug Treatment*. New York: Raven Press, 1984.

Bennett WM, Porter GA, Bagby SP, McDonald WJ. *Drugs and Renal Disease*. New York: Churchill Livingstone, 1978.

Bevan DR, Bevan JC, Donati F. Pharmacokinetic principles. In: *Muscle Relaxants in Clinical Anesthesia*. Chicago: Year Book Medical Publishers, 1988: 100–132.

Bischoff KB, Dedrick RL. Thiopental pharmacokinetics. *Journal of Pharmaceutical Sciences* 1968; **57** 1346–1351.

Blaschke TF. Protein binding and kinetics of drugs in liver diseases. *Clinical Pharmacokinetics* 1977; **2**: 32–44.

Boobis AR, Davies DS. Pharmacokinetics. *Hospital Update* 1981; **7**: 453–460.

Calvey TN, Williams NE, Muir K, Barber HE. Plasma concentration of edrophonium in man. *Clinical Pharmacology and Therapeutics* 1976; **19**: 813–820.

Creasy WA. *Drug Disposition in Humans*. Oxford: Oxford University Press, 1979.

Curry SH. *Drug Disposition and Pharmacokinetics*. Oxford: Blackwell Scientific Publications, 1974.

Dost FH. *Der Blutspiegel: Kinetic der Konzentrations-Abläufe in der Kreislaufflüssigkeit*. Leipzig: Thieme, 1953.

Galeazzi RL, Benet LZ, Sheiner LB. Relationship between the pharmacokinetics and pharmacodynamics of procainamide. *Clinical Pharmacology and Therapeutics* 1979; **20**: 278–289.

Gibaldi M. *Biopharmaceutics and Clinical Pharmacokinetics*, 3rd edn. Philadelphia: Lea & Febiger, 1984.

Gibaldi M, Levy G, Hayton W. Kinetics of the elimination and neuromuscular blocking effect of *d*-tubocurarine in man. *Anesthesiology* 1972; **36**: 213–218.

Gibaldi M, McNamara PJ. Tissue binding of drugs. *Journal of Pharmaceutical Sciences* 1977; **66**: 1211–1212.

Gibaldi M, McNamara PJ. Apparent volumes of distribution and drug binding to plasma proteins and tissues. *European Journal of Clinical Pharmacology* 1978; **13**: 373–378.

Gibaldi M, Perrier D. *Pharmacokinetics*, 2nd edn. New York: Marcel Dekker, 1982.

Gillis PP, De Angelis RJ, Wynn RL. Nonlinear pharmacokinetic model of intravenous anesthesia. *Journal of Pharmaceutical Sciences* 1976; **65**: 1001–1006.

Goldstein A, Aronow L, Kalman SM. *Principles of Drug Action: The Basis of Pharmacology*. New York: John Wiley, 1974; 301–355.

Greenblatt DJ, Koch-Weser J. Clinical pharmacokinetics. *New England Journal of Medicine* 1975; **293**: 702–705 and 964–970.

Greenblatt DJ, Smith TW, Koch-Weser J. Bioavailability of drugs: the digoxin dilemma. *Clinical Pharmacokinetics* 1976; **1**: 36–51.

Himmelstein KJ, Lutz RJ. A review of the applications of physiologically based pharmacokinetic modeling. *Journal of Pharmacokinetics and Biopharmaceutics* 1979; **7**: 127–145.

Hull CJ. Pharmacokinetics and pharmacodynamics. *British Journal of Anaesthesia* 1979; **51**: 579–594.

Hull CJ, Van Beem HBH, McLeod K, Sibbald A, Watson MJ. A pharmacodynamic model for pancuronium. *British Journal of Anaesthesia* 1978; **50**: 1113–1123.

Hunter JM, Jones RS, Utting JE. Use of atracurium in patients with no renal function. *British Journal of Anaesthesia* 1982: **54**: 1251–1258.

Hunter JM, Jones RS, Utting JE. Comparison of vecuronium, atracurium and tubocurarine in normal patients and in patients with no renal function. *British Journal of Anaesthesia* 1984; **56**: 941–951.

Kaplan SA, Jack ML, Alexander K, Weinfeld RE. Pharmacokinetic profile of diazepam in man following single intravenous and oral and chronic oral administrations. *Journal of Pharmaceutical Sciences* 1973; **62**: 1789–1796.

Klotz U. Pathophysiological and disease-induced changes in drug distribution volume; pharmacokinetic implications. *Clinical Pharmacokinetics* 1976; **1**: 204–218.

Koch-Weser J. Serum drug concentrations as therapeutic guides. *New England Journal of Medicine* 1972; **287**: 227–231.

Labaune J-P. *Textbook of Pharmacokinetics.* Chichester: Ellis Horwood, 1989.

Lalka D, Feldman H. Absolute drug bioavailability. Approximation without comparison to parenteral dose for compounds exhibiting perturbable renal clearance. *Journal of Pharmaceutical Sciences* 1974; **63**: 1812.

Levy G. Pharmacokinetics of salicylate elimination in man. *Journal of Pharmaceutical Sciences* 1965; **54**: 959–967.

Levy G. Kinetics of pharmacological activity of succinylcholine in man. *Journal of Pharmaceutical Sciences* 1967; **56**: 1687–1688.

Levy G. Pharmacokinetics of succinylcholine in newborns. *Anesthesiology* 1970; **32**: 551–552.

Levy G, Tsuchiya T, Amsel LP. Limited capacity for salicyl phenolic glucuronide formation and its effect on the kinetics of salicylate elimination in man. *Clinical Pharmacology and Therapeutics* 1970; **13**: 258–268.

Loo JCK, Riegelman S. Assessment of pharmacokinetic constants from post-infusion blood curves obtained after IV infusion. *Journal of Pharmaceutical Sciences* 1970; **59**: 53–55.

Lundquist F, Wolthers H. The kinetics of alcohol elimination in man. *Acta Pharmacologica et Toxicologica* 1958; **14**: 265–289.

Michaelis M, Menten ML. Die Kinetik der Invertinwirkung. *Biochemische Zeitschrift* 1913; **49**: 333–369.

Mikus G, Fischer C, Heuer B, Langen C, Eichelbaum M. Application of stable isotope methodology to study the pharmacokinetics, bioavailability and metabolism of nitrendipine after i.v. and p.o. administration. *British Journal of Clinical Pharmacology* 1987; **24**: 561–569.

Milne L, Williams NE, Calvey TN, Murray GR, Chan K. Plasma concentration and metabolism of phenoperidine in man. *British Journal of Anaesthesia* 1980; **52**: 537–540.

Nagashima R, Levy G, O'Reilly RA. Comparative pharmacokinetics of coumarin anticoagulants. IV. Application of a three compartment model to the analysis of the dose-dependent kinetics of bishydroxycoumarin elimination. *Journal of Pharmaceutical Sciences* 1968; **57**: 1888–1895.

Notari E. *Biopharmaceutics and Clinical Pharmacokinetics: an Introduction.* 3rd edn. New York: Marcel Dekker, 1980.

Paxton JW. Elementary pharmacokinetics in clinical practice; 3, Practical pharmacokinetic applications. *New Zealand Medical Journal* 1981; **94**: 381–384.

Peck CC, Barrett BB. Nonlinear least squares regression programs for microcomputers. *Journal of Pharmacokinetics and Biopharmaceutics* 1979; **5**: 537–541.

Price HL, Kovnat PJ, Safer JN, Conner EH, Price ML. The uptake of thiopental by body tissues and its relation to the duration of narcosis. *Clinical Pharmacology and Therapeutics* 1960; **1**: 16–22.

Prys-Roberts C, Hug CC (eds). *Pharmacokinetics of Anaesthesia.* Oxford: Blackwell Scientific Publications, 1984.

Riegelman S, Loo JCK, Rowland M. Shortcomings in pharmacokinetic analysis by conceiving the body to exhibit properties of a single compartment. *Journal of Pharmaceutical Sciences* 1968; **57**: 117–123.

Rowland M, Benet LZ, Graham GG. Clearance concepts in pharmacokinetics. *Journal of Pharmacokinetics and Biopharmaceutics* 1973; **1**: 123–136.

Rowland M, Tozer TN. *Clinical Pharmacokinetics: Concepts and Applications.* Philadelphia: Lea & Febiger, 1980.

Saidman LJ, Eger EI II. The effect of thiopental metabolism on duration of anesthesia. *Anesthesiology* 1966; **27**: 118–126.

Shand DG. Clinical pharmacokinetics. *Recent Advances in Clinical Pharmacology.* Edinburgh: Churchill Livingstone, 1978; 1–11.

Shaw TRD, Howard MR, Hamer J. Variation in the biological availability of digoxin. *Lancet* 1972; **2**: 303–307.

Sheiner LB, Stanski DR, Vozeh S, Miller RD, Ham J. Simultaneous modeling of pharmacokinetics and pharmacodynamics: application to *d*-tubocurarine. *Clinical Pharmacology and Therapeutics* 1979; **215**: 358–371.

Somani SM, Chan K, Dehghan A, Calvey TN. Kinetics and metabolism of intramuscular neostigmine in myasthenia gravis. *Clinical Pharmacology and Therapeutics* 1980; **28**: 64–68.

Stanski DR, Mihm FG, Rosenthal MH, Kalman SM. Pharmacokinetics of high-dose thiopental used in cerebral resuscitation. *Anesthesiology* 1980; **53**: 169–171.

Stanski DR, Watkins WD. *Drug Disposition in Anesthesia*. New York: Grune & Stratton, 1982.

Teorell T, Dedrick RL, Condliffe PG (eds). *Pharmacology and Pharmacokinetics*. New York: Plenum Press, 1974.

Tozer TN. Concepts basic to pharmacokinetics. *Pharmacology and Therapeutics* 1981; **12**: 109–131.

Tyrer JH, Eadie MJ, Sutherland JM, Hooper WD. Outbreak of anticonvulsant intoxication in an Australian city. *British Medical Journal* 1970; **4**: 271–273.

Van Rossum JM. Significance of pharmacokinetics for drug design and the planning of dosage regimes. In: Ariens EJ (ed.) *Drug Design*, Vol. 1. New York: Academic Press, 1971; Chapter 7.

Wagner JG. *Biopharmaceutics and Relevant Pharmacokinetics*, 1st edn. Hamilton, Illinois: Drug Intelligence Publications, 1971.

Ward S, Boheimer N, Weatherley BC, Simmonds RJ, Dopson TA. Pharmacokinetics of atracurium and its metabolites in patients with normal renal function and in patients in renal failure. *British Journal of Anaesthesia* 1987; **59**: 697–706.

Waud BE, Waud DR. Dose–response curves and pharmacokinetics. *Anesthesiology* 1986; **65**: 355–358.

Wilkinson GR, Shand DG. A physiologic approach to hepatic drug clearance. *Clinical Pharmacology and Therapeutics* 1975; **18**: 377–390.

Wood AJJ. Drug disposition and pharmacokinetics. In: Wood M, Wood AJJ (eds). *Drugs and Anesthesia: Pharmacology for Anesthesiologists*. Baltimore: Williams & Wilkins, 1982.

THREE

Drug Action

Drugs produce a wide range of varied responses in man. These usually depend on the modification of cellular or subcellular function by agents with a relatively simple chemical structure. In some instances (e.g. with inhalational anaesthetics, local anaesthetics, and non-depolarizing muscle relaxants) there is a reasonably close relationship between chemical structure or physicochemical properties and the effects of drugs. By contrast, compounds that are closely related chemically (e.g. promazine and promethazine) may produce quite different pharmacological effects. The relation between chemical structure and biological activity was a central theme of experimental research for many years; indeed, this relationship played an important part in the development of the concept of drug receptors by John Newport Langley and Paul Ehrlich.

RELATION BETWEEN DRUG DOSAGE AND RESPONSE

Pharmacological effects or responses are usually related to drug dosage or concentration by means of dose–response curves. In intact animals and in man, the concentration of drugs at their site of action is dependent on the processes of drug absorption, distribution, metabolism and excretion, and it may be difficult to determine the precise relationship between drug concentration in tissues and the pharmacological response. In experimental animals, the observation and analysis of the effects of drugs can be simplified by the use of *in vitro* preparations (for instance, the frog rectus abdominis muscle, the rat phrenic nerve–diaphragm preparation, and the guinea-pig ileum). In these isolated tissue preparations, a defined concentration of the drug can be added to a tissue bath, and the response obtained can be directly measured by appropriate techniques. Many of the effects of drugs that produce observable and measurable responses ('agonists') were originally assessed in these experimental conditions. Isolated human tissues removed during surgical operations are sometimes used to obtain dose–response curves in man.

In these *in vitro* preparations, the relationship between drug dosage and the biological response obtained is often described by a hyperbolic curve. The relationship can be represented graphically as a dose–response curve or a log dose–response curve (Fig. 3.1). The use of a sigmoid or S-shaped log dose–response curve (rather than the hyperbolic dose–response relationship) has a number of advantages; in particular, it is linear for most of its course (i.e. between 20 and 80% of the maximum response), and it permits the simultaneous comparison and assessment of drugs with large differences in potency. As shown in Fig. 3.1, incremental dosage progressively increases the response obtained. As the dose is further increased the proportional response diminishes, and eventually a maximum effect is obtained which cannot be exceeded irrespective of the dose. Highly potent agents (i.e. agents that produce a given biological response at a relatively low dose level) have a log dose–response curve which is displaced to the left (i.e. towards the ordinate or *y* axis). By contrast, drugs of lower potency have a log dose–response curve that is displaced to the right.

The relationship between drug concentration and response can also be represented by the Hill plot. This method was first used by A.V. Hill at the turn of the century, during his studies on the relation between the partial pressure of oxygen and the percentage saturation of haemoglobin. The Hill plot depends on relating the logarithm of drug dosage or concentration (*x* axis) to the value $\log E/(E_{max} - E)$ (*y* axis), where E_{max} is the maximum effect observed and E is the response obtained at different dose levels or concentrations (Fig. 3.2). If the relation between drug concentration and response is represented by a hyperbolic curve (Fig. 3.1), the Hill plot is usually linear and has a slope of +1 (the Hill coefficient). The linear relationship between the variables in the Hill plot considerably simplifies the statistical analysis of the results.

This type of dose–response relationship measures a graded response in isolated

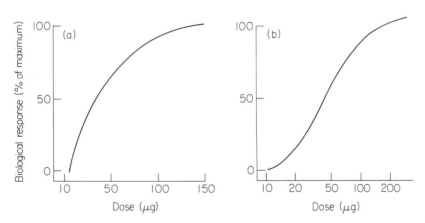

Fig. 3.1 The relation between drug dosage and response. In (a) the dose is plotted on a linear scale, giving a hyperbolic curve. In (b) the dose is plotted on a logarithmic scale, giving a sigmoid curve that is linear for most of its length.

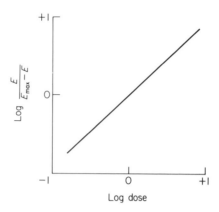

Fig. 3.2   A Hill plot relating the logarithm of drug dosage to the logarithm of $E/(E_{max} - E)$, where E_{max} is the maximum effect and E is the observed effect at different dose levels. The Hill coefficient in the example shown is $+1.0$.

tissue preparations, rather than an all or none ('quantal') response. (Quantal responses are widely used in experimental pharmacology; for instance, they are commonly used in the estimation of the median lethal dose or LD_{50}.) In intact animals or in man, the relation between drug dosage and response may be complex, and is often modified by pharmacokinetic processes. For these reasons, the plasma concentration of drugs (rather than their dosage) is usually related to their pharmacological effects in man. In these conditions, the slope of the plasma level–response curve may indicate the potential safety margin of a drug. When a relatively steep plasma level–response relationship is present, toxic effects may be produced after small increments in dosage. By contrast, if drugs have a more graded plasma level–response relationship, incremental increases in dosage are usually less hazardous.

THE BASIS OF DRUG ACTION

In general, drugs produce their pharmacological effects in three main ways. Firstly, the effects of drugs may be related to their physicochemical properties, or the chemical combination with other agents or trace elements. Secondly, they may act by inhibiting enzymes concerned with normal metabolic processes. Thirdly, drugs may act on receptor sites in cells or subcellular structures. In recent years, the nature of many drug–receptor reactions and the processes involved in the subsequent generation of drug responses have been extensively studied at a molecular level. These studies suggest that a small number of cellular and molecular mechanisms may mediate a wide range of different responses to drugs, hormones and other endogenous compounds.

Actions dependent on chemical or physicochemical properties

The effects of some drugs are directly dependent on their chemical properties. Thus, antacids primarily act by neutralizing gastric acid; similarly, alterations in systemic or urinary pH are produced by many acids and bases, due to the addition or removal of hydrogen ions from body fluids. The effects of chelating agents are also due to their chemical properties. These drugs combine with certain metallic ions (e.g. arsenic, lead, copper, zinc, mercury, silver and gold), and are sometimes used to remove these elements from the body. Chelating agents that are used in medicine include penicillamine, sodium calcium edetate, dicobalt edetate, desferrioxamine and the tetracyclines.

Penicillamine (dimethylcysteine) increases the elimination of lead, copper and mercury by combining with them and enhancing their urinary excretion. It is used for this purpose in the management of heavy metal poisoning and in the treatment of Wilson's disease (in which copper deposition occurs in the liver, the basal ganglia and the cornea). Although it has other therapeutic applications (e.g. in rheumatoid arthritis and cystinuria), these are not dependent on chelation. Penicillamine is a normal breakdown product of penicillin.

Sodium calcium edetate chelates lead (and certain other heavy metals) and is used in the management of lead poisoning and encephalopathy. It is usually administered by slow intravenous infusion; the presence of calcium prevents the development of hypocalcaemia. A related drug (calcium trisodium pentetate) has a greater affinity for heavy metals, and is sometimes used in lead or iron poisoning. Sodium edetate preferentially removes calcium ions from extracellular fluid; when injected intravenously it may cause severe hypocalcaemia. It is used *in vitro* as an anticoagulant. Sodium hydrogen citrate also chelates calcium ions (forming a calcio-citrate) and is used to prevent coagulation in stored blood. When large amounts of blood are given (or the rate of infusion is rapid) hypocalcaemia may occur; this complication can be prevented by calcium gluconate (1 g intravenously).

Dicobalt edetate chelates cyanide ions, and is now the treatment of choice in cyanide poisoning. It can also be used to remove cyanide ions which sometimes cumulate during the infusion of sodium nitroprusside. Dicobalt edetate is a relatively toxic drug, and cyanide poisoning must be unequivocally established before its use is considered.

Desferrioxamine is a specific chelating agent for iron, and is used in the treatment of iron poisoning and in the management of haemochromatosis. This drug has a high affinity for the iron in ferritin and haemosiderin; it has little effect on iron that is bound to transferrin or contained in myoglobin, haemoglobin, or the cytochrome enzymes.

The tetracyclines are potent chelating agents, and readily combine with iron, calcium, magnesium, and aluminium ions; when given orally with compounds containing these elements (e.g. antacids and iron salts), the absorption of tetra-cyclines may be impaired. The ability of tetracyclines to chelate calcium and magnesium ions may be partly responsible for their bacteriostatic effects.

The action of some other drugs may be dependent on their physicochemical properties. Both local anaesthetics and inhalational anaesthetics may act by producing non-specific changes in the lipid or protein components of neuronal membranes. These changes affect the diameter of minute channels or pores in the membrane that are concerned with ion transport. Nevertheless, recent evidence suggests that local and inhalational anaesthetics act on the nervous system in a more specific manner. Local anaesthetics may combine with receptors at the internal aspect of sodium channels, causing a decrease in their diameter. In these conditions, sodium conductance is reduced below the threshold required for de-polarization. Inhalational anaesthetics are generally considered to interact with non-polar sites associated with membrane proteins or phospholipids. Alternative-ly, they may affect certain proteins in the brain in a relatively selective manner, since they can combine with and inhibit purified enzymes (luciferases) at con-centrations that are present during general anaesthesia.

Actions dependent on enzyme inhibition

The action of many drugs is dependent on the inhibition of enzymes concerned with normal metabolic processes (Table 3.1). Drugs that act by enzyme inhibition are often chemically related to natural substrates that are normally metabolized by the enzyme or enzyme system. Thus, allopurinol is a close chemical analogue of the purine compounds xanthine and hypoxanthine, which are normally con-verted by xanthine oxidase to uric acid. The antimetabolite drug mercaptopurine is also metabolised to thiouric acid by xanthine oxidase. Similarly, sulphanilamide and other sulphonamides are closely related to *para*-aminobenzoic acid, and prevent the conversion of this compound to folic acid by the enzyme folate synthetase.

Drugs may inhibit enzymes in a reversible or an irreversible manner. Rever-sible enzyme inhibitors (e.g. edrophonium, allopurinol, and the sulphonamides) generally compete with natural substrates for enzymes, and their effects do not depend on the formation of stable chemical bonds. The reaction can be expressed as:

$$\text{inhibitor} + \text{enzyme} \rightleftharpoons \text{enzyme--inhibitor complex.}$$

The plasma or tissue concentration of reversible inhibitors may be related to the degree of enzyme inhibition. As these drugs are eliminated from the body, their plasma concentration falls and enzyme inhibition decreases. Since their action is not dependent on the formation of stable chemical bonds, their effects are usually brief and evanescent, and probably reflect the presence of drugs or their active

Table 3.1 Commonly used drugs whose effects are partly or totally due to enzyme inhibition.

Drug	Enzyme inhibited
Allopurinol	Xanthine oxidase
Aminophylline	
Enoximone	Phosphodiesterase
Peroximone	
Acetylsalicylic acid (and other NSAIDs)	Prostaglandin synthetase
Captopril	
Enalapril	Angiotensin-converting enzyme
Benserazide	
Carbidopa	Dopa decarboxylase
Chlorophenylalanine	Tryptophan hydroxylase
Disulfiram	Aldehyde dehydrogenase
Methotrexate	
Trimethoprim	Dihydrofolate reductase
Pyrimethamine	
Methyldopa	Amino acid decarboxylase
Mercaptopurine	
Thioguanine	Phosphoribosylphosphate amidotransferase
Neostigmine	
Pyridostigmine	Acetylcholinesterase
Physostigmine	Plasma cholinesterase
Organo-phosphorus compounds	
Penicillin	Bacterial wall transpeptidase
Phenelzine	
Tranylcypromine	Monoamine oxidase
Sulphonamides	Folate synthetase

In some instances, enzyme inhibition is dependent on the formation of drug metabolites.

metabolites in the immediate environment of the enzyme. Neostigmine, pyrido-stigmine, and physostigmine are usually also classified as reversible enzyme inhibitors; nevertheless, this is only partially correct. Although they initially combine in a reversible manner with plasma cholinesterase and acetylcholinesterase, their action is dependent on the formation of a covalent chemical bond resulting in carbamylation of the enzyme. This covalent bond is slowly hydrolysed in the body, and the enzyme is gradually regenerated (Chapter 9).

Irreversible enzyme inhibition usually depends on the formation of a stable chemical complex between the inhibitor and the enzyme. In these conditions, regeneration of the inhibited enzyme is often impossible and a latent period is required for resynthesis of the enzyme before its function is restored. Drugs that act by irreversible enzyme inhibition include organophosphorus compounds (e.g. ecothiopate), methotrexate and most potent monoamine oxidase inhibitors. These drugs have an extremely long duration of action, and they may produce effects for days or weeks after they are eliminated from the body.

In some instances, inhibitors that are closely related to natural substrates are metabolized by enzyme systems to compounds that interfere with or prevent normal cellular function. For instance, the cytotoxic drug fluorouracil competes with uracil for enzymes that normally synthesize ribonucleic acid (RNA); metabolites of fluorouracil are formed and incorporated into RNA, preventing protein synthesis. Similarly, methyldopa is converted to methyldopamine and methylnoradrenaline by both central and peripheral sympathetic neurones. These drug metabolites replace the physiological neurotransmitter in sympathetic nerve endings.

Actions dependent on combination with receptors

Many drugs produce their effects by combining with macromolecular sites known as drug receptors. These receptor sites are closely related to tissue cells that mediate the effects of drugs (effector cells). The concept of receptors was originally introduced by J.N. Langley, in order to account for the remarkable specificity and antagonism of certain drugs on physiological systems (e.g. the effects of pilocarpine and atropine on salivary secretion, and the action of nicotine and curare on neuromuscular transmission). The German physician Paul Ehrlich also played an important part in the development and acceptance of the concept of chemoreceptors associated with cells. Ehrlich was clearly influenced by the work of Langley, and by his own studies concerned with the development of cross-resistance to antitrypanosomal drugs with a similar chemical structure. The quantitative aspects of drug–receptor reactions and drug responses were developed later by A.J. Clark and J.H. Gaddum.

In subsequent work between 1930 and 1960, the nature and properties of drug receptors were mainly inferred from the investigation of structure–activity relationships. In these studies, the response of isolated tissues to a series of drugs with related chemical structures was analysed (e.g. the response of smooth muscle preparations to a series of choline esters). Although this work was of considerable value, it represented a relatively indirect approach to the study of drug–receptor reactions.

Since 1965, it has been possible to isolate certain receptors from tissues, or to study their properties in cell membrane preparations *in vitro*. These studies have been facilitated by the development of radio-labelled compounds (radioligands) with a high affinity for specific receptors. For instance, α-bungarotoxin (a polypeptide present in sea-snake venom) and cobra toxin are selectively bound by nicotinic receptors at the motor endplate. These radiolabelled neurotoxins have been widely used to isolate acetylcholine receptors from the synaptic junctions of electric fishes, and from the vertebrate neuromuscular junction. Muscarinic receptors in the heart, the small intestine, sympathetic ganglia, and the brain have also been identified by radiolabelled irreversible antagonists (e.g. ^{3}H-quinnucli-dinyl benzilate). Similarly, dopamine receptors have been identified and isolated from a number of sites in the CNS (e.g. the substantia nigra, the corpus striatum, the limbic system, the chemoreceptor trigger zone, and the pituitary gland), using radiolabelled dopamine antagonists (e.g. ^{3}H-haloperidol, ^{3}H-spiperone, and ^{3}H-flupenthixol). Dopamine receptors can also be identified in vascular smooth muscle (e.g. in the renal and the mesenteric circulation), and in sympathetic ganglia.

Both α- and β-adrenoceptors can also be specifically labelled and identified by different radioligands, which may be agonists (e.g. ^{3}H-hydroxybenzylisoprenaline) or antagonists (e.g. ^{3}H-prazosin or ^{3}H-dihydroalprenolol). The binding of radio-ligands to adrenergic receptors has been extensively studied *in vitro*; in these conditions, radiolabelled drugs have a high receptor affinity, and their binding to receptors is saturable, specific, and competitive (i.e. they can be readily displaced by other agonists or antagonists). Adrenergic receptors are widely distributed in the body; in some instances (e.g. $α_2$-receptors in platelets, or $β_2$-receptors in vascular smooth muscle) their presence is not associated with a nerve supply. Adrenergic receptor density is modified in various pathological conditions (e.g. bronchial asthma, congestive cardiac failure, and thyrotoxicosis). In general, high catecholamine concentrations reduce the number and density of adrenergic re-ceptors ('down regulation'). This phenomenon is partly due to the sequestration ('internalization') of receptors within cells, although receptor affinity may also be modified. By contrast, any fall in circulating adrenaline and noradrenaline, either produced by drugs or by sympathetic denervation, increases the number of receptors ('up regulation'). Similar changes in receptor density are prob-ably produced by most neurotransmitters that act at synapses and neuro-effector junctions.

In some situations, an increase in the number of receptors may be partly responsible for the phenomenon of denervation supersensitivity. After peripheral denervation or damage to skeletal muscle, the response to acetylcholine and other depolarizing agents is increased, due to 'up regulation'. Extrajunctional receptors develop on the surface of the muscle fibre, outside the motor endplate; the total number of nicotinic acetylcholine receptors may increase 100 times. In these conditions, the ionic changes associated with depolarization and repolarization may produce significant hyperkalaemia (e.g. when suxamethonium is given to patients with burns or some neurological conditions). Sympathetic denervation also increases peripheral responses to noradrenaline (and to a lesser extent, to adrenaline). In these circumstances, the increased response is mainly related to the impairment of neuronal uptake of the sympathetic neurotransmitter. Any increase in the number of adrenergic receptors due to 'up regulation' probably plays a less important part.

The identification of macromolecular sites that bind drugs as drug receptors depends on their association with a pharmacological effect or response. In addition, many receptor systems demonstrate the properties of sensitivity, specificity, and saturability. Most receptors are extremely sensitive to naturally occurring agonists, and only small concentrations are required to produce a significant response. Consequently, considerable amplification or enhancement of the initial stimulus may be required to generate pharmacological effects. In addition, many receptor systems show considerable selectivity; they characteristically respond to a limited range of chemical agents with a defined structure, which are often closely related to naturally occurring neurotransmitters or hormones. Finally, drug receptors usually have a finite binding capacity. The number of receptors associated with cells is usually constant (although it can be modified by physiological or pharmacological factors). In consequence, the binding of many radiolabelled ligands and drugs by authentic receptors is a competitive and saturable process. Drug receptors characteristically show a high affinity and a low capacity for specific agonists and antagonists; by contrast, non-specific binding is a low-affinity, high-capacity phenomenon.

Most receptors that have been studied and isolated are present on the external surface of cells. An important exception are receptors for steroid hormones, which are present in the cytoplasm or nucleus of certain cells (target cells). Specific receptor proteins are bound to, and activated by steroid hormones; the resulting complex indirectly affects ribosomal protein synthesis by modifying messenger RNA. Almost all other receptors that have been identified are associated with, or present on the cell membrane.

The most generally accepted theory of drug action suggests that the reversible combination of the agonist with the receptor (i.e. receptor occupancy) is the primary event that initiates a sequence of biophysical and biochemical reactions (e.g. ion transport, enzyme activation, and protein synthesis) which results in the response. These reactions may be expressed in the following manner:

$$
\begin{array}{l}
\text{drug} + \text{receptor} \\
\quad \uparrow \downarrow \\
\text{drug–receptor complex} \\
\quad \downarrow \\
\text{drug–activated receptor complex} \rightarrow \text{drug} + \text{receptor} \\
\quad \downarrow \\
\text{biophysical or biochemical change} \\
\quad \downarrow \\
\text{drug response.}
\end{array}
$$

In general, there are three types of biophysical or biochemical changes produced by receptor activation:

1   Direct changes in ionic permeability.

2 Accumulation of 'intermediate messengers'.
3 Modification of nucleic acid synthesis.

1 Direct changes in ionic permeability

In some instances, receptor activation directly affects ion channels in synaptic membranes, resulting in a selective or non-selective increase in ionic permeability. In these conditions, receptors and ion channels usually form part of the same macromolecular complex (i.e. the receptor is the ion channel). The increase in ionic permeability produced by receptor activation is usually rapid and evanescent; a maximal response may occur within microseconds, and only last for several milliseconds. Some neurotransmitters (e.g. acetylcholine, γ-aminobutyrate, glutamate and glycine) act in this manner, and directly increase the ionic permeability of the postsynaptic membrane.

Neuromuscular transmission is a well-known example of a direct response to receptor activation. Acetylcholine is released from the motor nerve terminal and combines with receptors containing non-selective ion channels. The nicotinic receptor at the neuromuscular junction is an integral membrane protein with a molecular weight of approximately 250 kDa; it consists of five subunits (α, α, β, γ, and δ) which traverse the postsynaptic membrane and surround the ion channel or ionophore. Two of these subunits (the α units) have a molecular weight of approximately 40 kDa and contain acetylcholine binding sites (at Cys 192–Cys 193). Combination of the neurotransmitter with these binding sites results in conformational changes that open the ion channel; the probability of this occurring is considerably increased when both sites are occupied by acetylcholine. Ion channel opening is an extremely rapid all-or-none phenomenon which lasts for 1–3 milliseconds, and causes a non-specific increase in permeability to small ions (mainly sodium, potassium, and calcium ions). In experimental conditions, it has been estimated that acetylcholine causes the transfer of 10 000 ions per ionophore during each millisecond that the channel is open. These changes result in a localized endplate potential; if this reaches a threshold amplitude, an action potential is conducted along the muscle fibre (Chapter 10).

Other neurotransmitters also activate receptors that are directly linked to ion channels. GABA (γ-aminobutyrate) is probably the main inhibitory neurotransmitter in the CNS, and is believed to mediate both presynaptic (axo-axonal) and postsynaptic (axo-dendritic or axo-somatic) inhibition at 20–40% of all synapses. Many responses that are mediated by GABA depend on a directly induced, selective increase in permeability to chloride ions, rather than the non-selective response that occurs at the motor endplate. Receptor activation allows ions to diffuse from the external environment into the neurone, resulting in hyperpolarization and decreased neuronal excitability. There are at least two binding sites for GABA on each receptor macromolecule; these are closely associated with chloride channels.

2 Accumulation of 'intermediate messengers'

In many cells, receptor activation does not directly cause changes in ionic permeability or other drug responses. Many drugs are extremely potent substances, and enhancement or amplification of the initial stimulus is essential in order to produce a significant response. In these conditions, receptor activation increases the activity of specific enzymes, resulting in the accumulation of intracellular metabolites that act as 'intermediate messengers'. (They are more commonly known as 'second messengers'; nevertheless, intermediate messengers is a better term, since more than one intracellular metabolite may be involved in drug responses.)

At least three intermediate messengers are known to play an important role in mediating responses to receptor activation. These are (1) cyclic adenosine monophosphate, (2) cyclic guanosine monophosphate, and (3) calcium ions. Although other intermediate metabolites may be involved in the transduction of drug responses, they have not been unequivocally identified.

Cyclic adenosine monophosphate (cAMP)

Activation of receptors on the external surface of cells may result in the synthesis of cAMP. This intracellular metabolite is formed from adenosine triphosphate (ATP) by the enzyme adenylate cyclase (Fig. 3.3). Cyclic AMP subsequently activates protein kinases, resulting in the phosphorylation of membrane proteins by ATP. These changes lead to other biophysical or biochemical effects (e.g. alterations in ionic permeability resulting in the depolarization or hyperpolarization of effector cells, or the translocation of calcium ions). Cyclic AMP is rapidly metabolized intracellularly by the enzyme phosphodiesterase (Fig. 3.3). A number of drugs (e.g. theophylline and its derivatives, and azothioprine) inhibit this enzyme, and may prolong and enhance the effects of receptor activation. In many cells, there are multiple forms of phosphodiesterase with different sensitivities to enzyme inhibition by drugs.

The effects of many drugs are dependent on the activation of adenylate cyclase and the subsequent synthesis of cAMP. All the β-adrenergic effects of catecholamines are mediated by this pathway; indeed, the significance of cAMP was first recognized by Sutherland and Rall during their studies on the effects of adrenaline on glycogenolysis in isolated liver cells. More recently, it has been recognized that cAMP mediates the effects of many hormones and other endogenous compounds (Table 3.2). In addition, the adenylate cyclase–cAMP system may play a crucial role in neuromuscular transmission. The release of

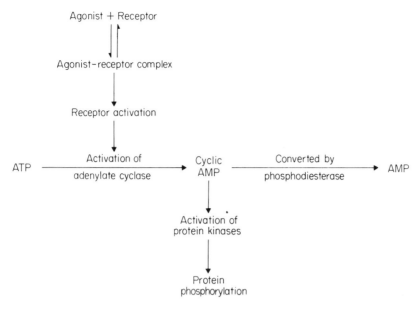

Fig. 3.3 The synthesis of cAMP by adenylate cyclase. After the synthesis of cAMP from ATP by adenylate cyclase, the second messenger is rapidly destroyed by phosphodiesterase.

acetylcholine from the motor nerve may be dependent on the generation of cAMP in the neuronal membrane, which then activates protein kinases that are coupled to a calcium ionophore. The entry of calcium ions into the nerve terminal results in the release of acetylcholine from the synaptic vesicles (Chapter 9). In experimental conditions, other drugs may affect the activity of adenylate cyclase and protein kinase; the practical significance of these effects is a matter of conjecture.

In some tissues, responses to receptor activation by hormones and drugs are dependent on the attenuation or inhibition of adenylate cyclase, and a subsequent reduction in the intracellular concentration of cAMP. The effects of noradrena-

Table 3.2 Hormones and endogenous compounds whose effects are dependent on activation of adenylate cyclase and enhanced synthesis of cAMP.

Adrenaline	β effects
Noradrenaline	β effects
Dopamine	D_1 effects
Histamine	H_2 effects
Hydroxytryptamine	
Glucagon	
Vasopressin	
ACTH	

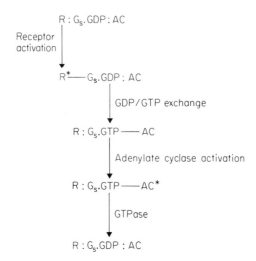

Fig. 3.4   The role of regulatory proteins (G_s) in the activation by receptors (R) of adenylate cyclase (AC); R^* and AC^* are the activated forms. In the inactive state, the regulatory protein G_s is bound to GDP. Receptor activation results in the binding of G_s.GDP by the receptor, followed by GDP/GTP exchange (i.e. GDP dissociates from G_s, and is replaced by GTP). The regulatory protein G_s.GTP is then transferred from the receptor to adenylate cyclase; the enzyme is activated and converts ATP to cAMP. Subsequently, GTP is hydrolysed and G_s. GDP dissociates from adenylate cyclase. A similar mechanism may be responsible for the inhibition of adenylate cyclase by the regulatory protein G_i. The activation of different receptor sites by agonists may result in competition for G_s and G_i, and this phenomenon will be reflected by the activity of adenylate cyclase and the subsequent production of cAMP. Certain toxins are selectively bound by regulatory proteins, and can prevent the conversion of G_s.GTP and G_i.GTP to their inactive states. Cholera toxin is bound by G_s, and prevents the hydrolysis of GTP; consequently, cAMP is continuously synthesized, and accumulates intracellularly. Conversely, one of the pertussis toxins (islet activating protein) is bound by G_i, and prevents the breakdown of G_i.GTP.

line on α_2-receptors (e.g. in postganglionic sympathetic nerve terminals, platelets, and fat cells), the degranulation of mast cells induced by Type 1 hypersensitivity, and the effects of acetylcholine on muscarinic receptors in the heart may be dependent on the inhibition of adenylate cyclase and the subsequent decrease in cAMP. In certain conditions, opioids, dopamine, adenosine, and somatostatin produce effects at receptors that are mediated by the attenuation of adenylate cyclase activity. In some instances, opposing or complementary physiological responses may be dependent on the activation and inhibition of adenylate cyclase (e.g. the effects of increased sympathetic and vagal tone on heart rate and cardiac contractility).

Receptor systems that modify adenylate cyclase activity are coupled to the enzyme by the regulatory proteins G_s or G_i. Receptor activation results in the binding of GTP by the regulatory protein, which is then transferred from the receptor to adenylate cyclase; the enzyme is then activated (G_s) or inhibited (G_i)

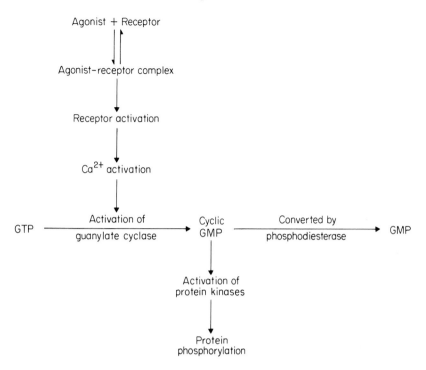

Fig. 3.5 The synthesis of cGMP by guanylate cyclase. Activation of the enzyme is usually dependent on the translocation of calcium ions.

(Fig. 3.4). Regulatory proteins that bind guanyl nucleotides play an important role in other cellular systems; they are closely related to oncogene products, are involved in the receptor-mediated breakdown of phosphoinositides, and may play an important part in the phenomenon of desensitization.

Cyclic guanosine monophosphate (cGMP)

Cyclic GMP may act as an intermediate messenger in certain cells. Its synthesis is dependent on the activation of guanylate cyclase, which is directly controlled by regulatory proteins that bind GDP and GTP. The formation of cGMP often appears to be dependent on the intracellular sequestration or translocation of calcium ions. In many ways, the synthesis of cAMP and cGMP are similar (Figs 3.3 and 3.5). Both of these second messengers are broken down by phospho-diesterase; similarly, cGMP (like cAMP) produces its effects by activating protein kinases that are specifically dependent on the cyclic nucleotide. Cyclic GMP may mediate some of the muscarinic effects of acetylcholine, as well as the response to histamine at H_1-receptors. Recent evidence suggests that 'endothelium-derived relaxing factor' (i.e. nitric oxide) and drugs that are metabolized to nitric oxide (e.g. glyceryl trinitrate and sodium nitroprusside) cause relaxation of vascular smooth muscle by increasing intracellular cGMP.

Calcium ions

Calcium ions probably play an important and ubiquitous role in the mediation of cellular responses to receptor activation. Indeed, calcium has been described as a universal second messenger responsible for regulating all forms of cellular activity. In recent years, it has become apparent that many agonists act by modifying the intracellular release or translocation of calcium ions. These effects are associated with the hydrolysis of a group of phospholipids in cell membranes (the phosphatidylinositols).

Receptor occupation by agonists activates the enzyme phospholipase C (Fig. 3.6). As in the case of adenylate cyclase and guanylate cyclase, phospholipase activation is dependent on a regulatory protein that can bind guanine nucleotides. Phospholipase C hydrolyses the membrane lipid phosphatidylinositol bisphosphate (PIP_2) to diacylglycerol (DAG) and inositol trisphosphate (IP_3). Both products of this reaction act as intermediate messengers. DAG activates a protein kinase (protein kinase C) resulting in the phosphorylation of intracellular proteins. By

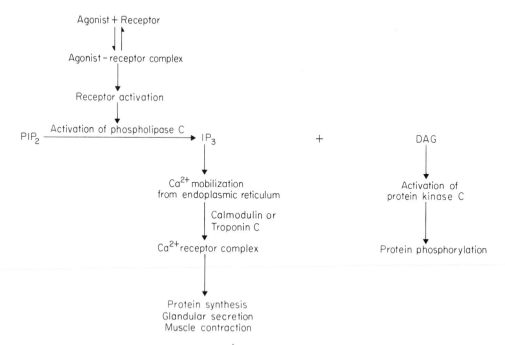

Fig. 3.6 The intracellular mobilization of calcium ions by inositol trisphosphate. PIP_2 = phosphatidylinositol 4,5-bisphosphate; IP_3 = inositol 1,4,5-trisphosphate; DAG = diacylglycerol.

contrast, IP_3 causes the intracellular mobilization of calcium ions from the endoplasmic reticulum (Fig. 3.6).

In many cells, IP_3 plays a crucial role as an intermediate messenger. Intracellular calcium concentrations are normally extremely low (approximately 100 nmol litre^{-1}); any increase in internal calcium causes profound changes in cellular activity. Calcium ions released from the endoplasmic reticulum by IP_3 combine with specific calcium-binding proteins (which can be considered as internal receptors for calcium ions). Calmodulin is the main calcium-binding protein in smooth muscle and all non-muscular tissue; the related protein troponin C plays an equivalent role in cardiac and skeletal muscle. The combination of calcium ions with calmodulin causes conformational changes in the protein, which can result in a wide range of pharmacological responses (e.g. protein synthesis, changes in ionic permeability, glandular secretion, and muscle contraction).

In skeletal and cardiac muscle, the sequestration of calcium ions by troponin C plays a crucial role in excitation–contraction coupling. When calcium ions are released from the sarcoplasmic reticulum and bound by the troponin–tropomyosin complex, myosin ATPase is activated and ATP is hydrolysed. Cross-bridges form between the myosin and actin filaments in the myofibril resulting in muscle contraction. IP_3 may play an important part in calcium release in cardiac and skeletal muscle; circumstantial evidence suggests that it may provide the connection between depolarization of T-tubules and the release of calcium ions from the sarcoplasmic reticulum. In addition, IP_3 (or closely related inositol phosphates) may regulate calcium entry into cells.

Although cAMP, cGMP, and calcium ions can be considered as independent intermediate messengers, there is considerable evidence that their effects are interrelated. Both cAMP and cGMP may affect and modify the response to calcium ions. For instance, in skeletal muscle calcium activates the enzyme phosphorylase kinase, causing glycogenolysis. Phosphorylation of the enzyme by cAMP results in a significant increase in its sensitivity to calcium ions.

3 Modification of nucleic acid synthesis

Steroid hormones and their synthetic analogues produce their effects by combining with intracellular receptors and indirectly affecting protein synthesis. Consequently, the onset of action of steroids is usually relatively slow. Steroid receptors are intracellular proteins that are mainly associated with nuclear chromatin (although some low affinity binding sites may also be present in the cytoplasm). Lipid-soluble steroids (e.g. oestrogens, progestogens, androgens, and glucocorticoids) readily diffuse across cellular membranes, and are then bound by unoccupied steroid receptors in the nucleus, resulting in the formation of activated steroid–receptor complexes. These complexes are then bound by specific high affinity binding sites on DNA ('steroid regulatory elements'). Genes

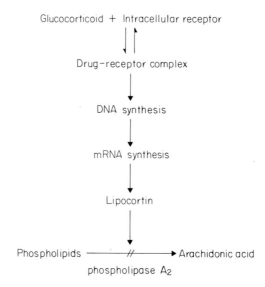

Glucocorticoid + Intracellular receptor

Drug–receptor complex

DNA synthesis

mRNA synthesis

Lipocortin

Phospholipids ⟶ // ⟶ Arachidonic acid

phospholipase A₂

Fig. 3.7   The effects of glucocorticoids on the formation of lipocortin and the synthesis of arachidonic acid by phospholipase A$_2$. ↛ represents enzyme inhibition.

in the immediate vicinity of the steroid regulatory elements are activated, resulting in the increased synthesis of messenger RNA and enhanced ribosomal protein synthesis. The diverse and ubiquitous nature of many of the cellular effects of steroids may be dependent on the synthesis of proteins by responsive tissues. Thus, the anti-inflammatory effects of glucocorticoids are mainly due to their combination with intracellular steroid receptors. The activation of these receptors by glucocorticoids modifies DNA and RNA synthesis, and indirectly increases the formation of an intracellular glycoprotein (lipocortin). This protein inhibits the enzyme phospholipase A$_2$, which normally mediates the conversion of membrane phospholipids to arachidonic acid (Fig. 3.7). In this manner, the formation of prostaglandins by inflammatory cells is reduced.

KINETICS OF DRUG–RECEPTOR REACTIONS

The classical analysis of drug responses in terms of the combination of agonists with receptors ('occupation theory') was introduced by A.J. Clark in the 1930s. It depends on the assumption that each drug molecule combines with a receptor in a reversible manner, forming a drug–receptor complex, i.e.

$$D + R \underset{k_2}{\overset{k_1}{\rightleftharpoons}} DR$$

where D is the number of free (unbound) drug molecules, R is the number of free receptors, DR is the number of occupied receptor sites, k_1 the association rate constant, and k_2 the dissociation rate constant. At equilibrium, the rates of association and dissociation are equal; if D, R, and DR are expressed as molar concentrations (i.e. $[D]$, $[R]$, and $[DR]$), then

$$k_1[D][R] = k_2[DR]$$

and

$$\frac{k_2}{k_1} = \frac{[D][R]}{[DR]} = K_d,$$

where K_d is the dissociation constant at equilibrium, and reflects the affinity with which drugs bind to receptors. When K_d is high, there is a low affinity for drug receptors; when K_d is low, there is high receptor affinity. In numerical terms, K_d represents the concentration of the drug required to occupy half the receptor sites at equilibrium. If R_t is the total number of receptors,

$$[R_t] = [R] + [DR]$$

and

$$[R] = [R_t] - [DR]$$

thus

$$K_d = \frac{[D][R]}{[DR]} = \frac{[D]([R_t] - [DR])}{[DR]}$$

and

$$[D]([R_t] - [DR]) = K_d[DR]$$

thus

$$[D][R_t] = K_d[DR] + [D][DR]$$

thus

$$[D][R_t] = K_d[DR] + [D][DR]$$
$$= [DR](K_d + [D])$$

and

$$\frac{[DR]}{[R_t]} = \frac{[D]}{K_d + [D]}.$$

Since the fraction of receptors occupied (f) $= [DR]/[R_t]$,

$$f = \frac{[D]}{K_d + [D]}.$$

This equation (the Langmuir equation) was originally derived by A.V. Hill in 1909; a similar relationship was used by Langmuir to characterize the absorption of gases to metal surfaces.

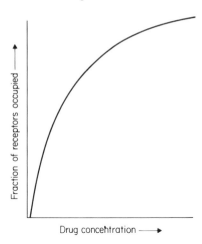

Fraction of receptors occupied ⟶

Drug concehtration ⟶

Fig. 3.8 The hyperbolic relationship between drug concentration and the fraction of receptors occupied by the drug. It is assumed that each drug molecule combines with a receptor in a non-cooperative manner.

If the total number of receptors remains constant, the Langmuir equation corresponds to a rectangular hyperbola; as the concentration of the drug is increased, the fraction of receptors that are occupied will rise progressively and approach the asymptote f = 1 at high drug concentrations (Fig. 3.8). If the pharmacological response is proportional to the fraction of receptors occupied, there will also be a hyperbolic relationship between drug dosage and response. As previously mentioned (p. 71), this type of relationship may be observed (Fig. 3.1), and in these circumstances the Hill plot (Fig. 3.2) has a coefficient of unity. If the number of drug binding sites on each unit of the receptor macromolecule is represented by n, a Hill plot with a coefficient n should be obtained.

Approximately 30 years ago, Stephenson pointed out the presence of several apparent anomalies in the currently accepted concepts of drug–receptor interactions. For instance, the assumption that drug responses were proportional to the fraction of the total receptors occupied by the drug was not consistent with the results of many experimental studies. In some instances, the relation between drug concentration and the pharmacological response is an S-shaped (sigmoid) curve rather than a rectangular hyperbola; a Hill plot relating the logarithm of drug concentration to the logarithm [observed effect/(maximum effect − observed effect)] often produced a non-integral coefficient greater than unity. It is now recognized that occupation theory represents a simplistic approach to the phenomenon of drug response, and that many pharmacological effects are a complex and non-linear function of receptor occupation. Many responses in *in vivo* conditions may reflect drug activity on different types or subtypes of receptors, and may be modified by reflex effects. Similarly, the relation between the plasma or tissue bath concentration of drugs and their concentration at receptor sites may be uncertain or unknown. In addition, Hill plots with non-integral coefficients greater than unity may be explained by the presence of multiple receptor sites for agonists on a single macromolecular complex. The binding of a molecule of the drug by one receptor site may produce conformational (allosteric) changes that alter the affinity of other receptor sites for the drug. In these conditions, the affinity of other receptor subgroups for the drug may be increased or decreased. This phenomenon, which is sometimes referred to as cooperativity, was originally advanced by Monod, Wyman and Changeux in the mid-1960s in order to explain the allosteric properties of enzymes. Certain protein molecules (e.g. haemoglobin) are known to combine with their substrates (oxygen) in this manner; the combination of haemoglobin with oxygen affects the affinity of the protein for additional molecules of the substrate. Similarly, other substances (e.g. 2,3-diphosphoglycerate) may bind to haemoglobin at different sites but significantly decrease its affinity for oxygen.

A comparable phenomenon probably occurs during neuromuscular transmission. When the effects of acetylcholine or other agonists on neuromuscular function are studied, the relationship between drug concentration and response is usually sigmoid, and the Hill plot characteristically has a slope (the Hill coefficient) of 1.5 or more. This is consistent with the presence of two agonist binding sites on each receptor macromolecule, which are present on the two α-subunits of the nicotinic receptor (p. 260). The Hill coefficient may reflect the increased probability of ion channel opening when both sites are occupied, as well as positive cooperativity.

For other reasons, the magnitude of pharmacological responses may not be predictably related to the proportion of receptors occupied by drugs. When highly potent drugs produce a maximal response, they may also occupy a relatively small proportion of the total population (i.e. 1% or even less). The presence of these 'spare receptors' in excess of the numbers required to produce a maximum response probably ensures that adequate pharmacological effects can be produced by relatively low concentrations of drugs or transmitters. There is considerable evidence that spare receptors are present at the neuromuscular junction. Only 25% of the receptor population at the motor endplate is required to produce a maximal twitch response to indirect stimulation, and only 50% is required to produce a sustained tetanic response. Consequently, non-depolarizing neuromuscular blockade may require the occupation of significant numbers of receptors before any effect on myoneural function is apparent.

DRUG ANTAGONISM

Drug antagonists characteristically prevent or decrease pharmacological responses to agonists. Drug antagonism can be classified in the following manner:

1 Reversible competitive antagonism.
2 Irreversible competitive antagonism.
3 Non-competitive antagonism.

1 Reversible competitive antagonists

The ability of drugs to combine with receptors ('affinity') is determined by simple intermolecular forces; this is usually considered to be distinct from their capacity to produce receptor activation ('intrinsic activity'). Agonists combine with receptors and induce a pharmacological response, i.e. they possess both receptor affinity and intrinsic activity.

By contrast, reversible competitive antagonists combine with the same receptors as agonists but do not induce a pharmacological response, i.e. they possess receptor affinity but no intrinsic activity. Consequently they do not cause receptor activation and induce the sequence of biochemical and biophysical changes that result in drug response. Reversible competitive antagonists can be completely displaced from receptors by a sufficiently high concentration of any agonist that acts on the same receptor system. They characteristically displace the log-dose–response curve to the right in a parallel manner, although the maximum response obtained is unaffected (Fig. 3.9). This is the essential feature of reversible competitive antagonism.

Reversible competitive antagonists that are commonly used in anaesthetic practice are shown in Table 3.3. In experimental conditions, they are often characterized by the dose ratio (i.e. the ratio between the doses of the agonist required to produce an equivalent response in the presence and absence of the antagonist). It can be shown that

$$\text{Dose ratio} - 1 = \frac{[A]}{K_a}$$

where $[A]$ is the molar concentration of the antagonist and K_a is the dissociation constant of the drug–antagonist complex at equilibrium. It is comparable with the dissociation constant of the drug–receptor complex K_d (p. 87), and is a measure of the affinity with which antagonists bind to receptors. The potency of reversible competitive antagonists can be conveniently compared by means of their pA_2 values; this parameter represents the negative logarithm of the molar dose of antagonist required to produce a dose ratio of 2 (i.e. in which the ratio of equieffective doses in the presence and absence of the antagonist is 2 : 1). In these conditions, $K_a = [A]$. The pA_2 values of some anticholinergic (antimuscarinic) drugs are shown in Table 3.4. These values were obtained from experiments in which acetylcholine was used as an agonist in an isolated tissue preparation (the guinea-pig ileum). Determination of the pA_2 is an extremely useful way of comparing the potency of a series of reversible competitive antagonists; the most

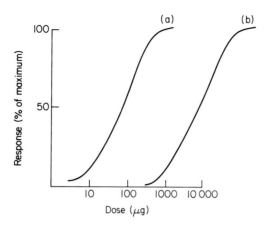

Fig. 3.9 The effect of competitive antagonists on the log-dose–response relationship, (a) in the absence of a competitive antagonist, and (b) in the presence of a competitive antagonist.

potent compounds have the highest pA_2 value. These parameters are entirely independent of the characteristics and the relative potency of the agonist, as long as different agonists compete with the antagonist for the same receptor population.

Table 3.3 Reversible competitive antagonists used in anaesthetic practice.

Drug	Endogenous compound antagonized
Atropine Hyoscine Glycopyrrolate	Acetylcholine (at muscarinic sites)
Tubocurarine Pancuronium Alcuronium Atracurium Vecuronium	Acetylcholine (at the motor endplate)
Trimetaphan Tubocurarine	Acetylcholine (at autonomic ganglia)
Propranolol Metoprolol Labetalol	Adrenaline and noradrenaline (β effects)
Metoclopramide Chlorpromazine Perphenazine Prochlorperazine	Dopamine
Naloxone Naltrexone Nalmefene	Endorphins
Flumazenil	?Endogenous benzodiazepines

Table 3.4 The pA_2 values of some drugs with anticholinergic properties, obtained using the guinea-pig ileum preparation.

Drug	pA_2 value
Hyoscine	9.5
Glycopyrrolate	9.5
Atropine	9.0
Promethazine	7.7
Chlorpromazine	7.5
Amitriptyline	6.7
Pethidine	5.3
Sotalol	5.1
Propranolol	5.0
Imipramine	3.4

2 Irreversible competitive antagonists

Irreversible competitive antagonists compete with agonists for receptors but only slowly dissociate from receptor sites, so that the total number of receptors that are available for combination with agonists is reduced. This type of competitive antagonism is usually due to the formation of stable chemical bonds between the agonist and the receptor (or to the disorientation and distortion of the receptor molecule). Irreversible competitive antagonists characteristically displace the log-dose–response curve to the right in a non-parallel manner, and also prevent the subsequent attainment of a maximal response to the agonist (even at extremely high concentrations). They often have a long duration of action, and their effects are usually unrelated to their plasma concentration. Examples of irreversible competitive antagonism include the effects of phenoxybenzamine on α-receptors, and the action of α-bungarotoxin on acetylcholine receptors at the neuromuscular junction.

In experimental conditions, a precise distinction between reversible and irreversible competitive antagonism is not always possible. Although irreversible competitive antagonists compete with agonists and reduce the total number of available receptor sites, many tissues contain significant numbers of 'spare receptors' (i.e. a receptor reserve that allows a maximum response to be obtained at a relatively low receptor occupancy). In these conditions, a reduction in the total number of receptor sites may not impair the maximal response, and low concentrations of irreversible competitive antagonists may produce effects consistent with reversible antagonism.

3 Non-competitive antagonists

All other types of drug antagonism can be described as non-competitive antagonism, since they do not directly depend on competition between agonists and antagonists for the same receptor population. Nevertheless, some types of non-competitive antagonism may be mediated by receptor systems or receptor mechanisms. For instance, the effects of gallamine on heart rate may be due to a reduction in the affinity of cardiac muscarinic receptors for acetylcholine, resulting in tachycardia.

Chemical antagonism is based on direct combination between the antagonist and the agonist, so that the effects of the agonist are prevented or diminished. For instance, the effects of some metallic ions (e.g. arsenic, copper, gold, lead, mercury, silver and zinc) can be neutralized by various chelating agents, and this type of chemical antagonism is widely used in the management of heavy metal poisoning. Similarly, heparin can be neutralized by the basic low molecular weight protein protamine, resulting in the formation of a stable salt. Heparin is an extremely acidic drug, due to the presence of large numbers of sulphate groups.

Functional antagonism or physiological antagonism is sometimes used to describe the effects of drugs on two independent receptor systems that normally mediate opposing responses. For example, histamine causes contraction of bronchial smooth muscle, while adrenaline causes relaxation; thus adrenaline can be considered to be a functional antagonist of histamine. In some instances, this type of antagonism occurs physiologically, and is responsible for the opposite effects of sympathetic and parasympathetic tone in many effector systems. In these situations, noradrenaline is a functional antagonist of acetylcholine.

Finally, pharmacokinetic interactions that reduce the plasma concentration and activity of other drugs by affecting the processes of absorption, distribution, metabolism and excretion can be considered to be a type of non-competitive antagonism that only occurs in *in vivo* conditions. Drug interactions are considered in Chapter 4.

PARTIAL AGONISTS

As mentioned previously, agonists can be considered to have two properties or characteristics: (1) they have the capacity to combine with receptors ('receptor affinity'), and (2) they have the ability, when combined with receptors, to cause receptor activation ('intrinsic activity'). Reversible competitive antagonists possess a variable receptor affinity, as reflected in their pA_2 value, but little or no intrinsic activity. Partial agonists (originally known as 'dualists') are drugs that possess considerable receptor affinity (and will therefore compete in appropriate concentrations with both agonists and reversible competitive antagonists) but also have some degree of intrinsic activity. This is intermediate between the intrinsic activity of reversible competitive antagonists (zero) and full agonists (unity). In consequence, partial agonists may produce either agonist or antagonist effects, depending on the circumstances in which they are used. In low doses or concentrations, they tend to produce agonist effects; in the presence of small concentrations of a full agonist, additive effects may be observed. When the response to the full agonist equals the maximum response to the partial agonist, the latter has no apparent action; in the presence of the full agonist, it produces neither agonist or antagonist effects. When high concentrations of the full agonist are present, the partial agonist acts as a reversible competitive antagonist and reduces the response to the agonist (Fig. 3.10). At least two groups of drugs are known to have some partial agonist activity which may be of clinical significance in man. These are (1) β-adrenoceptor antagonists, and (2) opioid analgesics.

β-adrenoceptor antagonists possess a variable degree of partial agonist activity (which is often referred to as intrinsic sympathomimetic activity). Propranolol has only minimal partial agonist activity and primarily induces β-adrenoceptor blockade; by contrast, pindolol possesses significant partial agonist activity and may produce sympathomimetic effects (Table 3.5). Other drugs that are partial agonists at β-adrenoceptors (i.e. xamoterol) are sometimes used as positive inotropic agents in intensive care. Partial agonist activity may be important when β-adrenoceptor antagonists are used in the management of patients with borderline congestive cardiac failure.

Some synthetic opioid analgesics are partial agonists at opioid receptors (Chapter 10). In consequence, they may show either agonist or antagonist activity, depending on the circumstances in which they are used. They are sometimes referred to as agonist/antagonists (or antagonist/agonists), although this term may also be applied to drugs with agonist and antagonist effects at different types of

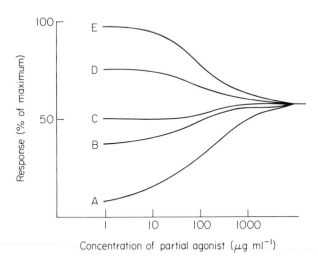

Fig. 3.10 Dose–response relationship for a partial agonist in the presence of increasing concentrations of a full agonist (represented by the curves A, B, C, D, and E). At lower concentrations of the full agonist (A and B), the partial agonist has additive effects; at higher concentrations of the full agonist (D and E), the partial agonist has antagonist effects. When the response to the full agonist equals the maximum response to the partial agonist alone (C), little or no effect is observed.

Table 3.5 The partial agonist activity ('intrinsic sympathomimetic activity') of some β-adrenoceptor antagonists.

Drug	Partial agonist activity
Acebutolol	+
Alprenolol	++
Atenolol	−
Metoprolol	−
Oxprenolol	++
Pindolol	+++
Propranolol	−
Sotalol	−
Timolol	+

− Absent or minimal; + slight; ++ moderate; +++ marked.

Table 3.6 Opioid analgesics with partial agonist activity at μ or κ receptors.

Drug	Partial agonist activity at opioid receptors	
	μ receptors	κ receptors
Nalorphine		+
Levallorphan		+
Pentazocine		++
Cyclazocine		++
Butorphanol		+++
Nalbuphine		++
Buprenorphine	++	

+ Slight; ++ moderate; +++ marked.

opioid receptor. Thus, nalorphine, levallorphan, pentazocine, cyclazocine, butorphanol, nalbuphine and buprenorphine have significant agonist and/or antagonist activity at one or more than one opioid receptor; this is least marked with nalorphine and levallorphan, which are primarily opioid antagonists with slight agonist activity (Table 3.6). Their partial agonist activity at opioid receptors may have some clinical implications. Firstly, the analgesic effects of full agonists (e.g. morphine, pethidine, dipipanone and fentanyl) may not be enhanced by partial agonists; indeed, their effects may possibly be antagonized. Secondly, partial agonists may not effectively antagonize the effects of other partial agonists, either at the same receptor, or at different opioid receptors. The drugs of choice in the management of narcotic overdosage are naloxone, naltrexone and nalmefene, which are 'pure' reversible competitive antagonists that are devoid of any agonist activity. These drugs (particularly naloxone) are the only antagonists that will reverse the respiratory depression or dysphoria induced by pentazocine (Chapter 11).

DESENSITIZATION, TACHYPHYLAXIS AND TOLERANCE

The repeated or continual, use of drugs sometimes leads to a progressive decrease in the observed response. This phenomenon is usually referred to as desensitization, tachyphylaxis, or tolerance, although these terms are usually applied in different circumstances.

Desensitization can be defined as a decrease in cellular sensitivity or responsiveness due to the continuous or repeated exposure to agonists. It is usually observed in *in vitro* conditions (in particular, in isolated tissues or cell preparations).

Acute desensitization usually occurs rapidly and is readily reversible. It was first described 30 years ago by Katz and Thesleff in relation to the effects of agonists on the motor endplate and skeletal muscle. This type of acute desensitization can be explained by the existence of a receptor population in three states: a resting state (R), an activated state (R^*), and a desensitized state (R^-). At the motor endplate, an increase in ionic permeability only occurs when the receptor is in the activated (R^*) state, as shown in the following model. (D represents the active drug or agonist.)

$$D + R \rightleftharpoons DR$$
$$\text{\Updownarrow} \qquad\qquad DR^* \rightarrow \text{response.}$$
$$D + R^- \rightleftharpoons DR^-$$

Certain antagonists may have a preferential affinity for the desensitized receptor ('metaphilic antagonists'). Acute desensitization may also occur with receptors that are linked to adenylate cyclase. Alternatively, it is sometimes due to secondary ionic changes that result in hyperpolarization of excitable membranes (particularly in smooth muscle preparations).

Chronic desensitization is a different phenomenon; as its name implies, it usually develops slowly and is less readily reversible. It is often associated with the loss of receptors from effector cells due to endocytosis ('internalization'), irreversible conformational changes, or receptor degradation. A chronic increase in hormonal or transmitter release frequently causes receptor loss or 'down regulation'; this can occur at both cholinergic and adrenergic synapses. Similarly, receptor loss and chronic desensitization often occurs when effector cells are exposed to excess concentrations of agonists (e.g. when bronchial smooth muscle cells are exposed to sympathomimetic amines with β_2-adrenergic effects). Chronic desensitization due to receptor loss may also occur in pathological conditions associated with autoimmune processes (e.g. myasthenia gravis).

Tachyphylaxis can be defined as a rapid decrease or diminution in the magnitude of pharmacological responses. It is sometimes applied to the phenomenon of acute desensitization or described as rapid tolerance. Nevertheless, it is probably best restricted to describe the effects of drugs that act by releasing endogenous transmitters from cells or nerve endings. In these conditions, the response to repeated doses of the drug rapidly declines, due to transmitter exhaustion. Tachyphylaxis is classically observed after the administration of indirectly acting sympathomimetic amines (e.g. tyramine, ephedrine or amphetamine); it may also occur with drugs that release dopamine (e.g. amantidine and tetrabenazine) or histamine.

Tolerance is a chronic phenomenon, and is usually restricted to *in vivo* situations in which increasing drug dosage is required to produce the desired therapeutic effect. It classically occurs with opioid analgesics and ganglion blocking agents (e.g. trimetaphan). Tolerance to opioid analgesics may be related to the modification of the synthesis or release of endorphins, resulting in the altered responsiveness of cells in the CNS. Clearly, drug tolerance in these conditions may encompass the phenomena of receptor loss and chronic desensitization. In other situations (e.g. with tolerance to barbiturates) increased metabolism due to the induction of hepatic enzymes may play an important contributory role.

FURTHER READING

Ariëns EJ. Affinity and intrinsic activity in the theory of competitive inhibition. Part I. Problems and theory. *Archives Internationales de Pharmacodynamie et de Therapie* 1954; **99**: 32–49.

Ariëns EJ. Receptors: from fiction to fact. *Trends in Pharmacological Sciences* 1979; **1**: 11–15.

Ariëns EJ, van Rossum JM, Simonis AM. A theoretical basis of molecular pharmacology. Part II. Interactions of one or two compounds with two interdependent receptor systems. *Arzneimittel-Forschungen* 1956; **6**: 611–621.

Axelrod J, Gordon E, Hertting G, Kopin IJ, Potter LT. On the mechanism of tachyphylaxis to tyramine in the isolated rat heart. *British Journal of Pharmacology* 1962; **19**: 56–63.

Barnes PJ. Radioligand binding studies of adrenergic receptors and their clinical relevance. *British Medical Journal* 1981; **282**: 1207–1210.

Berridge MJ. Inositol trisphosphate and diacylglycerol as second messengers. *Biochemical Journal* 1984; **220**: 345–360.

Berridge MJ. Inositol trisphosphate and diacylglycerol: two interacting second messengers. *Annual Review of Biochemistry* 1987; **56**: 159–193.

Budd K. Clinical use of opioid antagonists. *Clinics in Anaesthesiology* 1987; **1**: 993–1011.

Calvey TN. Side-effect problems of μ and ϰ agonists in clinical use. *Clinics in Anaesthesiology* 1987; **1**: 803–827.

Calvey TN, Williams NE, Muir KT, Barber HE. Plasma concentration of edrophonium in man. *Clinical Pharmacology and Therapeutics* 1976; **19**: 813–820.

Changeux J-P, Giraudat J, Dennis M. The nicotinic acetylcholine receptor: molecular architecture of a ligand-regulated ion channel. *Trends in Pharmacological Sciences* 1987; **8**: 459–465.

Changeux J-P, Thiéry J, Tung Y, Kittel C. On the cooperativity of biological membranes. *Proceedings of the National Academy of Sciences* 1967; **57**: 335–341.

Chenoweth MB. Clinical uses of metal-binding drugs. *Clinical Pharmacology and Therapeutics* 1968; **9**: 365–387.

Chuang DM, Costa E. Evidence for internalization of the recognition site of β-adrenergic receptors during receptor subsensitivity induced by (−) isoproterenol. *Proceedings of the National Academy of Sciences of the USA* 1979; **76**: 3024–3028.

Clark AJ. *Mode of Action of Drugs on Cells*. London: Edward Arnold, 1933.

Clark AJ. General Pharmacology. In: *Heffter's Handbuch der Experimentellen Pharmakologie, Ergänzungswerk*. Berlin: Springer-Verlag, 1937; **4**: 1–223.

Clark BJ, Menninger K, Bertholet A. Pindolol — the pharmacology of a partial agonist. *British Journal of Clinical Pharmacology* 1982; **13**: 149–158S.

Cooper JR, Bloom FE, Roth RH. *The Biochemical Basis of Neuropharmacology*, 3rd edn. New York: Oxford University Press, 1978.

Dretchen KL, Standaert FG, Skirboll LR, Morgenroth VH III. Evidence for a prejunctional role of cyclic nucleotides in neuromuscular transmission. *Nature* 1976; **264**: 79–81.

Ehrlich P. Chemotherapeutics: scientific principles, methods, and results. *Lancet* 1913; **ii**: 445–451.

Endo M. Calcium release from the sarcoplasmic reticulum. *Physiological Reviews* 1977; **57**: 71–108.

Fambrough DM. Control of acetylcholine receptors in skeletal muscle. *Physiological Reviews* 1979; **59**: 165–216.

Flower RJ. Lipocortin and the mechanism of action of the glucocorticoids. *British Journal of Pharmacology* 1988; **94**: 987–1015.

Gaddum JH. Theories of drug antagonism. *Pharmacological Reviews* 1957; **9**: 211–218.

Galant SP, Duriseti L, Underwood S, Insel PA. Decreased β-adrenergic receptors on polymorphonuclear leukocytes after adrenergic therapy. *New England Journal of Medicine* 1978; **299**: 933–936.

Gilman AG. G proteins: transducers of receptor-generated signals. *Annual Review of Biochemistry* 1987; **56**: 615–649.

Goldberg LI. Monoamine oxidase inhibitors. Adverse reactions and possible mechanisms. *Journal of the American Medical Association* 1964; **190**: 456–462.

Graziano MP, Gilman AG. Guanine nucleotide-binding regulatory proteins: mediators of transmembrane signaling. *Trends in Pharmacological Sciences* 1987; **8**: 478–481.

Griffiths TM, Edwards DH, Lewis MJ, Henderson AH. Evidence that cyclic guanosine monophosphate (cGMP) mediates endothelium-dependent relaxation. *European Journal of Pharmacology* 1985; **112**: 195–202.

Helmreich EJM, Pfeuffer T. Regulation of signal transduction by β-adrenergic hormone receptors. *Trends in Pharmacological Sciences* 1985; **6**: 438–442.

Hill AV. The possible effect of the aggregation of the molecules of haemoglobin on its dissociation curves. *Journal of Physiology* 1910; **40**: iv–vii.

Holmstedt B. Pharmacology of organophosphorus cholinesterase inhibitors. *Pharmacological Reviews* 1959; **11**: 567–688.

Huganir RL, Greengard P. Regulation of receptor function by protein phosphorylation. *Trends in Pharmacological Sciences* 1987; **8**: 472–477.

Karlin A, Kao PN, DiPaola M. Molecular pharmacology of the nicotinic acetylcholine receptor. *Trends in Pharmacological Sciences* 1986; **7**: 304–308.

Katz B, Thesleff S. A study of the 'desensitization' produced by acetylcholine at the motor endplate. *Journal of Physiology* 1957; **138**: 63–80.

Lamble JW (ed.) *Towards Understanding Receptors*. Amsterdam: Elsevier/North-Holland Biomedical Press, 1981.

Lamble JW, Abbott AC (eds) *Receptors Again*. Amsterdam: Elsevier Science Publishers, 1984.

Langley JN. On the physiology of the salivary secretion. Part II. On the mutual antagonism of atropin and pilocarpin, having especial reference to their relations in the sub-maxillary gland of the cat. *Journal of Physiology* 1878; **1**: 339–369.

Langley JN. On the reaction of cells and of nerve-endings to certain poisons, chiefly as regards the reaction of striated muscle to nicotine and to curari. *Journal of Physiology* 1905; **33**: 374–413.

Levine RR, Birdsall NJM, North RA, Holman M, Watanabe A, Iversen L L (eds) *Subtypes of Muscarinic Receptors*. Cambridge: Elsevier Publications, 1987.

Michell RH. Inositol phospholipids and cell surface receptor function. *Biochimica et Biophysica Acta* 1975; **415**: 81–147.

Miller KW. The nature of the site of general anesthesia. *International Review of Neurobiology* 1985; **27**: 1–60.

Monod J, Wyman J, Changeux J-P. On the nature of allosteric transitions: a plausible model. *Journal of Molecular Biology* 1965; **12**: 88–118.

Mukherjee C, Caron MG, Lefkowitz RJ. Regulation of β-adrenergic receptors by β-adrenergic agonists *in vivo*. *Endocrinology* 1976; **99**: 343–353.

Norman J. Drug–receptor interactions. *British Journal of Anaesthesia* 1979; **51**: 595–601.

Olsen RW. Drug interactions at the GABA receptor–ionophore complex. *Annual Review of Pharmacology* 1982; **22**: 245–277.

Palmer RMJ, Ferrige AG, Moncada S. Nitric oxide accounts for the biological activity of endothelium-derived relaxing factor. *Nature* 1987; **327**: 524–526.

Parascandola J. Origins of the receptor theory. In: Lamble JW (ed.) *Towards Understanding Receptors*. Amsterdam: Elsevier/North-Holland Biomedical Press, 1981; 1–7.

Paton WDM, Waud DR. The margin of safety of neuromuscular transmission. *Journal of Physiology* 1967; **191**: 59–90.

Putney JW. Calcium-mobilizing receptors. *Trends in Pharmacological Sciences* 1987; **8**: 481–486.

Rance MJ. Multiple opiate receptors — their occurrence and significance. *Clinics in Anaesthesiology* 1983; **1**: 183–200.

Rees DD, Palmer RMJ, Hodson HF, Moncada S. A specific inhibitor of nitric oxide formation from L-arginine attenuates endothelium-dependent relaxation. *British Journal of Pharmacology* 1989; **96**: 418–424.

Ringold GM. Steroid hormone regulation of gene expression. *Annual Review of Pharmacology and Toxicology* 1985; **25**: 529–566.

Schild HO. pA, a new scale for measurement of drug antagonism. *British Journal of Pharmacology* 1947; **2**: 189–206.

Schild HO. Drug antagonism and pA_x. In: Symposium on Drug Antagonism. *Pharmacological Reviews* 1957; **9**: 242–246.

Schleimer RP. The mechanisms of anti-inflammatory steroid action in allergic diseases. *Annual Review of Pharmacology and Toxicology* 1985; **25**: 381–412.

Stephenson RP. A modification of receptor theory. *British Journal of Pharmacology* 1956; **11**: 379–393.

Strichartz GR, Ritchie JM. The action of local anesthetics on ion channels of excitable tissues. In: Strichartz GR (ed.) *Handbook of Experimental Pharmacology, Vol. 81, Local Anesthetics*. Heidelberg: Springer-Verlag, 1987; 21–52.

Study RE, Barker JL. Cellular mechanisms of benzodiazepine action. *Journal of the American Medical Association* 1982; **247**: 2147–2151.

Sutherland EW, Rall TW. The relation of adenosine-3′, 5′-phosphate and phosphorylase to the actions of catecholamines and other hormones. *Pharmacological Reviews* 1960; **12**: 265–299.

Van Rossum JM (ed.) *Kinetics of Drug Action. Handbook of Experimental Pharmacology*, Volume 47. Heidelberg: Springer-Verlag, 1977.

Vane JR, Gryglewski RJ, Botting RM. The endothelial cell as a metabolic and endocrine organ. *Trends in Pharmacological Sciences* 1987; **8**: 491–496.

Werkheiser WC. The biochemical, cellular, and pharmacological action and effects of the folic acid antagonists. *Cancer Research* 1963; **23**: 1277–1285.

Whittaker VP. The storage and release of acetylcholine. *Trends in Pharmacological Sciences* 1986; **7**: 312–315.

Wildsmith JAW. Peripheral nerve and local anaesthetic drugs. *British Journal of Anaesthesia* 1986; **58**: 692–700.

Wilson IB, Hatch MA, Ginsburg S. Carbamylation of acetylcholinesterase. *Journal of Biological Chemistry* 1960; **235**: 2312–2315.

Woods DD. The biochemical mode of action of the sulphonamide drugs. *Journal of General Microbiology* 1962; **29**: 687–702.

FOUR

Drug Interaction

Drug interaction is the modification of the effects of one drug by another. Many of these reactions are clinically unimportant or harmless, while others form an integral part of medical or anaesthetic practice. A familiar example is the use of neostigmine to antagonize the effects of competitive neuromuscular blocking agents at the motor endplate and the concomitant use of atropine to prevent muscarinic activity due to the anticholinesterase. However, a small minority of interactions are hazardous or potentially fatal, and it is therefore important for the anaesthetist to be aware of their possible occurrence. Interactions may occur between drugs which are administered concurrently during anaesthesia; alternatively, reactions may occur with prescribed drugs or self-medication. It is thus essential for a full drug history to be available prior to the administration of anaesthesia.

Nevertheless, the assessment of drug interactions in man must be undertaken with a sense of balance. Reports of adverse effects based on single case histories or circumstantial and anecdotal evidence are of little value, particularly when the mechanisms involved are obscure or poorly understood.

In general medical practice, between 6 and 30% of adverse reactions to drugs are probably due to drug interactions. Comparable figures for anaesthetic practice are not available. However, most of the interactions that may occur in anaesthesia are well known and are usually predictable from an appreciation of the pharmacology of the drugs concerned.

In this chapter, a general account is given of the pharmacological mechanisms that are usually responsible for drug interactions in man. Reactions with specific groups of drugs that are commonly used in anaesthetic practice are then considered in detail.

Mechanisms of drug interactions may be described in three groups:
1 Pharmaceutical interactions which can occur *in vitro*.
2 Pharmacokinetic interactions which are due to the alteration of the disposition of one drug by another.

3 Pharmacodynamic interactions which are due to interference with the effects of drugs at tissue sites.

PHARMACEUTICAL INTERACTIONS

Some drug interactions are due to the mixing of drugs or incompatible solutions outside the body. These interactions may be responsible for the loss of activity of drugs, or for their aggregation or precipitation in solution, and this occasionally has serious consequences. Pharmaceutical interactions are divided into two groups, chemical and physical.

Chemical

Most drugs, including anaesthetic agents, inevitably have to be stored prior to use and in many instances may undergo deterioration during storage. When stored in a powder or solid form decomposition tends to occur more slowly. The addition of water or a mixing agent may accelerate the rate of decomposition of a drug (e.g. barbiturates for i.v. use), particularly when more concentrated solutions are formed, or when dextrose or saline are used as solvents. Other drugs (e.g. halothane or catecholamines) are decomposed by light or are sensitive to changes in temperature (e.g. isoflurane and enflurane).

Mixing of solutions with different pH values may result in drug precipitation. Weak acids (e.g. i.v. barbiturates and thiobarbiturates) are usually administered as their sodium salts and are only ionized and water soluble in alkaline conditions (pH 10–11). Similarly, many other drugs (e.g. local anaesthetics, analgesics and most sympathomimetic amines) are weak bases which can only exist in aqueous solutions as acid salts (e.g. sulphates or hydrochlorides with a pH 4–5). Mixing such dissimilar solutions in the same syringe or in an infusion set usually causes precipitation of free acid and base. The addition of drugs such as suxamethonium to a solution of thiopentone results in rapid alkaline hydrolysis, and thus inactivation of the muscle relaxant.

Direct chemical combination may also produce drug interaction *in vitro*. The addition of calcium salts to infusion lines containing bicarbonate solutions will result in significant precipitation of the insoluble salt, calcium carbonate. The use of trichlorethylene in anaesthetic circuits incorporating soda lime may lead to the production of the potentially neurotoxic vapour, dichloracetylene. When penicillin derivatives are added to infusion fluids containing amino acids, drug–protein complexes are formed that can induce the formation of cytophilic antibodies (IgE). Alternatively, the individual components of mixtures of drug solutions may be precipitated. Thus, the addition of drugs or electrolytes to fat emulsions (e.g. intralipid) or concentrated solutions (e.g. 20% mannitol) may result in the aggregation or precipitation of the mixture.

Epimerization or racemization of molecules in solutions also occurs. This may involve a change in the steric configuration of the molecule, as in the conversion of adrenaline from an *l* to a *d* form, which occurs with a pH change in solution. The Maillard reaction involves an interaction between dextrose and amino acid solutions. This results in a colour change and precludes the storage of combined parenteral nutrition mixtures. Although this reaction is minimal at room temperature it becomes important if the mixture is heat treated.

Physical

A difference in the osmolarity of infusion fluids may lead to interactions which occur during administration. The concurrent infusion of blood with either 5% dextrose or mannitol may result in significant damage to the blood. Solvent system polarity (the solubility of a drug in aqueous solution) may be important when relatively insoluble agents such as diazepam or propofol are presented in organic solvents which are subsequently added to aqueous solutions. The degree of precipitation will depend upon relative volume and concentration of both drug and aqueous solution.

Drugs may also interact with administration sets through which they are given. *Sorption* is best exemplified by nitroglycerine and refers to the lipophilicity and polarity of the solution which causes the subsequent binding to different types of plastic. *Adsorption* refers to the tendency of a drug to adhere to the surface of a container, as may occur with insulin in glass or plastic syringes.

Other physical phenomena which may occur include 'salting out' which results when electrolytes are added to supersaturated solutions such as mannitol, and 'emulsion cracking' which can ensue when calcium salts are added to fat emulsions. In the latter instance the surface charge on the fat globules which repels similar particles (the zeta potential) is reduced in the presence of additional cations and this will allow the globules to coalesce.

Pharmaceutical interactions are often predictable and are not usually an important cause of complications in anaesthetic practice. Their occurrence can be minimized by a number of simple precautions. If possible, only one drug should be added to each unit of a crystalloid solution, except in special circumstances. No additives should be incorporated in infusions of blood, blood products, lipid emulsions, amino acid preparations or hypertonic fluids. The addition of drugs to acid or alkaline solutions should be avoided. Solutions must be thoroughly mixed before administration and this is particularly important when potassium salts are added to intravenous fluids. Solutions containing additives are preferably prepared in the pharmacy and should be clearly labelled. When additives are used in the wards or theatre, the manufacturer's data sheet or a table of drug incompatibilities should be consulted. Cases of doubt can usually be resolved by a pharmacist or drug information centre.

PHARMACOKINETIC INTERACTIONS

Pharmacokinetic interactions occur in the body and are due to an alteration in the disposition of one drug by another. In these circumstances, the concentration of a drug at its site of action may be modified. According to the mechanisms involved, these interactions can be classified as those affecting:

1 Dissolution or absorption.
2 Distribution (including protein binding).
3 Metabolism.
4 Elimination.

Dissolution or absorption

These drug interactions usually occur in the stomach or upper intestine, and may concern the anaesthetist when premedicant drugs are given by this route. When drugs are administered orally in the form of capsules, they must be present in solution before absorption can occur. Drug dissolution usually takes place in the stomach, and the solubility of some drugs such as the tetracyclines is critically dependent on acid conditions. In these circumstances, drugs which affect gastric pH (e.g. antacids and H_2-receptor antagonists) will influence the degree of absorption. Most drugs, however, are absorbed in the more alkaline medium of the small intestine; thus those agents which affect the speed of gastric emptying will alter the rate of delivery of other drugs to the site of absorption and thus influence uptake. Metoclopramide stimulates gastric emptying and increases the speed of uptake of many drugs administered orally, whereas narcotic analgesics and anticholinergic agents will exert a converse effect.

   Drug interactions in the small intestine may decrease absorption when chelates or other insoluble complexes are formed. Thus the absorption of tetracyclines is reduced by the simultaneous administration of calcium, magnesium, or iron salts, and the resin cholestyramine may decrease the absorption of many other drugs (e.g. warfarin, aspirin and phenylbutazone).

   The absorption of drugs administered by subcutaneous or intramuscular injection is determined by the aqueous solubility of the drug at tissue sites, the extent of biotransformation locally and by the efficiency of peripheral blood flow. Drugs which are prepared in solvents (e.g. diazepam, phenytoin) may precipitate out in tissues, and this may account for the decrease in bioavailability (compared to that attained by oral administration). Various drugs exhibiting autonomic activity (e.g. sympathomimetic amines and α-adrenoceptor blocking agents) can significantly modify skin and muscle blood flow. If tissue blood flow is decreased by these mechanisms and extensive biotransformation of the parenterally administered drug occurs at tissue sites, bioavailability will be affected.

Distribution

Following administration and absorption, drugs are present in plasma either in simple solution or bound to carrier proteins or erythrocytes, whence they are conveyed to organs and tissues by the vascular system. The uptake and subsequent distribution of inhalational agents is primarily influenced by minute ventilation and cardiac output. The rate of rise of alveolar concentration, which correlates with the induction of anaesthesia, is largely determined by ventilatory activity; thus respiratory depressants (e.g. narcotic analgesics and barbiturates) may slow the rate of onset of anaesthesia. Conversely, drugs which reduce cardiac output (e.g. intravenous induction agents and β-adrenoceptor blocking agents) will allow an increased rate of rise of alveolar concentration and by reflex vasoconstrictor effects will lead to enhanced cerebral perfusion; the rate of induction of anaesthesia may thus be increased.

Protein binding

In many instances, the transport of drugs in the circulation necessitates binding to plasma proteins. Most acidic drugs (e.g. penicillins, salicylates, barbiturates) bind to albumin, whilst in general basic drugs (e.g. narcotic analgesics and local anaesthetic agents) bind to other plasma protein constituents such as lipoproteins, α_1-acid glycoprotein and γ-globulin.

Some drugs (e.g. oral anticoagulants) are extensively bound by albumin at therapeutic concentrations, so that only 1–2% of the total in plasma is available for diffusion into tissues. In consequence, drugs that displace oral anticoagulants from plasma proteins (e.g. phenylbutazone, mefenamic acid and some sulphonamides) may significantly increase the unbound fraction of the anticoagulant present in plasma and could enhance its therapeutic and toxic effects. However, it is doubtful whether displacement from plasma proteins is an important factor in the causation of drug interactions in man. Any increase in the concentration of unbound drug in plasma will usually be compensated by its increased renal and hepatic clearance, so that a new steady-state is established and drug distribution to the site of action is not significantly enhanced. Drugs that lead to clinical interactions with warfarin, such as phenylbutazone, will also affect its metabolism presumably by competing at enzymatic sites, whose protein configuration may be important. Certain sulphonamides have been considered to prolong the action of thiopentone by competing for binding on albumin, although it is extremely doubtful whether this interaction is of any clinical significance.

Some drugs are also extensively bound by proteins in tissues. The antimalarial drugs mepacrine and pamaquin are both bound by hepatic proteins, and may displace each other into extracellular fluid. It is unclear whether this phenomenon is responsible for clinically significant drug interactions in man. In general, little is known of the possible importance of the binding of drugs to cell and tissue proteins.

Metabolism

Drug interactions affecting metabolism mainly occur in the liver, and may be due to interference with several different physiological or biochemical processes. Following oral administration, some drugs are highly extracted and extensively metabolized by the liver before they gain access to the systemic circulation. This 'first pass effect' may be an important cause of the diminished response to certain drugs (e.g. narcotic analgesics) when given by the oral route. In the case of drugs which are extensively cleared by the liver (i.e. those with a high extraction ratio), the magnitude of the first pass effect is dependent on liver blood flow; in consequence, drugs that modify hepatic perfusion may affect the proportion of the oral dose that enters the systemic circulation. Thus the oral bioavailability of drugs such as lignocaine and some narcotic analgesics may be affected by drugs that reduce liver blood flow (e.g. propranolol and volatile anaesthetic agents).

Alternatively, drug interaction in the liver may be due to effects on enzymes that are responsible for drug metabolism. The oxidative metabolism of many drugs and some endogenous hormones is dependent on the activity of microsomal enzyme systems associated with the smooth endoplasmic reticulum of liver cells. One of the most important of these enzymes is a mixed function oxidase (cytochrome P-450) whose activity is enhanced by many drugs (e.g. barbiturates, some anticonvulsants, insecticides and polycyclic hydrocarbons). In some instances, the activity of other microsomal enzymes (e.g. glucuronyl transferase) is also increased. The phenomenon of enzyme induction is a common and important cause of drug interaction in man. Barbiturates, for example, may increase the metabolism of many other drugs (e.g. oral anticoagulants, anticonvulsants, antidepressants and glucocorticoids); enzyme induction reduces the plasma concentration and the pharmacological effects of these drugs. Conversely, withdrawal of the inducing drug will lead to a regression of the enzyme system to its original state. The serum concentration and plasma half-life will thus increase and toxicity will result if appropriate adjustment of dosage is not made. Phenobarbitone may induce enzymes and alter the rate of metabolism of other drugs within 2 days of commencing administration, with further increasing effects over the following weeks. As yet it is not clear whether the repeated use of barbiturates as intravenous anaesthetic agents can lead to significant enzyme induction.

In addition to inducing and enhancing enzyme activity in the liver, some drugs inhibit enzymes that are concerned with drug metabolism. Thus monoamine oxidase inhibitors *para*-aminosalicylate, isoniazid, verapamil, chloramphenicol and cimetidine may inhibit some enzyme systems and thus increase the activity of other drugs. Some compounds (e.g. suxamethonium and procaine) are not metabolized by hepatic enzymes but are broken down by a cholinesterase (ChE) present in plasma. Drugs that react with this enzyme (e.g. ecothiopate, neostigmine, pyridostigmine and cyclophosphamide) may prolong the effect of the depolarizing agent or possibly of local anaesthetic esters.

Elimination

The principal sites at which drugs are eliminated from the body are the liver, kidney, lungs, and gastrointestinal tract. Drug interactions are possible when any of these routes are involved.

Compounds that alter the pH of urine may influence the rate and extent of elimination of other drugs. The duration of drug action and the proportion of the dose metabolized by the liver may also be modified. In general, drugs that are weak acids or weak bases may be present in solution in both ionized and non-ionized forms and the relative proportions of the two forms is dependent on pH. In alkaline urine, significant amounts of some weak acids are ionized; in this state, they cannot readily diffuse back into the plasma across the renal tubule, and are therefore eliminated in the urine (Fig. 4.1). By contrast, in neutral or acid urine, a higher proportion of the acidic drug is non-ionized; diffusion back into plasma is thus facilitated and excretion accordingly reduced. Conversely, weak bases (e.g. tricyclic antidepressants, narcotic analgesics and local anaesthetics) are more

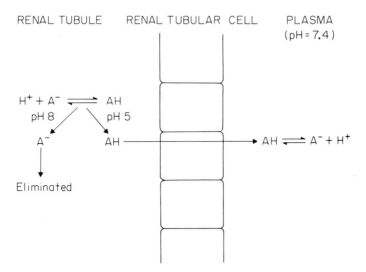

Fig. 4.1 Elimination of weak acids in alkaline and acid urine. Weak acids are present in plasma and the renal tubule in two forms (A$^-$ and AH); only AH can diffuse across renal tubular cell membranes. At pH 8, most of the drug in the renal tubule is present as A$^-$ and is eliminated in urine. At pH 5, more of the drug is present in a non-ionized form (AH), which can back-diffuse across the renal tubule and is eliminated to a lesser extent. Similar factors apply to the elimination of weak bases.

highly ionized in acidic urine and their elimination under these circumstances is enhanced whereas the presence of an alkaline urine will promote reuptake of the basic drug in the renal tubule.

These effects may be of value in the treatment of drug overdosage. Forced alkaline diuresis is useful in the management of salicylate or phenobarbitone poisoning, whilst an acid diuresis is sometimes used in the treatment of amphetamine, quinine, fenfluramine and phencyclidine poisoning. Although modification of the pH of urine may lead to other interactions, these are not usually of clinical significance.

Alternatively, drug interaction in the kidney may be related to competition for active transport. Both acid and basic drugs and their metabolites are partially eliminated from plasma by secretion in the proximal renal tubule. This process is competitive and may be subject to interference by other drugs. Thus, benzylpeni-cillin is a weak acid that is actively secreted by the proximal renal tubule; in consequence, it has a relatively short half-life (30–40 min) which can be prolonged by other drugs competing for active transport mechanisms (e.g. probenecid, NSAIDs and most diuretics). The elimination of endogenous substances can similarly be inhibited by drugs. Many thiazide diuretics compete for tubular secretion; in these conditions, the plasma urate concentration may be raised and acute gout can be precipitated.

Similarly, drug interactions in the liver may be due to competition for biliary excretion. Both anions (e.g. ampicillin) and cations (e.g. tubocurarine) are concentrated and excreted in the bile by transport mechanisms which require cellular enzymes; these are saturable systems at which other anions and cations may compete and reduce their transport. This interaction is rarely of practical significance.

The rate of removal of inhalational anaesthetic agents is principally deter-mined by minute ventilation and cardiac output, which lead to a fall in alveolar concentration. Drugs which affect either of these factors (e.g. respiratory depressants and some antiarrhythmic agents) will again influence the rate of elimination of volatile and gaseous agents.

Some highly basic and lipid soluble drugs (e.g. pethidine and fentanyl) may diffuse from plasma into the stomach, and subsequent reabsorption from the small intestine may result in a 'secondary peak' effect. This gastroenteric recirculation process may be modified by drugs which either influence splanchnic blood flow or produce changes in gastric pH.

PHARMACODYNAMIC INTERACTIONS

Pharmacodynamic interactions are due to interference with the effects of drugs at their sites of action in tissues. Drug interactions of this type may produce additive, synergistic, potentiating or antagonistic effects. Such interactions are frequently beneficial (e.g. the use of protamine to reverse the anticoagulant effects of heparin or the use of anticholinesterase drugs to antagonize the action of muscle relaxants at the neuromuscular junction). Alternatively, adverse interactions can occur; for instance, chlorpromazine and related drugs block α-adrenergic receptors, and may therefore potentiate the hypotensive effect of other drugs (e.g. tubocurarine and halothane). Some pharmacodynamic interactions are related to the additive effects of drugs on the CNS (e.g. barbiturates, benzodiazepines and phenothiazines), the autonomic nervous system (e.g. atropine, tricyclic antidepressants and antiparkinsonian drugs) or the cardiovascular system (e.g. β-adrenoceptor antagonists, calcium channel blockers and other antiarrhythmic agents).

Not all adverse interactions can be attributed to effects on drug absorption, distribution, metabolism and excretion or to reactions at receptor sites. In some instances, the pharmacological basis of a drug interaction is unknown or obscure. From the anaesthetist's point of view, it is often more important to be aware of the more common established interactions that may be encountered or anticipated in the course of anaesthetic practice.

DRUG INTERACTIONS IN ANAESTHETIC PRACTICE

Drug interactions in anaesthetic practice may occur between pre-existing drug therapy and general or local anaesthetic agents, muscle relaxants, analgesics and drugs used in premedication. Interactions between anaesthetic agents and their adjuvants may also occur and are similarly discussed. The principal interactions are summarized in Table 4.1.

1 Interactions with general anaesthetic agents

Drug interactions may occur with both intravenous and inhalational agents. Although reactions due to drug incompatibility may occur with intravenous agents in *in vitro* conditions, these interactions are well known and are easily avoided. More serious interactions between general anaesthetics may occur *in vivo*.

Due to drug incompatibility

Solutions of thiopentone sodium and methohexitone sodium are alkaline (pH 10–11). When these intravenous barbiturates are mixed with other drugs or solutions of lower pH, they may precipitate them or be precipitated by them. This drug incompatibility occurs with a wide range of compounds, some of which are used in anaesthesia (e.g. pethidine hydrochloride, propranolol hydrochloride and suxamethonium bromide). In general, thiopentone and methohexitone should not be dissolved in or mixed with oxidizing agents, acidic solutions or with drugs normally administered as sulphates, chlorides or hydrochlorides.

Table 4.1 Interactions between the main groups of drugs.

General anaesthetics	Local anaesthetics	Muscle relaxants and their antagonists	Analgesics	Hypnotics and tranquillizers
Incompatible drugs in solution	Tricyclic antidepressants	General anaesthetics	Central depressants	Central depressants
Other centrally acting drugs	Muscle relaxants and their antagonists	Local anaesthetics	Monamine oxidase inhibitors	Enzyme inducing and inhibiting agents
Cardiovascular drugs	Sulphonamides	Drugs which modify electrolytes	Narcotic antagonists	Anticholinergic drugs
Drugs which modify electrolytes		Drugs that modify acid–base balance	Oral anticoagulants	Antiparkinsonian drugs
Muscle relaxants		Cholinesterase inhibitors	Hypoglycaemic agents	
Enzyme inducing effects		Antibiotics	Uricosuric agents	
Nephrotoxic agents		Calcium-channel blockers	Antihypertensive drugs	
			Diuretics	

Other centrally acting drugs

As mentioned previously, drugs with a significant respiratory depressant effect can modify the uptake, distribution and elimination of inhalational anaesthetic agents. However, once anaesthesia is established all drugs which exhibit respiratory depression are likely to have supra-additive effects; for example, the minimum alveolar concentration (MAC) value of halothane (which reflects the potency of this agent at steady-state conditions) is reduced by about 30% when diazepam is also administered and similar effects may be predicted when narcotic analgesics, hypnotics, tranquillizers, antidepressants, and certain antihypertensive agents have been given, or if other inhalational agents (e.g. nitrous oxide) are being used. Conversely, the concomitant use of CNS stimulants (e.g. amphetamines, β_2-adrenoceptor agonists) could predictably increase the anaesthetic requirement.

Antiarrhythmic and antianginal agents

Organic nitrates, β-adrenoceptor antagonists and calcium channel blocking agents are commonly used in the management of angina; the latter two groups of drugs are also effective antihypertensive and antiarrhythmic agents. Such therapy should always be continued up to the immediate preoperative period as the risks of rebound phenomena (e.g. worsening of angina symptoms, and reappearance of arrhythmias) far outweigh those due to drug interactions which may occur during anaesthesia. The percutaneous administration of glyceryl trinitrate is sometimes continued during anaesthesia, although the theoretical risk of potentiation of systemic hypotension or reflex tachycardia must be borne in mind.

β-adrenoceptor antagonists

Bradycardia is frequently encountered during anaesthesia in patients receiving β-adrenoceptor antagonists, particularly when halothane (which can exhibit considerable vagomimetic activity) is being administered in relatively high concentrations. Severe bradyarrhythmias may result in hypotension; such an effect has been observed following the absorption of timolol eye-drops.

Calcium-channel blockers

There is now considerable evidence that volatile anaesthetic agents can themselves exert either significant calcium-channel blocking activity or interference with the mobilization of intracellular calcium. Furthermore, verapamil has been shown in animal studies to reduce the MAC value for halothane by 25%. Supraadditive effects with these two groups of drugs are thus predictable. In consequence, a large number of studies have been undertaken, both in animals and in man, to assess the possibility of drug interactions. It would appear that clinical concentrations of volatile anaesthetic agents and therapeutic doses of calcium channel blockers do not produce significant additive effects. However, class 1 calcium-channel blockers such as verapamil may induce varying degrees of heart block and this effect is likely to be enhanced in the presence of halothane or enflurane. Furthermore, the summative effects which may be anticipated from combined therapy with β-adrenoceptor antagonists and calcium-channel blockers in the presence of these volatile agents suggests that special vigilance is necessary during anaesthesia. The use of alternative anaesthetic agents or techniques should be considered.

It must be remembered that both β-adrenoceptor antagonists and calcium-channel blockers can exert a myocardial depressant effect. The resultant decrease in cardiac output may also modify the pharmacokinetic behaviour of inhalational agents and effectively increase their potency by secondary reflex mechanisms which facilitate cerebral blood flow.

Sympathomimetic amines

Sympathomimetic amines with β-adrenergic activity may precipitate dangerous or fatal arrhythmias during inhalational anaesthesia with cyclopropane or halogenated hydrocarbons. In current clinical practice, tachyarrhythmias may be predicted due to the presence of endogenous or exogenous catecholamines during halothane anaesthesia. Some of these may be of the re-entrant type; since halothane slows the conduction of impulses and also probably increases the refractory period in conducting tissue it creates the conditions necessary for re-entry, namely a unidirectional block with slow retrograde conduction. Halothane may also increase the automaticity of the myocardium. Increased secretion of adrenaline due to surgical stimulation, hypoxia and hypercarbia can potentiate this risk. Ventricular arrhythmias, in particular multiple ectopic beats ('pulsus bigeminus') can be induced and may progress to tachycardia or even fibrillation. Injection of adrenaline is thus potentially hazardous; however the risk of arrhythmias is unlikely if the dose of adrenaline used for haemostasis is limited to 100 μg, a concentration of $10 \mu g\,ml^{-1}$ (1 in 100 000) is not exceeded and due consideration is given to ventilatory parameters and to the depth of anaesthesia. The presence of lignocaine in the vasoconstrictor solution may afford some protection. Dysrhythmias are less common with the anaesthetic ethers in common use (enflurane and isoflurane) (Table 4.2). Ketamine produces central stimulation of sympathetic activity, possibly by an effect on σ-receptors, and effects of exogenous adrenaline are theoretically potentiated.

Interactions with sympathomimetic amines are mainly encountered when these drugs are administered during anaesthesia. However, it is uncertain whether

Table 4.2 Doses of submucosal adrenaline required to induce ventricular extrasystoles in the presence of inhalational agents (ED_{50} at 1.25 MAC).

Halothane	2.1 μg/kg*
Isoflurane	6.7 μg/kg
Enflurane	10.9 μg/kg

* When given in a mixture with lignocaine, the ED_{50} increases to 3.7 μg/kg.

patients on oral sympathomimetic drugs such as ephedrine, phenylephrine and phenylpropanolamine (some of which are present in over-the-counter cold and cough remedies) are also at risk during general anaesthesia. Similarly, phenylephrine (10%) and neutral adrenaline (1%) eye-drops are sometimes used in ophthalmic practice. Small amounts of these agents are absorbed and may cause transient dysrhythmias on occasions; in these conditions, general anaesthesia with halogenated compounds may increase their effects on the heart. A similar phenomenon may be produced by large doses of oral fenfluramine, and this drug should be discontinued a week before surgery is contemplated, if this is possible.

Cardiovascular effects may occur during anaesthesia from the prior administration of levodopa. Such effects appear to be dose-related in that large doses of levodopa tend to produce tachyarrhythmias and vasoconstriction, presumably due to the metabolite dopamine; with smaller doses, vasodilatation usually predominates.

Arrhythmias induced by sympathomimetic amines during inhalational anaesthesia can usually be prevented or controlled by β-adrenoceptor antagonists. Propranolol (1 mg i.v.) is commonly used for this purpose. The dose may be repeated at 2 min intervals until a maximum of 5 mg has been administered. Propranolol may enhance the effects of the increase in vagal tone and the hypotension induced by most halogenated anaesthetics, and may cause bronchospasm (particularly in susceptible patients concurrently given histamine-releasing agents such as tubocurarine and morphine); atenolol may be a suitable alternative.

Antihypertensive agents

During general anaesthesia, hypotensive responses may be induced by a number of drug interactions. Most of these reactions are simply due to the additive effects of drugs that affect blood pressure. For instance, halothane and the intravenous barbiturates tend to lower blood pressure, and may interact with α- or β-adrenoceptor blocking agents or with other drugs that can produce vasodilatation (e.g. chlorpromazine, morphine and tubocurarine). These actions are predictable and may be desirable in normotensive patients during anaesthesia.

In hypertensive patients on drug therapy, severe hypotension may occur during general anaesthesia, or postural hypotension may be seen on recovery. Intravenous agents are particularly liable to induce such responses in treated hypertensive patients. Both thiopentone and methohexitone reduce cardiac output and often decrease blood pressure in both hypertensive and normotensive subjects. Similarly inhalational agents (via negative inotropic or chronotropic effects or by a reduction in peripheral resistance) may lead to falls in systemic pressure which may be exaggerated in the hypertensive patient. These reactions are predictable and can readily be explained on a physiological basis. As long as it is recognized that the treated hypertensive patient carries a greater risk of perioperative hypotension than the normotensive subject, and appropriate dose modification of the anaesthetic agents used is made, drug interaction should not be a major problem.

Drugs that modify electrolyte balance

Drugs affecting electrolyte balance may also predispose or contribute to the occurrence of cardiac arrhythmias during inhalational anaesthesia. For instance, drugs that lower serum potassium (e.g. most diuretics, corticosteroids, carbenoxolone, and insulin) may induce supraventricular or ventricular ectopic beats during inhalational anaesthesia, particularly in patients who are digitalized or have disorders of electrolyte balance. Conversely, drugs that induce hyperkalaemia (e.g. suxamethonium, potassium salts, and potassium-sparing diuretics) tend to impair cardiac conduction and may cause sinoatrial block. Agents that lower serum calcium (e.g. calcitonin and blood transfusions or intravenous infusions containing citrates, edetates or other chelating agents) depress cardiac contractility and may predispose to cardiac arrhythmias. Additional factors unrelated to drug administration may also be involved (e.g. stimulation during anaesthesia or surgery).

Muscle relaxants

Many inhalational agents increase the neuromuscular block induced by non-depolarizing muscle relaxants. Enhancement of myoneural blockade is dependent on the nature and concentration of the anaesthetic agent; enflurane and isoflurane (and probably diethylether) produce a greater degree of skeletal muscle relaxation than halothane at equivalent MAC values. The mechanism of this effect is not entirely clear; it may be due to central actions or to increased sensitivity of the postsynaptic receptor or the muscle cell membrane.

Volatile anaesthetics may also affect the kinetic disposition of muscle relaxants. For instance, when gradually increasing concentrations of halothane are administered, neuromuscular junction sensitivity also increases but the rate of equilibration between the plasma concentration of the relaxant and the onset of paralysis will decrease. This reflects decreased perfusion to the neuromuscular junction, causing a reduced rate of drug delivery.

In contrast, the action of a single dose of suxamethonium is not significantly affected by general anaesthetic agents in current use, although some enhancement of its effect was observed when the now obsolete intravenous induction agent, propanidid, which shared a common metabolic pathway, was used concomitantly. However, evidence suggests that the onset of 'dual block' when repeated doses of suxamethonium are used is more prevalent when volatile agents are being used concurrently.

Enzyme induction

Many agents used in anaesthesia (e.g. thiopentone, nitrous oxide, and halothane) have been shown to induce the activity of drug metabolizing enzymes. It is thus possible that the plasma concentration and therefore the pharmacological activity of certain other drugs concurrently used (e.g. steroids, anticoagulants, and anti-convulsants) could be reduced; alternatively, an increase in the production of toxic metabolites of certain agents (e.g. isoniazid) might be envisaged. The problem is complicated by the fact that the underlying disease and associated trauma may have a depressant effect on drug metabolism and lead to higher plasma concentrations of drugs administered in the postoperative period. Studies using antipyrine clearance as an index of the efficiency of drug metabolizing enzymes have shown that short procedures are followed by increased enzyme activity, but in protracted operations activity is diminished.

Nephrotoxic agents

The use of methoxyflurane, a halogenated ether which has now been withdrawn, was not uncommonly associated with the development of impaired renal function, and was related to the increased elimination of the main metabolite, inorganic fluoride. A limited increase in the urinary excretion of fluoride ions follows the administration of enflurane, and there is a slight risk of renal damage, particularly when other nephrotoxic agents (e.g. tetracyclines) are being used concomitantly.

2   Interactions with local anaesthetic agents

Although local anaesthetics are extensively used in current practice, undesirable or adverse drug reactions are uncommon. Nevertheless, interactions involving local anaesthetic solutions are a potential risk when they are administered to patients who are taking certain other drugs. Preparations of local anaesthetics often contain vasoconstrictors, and drug interaction can occur with either the vasoconstrictor or the local anaesthetic agent. Other constituents of local anaes-thetic solutions (reducing agents, preservatives and fungicides) have not been incriminated in drug interactions.

Tricyclic antidepressants and related drugs

Endogenous noradrenaline which is released in response to sympathetic nerve stimulation is partly removed from the synaptic cleft by active transport back into the nerve terminal — this process is known as $Uptake_1$ or the amine pump (Chapter 11). Exogenous noradrenaline (and to a lesser extent, adrenaline) are removed from the circulation in a similar manner. This mechanism can be blocked by most tricyclic antidepressant drugs and their derivatives, which compete with the catecholamines for axonal transport. The pressor response to noradrenaline is potentiated four to nine times in the presence of tricyclic agents, whilst the effect of adrenaline is increased by two to three fold. Deaths have occurred in patients receiving tricyclic antidepressants to whom local anaesthetics containing nor-adrenaline were administered. Such solutions are no longer commercially avail-able in the UK. Infusion or injection of noradrenaline or other α-receptor agonists such as methoxamine or phenylephrine to patients on tricyclic antidepressants may cause a marked rise in blood pressure that can precipitate subarachnoid haemorrhage. There is some evidence that pancuronium may also sensitize tissues to adrenaline and noradrenaline by a similar mechanism and special care should be taken when these substances or other pressor amines are administered in the presence of this muscle relaxant.

Reservations have long been expressed concerning the use of adrenaline-containing solutions of local anaesthetics in patients receiving tricyclic antide-pressants. Current opinion suggests that, providing proper attention is given to dosage and technique, clinically significant drug interaction will not ensue. Similar considerations should also be given to other drugs which can compete for or inhibit $Uptake_1$ (e.g. phenothiazines and adrenergic neurone-blocking agents) when local anaesthetics containing vasoconstrictors are being used. Local anaesthetics containing catecholamines are perhaps more dangerous in patients with ischaemic heart disease or significant hypertension. A suitable alternative preparation is prilocaine hydrochloride (3%) and felypressin (0.03 iu ml^{-1}). Felypressin is a polypeptide which produces vasoconstriction but which is not dependent on the amine pump for its removal from the circulation; drug interac-tions with the use of this vasoconstrictor have not been reported.

Muscle relaxants and their antagonists

Local anaesthetics can enhance the effects of both depolarizing and competitive muscle relaxants on neuromuscular transmission. In high concentrations, local anaesthetics of the ester group (e.g. procaine and amethocaine) can compete with suxamethonium for plasma ChE; in these conditions, they may prevent the hydrolysis of suxamethonium and enhance depolarizing block. Conversely, the effects of local anaesthetic esters may themselves be prolonged by drugs that inhibit, compete for, or degrade ChE. Interactions of this type may occur between ester anaesthetics and neostigmine, pyridostigmine, suxamethonium, ecothiopate and cytotoxic drugs.

Many local anaesthetics may also augment competitive block, although their mechanism of action is uncertain. Local anaesthetics decrease acetylcholine release from the nerve terminal, and stabilize the postsynaptic receptor and the muscle cell membrane. These effects can clearly contribute to and enhance non-depolarizing blockade.

Sulphonamides

Some local anaesthetics antagonize the actions of sulphonamides in both *in vivo* and *in vitro* conditions. The antibacterial effects of sulphonamides are dependent on the antagonism of *para*-aminobenzoate, which is essential for nucleic acid synthesis in certain organisms. Drugs that release *para*-aminobenzoate in tissues, such as procaine and related esters, can overcome this antagonism and prevent the bacteriostatic effects of sulphonamides. Since local anaesthetics and their metabolites are rapidly removed from the circulation, antagonism of sulphonamide-induced bacteriostasis only occurs at the site of injection. Instances of this interaction have only rarely been reported, and its significance is now mainly of historical interest. Nevertheless, local anaesthetic solutions or sprays containing procaine or amethocaine should be avoided in patients with infections that are being concurrently treated with sulphonamides or sulphonamide combinations (e.g. co-trimoxazole).

3   Interactions with muscle relaxants and their antagonists

The effects and duration of action of depolarizing and competitive neuromuscular blocking agents may be modified by many other drugs. These can affect transmitter release, modify the enzymic hydrolysis of acetylcholine, act on the postsynaptic receptor or directly affect the voluntary muscle cell. Interactions of this type may be associated with prescribed or self-administered oral therapy, with parenteral or locally applied preparations or with agents concurrently administered in the course of anaesthesia.

General anaesthetics

Most inhalational agents will affect both the pharmacodynamic activity and the kinetic behaviour of competitive neuromuscular blocking agents. The enhanced and prolonged effects observed may be related to depression of the CNS decreased neurotransmitter release, reduced motor endplate sensitivity or to direct effects on the muscle membrane. Furthermore, the cardiovascular effects of most volatile agents may result in decreased tissue perfusion and thus influence the rate of uptake and subsequent removal of the muscle relaxants from their site of action. Interactions involving general anaesthetic agents and suxamethonium are unlikely to occur, except when the depolarizing agent is administered in repeated dosage.

Local anaesthetics

Most local anaesthetic agents enhance the effects of competitive blockers on neuromuscular transmission. Many other drugs, including phenothiazines, antihistamines, and antiarrhythmic drugs such as quinidine, procainamide and phenytoin have local anaesthetic or membrane-stabilizing properties, and may also augment competitive neuromuscular blockade. In addition, local anaesthetic esters may compete with suxamethonium for plasma ChE and prolong depolarization blockade.

Drugs that affect electrolyte balance

Drugs that modify electrolyte balance (in particular, those that affect the plasma concentration of magnesium, calcium and potassium ions) may profoundly influence neuromuscular transmission. Magnesium salts decrease acetylcholine release and the sensitivity of the motor endplate; in consequence, the amplitude of the endplate potential is reduced. In these conditions competitive blockade is augmented and depolarization is antagonized. In general, opposite effects are produced by calcium salts and by drugs that raise plasma calcium levels (e.g. parathormone and possibly thiazide diuretics); acetylcholine release is increased and excitation–contraction coupling is enhanced. Calcium ions also stabilize the postjunctional membrane.

    Drugs that increase plasma potassium (e.g. spironolactone, triamterene and amiloride) decrease the resting membrane potential of muscle and augment depolarization blockade, while drugs that induce hypokalaemia (e.g. carbenoloxone, thiazide diuretics and corticosteroids) increase the resting potential and enhance the effects of competitive agents. Changes in plasma potassium may also modify transmitter release. In the presence of hypokalaemia the dosage of competitive agents should be reduced; conversely the dose of suxamethonium may need to be increased.

Drugs that modify acid–base balance

Neuromuscular blockade can be modified by changes in acid–base balance. In particular, both respiratory acidosis and metabolic alkalosis appear to enhance and prolong competitive blockade. Any drug which induces respiratory acidosis (e.g. carbon dioxide, narcotic analgesics and barbiturates) or metabolic alkalosis (e.g. thiazide diuretics and certain antacids) may therefore enhance the response to competitive agents. The effect of other alterations in acid–base balance on neuromuscular blockade is less clear.

Potentiation of the response to muscle relaxants by respiratory acidosis and metabolic acidosis is probably due to changes in intracellular pH and potassium balance. During hypokalaemia, the resting membrane potential of excitable tissues is increased, resulting in an enhanced response to competitive blockers. Although pH changes can also affect binding of muscle relaxants and receptor ionization at the motor endplate, the role of these factors is uncertain.

In vitro studies suggest that changes in acid–base balance may also affect the ionization of certain muscle relaxants in *in vivo* conditions. Many of the experimental and clinical studies concerned with the modification of neuromuscular blockade have involved the use of *d*-tubocurarine. This drug is a monoquaternary amine, but also has a basic (tertiary amine) group that attracts H^+ during acidosis. In these conditions, *d*-tubocurarine has a similar configuration to bisquaternary amines which have a greater potency and activity at the neuromuscular junction. Other competitive agents do not have these pH dependent physicochemical properties, and changes in acid–base balance may affect their activity in a different manner.

Calcium channel blockers

The importance of calcium ions in the presynaptic release of acetylcholine and subsequent muscle contraction has already been considered. The potentiation of neuromuscular blockade by drugs which inhibit transmembrane calcium transport and intracellular calcium mobilization may thus be anticipated. The problem is likely to be enhanced in the presence of volatile anaesthetic agents; in this context isoflurane may cause particular problems.

Drugs that inhibit ChE

Such drugs may interact with both main groups of muscle relaxants. Many drugs are known to affect the enzymatic hydrolysis of suxamethonium. Thus drugs which compete for or inhibit plasma ChE such as neostigmine, edrophonium, organophosphorus compounds and local anaesthetic esters, or which interfere with the synthesis of the enzyme (certain cytotoxic agents such as cyclophosphamide and possibly thiotepa), can prolong the duration of action of suxamethonium. In the past, certain inhibitors of plasma ChE (particularly tetrahydroaminacrine and hexafluorenium) were deliberately used to prolong the action of suxamethonium; they are no longer commercially available in the UK. Pancuronium is a moderately potent inhibitor of plasma ChE, and it may prolong the action of drugs that are normally metabolized by the enzyme. Unpredictable effects are sometimes observed when certain ganglion-blocking agents (e.g. hexamethonium, trimetaphan) are used in the presence of muscle relaxants. Competition at both junctional enzymatic sites and at the postsynaptic receptor have been reported from animal studies; trimetaphan is also thought to inhibit plasma ChE.

The effects of all competitive muscle relaxants are antagonized ('reversed') by drugs which inhibit junctional acetylcholinesterase. In anaesthetic practice, neostigmine is commonly used for this purpose. Other drugs which inhibit this enzyme (e.g. pyridostigmine, physostigmine, organophosphorus compounds) may also modify competitive blockade. It is uncertain whether the reversal of neuromuscular block is directly due to enzyme inhibition or to other properties of the drug.

In some countries, drugs that release acetylcholine from nerve terminals such as 4-aminopyridine have been used to antagonize neuromuscular blockade. Although 4-aminopyridine has some advantages over the anticholinesterase drugs (e.g. the concurrent administration of atropine is not required) it enters the CNS and may cause cerebral excitation and convulsions.

Antibiotics

Some antibiotics can induce neuromuscular blockade and may potentiate the effects of competitive agents. Occasionally, depolarization block produced by suxamethonium or decamethonium is also enhanced. This phenomenon was first observed when antibiotic sprays containing streptomycin or neomycin were applied to the peritoneum after abdominal surgery; in these conditions hypoventilation may supervene postoperatively due to the local effects of the antibiotic on the diaphragm. Similar interactions after the systemic administration of antibiotics are relatively rare, and usually involve the aminoglycosides (e.g. neomycin, streptomycin, kanamycin, gentamicin, polymyxins, colistin, tetracyclines or lincomycin and clindamycin). In these circumstances, neuromuscular block is probably dependent on several factors which may vary with different antibiotics. Blockade induced by aminoglycoside antibiotics or tetracyclines is variably affected by anticholinesterase drugs and is more commonly antagonized by calcium salts (e.g. calcium gluconate $2-3\,mg\,kg^{-1}\,min^{-1}$ for 5 min).

It has been suggested that the neuromuscular blockade induced by these antibiotics is due to competition for calcium binding sites in the nerve terminal or the prejunctional membrane. By contrast, neuromuscular blockade which is induced by the polymyxins, colistin, lincomycin and clindamycin is usually unaffected by anticholinesterases and calcium salts. These interactions are usually managed by controlled ventilation until normal neuromuscular function is restored, although 4-aminopyridine is sometimes effective. Although potentiation of neuromuscular blockade usually occurs when competitive agents are administered to patients on antibiotics, similar effects may be induced when antibacterial drugs are given to patients with myasthenia gravis.

4 Interactions with analgesics

Narcotic analgesics

Narcotic analgesics are extensively used in anaesthesia, and drug interaction between them and other agents is of particular concern to the anaesthetist. In patients receiving certain other drugs (e.g. monoamine oxidase inhibitors) dangerous interactions may occur after single doses of some narcotic analgesics (e.g. pethidine). However, in most cases drug interactions with narcotic analgesics are readily predictable from a knowledge of the pharmacological effects of these agents.

Other central depressants

Effective analgesic doses of opiates tend to cause sedation and invariably produce some respiratory depression. Their depressant effects on ventilation may be enhanced by other drugs that affect medullary centres such as inhalational anaesthetics, intravenous induction agents and some hypnotics and tranquillizers. Tricyclic antidepressants may also enhance the depression produced by narcotic analgesics. Similarly, the administration of more than one opiate may cause summation of this depressant effect. Conversely, the respiratory depression induced by morphine and related compounds may decrease the rate of uptake and subsequent removal of general anaesthetics given by inhalational techniques.

Monoamine oxidase inhibitors

Although monoamine oxidase inhibitors primarily interfere with the metabolism of monoamines (e.g. tyramine and dopamine) they may also affect the breakdown of other drugs. In particular, dangerous interactions may occur between these agents and pethidine. Serious side-effects are considered to be due to the accumulation of the principal metabolite, norpethidine, and include mental confusion, cerebral excitation, hyperpyrexia and either hypertension or circulatory collapse. Although similar interactions have occasionally been reported with other opiates, they appear to be far less common. Pethidine should never be administered to patients receiving monoamine oxidase inhibitors; but buprenorphine and possibly fentanyl have been considered to be safe alternatives.

Narcotic antagonists

The effects of all narcotic analgesics may be modified by drugs that compete with them for opiate receptors in the CNS. Naloxone competitively antagonizes the effects of all narcotic analgesics; it is a pure narcotic antagonist and has no agonist activity. By contrast, other antagonists (e.g. nalorphine, levallorphan and pentazocine) also possess some agonist activity at opiate receptors. These drugs ('partial agonists') antagonize some of the effects of other narcotic analgesics, but also produce central effects of their own (e.g. dysphoria, analgesia, and respiratory depression) due to their intrinsic activity at opiate receptors.

Other interactions

Other interactions with narcotic analgesics are usually of little practical significance. Most narcotic analgesics may delay the oral absorption of other drugs by decreasing gastric motility and slowing down the rate of gastric emptying. The urinary elimination of some analgesics (e.g. pethidine, fentanyl, and phenoperidine) is increased by acids, or by drugs that increase acidosis. Since these drugs are extensively metabolized, their enhanced elimination in acid urine is of little value in the treatment of drug overdosage; it is sometimes of value in the detection of drug dependence. Nausea and vomiting are common side-effects of many narcotic analgesics; these effects may be modified by antiemetic drugs (e.g. chlorpromazine and the antihistamines).

Non-opioid analgesics

Non-opioid analgesics include aspirin and other NSAIDs (e.g. ibuprofen, mefenamic acid, and naproxen) and paracetamol. These drugs, which are being increasingly used in the perioperative period and in the management of chronic pain, are the commonest group of compounds involved in drug interactions in man.

In particular, aspirin and other salicylates have been associated with clinically significant interactions of this type. In most instances, these interactions have only been reported after large and repeated doses of these drugs; the possible effect of restricted administration or of single doses is more difficult to evaluate.

Aspirin and related compounds may induce drug interactions by two principal mechanisms. Firstly, aspirin-like drugs bind firmly to plasma proteins and thus can displace other drugs (e.g. warfarin anticoagulants, oral hypoglycaemic agents) from binding sites. The problem with warfarin is accentuated, because aspirin itself can cause gastric bleeding due to mucosal damage, inhibit platelet aggregation and in large doses reduce the synthesis of prothrombin. The use of aspirin should be avoided in patients receiving warfarin therapy. Paracetamol, which is devoid of such effects and does not compete for protein binding sites, is a suitable alternative.

Secondly, salicylates produce dose-dependent effects on tubular secretion in the kidney. Aspirin can decrease the urinary elimination of urates, and may antagonize the effects of uricosuric agents (e.g. probenecid, sulphinpyrazone) which are being administered concurrently. Furthermore, salicylates may interfere with the removal of other drugs which rely on active transport processes such as methotrexate and can potentiate their effects.

Certain NSAIDs (e.g. indomethacin) have been shown to inhibit the renal excretion of sodium and possibly antagonise the effects of other drugs used in the treatment of hypertension and heart failure. Aspirin and most other related drugs have been less commonly implicated; nevertheless this effect is worth remembering when refractory hypertension or oedema develops during treatment with NSAIDs and appropriate adjustment of dosage may be necessary.

Drug interactions involving paracetamol appear to be extremely uncommon. However, a number of compound preparations containing paracetamol may also include either codeine or dextropropoxyphene. Both these drugs are potential respiratory depressants and such effects may be enhanced by the concurrent administration of general anaesthetics, sedatives and tranquillizers. Dextropropoxyphene poisoning is not infrequently associated with excessive consumption of alcohol. Dextropropoxyphene may prolong and enhance the effects of oral anticoagulants; interactions between this drug and the anticholinergic compound orphenadrine have also been reported.

5   Interactions with hypnotics and tranquillizers

Agents which induce sleep (hypnotics) or which relieve anxiety and tension (tranquillizers) are closely related to each other and are probably the most frequently prescribed drugs in general medical practice. Benzodiazepines are commonly administered in the perioperative period. Diazepam is often used for premedication to allay anxiety prior to surgery, and temazepam may be prescribed as a hypnotic on the night before operation. In addition, intravenous benzodiazepines (e.g. diazepam, lorazepam, midazolam) are commonly used to induce sedation during endoscopy and minor surgical procedures. Other drugs with sedative or anticholinergic properties (e.g. antihistamine compounds, atropine or hyoscine) may also be used for premedication.

Other central depressants

Doses of tranquillizers or sedatives that relieve anxiety and tension may induce drowsiness and cause loss of concentration in susceptible subjects. These drugs should not be given to ambulant patients without warning them of the possible hazards of their administration, particularly in their relation to driving. Furthermore, all such drugs may interact with other agents which have depressant effects on the CNS (e.g. other sedatives, general anaesthetics and alcohol). Their effects may also be enhanced during the concurrent administration of antidepressant drugs, although authentic reports of this interaction are extremely rare. The effects of drugs that induce respiratory depression (e.g. intravenous barbiturates and narcotic analgesics) may also be potentiated.

Enzyme inducing and inhibiting agents

Some drugs which are used as hypnotics and sedatives (e.g. barbiturates, dichloralphenazone) can induce hepatic enzymes and stimulate the metabolism of other drugs such as warfarin and related anticoagulants and oral contraceptives; they are potentially capable of interactions with a wide range of other drugs.

Interactions of this type involving benzodiazepines are relatively rare, although both diazepam and chlordiazepoxide may inhibit the metabolism of phenytoin and increase its toxicity. In contrast, the H_2-receptor antagonist, cimetidine, binds to cytochrome P-450 and can inhibit the metabolism of diazepam and related compounds (as well as phenobarbitone, phenytoin, propranolol and imipramine).

Other interactions involving premedicant drugs

Drugs with significant anticholinergic properties that are used for premedication (e.g. atropine, hyoscine) can induce a marked antisialogogue effect and decrease the effect of other drugs which may be administered sublingually (e.g. glyceryl trinitrate, buprenorphine). Anticholinergic drugs may also antagonize the effects of certain antiemetic agents (e.g. domperidone, metoclopramide) on the gastrointestinal tract.

Phenothiazines and butyrophenones are often used during anaesthesia, principally for their antiemetic effect. In patients who are receiving levodopa, the action of these antiemetic drugs with central dopaminergic properties may be inhibited; conversely the mutual antagonism of these drugs and levodopa may result in an exacerbation of the extrapyramidal disorder.

Prevention of adverse drug interactions

Although adverse drug interactions cannot be entirely prevented, their incidence may be minimized by an appreciation of the factors which contribute to their occurrence. Firstly, many interactions occur with prescribed or self-administered oral therapy; it is therefore important to take a drug history before the administration of any other agent, and to be conversant with the effects of the drugs that are involved. Secondly, the possibility of adverse interactions rises exponentially as the number of drugs administered is increased (although only two agents are usually involved). Thirdly, drug interactions are more likely when drug elimination is prolonged, as in hepatic or renal disease. Finally, adverse interactions are more common with agents which have a relatively steep dose–response curve, or when there is little difference between the toxic and therapeutic doses of drugs.

FURTHER READING

Aronson JK, Grahame-Smith DG. Clinical pharmacology: adverse drug interactions. *British Medical Journal* 1981; **282**: 288–291.

Attia RR, Grogono AW. Drug and disease interactions In: *Practical Anaesthetic Pharmacology*. New York: Appleton County Croft, 1978; **15**: 243–261.

Baraka A. The influence of carbon dioxide on the neuromuscular block produced by tubocurarine chloride in the human subject. *British Journal of Anaesthesia* 1964; **36**: 272–278.

Bennett JA, Eltrincham RJ. Possible dangers of anaesthesia in patients receiving fenfluramine. Results of animal studies following a case of human cardiac arrest. *Anaesthesia* 1977; **32**: 8–13.

Bevan DR, Monks PS, Calne DB. Cardiovascular reaction to anaesthesia during treatment with levodopa. *Anaesthesia* 1973; **28**: 29–31.

Blackman JG, Gauldie RW, Milne RJ. Interaction of competitive antagonists. The anti-curare action of hexamethonium and other antagonists at the skeletal neuromuscular junction. *British Journal of Pharmacology* 1975; **54**: 91–100.

Bowman WC, Webb SN. Neuromuscular blocking and ganglion-blocking activities of some acetylcholine antagonists in the cat. *Journal of Pharmacy and Pharmacology* 1972; **24**: 262–272.

Calvey TN. Drugs affecting administration of anaesthetics. *British Dental Journal* 1980; **149**: 185–186.

Calvey TN, Milne LA, Williams NE *et al.* Effect of antacids on the plasma concentration of phenoperidine. *British Journal of Anaesthesia* 1983; **55**: 535–539.

Clive DM, Stoff JS. Renal syndromes associated with non-steroidal anti-inflammatory drugs. *New England Journal of Medicine* 1984; **310**: 563–572.

Conney AH. Pharmacological implications of microsomal enzyme induction. *Pharmacological Reviews* 1967; **19**: 317–366.

Conrad KA, Byers JM III, Finley PR, Burnham L. Lidocaine elimination. Effects of metoprolol and propranolol. *Clinical Pharmacology and Therapeutics* 1983; **33**: 133–138.

Csogor SI, Kerek SF. Enhancement of thiopentone anaesthesia by sulphafurazole. *British Journal of Anaesthesia* 1970; **42**: 988–990.

Dodson M. Drug interactions and anaesthesia. *Hospital Update* 1982; **8**: 57–68.

Durant NN, Nguyen N, Katz RL. Potentiation of neuromuscular blockade by verapamil. *Anesthesiology* 1984; **60**: 298–303.

Eger EI II. Ventilation, circulation and uptake. In: *Anaesthetic Uptake and Action*. Baltimore: Williams and Wilkins, 1974; 122–145.

Ellis CH, Wnuck AL, De Beer EJ, Foldes FF. Modifying actions of procaine on the myoneural blocking properties of succinylcholine, decamethonium and *d*-tubocurarine in dogs and cats. *American Journal of Physiology* 1953; **174**: 277–282.

Ellis GP. The Maillard Reaction. *Advances in Carbohydrate Chemistry* 1959; **14**: 63–134.

Enderby GEH. The use and abuse of trichlorethylene. *British Medical Journal* 1944; **ii**: 300–302.

Goldberg LI. Monoamine oxidase inhibitors: adverse reactions and possible mechanisms. *Journal of the American Medical Association* 1964; **190**: 456–462.

Grayson JG. Incompatibilities of multiple additives to intravenous infusion fluids. *Pharmaceutical Journal* 1971; **206**: 64–71.

Greenblatt DJ, Abernethy DR, Morse DS *et al*. Clinical importance of the interaction of diazepam and cimetidine. *New England Journal of Medicine* 1984; **319**: 1639–1643.

Grogono AW. Drug interactions in anaesthesia. *British Journal of Anaesthesia* 1974; **46**: 613–618.

Hart AP, Royster RL, Johnston WE. Cardiac conduction interactions of propranolol and verapamil with halothane in pentobarbitone anaesthetised dogs. *British Journal of Anaesthesia* 1988; **61**: 748–753.

Humphrey JH. McClelland M. Cranial nerve palsies with herpes following general anaesthesia. *British Medical Journal* 1944; **1**: 315–316.

Iversen LL. The inhibition of noradrenaline uptake by drugs. *Advances in Drug Research* 1965; **2**; 5–23.

Johnston RR, Eger EI II, Wilson C. A comparative interaction of epinephrine with enflurane, isoflurane and halothane in man. *Anesthesia and Analgesia* 1976; **55**: 709–712.

Johnstone M, Nisbet HIA. Ventricular arrhythmia during halothane anaesthesia. *British Journal of Anaesthesia* 1961; **33**: 9–16.

Karis JH, Gissen AJ, Nastuk WL. The effect of volatile agents on neuromuscular transmission. *Anaesthesiology* 1967; **28**: 128–134.

Katz RL, Katz GJ. Surgical infiltration of pressor drugs and their interaction with volatile anaesthetics. *British Journal of Anaesthesia* 1966; **38**: 712–718.

Koch-Weser J, Sellers EM. Drug interactions with coumarin anticoagulants. *New England Journal of Medicine* 1972; **285**: 487–498, 547–558.

Lynch C. Differential depression of myocardial contractility by halothane and isoflurane *in vitro*. *Anesthesiology* 1986; **64**: 620–631.

Macphee GIA, McInnes GT, Thompson GG. Verapamil potentiates carbamazepine neurotoxicity: a clinically important inhibitor interaction. *Lancet* 1986; **i**: 700–703.

Maze M, Mason DM. Verapamil decreases the MAC for halothane in dogs. *Anesthesia and Analgesia* 1983; **62**: 274.

Mazze RI. Fluorinated anaesthetic nephrotoxicity: an update. *Canadian Anaesthetists Society Journal* 1984; **31**: S16–22.

Merin M, Calcium channel blocking drugs and anaesthetics: is the drug interaction beneficial or detrimental? *Anesthesiology* 1987; **66**: 1111–1113.

Mishra P, Calvey TN, Williams NE. Intraoperative bradycardia associated with timolol and pilocarpine eye-drops. *British Journal of Anaesthesia* 1983; **55**: 897–899.

Nies AS, Shand DG, Wilkinson GR. Altered hepatic blood flow and drug disposition. *Clinical Pharmacokinetics* 1976; **1**: 135–155.

Pantuck EJ. Ecothiopate iodide eye-drops and prolonged response to suxamethonium. *British Journal of Anaesthesia* 1966; **38**: 406–407.

Perisho JA, Buechel DR, Miller RD. The effect of diazepam on minimal alveolar anaesthetic requirement in man. *Canadian Anaesthetists Society Journal* 1971; **18**: 536–540.

Pessane D, Allemand H, Benoist C *et al*. Effect of surgery under anaesthesia on antipyrine clearance. *British Journal of Clinical Pharmacology* 1978; **6**: 505–514.

Pittinger CB, Eryaza Y, Adamson R. Antibiotic-induced paralysis. *Anesthesia and Analgesia* 1970; **49**: 487–501

Prys-Roberts C, Greene LT, Meloche R, Foex P. Studies of anaesthesia in relation to hypertension II. Haemodynamic consequences of induction and endotracheal intubation. *British Journal of Anaesthesia* 1971; **43**: 531–547.

Riley BB. Incompatibilities in intravenous solutions. *Journal of Hospital Pharmacy* 1970; **28**: 228–240.

Sedman AJ. Cimetidine–drug interactions. *American Journal of Medicine* 1984; **76**: 109–114.

Serlin MJ, Breckenridge AM. Drug interactions with warfarin. *Drugs* 1983; **25**: 610–620.

Smith SE. Neuromuscular blocking drugs in man. In: Zaimis E (ed.) *Handbook of Experimental Pharmacology, Vol. 42, Neuromuscular Junction*. Heidelberg: Springer-Verlag, 1976; 593–660.

Sokoll MD, Gergis SD. Antibiotics and neuromuscular function. *Anesthesiology* 1981; **55**: 148–159.

Soni N. Mechanisms of drug interactions (Appendix III). In: Feldman S, Scurr CF, Paton W (eds) *Drugs in Anaesthesia: Mechanisms of Action*. London: Edward Arnold, 1987; 408–427.

Stack CG, Rogers P, Linter SP. Monoamine oxidase inhibitors and anaesthesia — a review. *British Journal of Anaesthesia* 1988; **60**: 222–227.

Stanski DR, Ham J, Miller RD *et al*. Pharmacokinetics and pharmacodynamics of *d*-tubocurarine during nitrous oxide–narcotic and halothane anaesthesia in man. *Anesthesiology* 1979; **51**: 235–241.

Stockley I. *Drug Interactions and their Mechanisms*. The Pharmaceutical Press, London. 1974; 1–78.

Stoelting RK, Longnecker DE. Influence of end-tidal halothane concentration on *d*-tubocurarine hypotension. *Anesthesia and Analgesia* 1972; **51**: 364–367.

Todd JG, Nimmo WS. Effect of premedication on drug absorption and gastric emptying time. *British Journal of Anaesthesia* 1983; **55**: 1189–1192.

Trissel LA. *Handbook on Injectable Drugs*, 3rd edn. Bethesda MD; American Society of Hospital Pharmacists, 1983.

Welling PG. Interactions affecting drug absorption. *Clinical Pharmacokinetics* 1984; **9**: 404–434.

Williams JS, Broadbent MP, Pearce AC, Jones RM. Verapamil potentiates the neuromuscular blocking effects of enflurane *in vitro*. *Anesthesiology* 1983; **59**: A276.

Zaimis E. The neuromuscular junction — areas of uncertainty. In: Zaimis E (ed.) *Handbook of Experimental Pharmacology*, *Vol. 42*, *Neuromuscular Junction*. Heidelberg: Springer-Verlag, 1976; 1–21.

Zink J, Sasyniuk BI, Dresel PE. Halothane–epinephrine-induced cardiac arrhythmias and the role of heart rate. *Anesthesiology* 1975; **43**: 548–555.

Zsigmond EK, Robins G. The effects of a series of anti-cancer drugs on plasma cholinesterase activity. *Canadian Anaesthetists Society Journal* 1972; **19**: 75–82.

FIVE

Variability in Drug Response

It has long been recognized and acknowledged that individual patients show a wide variability in response to the same drug or treatment modality. Drug effects are never identical in all patients, nor even in an individual patient on different occasions. A dose–response curve only applies to a single patient or reflects an average value. Using the logarithmic scale, a sigmoid dose–response curve can be plotted and illustrated to show four variables (Fig. 5.1). The vertical arrows illustrate that a range of effects may be observed in a group of patients after the same dose of drug is administered, whilst the horizontal arrows indicate that a range of doses may be required to produce a specific intensity of effect in all individuals.

When the dose requirements of a population sample (say 100) to produce a specific pharmacological effect have been elicited, the geometric mean (average log-dose), median (statistic of central tendency dividing the sample into two equally sized groups) and mode (the most commonly occurring value) can be calculated. These values in most cases are nearly coincident. The results can be plotted as a histogram, and a Gaussian distribution (normal) curve having the same mean and standard deviation as the sample imposed upon the data (Fig. 5.2). Correlation with these values or with the slope of the curve plotted as a cumulative frequency (Fig. 5.3) would suggest that the results reflected those which would be obtained from a much larger group.

The dose of a drug which is required to produce a specific intensity of effect in 50% of individuals is known as the median effective dose (ED_{50}). The median lethal dose (LD_{50}) is determined in laboratory studies and the LD_{50}/ED_{50} ratio gives the therapeutic index of the drug.

Some obvious factors may influence the variability in response to a drug. In most instances, little account is taken of the wide range of differences in body weight when drugs are prescribed, and predictable variations in response to some drugs (e.g. hypnotics and analgesics) may be observed.

Racial differences in drug response are not infrequently described. Whilst in the majority of these cases an underlying genetic cause, usually relating to the way

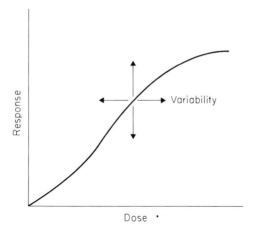

Fig. 5.1 Log-dose–response curve illustrating how variability may occur.

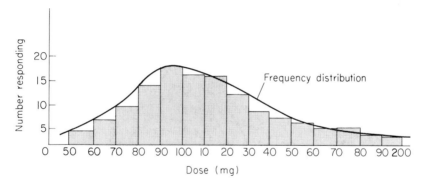

Fig. 5.2 Frequency distribution curve showing dose requirements to produce a quantal response in an experiment performed on 100 subjects.

in which the body handles the drug, has been determined, this is not always true. For example, patients of Chinese descent exhibit enhanced pharmacological effects to propranolol even though the rate of clearance is increased as compared with the Caucasian population. Similarly, Scandinavians and Chileans exhibit a higher incidence of cholestatic jaundice induced by oral contraceptives. There is also some anecdotal evidence that the effects of thiopentone, the action of which is terminated by distribution factors, is prolonged in Orientals.

A number of studies have suggested that women may be more susceptible than men to adverse drug reactions; particular examples include digoxin toxicity, the development of acute dystonic reactions following the administration of metoclopramide, and blood dyscrasias associated with phenylbutazone or

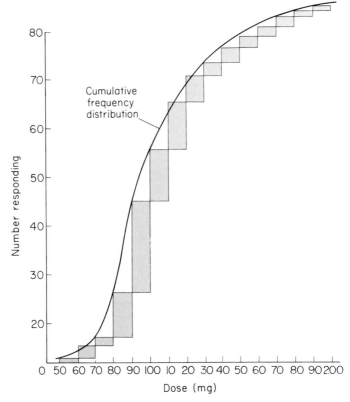

Fig. 5.3 Summated results in Fig. 5.2, expressed as a cumulative frequency distribution.

chloramphenicol. The underlying mechanisms that are associated with these observations are unclear.

Differences in bioavailability may be of considerable importance. Bioavailability has been defined as the rate and extent to which the therapeutic moiety is absorbed and becomes available at the site of action. This is normally estimated by its concentration in body fluids, rate of excretion and acute pharmacological effects. The concept of bioavailability is usually related in practice to drugs given by the oral route. The area under the plasma concentration versus time curve (AUC) between zero time and infinity is measured and compared with the AUC after i.v. administration (which assumes 100% bioavailability), thus:

$$\text{Absolute (oral) bioavailability (\%)} = \frac{\text{AUC following oral administration}}{\text{AUC following i.v. administration}} \times 100.$$

Comparison of oral formulations of the same drug may reveal differences in bioavailability which may reflect statistically significant differences (bioinequivalence), or clinically significant differences (therapeutic inequivalence). Differ-

Table 5.1 Principal factors associated with variability to drug response.

Physiological
   Age
   Pregnancy
   'Social' drugs (tobacco and alcohol)

Pharmacological
   Idiosyncracy
   Supersensitivity
   Tachyphylaxis and tolerance
   Hypersensitivity

Pathological
   Hepatic
   Renal
   Cardiovascular } disease
   Respiratory
   Neurological

ences in bioavailability are only likely to be of consequence for drugs with a steep dose–response curve (e.g. digoxin, phenytoin, cytotoxic agents) or with a narrow therapeutic index.

Clinical complications relating to variable responses to drugs which have been administered are not uncommon. While these are by no means always predictable, a further understanding of the problem may be gained by considering the possible mechanisms involved. These are summarized in Table 5.1

PHYSIOLOGICAL VARIABILITY

Considerable variations in response to drugs may occur at extremes of age.

Children

There are marked differences in the way that children and adults assimilate drugs. In the neonatal period absorption of drugs is slower because of longer gastric emptying and increased intestinal transit time, although more of the drug may be absorbed because of the greater time in contact with the mucosa. The gastric contents are less acidic and consequently some drugs (e.g. benzylpenicillin, ampicillin) will have greater overall absorption when swallowed. The vasomotor instability observed in the newborn period may result in unreliable absorption of drugs administered, by subcutaneous or intramuscular injection, at tissue sites.

The distribution process is influenced by a number of factors including tissue mass, fat content, blood flow, membrane permeability, and the degree of protein binding. Total body water as a percentage of body weight falls from 87% in the preterm baby to 73% at 3 months and 55% in the adult. Thus doses of water-soluble drugs calculated by scaling down adult doses in proportion to body weight can result in lower tissue concentrations. However, distribution will also be affected by the lower body fat content and by the increased permeability of the blood–brain barrier in the neonate; non-polar drugs may thus achieve relatively higher concentrations in the CNS. Furthermore, decreased plasma protein levels in the newborn will result in more unbound drug being available for both pharmacological activity and biotransformation. The lower plasma pH found in the neonate will influence the degree of ionization and subsequent membrane permeability of both acidic and basic drugs.

The rate of drug metabolism depends both on the size of the liver and the activity of the microsomal enzyme system. Enzyme activity is immature in the early newborn period until different enzyme pathways have been induced. In older children enzyme activity is similar to that of adults and (probably because of the greater liver volume) relatively faster rates of metabolism of most drugs are found.

Glomerular filtration rates comparable to those seen in the adult are achieved at about 4 months of age. In the neonatal period they are only 20–40% of adult rates, and drugs which are removed from the body by glomerular filtration (e.g. digoxin and gentamicin) are eliminated at relatively slow rates. These kinetic differences may have significant practical implications:

Neonates

In the neonate, weight-related doses of water-soluble, polar compounds (e.g. most antibiotics) produce lower tissue concentrations and thus a decreased pharmacological effect. Dose regimes which relate to body surface area are required to produce similar blood levels. However, the increased volume of distribution (V) and the decreased renal clearance (CL) will result in an increase in the elimination half-life ($t_{\frac{1}{2}\beta}$), thus dose intervals should be prolonged.

Conversely, the enhanced pharmacological effects of drugs which act on the CNS observed in neonates following their administration in labour (e.g. morphine, diazepam) is undoubtedly a result of an increased fraction of unbound drug, greater CNS permeability because of an immature blood–brain barrier and a delay in biotransformation.

For many years, neonates were regarded as being highly sensitive to the effects of competitive neuromuscular blocking agents, particularly in the first 10 days of life, whilst resistant to depolarizing agents. Such observations cannot be explained in terms of differences of body water volume which should make neonates resistant to all types of muscle relaxants. Electromyographic recordings suggested a qualitative difference, resembling that of myasthenia, at the postsynaptic membrane.

More recent studies have not confirmed these original observations. When tubocurarine is administered, neonates will exhibit equivalent neuromuscular depression to that seen in older children and adults at significantly lower plasma levels of the drug. Nevertheless, the greatly enhanced volume of distribution (V) of the muscle relaxant in the neonate in relative terms indicates that the initial dose requirements (in terms of body weight) are similar. However, the elimination half-life ($t_\frac{1}{2}$) of tubocurarine will be proportionally longer, and thus the interval between incremental doses should be greater. Similar studies using an atracurium infusion indicate that dose requirements in the neonate (in proportion to body weight) do not differ greatly from those at other ages. Any variations may be attributed to lower body temperatures in the newborn and subsequent effects on drug distribution.

Abnormal responses to the effects of opiates may be observed in the neonate. Experimental studies in newborn animals have demonstrated a relative insensitivity to morphine analgesia and a marked sensitivity to its respiratory depressant effects. It has been suggested that this may be due to a differing distribution of the two subtypes of μ receptors in the neonatal period.

Older children

In older children when protein binding characteristics, microsomal enzyme activity, renal function and the efficiency of the blood–brain barrier have reached adult proportions, differences in drug disposition are less likely. However, drug dosage is again best tailored to body surface area (because of the proportional increase in body water), while more frequent rates of administration, especially of the less polar compounds, may be necessary because of the relatively increased liver blood flow. Differences in pharmacodynamic activity are less easy to determine.

The elderly

There is a clinical impression that elderly patients often respond differently to standard adult doses of drugs and that they are more likely than the young to react adversely to drugs prescribed in hospital.

Failing memory, confusion and poor eyesight make compliance worse. However, after appropriate oral intake drug absorption is not appreciably altered, except for those substances which rely on active transport mechanisms (e.g. iron, thiamine and calcium).

In contrast to the neonate, total body water in proportion to body weight is reduced whilst there is a relative increase in body fat. Accordingly, the volume of distribution of water-soluble drugs will be reduced and tissue concentrations thus effectively increased. Albumin levels tend to fall with age, and the free fractions of certain drugs (e.g. phenytoin, phenylbutazone, carbenoxolone and tolbuta-mide) will increase, thus enhancing their rate of availability at cellular levels.

At the age of 65, hepatic blood flow is reduced by up to 45% of the rate at 25 years of age, and experimental evidence shows that the activity of the microsomal enzyme system similarly declines. Thus the systemic bioavailability of drugs which are subject to either high or low intrinsic clearance by the liver will be increased, with enhancement of pharmacological action. Similarly, glomerular filtration and tubular secretion will decline with age, making the elderly patient distinctly at risk from drugs with a low therapeutic index (e.g. digoxin, gentamicin and lithium).

Enhanced effects of drugs used in anaesthetic practice can therefore be anticipated. Dose–response studies have shown that thiopentone dose require-ments diminish with increasing age. Kinetic factors (decreased plasma protein binding, lowered volume of distribution and increased accumulation in fat) undoubtedly contribute. The free (unbound) fraction of pethidine will be four times higher in the elderly than in the young, indicating that the dose of this drug should be reduced in the aged.

There is some evidence that a change in receptor sensitivity may account for

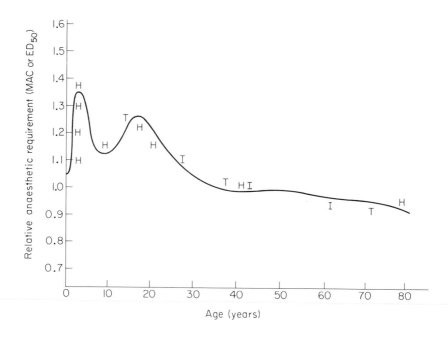

Fig. 5.4 Relative anaesthetic requirement expressed as a multiple of minimum alveolar concentration (MAC) or median effective dose (ED_{50}) for various inhalational and intravenous anaesthetic agents. Requirement normalized for established values for young healthy adults. H = halothane; I = isoflurane; T = thiopentone.

alteration in drug response in the elderly, for example in the increased degree of analgesia observed in elderly patients who have received morphine or pentazocine for the relief of postoperative pain. Altered sensitivity of the elderly to a given concentration of drug at receptor sites has been demonstrated for nitrazepam, warfarin and for β-adrenoceptor antagonists.

Studies at anaesthetic equilibrium such as those which measure minimum alveolar concentration (MAC) for inhalation anaesthetics leave little doubt that anaesthetic requirement is significantly, if not linearly, depressed with advancing age. Comparative data for intravenous induction agents can easily be superimposed graphically on the results of these studies (Fig. 5.4), suggesting that pharmacodynamic factors based upon underlying anatomical, biochemical or functional changes associated with the ageing process itself are primarily responsible.

Pregnancy

The absorption, distribution and elimination of a number of drugs may alter during pregnancy. Delay in gastric emptying will result in an increased rate of uptake of drugs absorbed in the stomach (e.g. diazepam) and a delay in those which are principally absorbed in the upper gastrointestinal tract (e.g. aspirin and paracetamol). Disturbances of gastrointestinal motility during pregnancy have been related to changes in the relative amounts of gastric acid and mucus secretion; the effects of increased progesterone levels have also been implicated.

The placenta contains a wide range of enzymes that are concerned with the metabolism of some neurotransmitters and other endogenous compounds. The decreased sensitivity to insulin which occurs in pregnancy is thought to be due to a placental lactogen (insulinase), a growth hormone-like substance. Other enzymes whose levels of activity in serum are increased in pregnancy include alkaline phosphatase and β-glucuronidase, which is secreted into the small intestine and hydrolyses glucuronide conjugates excreted in the bile. It is thus possible that the effects of some drugs (e.g. analgesics and antibiotics) may be potentiated in pregnancy due to increased enterohepatic shunting.

Plasma volume and cardiac output are both increased during pregnancy (by 50% and 30% respectively, with maximum values achieved at 30–34 weeks gestation). Clearance of many drugs (e.g. phenytoin) may be enhanced in pregnancy due to increased cardiac output and subsequent increases in hepatic and renal blood flow. The increase in cardiac output, associated with a degree of hyperventilation which normally occurs during pregnancy, will enhance both the rate of uptake and subsequent elimination of inhalational anaesthetic agents.

Conversely, the elimination half-life of theophylline has been shown to be prolonged during pregnancy, while the clearance rate remains unaffected. The resultant increase in the volume of distribution appears to be associated with decreased plasma protein binding. It has been shown that the binding of a number of drugs to albumin and globulins (e.g. diazepam, pethidine, and propranolol) is decreased during pregnancy, particularly during the last trimester. It is suggested that exogenous substances may interfere with drug binding. The pharmacokinetics of thiopentone in pregnant patients undergoing caesarean section has been studied. Plasma protein binding and clearance were not markedly altered, but the elimination half-life of thiopentone increased significantly, due to a larger volume of distribution at steady state.

Smoking

Cigarette smoking results in the induction of microsomal enzyme systems. The mean rates of elimination of drugs that are metabolized by this pathway are generally greater in smokers than in non-smokers, but there is a considerable overlap. The rates of metabolism of antipyrine, theophylline, imipramine and pentazocine would appear to be increased, whilst drugs such as diazepam, pethidine and warfarin are not significantly affected.

Clinical studies have shown that smokers may require more opioids to obtain relief from pain, may be less sedated by benzodiazepines and may obtain less antianginal effects from certain β-blockers and nifedipine. It is known that not all these differences arise from altered rates of drug metabolism, although the exact mechanism is unclear.

Alcohol

Chronic use of alcohol results in an increased capacity to metabolize alcohol. At the same time pharmacodynamic tolerance occurs, so that higher blood concentrations of alcohol are necessary to produce intoxication in tolerant than in normal individuals. Cross-resistance between a variety of sedative drugs, including the benzodiazepines, is known to occur, and is considered to result from both pharmacodynamic (CNS) tolerance and from more rapid metabolism. The resistance to thiopentone which is frequently encountered in chronic alcoholics is undoubtedly due to tolerance at a cellular level, as the duration of action of this induction agent is primarily determined by redistribution and not metabolism.

A change in the availability of γ-aminobutyric acid (GABA) with alteration in the receptor population for this neurotransmitter has been postulated. Similar concepts may also apply to the studies of reported tolerance of alcoholics to inhalational agents, although these do not take into account the state of agitation of the patient who may be on the edge of withdrawal symptoms.

It must be emphasized that the previous remarks only apply to patients in whom prolonged prior exposure to alcohol has occurred. Following acute ingestion of alcohol, the administration of other CNS depressants will lead to supra-additive effects. The half-life of barbiturates will also be increased, presumably due to competition with alcohol for microsomal enzymes.

PHARMACOLOGICAL VARIABILITY

Idiosyncracy

Idiosyncracy is correctly defined as a genetically determined abnormal reactivity to a drug. This may present in the form of extreme sensitivity to low doses, or marked insensitivity to high doses of the agent.

The term has also been used empirically to describe marked side-effects (e.g. dysphoria, nausea, vomiting and other gastrointestinal tract disturbances) which occur in patients who receive certain drugs (e.g. opiates and NSAIDs); these side-effects often disappear when closely related compounds are substituted. The underlying mechanisms are unclear, but may involve hypersensitivity responses.

Examples of genetically determined variability include:

1   The increased susceptibility to the haemolytic effects of certain drugs (e.g. antimalarial agents, sulphonamides, and NSAIDs) observed in those ethnic groups who exhibit a quantitative deficiency of glucose-6-phosphate dehydrogenase (6-GPD). Lack of this enzyme delays the regeneration of NADPH, which protects the erythrocyte from the injurious effects of oxidative drugs.

2   The prolonged activity of suxamethonium which may occur due to the presence of genetic variants of plasma cholinesterase. Polymorphism is displayed and four separate alleles for the enzyme occur at one locus. Ten genotypes, which exhibit a wide range of differing enzyme activity, will result. The topic is discussed more fully in Chapter 9.

3   A bimodal distribution in the rate of acetylation of isoniazid, as the metabolizing enzyme (*N*-acetyltransferase) also exhibits genetic polymorphism. Other drugs (e.g. hydralazine, phenelzine and certain sulphonamides) may be similarly affected, and toxic effects more usually occur in the 'slow' acetylators.

4   Hereditary resistance to oral anticoagulants has been detected in animals and man, and appears to be an autosomal dominant trait. The mechanism of action is obscure. One hypothesis is that a suppressor substance manufactured by mutant subjects has an altered reactivity with either vitamin K, the antagonists, or both. Alternatively, it has been suggested that the enzyme diaphorase (epoxide reductase), which reduces vitamin K to its active form, develops resistance to the oral anticoagulant.

5   The development of the rare but potentially fatal complication of anaesthesia, malignant hyperpyrexia. A strong family susceptibility to the disorder is apparent. A similar abnormality can be induced in some strains of the Landrace pig. An impaired ability of the sarcoplasmic reticulum to bind calcium, particularly in the presence of halothane, may be the primary, genetically determined, abnormality.

6   Attacks of acute hepatic porphyria (acute intermittent porphyria, variegate porphyria and hereditary porphyria) are commonly precipitated by drugs in susceptible individuals. Those agents commonly implicated are known inducers of the enzyme δ-aminolaevulinic acid (ALA) synthetase and their administration will lead to increased production and urinary excretion of the porphyrin derivatives of ALA and porphobilinogen (see also Chapter 6). Drug-induced porphyria is associated with the use of barbiturates, phenytoin, dichloralphenazone, alcohol, oral contraceptives and certain other steroid compounds, griseofulvin, sulphonamides, and sulphonylureas.

7   Other genetically determined disorders associated with drug administration include defective debrisoquine oxidation, where exaggerated hypotension after normal oral dosage will occur, the rise in intraocular pressure which may be detected in some patients following the long-term administration of steroid eye-drops and the intense facial flushing which is induced by alcohol in a significant number of patients receiving chlorpropamide.

Inherited characteristics which also appear to be linked to specific adverse reactions include HLA (human lymphocyte antigen) serotypes and toxic reactions to gold, levamisole and procainamide. The incidence of digoxin toxicity and of thromboembolism caused by oral contraceptives has also been linked to differences in ABO blood groups.

The term pharmacogenetics was originally introduced to describe the study of genetically determined variations that are initially revealed by the effects of drugs, but the term now usually involves the wider field of genetic determinants of drug action.

Temporal variability

Supersensitivity

Receptors are not only the determinants of acute regulation of physiological and biochemical function but are themselves subject to regulatory and homeostatic control. Continued stimulation of cells with an agonist appears to lead to a qualitative or quantitative diminution in receptor activity, and is exemplified by the refractory response which follows the repeated administration of β-adrenoceptor agonists in the treatment of bronchial asthma.

Conversely, a hyperreactivity to receptor agonists may be observed following a reduction in the chronic level of receptor stimulation. In such cases, supersensitivity may result from the synthesis of additional receptors. This phenomenon can explain the rebound effects which result from the sudden withdrawal of certain antihypertensive drugs (e.g. β-adrenoceptor antagonists, clonidine, minoxidil) following their long-term administration, and may account for the production of tardive dyskinesia by phenothiazines and potentiation of this side-effect by dopamine precursors. The exaggerated response to the administration of a vasopressor by patients receiving adrenergic neurone-blocking agents and the increased hyperkalaemia which occurs following the administration of suxamethonium to patients with severe burns or following spinal cord injuries are other manifestations of a variable response which is probably due to an 'up regulation' of receptors.

Tachyphylaxis and tolerance

In some instances, the repeated administration of the same dose of a drug will lead to a diminishing effect. Tachyphylaxis implies a fairly rapid diminution in responses, while tolerance usually describes a more gradual decrease in the activity of the drug concerned.

A number of mechanisms may be involved:

1 A slow rate of dissociation of the drug from its receptor, so that receptor occupancy remains high when a second dose of the drug is given; this is a possible explanation of the 'tachyphylaxis' sometimes observed during repeated administration of suxamethonium.

2 'Exhaustion' of endogenous transmitter availability which has been stimulated by exogenous agents; for instance noradrenaline stores following the administration of indirectly acting sympathomimetic amines (e.g. ephedrine and amphetamines), or dopamine stores following the use of amantadine, will be depleted and eventually lead to a reduced therapeutic effect.

3 Tolerance due to 'down regulation' of receptors has previously been mentioned with regard to sympathomimetic agonists. The tolerance (and subsequent dependence) which develops with the repeated use of hypnotics and narcotic analgesics may also relate to a quantitative or qualitative diminution of CNS receptors. However, in the case of narcotic drugs, in which experimental studies have shown that tolerance can develop within a matter of a few hours, a negative 'feedback' system involving endogenous opiates (enkephalins, endorphins) has also been postulated.

4 Tolerance also develops to the haemodynamic and anti-ischaemic effects of organic nitrates during continuous administration. One aspect of this phenomenon is the development of tolerance to the side-effects of nitrates which has been observed in individuals exposed to nitroglycerine in the manufacture of explosives. Workers in this industry experience headaches and dizziness on first exposure during their initial period of employment. These symptoms rapidly abate, but may reappear following a few days absence from work. Similarly, the use of intermittent regimes of drug therapy avoids the development of attenuation to their therapeutic effects, although it may expose the patient to further risk of anginal episodes during the nitrate-free period.

The underlying mechanism responsible for this effect has recently been clarified. Organic nitrates are lipid-soluble compounds which readily penetrate smooth muscle cells. They are metabolized intracellularly to nitric oxide, which combines with sulphydryl groups to form reactive intermediates (*S*-nitrosothiols). These compounds activate soluble guanylate cyclase, which converts GTP to cyclic GMP (cGMP); this in turn activates protein kinases, causing relaxation of vascular smooth muscle (Chapter 14). Tolerance may be due to the depletion of sulphydryl groups from vascular smooth muscle; this prevents the formation of *S*-nitrosothiols from nitric oxide. In some studies, the administration of sulphydryl donors such as *N*-acetylcysteine can delay or prevent tolerance to nitrates.

5   Increased drug metabolism due to auto-induction of microsomal enzymes (e.g. barbiturates, phenytoin, chlorpromazine).

This topic is also discussed in Chapter 3.

HYPERSENSITIVITY

Approximately 10% of adverse reactions to drugs result from immunological mechanisms and associated humoral responses. Most drugs are of low molecular weight and act as haptens to form fairly stable complexes involving conjugation with lysyl side-chains of tissue proteins.

Hypersensitivity reactions have been grouped into four main types, according to the disposition of the participating antigen and antibody.

Type 1

Anaphylactic reactions (immediate hypersensitivity)

These occur when the antigen has stimulated the production of reaginic antibody (IgE in man) which becomes fixed to circulating basophils and mast cells in tissues. Subsequent re-exposure to the antigen leads to cytoplasmic disruption of the cellular component of the antibody with the release of histamine, heparin, 5-hydroxytryptamine, slow-reacting substance of anaphylaxis and anaphylatoxin. It is considered that, for this reaction to occur, adjacently bound IgE molecules must become cross-linked by binding to the specific antigen. Thus Type 1 hypersensitivity should only be observed with those drugs which:

1   Form multivalent drug–carrier conjugates; or

2   Are inherently divalent because they have identical structural features in different regions of the molecule (e.g. most neuromuscular blocking agents)

Anaphylactic shock manifests as severe hypotension due to profound peripheral vasodilatation with peripheral 'pooling' and as bronchiolar constriction. Type 1 hypersensitivity responses are not uncommon with certain drugs (e.g. penicillin, sulphonamides, and salicylates) and many follow insect stings and the ingestion of certain food proteins. In some instances an exaggerated 'triple response' to histamine may result, the presenting sign being generalized urticaria or angioneurotic oedema.

An alternative mechanism for the production of hypersensitivity responses by salicylates and other NSAIDs has also been proposed. Inhibition of cyclo-oxygenase by this group of drugs may allow more arachidonic acid to be available for conversion by lipo-oxygenase. The end products of this enzymatic reaction are the leukotrienes which have been identified as the slow-reacting substance of anaphylaxis. Leukotrienes, along with chemotactic factors released from eosinophils and neutrophils (plus a platelet-activating factor), appear to be important mediators of attacks of bronchospasm which occur secondary to airway inflammation.

Type 2

Cytolytic reactions

Cytolytic reactions depend upon the reaction of circulating antibodies (IgG or IgM) with an antigen associated with a cell membrane. Formation of the antigen–antibody complex is followed by complement fixation and subsequent lysis of the cell. Incompatible blood transfusion is a classical Type 2 reaction, and this is also the mechanism of drug-induced depression of haemopoietic function, such as haemolytic anaemia, thrombocytopaenia or agranulocytosis which is associated with a variety of drugs (e.g. phenothiazines, phenylbutazone, and antithyroid agents).

Type 3

Immune complex mediated sensitivity

Immune complex mediated sensitivity results from the formation of a precipitin complex by the reaction of circulating antibodies with soluble antigens such as bacterial toxins. Normally, precipitin is removed by the reticulo-endothelial system, but when excess antigen is present, the complex formed may be deposited in the endothelial lining of small blood vessels, the glomerular membrane and the connective tissue of joints. Type 3 reactions form the basis of certain systemic diseases, such as acute glomerulonephritis, polyarteritis nodosa and rheumatoid arthritis. A localized type of inflammatory response which can occur 4–8 h after the administration of a drug or toxoid (Arthus phenomenon) is an example of Type 3 hypersensitivity. Similarly, injection of a large dose of antigen which remains in the circulation may produce serum sickness after 7–14 days. This is manifested by an urticarial rash, joint stiffness and swelling, albuminuria, and pyrexia, and may follow the administration of penicillin or sulphonamides. This phenomenon does not require previous exposure to the drug, but rather depends upon the continuous production of antibodies, notably IgG.

Type 4

Cell-mediated (delayed) hypersensitivity responses

These result from the combination of antigen with T-cell (killer) lymphocytes. The subsequent release of lymph node permeability factor, which promotes vascular leakage, results in erythema and induration due to accumulation of macrophages and lymphocytes at the site of injection; blistering and exfoliation will ensue. This response is typified by the Mantoux reaction and by certain forms of contact dermatitis, and may include the skin manifestations which sometimes occur after prolonged contact with local anaesthetic esters.

Anaphylactoid reactions

Anaphylactoid responses occur through a direct or non-immune mechanism, and may result from the release of vasoactive substances by circulating basophils following the intravenous administration of certain drugs. Various agents have been incriminated including intravenous induction agents, neuromuscular and ganglion-blocking compounds, certain contrast media and colloid infusions. Clinical reports suggest that such reactions are directly related to the dosage and rate of injection of the offending agent and that the effects are often transient. It has also been suggested that anaphylactoid reactions may occur when different drugs are administered into small infusion needles. Physicochemical combination may result in the production of colloid aggregates which could eventually be taken up at pulmonary sites; more serious sequelae may then be predicted.

Local evidence of histamine release is commonly observed after the intravenous administration of many narcotic analgesics and neuromuscular blocking agents. A similar disruptive effect on mast cells in the vessel walls is postulated; such an effect is unlikely to be of any clinical consequence.

Both Type 2 and Type 3 responses involve fixation of complement and activation of the complement cascade (C3 → C9), leading to opsonization of cellular debris and subsequent augmentation of the inflammatory response. A significant reduction in classical pathway activity has been demonstrated in patients undergoing anaesthesia and surgery (Fig. 5.5).

C3 function is particularly diminished, and its conversion to C3a and C3b with the subsequent release of C5a ('the alternate pathway') was principally associated with the use of two intravenous induction agents which have now been withdrawn (propanidid and Althesin). The ensuing release of histamine and other vasoactive peptides may lead to an effect not dissimilar to a Type 1 reaction but occurring

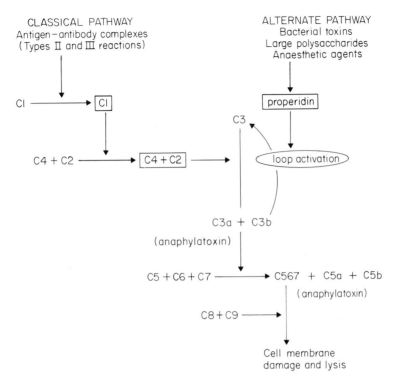

Fig. 5.5 Routes of activation of classical and alternate complement pathways. ⬜▭ indicate activated factors.

without previous exposure to the drug. The incriminating factor was undoubtedly Cremophor-EL, the solubilizing agent used with both drugs. Large polysaccharide molecules are also considered to activate the 'alternate' pathway and it is postulated that anaphylactoid responses occasionally observed following the administration of large molecular weight dextrans, hydroxyethyl starch and possibly heparin may result from a similar mechanism.

Hypersensitivity responses associated with anaesthesia

Such responses are not infrequent and occasionally result in a life-threatening problem. In many instances, commonly used drugs such as thiopentone, suxamethonium, alcuronium and morphine are involved and colloid infusions may have been administered. It can be particularly difficult to detect patients who are at risk from such responses, although those with a history of atopy (asthma, hay fever or eczema) or with a previous or family history of adverse reaction must be considered as vulnerable. It has been suggested that relatively 'safe' drugs in this context are etomidate, pancuronium, fentanyl and the amide group of local anaesthetic agents. Pretreatment with both H_1- and H_2- receptor antagonists (e.g. chlorpheniramine and cimetidine) may also confer considerable protection in this context.

It must be stated that not all the adverse responses to drugs that may occur in 'normal' individuals can be considered to be due to immunological mechanisms or to underlying genetic disorders. In some cases, the adverse responses observed are an extension of the pharmacological effects of the agent, or may reflect intrinsic toxicity which is primarily dependent on the chemical properties of the drug or its reactive metabolites. Such effects are dose dependent and can usually be reproduced in animals. Adverse responses of this type are becoming less of a problem because of an increased understanding of the structural features of drugs which contribute to their intrinsic toxicity and because such toxicities are frequently uncovered in preclinical trials.

Halothane 'hypersensitivity'

Much controversy has reigned over the last three decades with regard to the small number of patients who develop postoperative jaundice following halothane anaesthesia. The possible mechanisms involved may be summarized as:

1   *A coincidental effect*

In a number of these cases there was undoubtedly another cause for the hepatic dysfunction. Coexistent viral hepatitis, surgical trauma involving the common bile duct, haemolytic effects associated with massive transfusion and jaundice induced by other drugs have all been implicated.

2   *An intrinsic toxic effect*

A direct, non-immunologically mediated toxic effect on liver parenchymal cells may occur, due to halothane itself or more likely to one of its reductive metabolites. In these circumstances, jaundice would appear to be more prone to develop in those patients who: (a) receive repeated anaesthetics involving halothane; (b) are more liable to accumulate metabolites (e.g. those undergoing prolonged surgical procedures and obese subjects); and (c) are concurrently taking enzyme-inducing agents (e.g. barbiturates and alcohol) which will enhance the availability of metabolites.

In these instances, jaundice usually develops within 24 h of exposure to halothane, and the ensuing clinical manifestations are normally of a relatively mild nature.

3 *A true hypersensitivity response*

Immunochemical studies have demonstrated that sera from the majority of patients who develop halothane hepatitis contain antibodies of the IgG type. These antibodies can be shown to react with halothane–carrier conjugates produced in the liver of animals exposed to halothane and subsequently to mediate hepatocyte damage. An oxidative product of halothane metabolism (a trifluoroacetic acid radical) appears to act as a hapten and combine with microsomal liver proteins to form a neoantigen. A cytolytic (Type 2) response may then be induced by this mechanism; a clinically more severe form of hepatotoxicity may then be anticipated.

Current medicolegal opinion in the UK suggests that halothane should never be administered to patients at intervals of less than 3 months. This is obviously most sensible as regards to the possible development of intrinsic toxic effects of halothane and its reductive metabolites. However, it would appear that the immune-mediated (cytolytic) response can occur after initial exposure to the drug and it is interesting to note that there may be some cross-reactivity with certain metabolites of enflurane.

PATHOLOGICAL VARIABILITY

Liver disease

Liver disease can affect hepatic drug clearance by several mechanisms. There may be alterations in hepatic blood flow (both total flow and degree of intrahepatic shunting), plasma protein binding and intrinsic clearance. Severe liver disorders may also be associated with a reduction in renal blood flow.

Effects on drug disposition are complex and vary according to the type and duration of liver pathology. This is well exemplified by studies on pancuronium kinetics in different types of liver disease. Obstructive disorders lead to a decreased total body clearance of the muscle relaxant, presumably due to decreased elimination of pancuronium and its metabolites in the bile; clinically, a slower recovery from neuromuscular block will occur. When cirrhosis predominates, the increased volume of distribution, associated with changes in plasma binding, will result in a lower plasma concentration initially and thus a decreased rate of uptake at receptor sites. This apparent 'resistance' to the effects of the drug would correlate with original observations when *d*-tubocurarine was used in the presence of liver disease.

In chronic hepatic dysfunction a decreased thiopentone dose requirement to produce hypnosis, and a longer duration of effect has been observed. As the pharmacological effects of thiopentone are primarily determined by distribution, such findings would correlate with decreased protein binding of the drug, i.e. an increased fraction available to cross the blood–brain barrier associated with an increased distribution (and therefore redistribution) half-life.

General anaesthesia will undoubtedly influence hepatic clearance due to alterations in cardiac output and redistribution of regional blood flow. Splanchnic perfusion is invariably decreased and elimination of drugs with a high hepatic clearance (e.g. narcotic analgesics and β-adrenoceptor antagonists) will be reduced. The problem can be accentuated if there is pre-existing liver disease.

Renal disease

For most drugs, renal clearance is proportional to the glomerular filtration rate, of which the creatinine clearance provides a reliable index. Tubular processes of secretion and reabsorption are also proportional to the efficiency of the glomerular filtration process; thus renal efficiency is directly related to the number of functioning nephrons.

Most drugs and their metabolites are excreted partially or wholly by the kidneys. Enhanced and prolonged responses to many drugs, with increased toxicity due to the accumulation of metabolites, is thus predictable in renal failure. Nomograms for the adjustment of drug dosage have been developed, using creatinine clearance as a measure of renal function. Elimination of acidic drugs (e.g. penicillin, NSAIDs) may be further complicated by the accumulation in renal failure of fixed organic acids which compete for active tubular transport processes.

Alterations in protein binding may also occur in renal failure. It has been demonstrated that the binding of acidic drugs (which are normally bound to albumin) is generally decreased in plasma from uraemic patients. Basic drugs exhibit a more variable response, although an increase in the free fraction of some drugs (diazepam, morphine and chloramphenicol) has been shown. Endogenous binding inhibitors which accumulate in renal failure may be involved.

It is generally considered that dosage requirements of thiopentone are reduced in renal failure. It is unclear whether this is due to an increase in the free (unbound) fraction of the drug, an altered permeability of the blood–brain barrier, or to abnormal cerebral metabolism.

Renal clearance is the mode of removal of narcotic analgesics and their metabolites. Dose requirements are reduced in renal failure and the accumulation of active metabolites (e.g. glucuronide conjugates of morphine) and toxic metabolites (e.g. norpethidine) may be predicted. Fentanyl undergoes rapid and extensive hepatic metabolism. However, no activity or toxicity has been demonstrated in the metabolites, and fentanyl may thus have some advantages over other narcotic analgesics in this context.

Renal failure can have a profound effect on the pharmacokinetics of muscle relaxants. Apparent 'resistance' to the onset of neuromuscular blockade is sometimes observed clinically, and this may be related to altered distribution factors associated with changes in plasma protein binding. Renal elimination accounts for 40–50% of the clearance of pancuronium and *d*-tubocurarine, and 70–100% of the clearance of gallamine and will diminish proportionally with the decline in renal function. Tubocurarine may have some advantages in this context; when the renal route for elimination of this muscle relaxant is removed, a higher drug concentration in the liver results in a greater amount (12–40%) being excreted in the bile. Reparalysis due to the loss of effect of anticholinesterases is unlikely to occur in patients with renal failure, because the clearance and elimination half-life of cholinesterase inhibitors change in parallel with those values for competitive neuromuscular blocking agents.

The pharmacokinetic properties of atracurium are unaffected by renal failure because of endogenous metabolism due to Hoffman elimination. The duration of action of single and repeated doses is not prolonged.

Variability in response to suxamethonium in renal disease will only occur if there is concomitant hyperkalaemia. The duration of action of local anaesthetic blockade appears to be reduced in renal failure, possibly because drug removal from the site of action is facilitated by an associated increase in cardiac output. The elimination half-life of diazepam is actually reduced in chronic renal failure (from approximately 97 to 37 h). Less protein binding occurs, but the volume of distribution of the unbound fraction of the drug is decreased. The clinical significance of this is unclear. The elimination of active metabolites, such as nordiazepam and temazepam, is likely to be decreased and the sedative effect prolonged.

Respiratory disease

A variable response to a number of drugs used in anaesthesia and in other situations may be anticipated in patients with chronic respiratory disorders. In chronic obstructive airways disease (COAD), the respiratory centre may become insensitive to carbon dioxide levels and rely on the hypoxic drive. The respiratory depressant effects of narcotic analgesics and intravenous induction agents may thus be exaggerated. Furthermore, the administration of benzodiazepines in doses used for endoscopy to such patients may cause carbon dioxide narcosis. Acid–base changes and electrolyte imbalance associated with long-standing respiratory disorders may result in variable responses to muscle relaxants. Coexisting bronchospasm may lead to further problems when drugs with potential histamine-releasing properties (e.g. morphine and tubocurarine) or which alter the autonomic 'balance' in the bronchial musculature (e.g. propranolol and neostigmine) are administered.

Ventilation–perfusion abnormalities which occur during anaesthesia are likely to be enhanced with pre-existing respiratory disease. The rate of induction of anaesthesia with poorly soluble agents (e.g. nitrous oxide and cyclopropane) is liable to be delayed, but is usually not affected when more soluble agents such as diethyl ether are used, as compensatory increases in alveolar concentrations of the latter can be attained. When surgical anaethesia is achieved, hypoventilation can be a problem if spontaneous ventilation is maintained. 'Exaggerated' effects on respiratory function occur; the activity of the accessory muscles appears to be abolished at relatively light planes of anaesthesia. Further problems relating to the uptake and elimination of inhalational anaesthetic agents may thus occur.

Cardiac disease

Considerable alteration in the response to a number of drugs which may be administered to patients with pre-existing cardiovascular disease can be anticipated. The systemic disorder may present with one or more differing clinico-pathological patterns, such as congestive cardiac failure, fixed-output cardiac dysfunction, ischaemic heart disease, conduction defects and associated dysrhythmias and arterial hypertension.

Most general anaesthetics that are administered by intravenous or inhalational routes can induce depressant effects on different cardiovascular parameters (e.g. myocardial contractility, systemic vascular resistance, coronary blood flow, baroreceptor reflex activity and circulating catecholamine levels), and such effects may undoubtedly be enhanced in patients with diminished cardiac reserve. The resultant clinical manifestations are complex. In some cases they can be extremely hazardous; for instance, in patients with constrictive pericarditis the myocardial depressant effect of thiopentone can induce profound hypotension and pulmonary oedema. Alternatively, a beneficial effect is sometimes achieved, as demonstrated by the reduction in cardiac work and systemic afterload which occurs when moderate concentrations of halothane are administered to patients with congestive cardiac failure.

More specifically, pronounced differences with regard to distribution and elimination of drugs used in anaesthesia may occur in patients with low cardiac output states. Drugs with significant cardiac muscarinic effects (e.g. suxamethonium and halothane) can lower the sensitivity of the myocardium to circulating catecholamines and pre-existing dysrhythmias may be enhanced. Isoflurane, although a potent coronary vasodilator, may induce maldistribution of myocardial blood flow in the presence of ischaemic heart disease (the 'steal' effect). Exaggerated changes in blood pressure may be observed following the induction of anaesthesia in hypertensive patients. Although such effects are usually more pronounced when the hypertension is untreated, no specific anaesthetic agent has been incriminated and the mechanism of this response remains unclear.

Neurological disease

Many neurological diseases are associated with abnormal responses to muscle relaxants. In those conditions which primarily affect the neuromuscular junction (e.g. myasthenia gravis, Eaton–Lambert syndrome), a markedly increased sensitivity to competitive neuromuscular blocking agents occurs. In these circumstances, the response to depolarizing drugs is variable. Myasthenia gravis is an auto-immune disease in which there is a quantitative reduction in acetylcholine receptors. In untreated cases, apparent 'resistance' occurs following the administration of a single dose of suxamethonium or decamethonium, although there is an increased likelihood of the development of 'dual' block. In those patients who are receiving anticholinesterase therapy, the effect of suxamethonium will be prolonged due to inhibition of enzymatic hydrolysis. In the Eaton–Lambert syndrome, where there appears to be a deficiency of acetylcholine synthesis or release, increased sensitivity to suxamethonium is usually observed. Depolarizing agents are best avoided in diseases affecting the neuromuscular junction.

Dystrophia myotonica is an inherited disorder in which the prime defect is in the muscle fibre itself. A variety of signs and symptoms are usually associated with this condition including mental disturbances, cataracts, testicular atrophy, premature baldness and various endocrine disturbances. The underlying muscle dysfunction results in generalized muscular weakness (including those involved in respiration and deglutition) associated with prolonged contracture of the muscle after stimulation. The latter is particularly noticeable as difficulty in releasing the grip after shaking hands. There is a high incidence of cardiomyopathy with abnormalities of conduction linked with this disorder and this may also reflect the underlying muscle pathology. Prolonged and generalized myotonia has been reported following the administration of suxamethonium. Excessive quantities of potassium may be released from the 'damaged' muscle and enhance any existing dysrhythmia. Depolarizing agents are absolutely contraindicated in this condition. The response to competitive neuromuscular blocking agents is equally unpredictable. The duration of action may be normal or prolonged and reduced doses of these drugs are recommended to be used. Undue sensitivity to the effect of respiratory depressants (e.g. general anaesthetic agents, narcotic analgesics) may also be anticipated, whilst the administration of volatile agents such as halothane is likely to induce cardiotoxic effects.

In a number of neurological diseases in which muscle wasting is a predominant feature (e.g. motor neurone disease, long-standing spinal injuries, the advanced stage of multiple sclerosis), an increased sensitivity to the effects of suxamethonium may be predicted. Degeneration of the motor endplate appears to be followed by an 'up regulation' of receptor activity so that the whole muscle membrane will respond to the effects of an agonist. A greatly augmented potassium efflux may result with the likelihood of dysrhythmias or cardiac arrest ensuing. In some other neurological diseases (e.g. muscular dystrophies, Friedreich's ataxia and Huntington's chorea) unpredictable responses to both depolarizing and competitive agents have been reported. In Duchenne's progressive muscular dystrophy, hazards associated with induction and recovery have been reported; these are likely to be due to the associated cardiomyopathy. Furthermore, the development of a hyperpyrexia-like response has been associated with the use of suxamethonium.

In those neurological disorders which involve autonomic disturbances (e.g. diabetic autonomic neuropathy, acute polyneuritis, Shy–Drager syndrome) enhanced falls in arterial blood pressure can be predicted following the administration of most general anaesthetic agents or other drugs with significant cardiovascular effects (e.g. phenothiazines and tubocurarine). This is undoubtedly due to the inadequacy of compensatory baroreceptor mechanisms.

Endocrine disease

There have been suggestions that an increased response to drugs acting on the CNS, including narcotic analgesics and various general anaesthetic agents, may occur in patients with myxoedema. Various factors, including a decreased efficiency of microsomal enzyme systems, alterations in drug distribution due to associated bradycardia or congestive cardiac failure, prolonged gastrointestinal transit and changes in body temperature may be involved.

Thyrotoxicosis is well known to affect metabolism and more specific pharmacokinetic studies have shown enhancement of microsomal drug oxidation. Binding of both acidic and basic drugs to plasma proteins is decreased in hyperthyroidism. Evidence of sympathetic overactivity is an accompanying feature of uncontrolled thyrotoxicosis. A varying response to a number of drugs used during anaesthesia may thus be anticipated. Adrenocorticosteroids exert permissive effects on catecholamines. An exaggerated response to a variety of drugs with a propensity to reduce the systemic blood pressure may occur in patients with inadequate adrenal function, and adequate replacement therapy should always be provided.

In patients with a phaeochromocytoma, drugs with the ability to release histamine (e.g. morphine and tubocurarine) or to induce dysrhythmias (e.g. halothane and enflurane) may induce exaggerated hypertensive responses or disorders of cardiac conduction. Similarly, patients with carcinoid tumours are also at risk of developing tachyarrhythmias and hypertension when drugs with histamine provoking activity are administered.

FURTHER READING

Abbott TR. Anaesthesia in untreated myxoedema. *British Journal of Anaesthesia* 1967; **39**: 510–514.

Bentley JB, Borel JD, Nenad RE Jr, Gillespie TJ. Age and fentanyl pharmacokinetics. *Anesthesia and Analgesia* 1982; **61**: 968–971.

Bentley JB, Vaughan RW, Gandolfi J, Cork RC. Halothane bio-transformation in obese and non-obese patients. *Anesthesiology* 1982; **57**: 94–97.

Bush GH, Stead AL. The use of *d*-tubocurarine in neonatal anaesthesia. *British Journal of Anaesthesia* 1962; **34**: 721–728.

Christiensen JH, Andreasen F. Individual variation in the response to thiopental. *Acta Anaesthesica Scandinavica* 1978; **22**: 303–313.

Churchill-Davidson HC, Wise RP. Neuromuscular transmission in the newborn infant. *Anesthesiology* 1963; **24**: 271–278.

Cohen EN, Brewer HW, Smith D. The metabolism and elimination of *d*-tubocurarine-H3. *Anesthesiology* 1967; **28**: 309–317.

Crooks J, O'Malley K, Stevenson IH. Pharmacokinetics in the elderly. *Clinical Pharmacokinetics* 1976; **1**: 280–296.

Day RO, Brooks PM. Variations in response to non-steroidal anti-inflammatory drugs. *British Journal of Clinical Pharmacology* 1987; **23**: 655–658.

Dean G. *The Porphyrias—A Story of Inheritance and Environment*, 2nd edn. London: Pitman, 1971; 1–118.

Doenicke R, Grote B, Lorenz W. Blood and blood substitutes. *British Journal of Anaesthesia* 1977; **49**: 681–688.

Dundee JW, Gray TC. Resistance to *d*-tubocurarine chloride in the presence of liver damage. *Lancet* 1953; **ii**: 16–17.

Duvaldestin P, Agoston S, Henzel D *et al*. Pancuronium pharmacokinetics in patients with liver cirrhosis. *British Journal of Anaesthesia* 1978; **50**: 1131–1136.

Edwards R, Mosher VB. Alcohol abuse, anaesthesia and intensive care. *Anaesthesia* 1980; **35**: 474–489.

Eger EI II, Severinghaus JW. Effect of uneven pulmonary distribution of blood and gas on induction with inhalational anaesthetics. *Anesthesiology* 1964; **25**: 620–626.

Eichelbaum M. Drug metabolism in thyroid disease. *Clinical Pharmacokinetics* 1976; **1**: 339–350.

Evans DAP, Manley KA, McKusick VA. Genetic control of isoniazid metabolism in man. *British Medical Journal* 1960; **2**: 485–491.

Fisher DM, O'Keeffe C, Stanski DR *et al*. Pharmacokinetics and pharmacodynamics of *d*-tubocurarine in infants, children and adults. *Anesthesiology* 1982; **57**: 203–208.

Flaherty JT. Nitrate tolerance—a review of the evidence. *Drugs* 1989; **37**: 523–550.

Frederiksen MC, Ruo TI, Chow MJ, Atkinson AJ Jr. Theophylline pharmacokinetics in pregnancy. *Clinical Pharmacology and Therapeutics* 1986; **40**: 321–326.

Friis-Hansen B. Body water compartments in children. Changes during growth and related changes in body composition. *Pediatrics* 1961; **28**: 169–181.

Gell PGH, Coombes RRA. *Clinical Aspects of Immunology*, 2nd edn. Oxford: Blackwell Scientific Publications; 1968.

Gibaldi M. Drug distribution in renal failure. *American Journal of Medicine* 1977; **62**: 471–474.

Gregory GA, Eger EI II, Munson ES. The relationship between age and halothane requirement in man. *Anesthesiology* 1969; **30**: 488–491.

Gronert GA. Malignant hyperthermia *Anesthesiology* 1980; **53**: 395–423.

Hockings NF. Problems in prescribing for the elderly. *Hospital Update* 1981; **7**: 1201–1204.

Horowitz JD, Henry CA, Syrjanen ML *et al*. Combined use of nitroglycerin and acetylcysteine in the management of unstable angina pectoris. *Circulation* 1988; **77**: 787–794.

Hunter JM, Jones RS, Utting JE. Use of atracurium in patients with no renal function. *British Journal of Anaesthesia* 1982; **54**: 1251–1258.

Hurwitz N, Wade OL. Intensive hospital monitoring of adverse reactions to drugs. *British Medical Journal* 1969; **1**: 531–536.

James ML. Endocrine disease and anaesthesia. *Anaesthesia* 1970; **25**: 232–252.

Jusko WJ. Influence of cigarette smoking on drug metabolism in man. *Drug Metabolism Reviews* 1979; **9**(2): 221–236.

Koch-Weser J, Greenblatt DS *et al*. Drug disposition in old age. *New England Journal of Medicine* 1982; **306**: 1081–1082.

Krauer B, Krauer F. Drug kinetics in pregnancy. *Clinical Pharmacokinetics* 1977; **2**: 167–181.

Lewis RE, Cruse JM, Richley JV. Effects of anaesthesia and operation on the classical pathway of complement activation. *Clinical Immunology and Immunopathology* 1982; **23**: 666–671.

Lindenbaum J, Mellow MH, Blackstone MO *et al*. Variations in biological availability of digoxin from four preparations. *New England Journal of Medicine* 1971; **285**: 1344–1347.

Mather LE, Meffin PJ. Clinical pharmacokinetics of pethidine. *Clinical Pharmacokinetics* 1978; **3**: 352–368.

Morgan DJ, Blackman GL, Paull JD *et al*. Pharmacokinetics and plasma binding of thiopental: studies at cesarian section. *Anesthesiology* 1981; **54**: 474–480.

Muravchick S. Immediate and long-term nervous system effects of anaesthesia in elderly patients. *Clinics in Anaesthesiology* 1986; **4**: 1035–1048.

Neuberger J, Kenna JG. Halothane hepatitis: a model of immune mediated toxicity. *Clinical Science* 1987; **72**: 263–270.

Nightingale DA. Use of atracurium in neonatal anaesthesia. *British Journal of Anaesthesia* 1986; **58**: 32S–36S.

Park BK, Coleman JW, Kitteringham NR. Drug disposition and drug hypersensitivity. *Biochemistry and Pharmacology* 1987; **36**: 581–590.

Pickles H. Prescriptions, adverse reactions and the elderly. *Lancet* 1986; **ii**: 40–41.

Perucca E, Crema A. Plasma protein binding of drugs in pregnancy. *Clinical Pharmacokinetics* 1982; **7**: 336–352.

Radford SG, Lockyer JA, Simpson PJ. Immunological aspects of adverse reactions to anaesthesia. *British Journal of Anaesthesia* 1982; **54**: 859–864.

Ross EM, Gilman AG. Pharmacodynamics: mechanisms of drug action and the relationship between drug concentration and effect. In: Goodman LS, Gilman A, Rall TW, Murad F (eds) *The Pharmacological Basis of Therapeutics* 7th edn. New York: Macmillan, 1985; 35–48.

Rylance G. Drugs in children. *British Medical Journal* 1981; **282**: 50–51.

Sauder RA, Hirshman CA. Anaesthesia for the patient with reactive airway disease. *Current Opinions in Anaesthesiology* 1989; **2**: 776–781.

Sear JW. Adverse effects of drugs given by injection. In: Taylor TH, Major E (eds) *Hazards and Complications of Anaesthesia*. Edinburgh: Churchill-Livingstone, 1987; 213–236.

Sjöholm I, Kober A, Odar-Cederlöf I, Borga O. Protein binding of drugs in uremic and normal serum. The role of endogenous binding inhibitors. *Biochemical Pharmacology* 1976; **25**: 1205–1213.

Smith CL, Bush GH. Anaesthesia and progressive muscular dystrophy. *British Journal of Anaesthesia* 1985; **57**: 1113–1118.

Stevens WC, Dolan WM, Gibbons RT *et al*. Minimal alveolar concentration (MAC) of isoflurane with and without nitrous oxide in patients of various ages. *Anesthesiology* 1975; **42**: 197–200.

Tarlov AR, Brewer GJ, Carson PE, Alving AS. Primaquine sensitivity. *Archives of Internal Medicine* 1962; **109**: 209–234.

Vestal RE. Drug use in the elderly: a review of problems and special considerations. *Drugs* 1978; **16**: 358–362.

Watkins J. Intravenous therapy and immunological disasters. *Theoretical Surgery* 1986; **1**: 103–112.

West JR, Smith HW, Chasis H. Glomerular filtration rate, effective renal blood flow and maximal tubular excretory capacity in infants. *Journal of Pediatrics* 1948; **32**: 10–18.

Wilkinson GR, Shenker S. Drug disposition and liver disease. *Drug Metabolism Reviews* 1975; **4**: 139–175.

Williams RL, Mamelok RD. Hepatic diseases and drug pharmacokinetics. *Clinical Pharmacokinetics* 1980; **5**: 528–547.

Wooley PH, Griffin J, Panayi GS, Batchelor JR, Welsh KI, Gibson TJ. HLA-DR antigens and toxic reaction to sodium aurothiomalate and *d*-penicillamine in patients with rheumatoid arthritis. *New England Journal of Medicine* 1980; **303**: 300–302.

Zhang A-Z, Pasternak GW. Opiates and enkephalins: a common binding site mediates their analgesic action in rats. *Life Science* 1981; **29**: 843–847.

Zhou H-H, Koshakji RP, Silberstein DJ, Wilkinson GP. Racial differences in drug response: altered sensitivity to and clearance of propranolol in men of Chinese descent as compared with American Whites. *New England Journal of Medicine* 1989; **320**: 565–570.

SIX

Intravenous Anaesthetic Agents

Intravenous anaesthetic agents are usually defined as drugs that induce loss of consciousness in one arm–brain circulation time, when given in appropriate dosage. In the early years of anaesthesia, many drugs were administered intravenously in an attempt to produce rapid unconsciousness; these included several opiates, chloral hydrate, bromethol, infusions of chloroform and ether, and various intravenous preparations of the available barbiturate derivatives (e.g. amylobarbitone, butobarbitone, and pentobarbitone). Unfortunately, problems with the delayed onset and prolonged duration of anaesthesia, as well as the toxic effects of individual drugs, were frequently encountered.

In the early 1930s, a milestone in anaesthetic practice was achieved with the introduction of barbiturates with a rapid onset of hypnotic activity and an extremely short duration of action. In 1932, hexobarbitone was introduced by Weese and Scharpff in Germany; its rapid onset of action was responsible for its acceptance as an induction agent. It was soon superseded by thiopentone, which was independently studied by Lundy and Waters in the USA. The potential hazards of thiopentone (particularly when used alone in large doses) were not fully appreciated until the disaster at Pearl Harbour in 1941. In subsequent years, thiopentone became widely accepted as an intravenous induction agent; however, many thiobarbiturates have essentially similar properties, and in some respects it is remarkable that the drug has stood the test of time. Methohexitone, which became generally available in the UK in 1959, is the only other barbiturate derivative in current use.

Many steroid drugs can produce hypnosis, but their use as intravenous anaesthetics is precluded by their hormonal effects. Nevertheless, several steroids have been used as anaesthetic agents. Approximately 30 years ago, hydroxydione was introduced into anaesthetic practice; it had a high hypnotic potency, but no hormonal actions. Due to the poor solubility of the drug, administration was dependent on its continuous infusion in a large volume of saline, which delayed its onset of action. A polymerized, more concentrated preparation of the drug was subsequently introduced; unfortunately, this led to the frequent occurrence of thrombophlebitis, and the use of hydroxydione was discontinued.

More recently, Althesin (a combination of the steroids alphaxolone and alphadolone) has been used as an intravenous anaesthetic. Despite its many advantages, the occurrence of anaphylactoid or anaphylactic phenomena (particularly bronchospasm, hypotension, and vascular collapse) led to the withdrawal of the drug in 1984. These phenomena were probably related to the polyethoxylated castor oil ('Cremophor EL') which was used in Althesin to increase the solubility of the steroids. Minaxolone, a water-soluble steroid, has also been used in man as an intravenous induction agent. Unfortunately, its use was associated with a significant incidence of excitatory effects; in addition, it was shown to produce neoplasia in experimental animals, and its development was subsequently discontinued. Consequently, no steroid anaesthetics are currently available in the UK.

A number of derivatives of eugenol have also been used as intravenous anaesthetic agents. Eugenol is chemically related to phenoxyacetic acid, and is one of the main constituents of oil of cloves. The eugenol derivative propanidid was used as an occasional induction agent for approximately 20 years, but was withdrawn in 1983. Propanidid is an ester which is poorly soluble in water; preparations of the drug also contained 'Cremophor EL', and occasionally produced bronchospasm and profound hypotension during induction. In addition, propanidid caused various excitatory effects (e.g. hiccup, abnormal muscle movements and convulsive activity).

Other drugs that have been used as intravenous anaesthetic agents are structurally related to cyclohexamine. Approximately 30 years ago, its analogue phencyclidine was used as an induction agent; however, it was soon discarded due to the occurrence of severe psychotomimetic reactions. The related compound ketamine was introduced in 1970; although it does not produce loss of consciousness in one arm–brain circulation time, it is usually classified as an intravenous anaesthetic agent. In spite of several disadvantages, the drug has a definite but limited place in current anaesthetic practice.

In contrast, etomidate is an imidazole ester with hypnotic activity but little or no analgesic effects. Although etomidate has a high margin of safety, it has several disadvantages which have restricted its use as an intravenous agent.

Propofol is a recently introduced anaesthetic agent with a relatively short duration of action. Consequently, it can be used as an induction agent or for the maintenance of anaesthesia. It usually produces rapid symptom-free recovery, and undoubtedly has a place in current practice (particularly for day-case surgery).

All intravenous anaesthetics must be administered in aqueous solution or as an oil or emulsion that is readily miscible with plasma. In addition, they must be partially non-ionized and lipid-soluble in plasma at pH 7.4, in order to cross the blood–brain barrier and produce rapid loss of consciousness. These conflicting physicochemical requirements are usually resolved by the use of alkaline solutions, or by the administration of lipid-soluble drugs in water-miscible oils and emulsions. Consequently bases, buffers, or solubilising agents are frequently added to solutions of intravenous anaesthetic agents.

In this chapter, the following drugs will be considered as intravenous induction agents:

1 Barbiturates (thiopentone and methohexitone).
2 Etomidate.
3 Propofol.
4 Ketamine.

Although other drugs are occasionally used to induce anaesthesia (e.g. benzodiazepines, opioids, and neuroleptic agents), they do not produce rapid loss of consciousness and are not usually considered as intravenous anaesthetics.

BARBITURATES

Barbiturates are derivatives of barbituric acid, which can be regarded as a condensation product of urea and malonic acid:

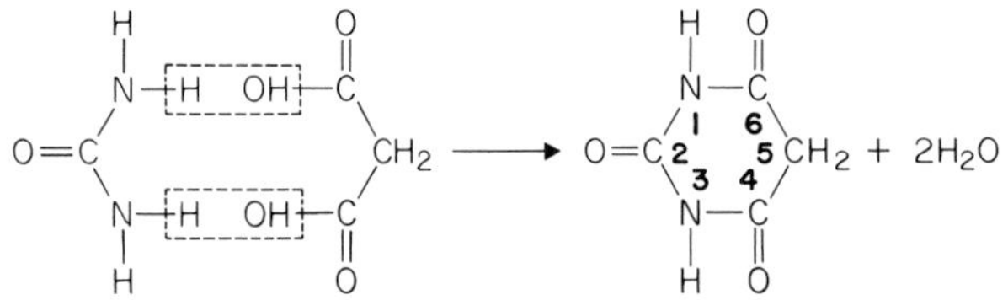

Although barbituric acid itself is inert, the substitution of both hydrogen atoms at the C5 position by organic groups produces compounds with hypnotic activity. These drugs are referred to as oxobarbiturates. An analogous series of compounds can be regarded as substitution products of thiobarbituric acid:

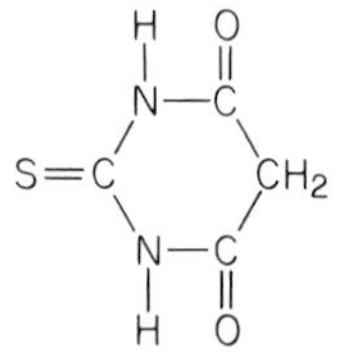

In general, thiobarbiturates (e.g. thiopentone) have a greater lipid solubility than their oxobarbiturate analogues (i.e. pentobarbitone); consequently, they cross the blood–brain barrier more rapidly. Most of the barbiturates which have been used as sedatives, hypnotics, or anticonvulsants contain two alkyl groups with 2–5 carbon atoms at the C5 position of the ring. Within certain limits, an increase in the length of these alkyl groups enhances hypnotic potency and activity. Substitution by extremely long alkyl groups decreases hypnotic activity and may be associated with convulsant properties. Similarly, *N*-methylation of the N1 or

N3 nitrogen atom produces compounds which may have excitatory or convulsant effects (e.g. methohexitone and methylphenobarbitone). Conversely, substitution by aromatic or heterocyclic groups at C5 is often associated with anticonvulsant effects (e.g. phenobarbitone).

Barbiturates are not readily soluble in water (except in alkaline solution). In aqueous conditions, their solubility is dependent on isomerism from the keto to the enol form, and their presence in solution as weak acids:

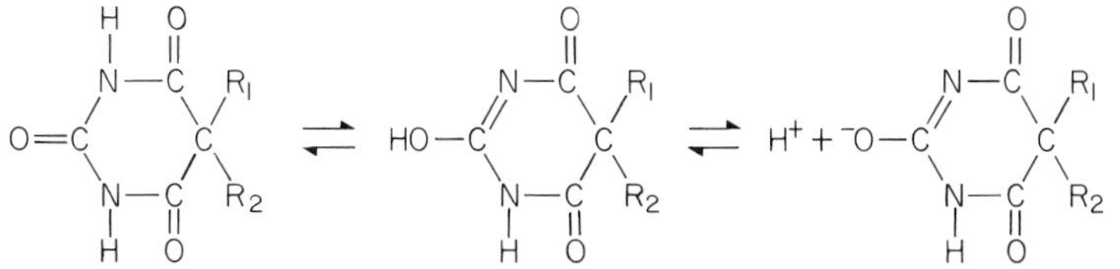

Isomerism from the keto to the enol form is pH-dependent, and readily occurs in alkaline solutions. The water solubility of sodium salts of barbituric acids is dependent on the presence of the enol form and its subsequent ionization in alkaline solution:

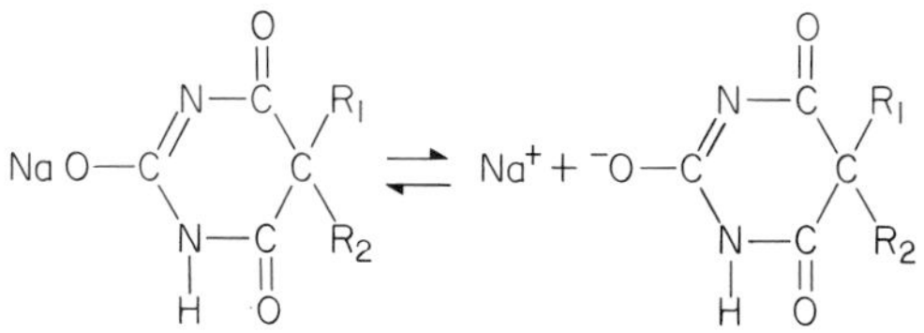

The dissociation constants of most barbiturates range from 7.3–8.0; consequently, in *in vivo* conditions the degree of ionization of different drugs is relatively constant.

In contrast, there are marked differences between the various barbiturates in lipid solubility, plasma protein binding, and the extent of drug metabolism. In general, thiobarbiturates have a high lipid solubility, are extensively bound to plasma proteins (usually 60–90%), and are completely metabolized by liver enzymes. Some oxobarbiturates (e.g. cyclobarbitone and pentobarbitone) are 20 times less lipid-soluble, moderately bound to plasma proteins (i.e. 30–50%), and are mainly eliminated by hepatic metabolism; other oxobarbiturates (e.g. barbitone and phenobarbitone) are approximately 200 times less lipid-soluble, only slightly bound to plasma proteins (i.e. less than 20%) and are almost entirely excreted unchanged in urine. Consequently, barbitone and phenobarbitone have a relatively long terminal half-life.

Although barbiturates have depressant effects on cellular function in many tissues and organs, the CNS is particularly sensitive to their effects. Early neurophysiological studies suggested that the effects of barbiturates were dependent on the suppression of the midbrain reticular formation (the reticular activating system). Thus, barbiturates modified sensory and auditory cortical evoked responses, and depressed the electro-encephalographic and arousal response to reticular stimulation. These effects were generally considered to be due to the modification of synaptic activity.

It was subsequently shown that excitatory neurotransmission (and excitatory postsynaptic potentials) were depressed by barbiturates while inhibitory transmission was unaltered or enhanced. These effects were initially believed to be related to actions on cellular metabolism; thus barbiturates decrease cerebral oxygen consumption and mitochondrial respiration, increase glycogen and phosphate levels, reduce acetylcholine release, and depress dopamine, noradrenaline, and 5-hydroxytryptamine turnover in certain areas of the brain. It is now considered that these changes represent indirect and secondary effects of barbiturates on the CNS.

During the past decade, it has been shown that barbiturates primarily affect GABA-dependent chloride channels in the brain. Gamma-aminobutyric acid (GABA) is probably the main inhibitory neurotransmitter in the CNS, and is believed to mediate both presynaptic and postsynaptic inhibition at 20–40% of all synapses. In the presence of GABA, chloride channels in neuronal membranes open, and chloride ions can diffuse into the neurone; this results in hyperpolarization and decreased neuronal excitability (i.e. inhibition). Barbiturates primarily act by increasing the duration of GABA-dependent chloride channel opening; the resultant hyperpolarization decreases excitability at all neuronal sites where GABA is an inhibitory neurotransmitter. Barbiturates also inhibit the binding of radiolabelled picrotoxin analogues at sites related to chloride channels, and the chronic administration of phenobarbitone increases GABA levels in all regions of the CNS. These neurochemical phenomena may well account for most of the electrophysiological effects of barbiturates on the brain.

Barbiturates have been widely used as sedatives and hypnotics for many years, and proprietary preparations of amylobarbitone, butobarbitone, cyclobarbitone, pentobarbitone, and quinalbarbitone are still available in the UK. Although they are currently classified as controlled drugs, they are sometimes used to induce sleep. In some patients with long-standing and intractable insomnia, they may produce more predictable and reliable effects than the benzodiazepines. Nevertheless, there are many disadvantages associated with their use. Like other hypnotic drugs, they impair judgement and increase reaction time; ambulant patients should always be warned of their hazards in relation to car driving, working at heights, and operating dangerous machinery. All barbiturates may impair psychomotor performance or produce hangover effects on the day after their administration. In addition, hypnotic doses may affect respiration; accidental or intentional barbiturate overdosage is classically associated with severe respiratory depression. Barbiturates may interact with other central depressants, including ethyl alcohol, and are particularly dangerous in patients with pulmonary disease (e.g. chronic bronchitis and asthma). They induce hepatic enzymes concerned with drug metabolism, and may affect the breakdown of other drugs (e.g. oral anticoagulants, tricyclic antidepressants, anticonvulsants, and oral contraceptives). They also may precipitate acute porphyria in genetically susceptible patients (p. 165). The elimination of barbiturates may be compromised in hepatic and renal impairment, and in patients over 60 years old. In general, they are poorly tolerated by elderly patients, and drowsiness, disorientation, and unsteadiness may result in slurred speech, falls and fractures, poor memory, and acute confusional states. The increased susceptibility of elderly patients is partly due to pharmacokinetic factors (i.e. decreased hepatic oxidative drug metabolism), and partly to enhanced sensitivity at neuronal sites in the CNS. Continuous or long-term barbiturate administration commonly causes drug tolerance, due to hepatic enzyme induction ('pharmacokinetic tolerance') as well as decreased neuronal sensitivity ('pharmacodynamic tolerance'). Barbiturates may antagonize the effects of analgesics, and may induce physical and psychological dependence. Consequently, barbiturate abuse is not uncommon. Central and peripheral adverse effects are not infrequent, and benzodiazepines are safer hypnotic drugs.

In addition to their use as hypnotics, some barbiturates (particularly phenobarbitone, methylphenobarbitone, and primidone) have been used as anticonvulsant drugs. Only two barbiturates (i.e. thiopentone and methohexitone) are currently used as intravenous anaesthetic agents.

THIOPENTONE

Thiopentone (5-ethyl-5'-(1-methylbutyl)-2-thiobarbituric acid; Fig. 6.1) is the sulphur analogue of the oxobarbiturate pentobarbitone. The sodium salt is a pale yellow powder with a bitter taste which is readily soluble in water. The solution commonly used to induce anaesthesia (2.5% w/v) has a pH of approximately 10.5, for two reasons:

1   All salts of weak acids form alkaline solutions when dissolved in water. In these conditions, sodium thiopentone ($pK_a = 7.6$) ionizes and the thiopentone anion can attract H^+, forming an undissociated weak acid. Consequently, the resultant solution is alkaline:

$$R_1{-}S{-}Na \rightleftharpoons Na^+ + R_1{-}S^-$$
$$H_2O \rightleftharpoons OH^- + H^+$$
$$\rightleftharpoons R_1{-}S{-}H + Na^+ + OH^-$$

Thiopentone

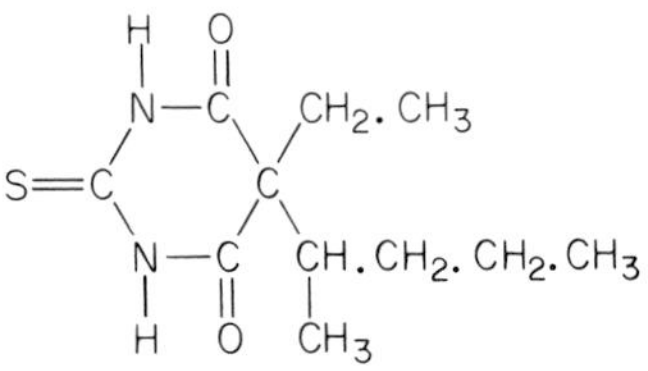

Methohexitone

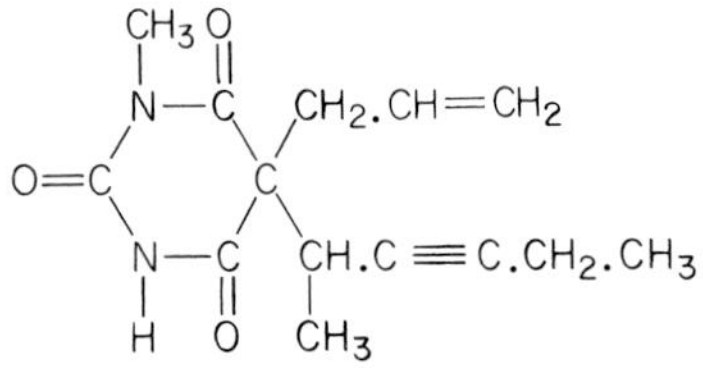

Etomidate

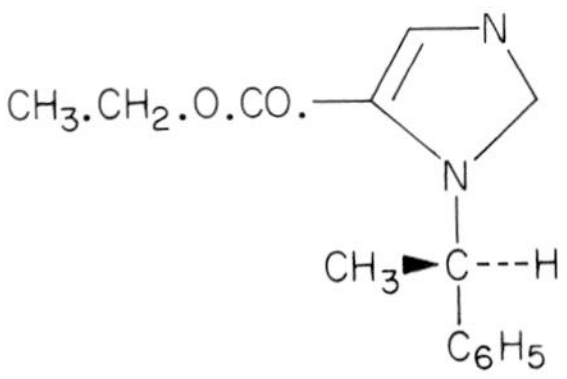

Propofol

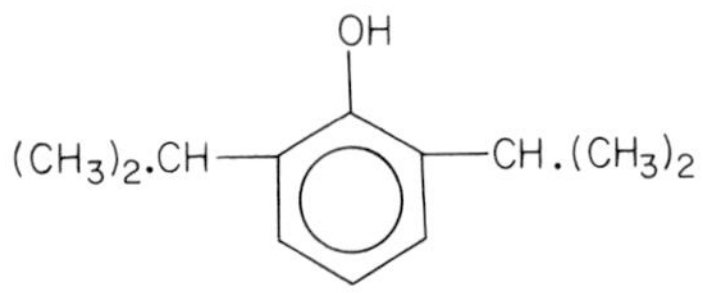

Ketamine

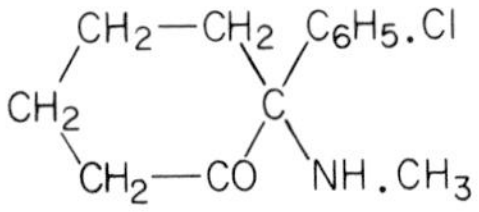

Fig. 6.1 Chemical structure of intravenous anaesthetics.

Nevertheless, the extent to which this occurs is limited, due to the small concentration of H^+ in solution. At pH 10.5, approximately 99.9% of thiopentone is still present in the ionized form R_1–S^-. The solubility of the non-ionized form R_1–S–H in water is extremely low, and in concentrations above 0.003% (30 µg/ml^{-1}) it readily precipitates from solution.

2   Commercial preparations of thiopentone sodium contain six parts of sodium carbonate to 100 parts of barbiturate (by weight). Sodium carbonate produces

free hydroxyl ions in solution, and is added to prevent the precipitation of the insoluble free acid (R_1–S–H) by atmospheric carbon dioxide. Solutions of thiopentone sodium may remain stable at room temperature for up to 2 weeks (and for rather longer at 4°C), but should be immediately discarded if they become cloudy. They are not normally used more than 48 hours after their preparation.

Due to their alkaline pH, 2.5% solutions of thiopentone are usually bacteriostatic, but may be incompatible with many basic drugs. In general, thiopentone should not be mixed with oxidizing agents, acidic solutions, or drugs normally administered as sulphates, chlorides, or hydrochlorides.

Effects on the CNS

The effects of thiopentone on the CNS are closely related to the dose and the rate of administration of the drug. They are mainly due to prolonged opening of GABA-dependent chloride channels, which produces hyperpolarization at many sites in the CNS (p. 158). After a normal induction dose of thiopentone (3–5 mg kg^{-1}), the rapid loss of consciousness is mainly due to two factors. In the first place, brain tissue is extremely vascular, and normally receives approximately 25% of the cardiac output. Secondly, thiopentone is highly lipid-soluble (oil/water solubility coefficient = 500–700) and more than 90% of the drug in the cerebral capillaries immediately crosses the blood–brain barrier. At pH 7.4, 39% of the drug is ionized (pK_a = 7.6) and approximately 80% is bound to plasma albumin; these factors do not significantly restrict the transfer of thiopentone into the brain. The initial loss of consciousness is usually smooth, and excitatory effects are rare. It is frequently preceded by one or more deep breaths, and may be associated with rapid eye movements and electroencephalographic changes. Characteristically, the EEG shows a variable amplitude and high frequency pattern (predominantly at 20–30 Hz); this is usually replaced by slow wave activity as anaesthesia deepens. The high frequency response may be due to the selective depression of inhibitory neurones in the reticular formation (probably at the pontomedullary level). It may correspond to the second stage of anaesthesia described by Guedel (excitement stage); it could account for an enhanced reflex response to surgical stimulation, increased vagal activity and laryngospasm, and hyperalgesia (a decreased threshold for the appreciation of a painful stimulus). These effects can be shown to occur when small doses of thiopentone are administered, or they may be observed clinically during recovery from barbiturate anaesthesia.

As anaesthesia deepens due to the increased cerebral uptake of thiopentone, cortical responsiveness declines, and EEG waveforms of low voltage become predominant. As the dose of thiopentone is increased, effects on the brainstem are produced. Respiratory depression is due to a direct action on the respiratory centre and its pontine connections; the sensitivity to carbon dioxide is decreased in proportion to the depth of anaesthesia. Consequently, $Paco_2$ increases, pH falls, and apnoea may occur. In deep barbiturate anaesthesia, hypoxic drive mediated by the aortic and carotid chemoreceptors may play an important part in the maintenance of respiration. Fetal respiration is particularly sensitive to thiopentone. In contrast to the opiates, barbiturates predominantly affect the depth rather than the rate of respiration. In clinical practice, the respiratory effects of thiopentone may be considerably modified by the degree of surgical stimulation and by the concomitant use of other central depressant drugs (particularly inhalational anaesthetics and opiates). Patients with impaired cardiovascular and respiratory function may be particularly sensitive to the effects of thiopentone.

A phenomenon described as 'acute tolerance' may occur with thiopentone. After the administration of different doses, the plasma concentration at the time of recovery is directly related to the dose (i.e. CNS sensitivity declines as the dose of thiopentone is increased). The earlier return of consciousness has also been related to the increased rate of injection of a given dose of the drug. It is unclear whether this phenomenon truly reflects an alteration in CNS sensitivity to thiopentone (i.e. a pharmacodynamic phenomenon), or may be explained by distribution dysequilibrium ('hysteresis'; a pharmacokinetic phenomenon). Indeed, the concept of acute tolerance to thiopentone has recently been challenged.

Thiopentone and other barbiturates also decrease cerebral metabolism and reduce oxygen consumption (see p. 158). Cerebral blood flow, cerebral blood volume, and CSF pressure also fall during barbiturate anaesthesia, possibly due to the decreased production of carbon dioxide. Consequently, thiopentone is sometimes used for cerebral resuscitation, or to reduce raised intracranial pressure. These effects may be modified by any changes in systemic $Paco_2$ produced by respiratory depression, which will have opposite effects on cerebrovascular tone and CSF pressure.

Effects on the cardiovascular system

In healthy patients, the plasma concentration of thiopentone associated with surgical anaesthesia causes minimal cardiovascular depression. Nevertheless, normal induction doses commonly cause a variable degree of hypotension. Particular problems may occur in hypovolaemic states, in patients with cardiovascular disease or cardiac insufficiency (including hypertension), or in patients who are being concurrently treated with drugs that affect the sympathetic nervous system (e.g. vasodilators and β-adrenoceptor antagonists). In these conditions, the ability of the cardiovascular system to compensate for the haemodynamic effects of thiopentone is impaired, and dose requirements are reduced. The reduction in blood pressure produced by thiopentone is primarily due to decreased stroke volume and cardiac output; indeed, there may be a compensatory reflex increase in systemic vascular resistance. The changes in cardiac output may be due to several factors. In the first place, the vasomotor centre and the hypothalamic nuclei controlling the force of cardiac contraction may be depressed by thiopentone. In addition, ganglionic transmission and the contractility of vascular smooth muscle may be impaired, causing venous dilatation, the peripheral pooling of blood, and a reduction in venous return. High doses and high concentrations may directly depress cardiac contractility, probably due to the local anaesthetic (membrane stabilizing) effects of thiopentone.

Renal effects

During thiopentone anaesthesia, glomerular filtration rate, renal plasma flow, and electrolyte and water excretion are decreased. These effects may be partly due to the reduction in renal blood flow produced by hypotension, but are mainly related to the increased release of antidiuretic hormone from the posterior lobe of the pituitary gland. Secretion of antidiuretic hormone is dependent on the activity of hypothalamic nuclei and the integrity of the hypophyseal tract. Inhibition of inhibitory pathways affecting hypothalamic nuclei (particularly the supra-optic nucleus) increases the secretion of antidiuretic hormone. Consequently, urine output during thiopentone anaesthesia is approximately $0.1 \, \text{ml} \, \text{min}^{-1}$ (about 10% of normal). In uraemic patients, a decrease in the protein binding of thiopentone may occur causing potentiation of its effects.

Hepatic effects

There is little or no definite evidence that normal induction doses of thiopentone cause any impairment of hepatic function. Nevertheless, respiratory depression (producing hypoxia and hypercarbia), as well as some systemic and hepatic diseases, may adversely affect liver blood flow and hepatocellular function; this may explain the occasional association of thiopentone with toxic jaundice and abnormal liver function tests. In common with most other barbiturates, thiopentone may induce hepatic enzymes, increasing the activity of the mixed function oxidase system (cytochrome P-450) in the smooth endoplasmic reticulum. Enzyme activity may be increased following anaesthesia with thiopentone (although other agents, such as nitrous oxide and halothane, have also been shown to stimulate enzyme activity). Thiopentone may also precipitate acute intermittent porphyria, and its use (as well as that of all other barbiturates) is absolutely contraindicated in this condition (p. 165).

In chronic hepatic dysfunction, the effects of thiopentone may be prolonged, and slower recovery of consciousness may be anticipated. In liver disease, the protein binding of thiopentone may be modified by a reduction in albumin synthesis.

Pharmacokinetics

The rapid onset of action of thiopentone is due to the immediate uptake of non-ionized and non-protein bound drug by the brain. At pH 7.4, 75–80% of thiopentone is bound to plasma albumin, and 61% of the non-protein bound drug is non-ionized; consequently, alterations in extracellular pH and plasma protein binding may affect the uptake of thiopentone by the brain. In experimental conditions, the plasma concentration of thiopentone at pH 6.8 is reduced by 40%, presumably due to the enhanced uptake of non-ionized drug by the tissues. Similarly, alkalosis (e.g. hyperventilation) may increase the concentration and the proportion of ionized thiopentone in plasma, and diminish the effects of a given dose. In addition, protein-binding sites on plasma albumin may be occupied by other drugs (e.g. probenecid and iodine-containing contrast media); their prior administration may enhance the effects of thiopentone. In *in vitro* conditions, high concentrations of many non-steroidal anti-inflammatory drugs (e.g. indomethacin, phenylbutazone, acetylsalicylic acid and naproxen) displace thiopentone from albumin; the clinical significance of this phenomenon is a matter of conjecture.

High concentrations of thiopentone are present in the brain and other well-perfused tissues within 1 min of intravenous administration. The rapid emergence from sleep after single dose thiopentone anaesthesia is due to redistribution from the brain to less vascular regions (particularly muscle and skin). These tissues become saturated with thiopentone within 15–30 min; as thiopentone is taken up, the plasma concentration rapidly falls and the drug diffuses out of the brain. In contrast, the fat depots, which have a poor blood supply, may require several hours to take up significant amounts of thiopentone and reach saturation. The concentration of thiopentone in blood, skeletal muscle and subcutaneous fat at various times after its administration is consistent with a physiological pharmacokinetic model with a central blood pool and six tissue compartments (Chapter 2). The model supports the concept that thiopentone is primarily removed from the brain by lean body tissues (e.g. muscle), and that subcutaneous fat only plays a small part in the termination of its anaesthetic effects.

After intravenous administration of thiopentone, there is a triexponential decline in the plasma concentration of the drug. The initial rapid disposition phase (half-life = 2–4 min) presumably reflects the distribution of the drug to well-perfused organs (e.g. brain and hepatorenal tissues); this is followed by a slower disposition phase (half-life = 45–60 min), due to the uptake of thiopentone by muscle and skin. Finally, the elimination of the drug from the body is reflected by the terminal decline in plasma concentration (half-life = 5–10 h). The volume of distribution of thiopentone at steady state is slightly greater than total body water (1–4 litres kg^{-1}), while its clearance is approximately 10–20% of liver blood flow (i.e. 1–5 ml min^{-1} kg^{-1}). The low hepatic extraction ratio of thiopentone is consistent with capacity-limited elimination by the liver, and will be sensitive to changes in plasma protein binding. The clearance of thiopentone is greater in infants and children than in adults; it is significantly decreased in obese patients, and in elderly subjects.

Since thiopentone is highly lipid-soluble, it is extensively metabolized by the liver (and possibly by other tissues). Only trace amounts are eliminated unchanged in urine (normally less than 1% of the dose). Although metabolism only plays a limited part in recovery from the effects of thiopentone, it is eventually entirely responsible for the elimination of the drug from the body. Drug metabolism is relatively slow ($6-15\%\ h^{-1}$) and is mainly due to ω-oxidation of thiopentone to the inactive metabolite thiopentone carboxylic acid (ω-oxidation refers to oxidation of the terminal methyl group on the l-methylbutyl side-chain to the corresponding carboxylic acid). To some extent, thiopentone is also metabolized by (ω-1) oxidation to hydroxythiopentone, and by desulphuration to its oxobarbiturate analogue pentobarbitone. This compound has a longer half-life than thiopentone ($20-50\,h$), and is itself metabolized to inactive products (e.g. pentobarbitone carboxylic acid and hydroxypentobarbitone). When large doses of thiopentone are used in cerebral resuscitation, thiopentone metabolism becomes non-linear (zero-order), due to saturation of hepatic enzyme systems. In these conditions, significant concentrations of thiopentone are present in plasma and may contribute to delayed recovery.

Unwanted effects

Thiopentone is undoubtedly a safe and reliable intravenous induction agent, as long as certain precautions are observed. Facilities for artificial ventilation and oxygenation must always be available. Deep thiopentone anaesthesia can reduce smooth muscle tone in the gut and reflex laryngeal activity, and the risk of the aspiration of gastric contents must always be recognized. In particular, the dose usually recommended ($4-5\,mg\ kg^{-1}$) may need to be considerably reduced in elderly, debilitated, and hypovolaemic patients.

In subjects with acute intermittent porphyria and porphyria variegata, thiopentone increases the synthesis of cytochrome P-450 from haem, and thus induces ('derepresses') the enzyme δ-aminolaevulinic acid synthetase (δ-ALA-synthetase). This enzyme plays a crucial role in porphyrin synthesis by the liver and other tissues. Increased synthesis of porphobilinogen and other porphyrins may cause progressive demyelination and neuropathy, voluntary muscle weakness and paralysis, abdominal pain, or psychiatric sequelae. The urine usually contains porphobilinogen and uroporphyrin, and may turn red when allowed to stand in daylight for several hours. Some types of porphyria (e.g. erythropoietic porphyria and porphyria cutanea tarda) are not adversely affected by thiopentone; even in acute intermittent porphyria, barbiturates do not always induce an acute attack.

Nevertheless, the precipitation of acute porphyria may be fatal, and all barbiturates should be completely avoided in all forms of porphyria.

Thiopentone may induce transient urticarial or erythematous rashes (and occasionally other types of cutaneous reactions). Urticarial responses are usually related to histamine release from mast cells, and may be associated with raised plasma histamine concentrations. This may be related to the dose and the speed of injection. True hypersensitivity or anaphylactic responses (i.e. reactions involving immunoglobulins or T-lymphocytes) appear to be extremely rare, with a presumed incidence of 1 in 30 000 to 1 in 100 000. They usually present as bronchospasm, hypotension, generalized oedema, or peripheral vascular collapse, and may be associated with a significant mortality.

The relatively slow elimination of thiopentone (terminal half-life $= 5-10 \, h$) necessitates care and supervision during the prolonged recovery period. Patients must be advised against driving, working at heights, or operating machinery within the following 24 hours. Possible drug interactions with other sedatives and hypnotics (particularly ethyl alcohol and the benzodiazepines) should be avoided.

Although intravenous thiopentone is usually painless, inadvertent extravascular administration can cause significant adverse effects. Subcutaneous or perivenous injection may produce local complications, ranging from slight pain to extensive tissue necrosis. They are far less frequent with dilute thiopentone (2.5%) than with more concentrated solutions (e.g. 5%, which was at one time widely used). These effects are probably due to local tissue irritation, produced by precipitation of insoluble non-ionized thiopentone acid at the pH of extracellular fluid. They are unlikely to be primarily related to the pH of solutions of thiopentone, since they are less frequently observed when the slightly more alkaline solution of methohexitone (1%) is used. Dispersal of thiopentone by local injection of hyaluronidase and topically applied demulcents may be useful in the symptomatic treatment of local complications.

The intra-arterial injection of thiopentone causes an immediate, severe, and agonizing shooting pain in the arm, which is usually followed by signs of arterial spasm, with blanching of the limb, increasing cyanosis, and disappearance of the radial pulse. The onset of unconsciousness may be delayed. When more dilute solutions are used, the incidence and severity of the sequelae are reduced, but untreated cases may develop gangrene.

The precise explanation for these complications due to accidental intra-arterial administration is unclear. Arterial injection is rapidly followed by the precipitation of insoluble thiopentone acid crystals (which have a maximum solubility of 0.003% or $30 \, \mu g \, ml^{-1}$ at pH 7.4); these are transported in a progressively narrowing arterial vasculature (where there is no opportunity for dilution), and aggregate in small arterioles. Initial vascular spasm may be due to the local release of noradrenaline from the arterial or arteriolar wall. This is followed by an intense chemical endarteritis, which rapidly involves the endothelium and periendothelial tissues. In addition, blood vessels may be occluded by crystals of thiopentone and by erythrocyte and platelet aggregation, resulting in arterial thrombosis and gangrene. The important factor in the pathogenesis of the condition is the injection of thiopentone into the arterial tree where the drug is neutralized but is not immediately diluted. Although crystal formation may occur immediately after intravenous injection due to the alteration in pH, it is of little or no importance since the drug is rapidly diluted within 1–2 seconds by the collateral venous return.

After intra-arterial injection of thiopentone, immediate treatment is necessary. If the needle is still *in situ* in the artery, injection of a vasodilator (e.g. papaverine or procaine, 80–120 mg, or possibly a calcium antagonist) is required. Temporary sympathetic blockade by continuous axillary block or repeated stellate ganglion block will open up the collateral circulation, and heparin is often useful.

The pharmacological properties and pharmacokinetics of thiopentone are summarized in Tables 6.1 and 6.2.

METHOHEXITONE

Methohexitone is l-methyl-5-allyl-5'-(l-methyl-2-pentynyl)-2-barbituric acid (Fig. 6.1). There are four possible optically active isomers of the compound; a racemic mixture of two of these stereoisomers (α-*d*-methohexitone and α-*l*-methohexitone) is used clinically to induce anaesthesia. The sodium salts of both these enantiomorphs are white powders, which are readily soluble in water. Commercial preparations of methohexitone also contain six parts of sodium carbonate to 100 parts of barbiturate (by weight), and the drug is usually prepared as a 1% solution with a pH of approximately 11. Aqueous solutions of methohexitone, when maintained at room temperature, have a shelf-life of at least 6 weeks; if other media (e.g. dextrose and saline) are used for the continuous infusion of methohexitone, solutions may become unstable within 24 hours. Solutions of methohexitone are usually bacteriostatic, due to their alkaline pH, and are often incompatible with solutions of many basic drugs.

Methohexitone is approximately three times as potent as thiopentone (usual induction dose = 1–2 mg kg^{-1}), but has a similar profile of pharmacological activity. The rapid onset of action of methohexitone is due to its high lipid solubility (oil/water solubility coefficient = approximately 300) and the extensive blood supply of the brain, which normally receives 25% of the cardiac output. The short duration of unconsciousness reflects the redistribution of the drug from the brain to less well-perfused organs and tissues, such as muscle and subcutaneous fat. In most respects (e.g. its effects on the CNS, the cardiovascular system, renal and hepatic function, as well as its propensity to induce hepatic enzymes, acute intermittent porphyria, and undesirable systemic reactions),

Table 6.1 Pharmacological properties of intravenous anaesthetic agents.

	Onset of action	Recovery	Cardiovascular effects	Other effects
Thiopentone	Rapid	Relatively rapid; complete recovery delayed	BP ↓ CO ↓	Extravascular complications Arterial thrombosis Laryngospasm and bronchospasm Enzyme induction ↑ ↓ intracranial pressure
Methohexitone	Rapid	Rapid	BP ↓ CO ↓ HR ↑	Pain on injection Excitatory effects Abnormal muscle movement Cough and hiccup
Etomidate	Rapid	Moderately rapid	Minimal	Pain on injection Excitatory effects Adrenocortical suppression
Propofol	Rapid	Rapid	BP ↓ CO ↓	Pain on injection Delayed recovery after prolonged administration
Ketamine	Slow	Slow	BP ↑ CO ↑ HR ↑	Analgesia ↑ intracranial pressure Psychotomimetic effects

BP = blood pressure; CO = cardiac output; HR = heart rate.

Table 6.2 Pharmacokinetics and metabolism of intravenous anaesthetic agents.

	Terminal half-life (min)	Clearance (ml min^{-1} kg^{-1})	Apparent volume of distribution (l kg^{-1})	Metabolites
Thiopentone	300–600	1.4–5.7	1.0–4.0	Thiopentone carboxylic acid Hydroxythiopentone Pentobarbitone
Methohexitone	90–250	10.0–13.0	1.2–2.2	Hydroxymethohexitone Hydroxymethohexitone glucuronide
Etomidate	60–90	10.0–24.3	2.2–4.3	Ethyl alcohol 1-(α-methylbenzyl)-imidazole-5-carboxylic acid
Propofol	300–700	21.4–28.6	3.3–5.7	2,6-diisopropylphenol glucuronide 2,6-diisopropylquinol glucuronide
Ketamine	150–200	17.1–20.0	2.9–3.1	Norketamine Hydroxynorketamine Hydroxyketamine glucuronide Hydroxynorketamine glucuronide

methohexitone is generally similar to thiopentone (Table 6.1). Nevertheless, there are several important differences between the two drugs:

1 There is less danger of tissue damage and vascular complications when methohexitone is injected subcutaneously or intra-arterially. This appears to be directly related to the lower concentration of methohexitone in solutions of the drug. As discussed previously (p. 166), the complications produced by sub-cutaneous and intra-arterial thiopentone are commoner and more serious when concentrated solutions of the drug are injected. Most of the evidence suggests that these complications are dependent on the precipitation of insoluble barbiturate crystals at pH 7.4, and that this is increased when concentrated solutions are used. Administration of dilute solutions appears to be the main factor that limits the complications of crystal formation when the drug is injected into a progressively narrower arterial tree (where no further dilution can occur). Other properties of barbiturates appear to be of little importance. Experimental studies suggest that high concentrations of methohexitone injected intra-arterially produce similar effects to thiopentone. Paradoxically, localized pain on injection of 1% methohexitone is more frequent than with 2.5% thiopentone. The explanation for the differential effects of intravenous barbiturates on the occurrence of local pain is unknown.

2 Methohexitone (and other barbiturates that are methylated at the N1 position of the oxobarbiturate ring, e.g. methylphenobarbitone) may cause excitatory side-effects. Although these occasionally occur with thiopentone, they are much more frequently observed after the use of methohexitone. Spontaneous involuntary muscle movements, tremor, hypertonus, coughing, and hiccuping may occur in up to 80% of patients. Their incidence is dependent on the dose and the rate of administration of methohexitone and may be modified by appropriate premedication. Similarly, it is usually considered unwise to administer methohexitone to patients with a history of epilepsy. The drug can precipitate convulsive activity in patients with an abnormal EEG or a history of focal epilepsy (indeed, it has been used for this specific purpose during neurosurgery). Nevertheless, the use of methohexitone in patients with epilepsy is controversial, and some authorities consider that the drug can be used safely in patients with convulsive disorders.

3 Methohexitone may produce less hypotension than thiopentone, and many anaesthetists prefer to use the drug in patients in shock. The reduced incidence of hypotension may be related to the tachycardia produced by methohexitone (which may be a feature of intravenous anaesthesia with methylated barbiturates). Similarly, ECG changes are less commonly seen during anaesthesia with methohexitone. It is unclear whether these effects are primarily related to barbiturate administration, or whether they reflect other haemodynamic changes during anaesthesia.

4 Although equivalent doses of thiopentone and methohexitone produce hypnosis for a similar duration of time, complete recovery from the effects of anaesthesia is significantly quicker after methohexitone. Similarly, when given by intermittent or multiple intravenous injection, methohexitone is less liable to cumulate than thiopentone. Consequently, methohexitone is more suitable for day case or out-patient surgery, and complete recovery from its effects usually occurs within 6–8 h. These differences between thiopentone and methohexitone are related to the different pharmacokinetics of the two drugs (Table 6.2). After intravenous injection of single doses of methohexitone, there may be a biexponential or a triexponential decline in the plasma concentration of the drug. An initial rapid distribution phase (half-life = 5–6 min) is due to the distribution of methohexitone to well-perfused tissues; this may be followed by a slower disposition phase (half-life = 60 min) which presumably reflects the uptake of the drug by less well-perfused tissues, such as muscle and subcutaneous fat. Finally, the elimination of methohexitone from the body is reflected by the terminal decline in the plasma concentration (elimination half-life = 1.5–4 h). Thus the terminal half-life of methohexitone is significantly less than thiopentone (Table 6.2). These differences in the elimination half-lives of the two intravenous barbiturates are mainly due to the more extensive clearance of methohexitone by the liver; the apparent volumes of distribution of the drugs are similar (Table 6.2). The clearance of methohexitone is approximately 50% of liver blood flow, and the relatively high extraction ratio is consistent with flow-limited hepatic elimination. Consequently, the clearance of methohexitone may be modified by changes in hepatic blood flow, but is unaffected by changes in protein binding or by alterations in hepatic enzyme activity. Both thiopentone and methohexitone are approximately 80% bound at physiological pH values (mainly to plasma albumin).

Methohexitone is almost entirely eliminated from the body by hepatic metabolism; only trace amounts of the unchanged drug are present in bile and urine. Methohexitone is metabolized by (ω-1) oxidation to hydroxymethohexitone, which may also have some hypnotic activity. (ω-1) oxidation refers to oxidation of the penultimate group on the substituted pentynyl side-chain (Fig. 6.1). Hydroxymethohexitone may be eliminated in urine as a glucuronide metabolite.

USES OF INTRAVENOUS BARBITURATES

Both thiopentone and methohexitone are widely used as induction agents in anaesthesia. Methohexitone has been widely used in obstetric anaesthesia and in out-patient anaesthesia (particularly in dental practice). Thiopentone is preferred in most other situations. Both drugs (particularly methohexitone) have been used by continuous intravenous infusion to supplement nitrous oxide anaesthesia. Pharmacokinetic models can be used to determine the dose and the required infusion rate.

When facilities for controlled ventilation are available, thiopentone may be the drug of first choice for the treatment of status epilepticus. In these conditions, it has a more rapid onset of action than diazepam, and this can be a considerable advantage. In addition, the drug can be extremely useful in the management of status epilepticus which does not respond to conventional anticonvulsant therapy, particularly when controlled ventilation under neuromuscular blockade is practicable. Thiopentone, and other barbiturates, have been used to protect the brain from the effects of hypoxia after stroke and head injury. The haemodynamic effects of the barbiturates may tend to reduce cerebral blood flow. Nevertheless, the depression of cerebral metabolism reduces brain oedema and intracranial pressure, so that cerebral perfusion actually improves. For such therapeutic procedures, meticulous care of the airway, monitoring of cardiovascular parameters, and measurement of intracranial pressure (when possible) are indicated. In the UK, the use of barbiturates for cerebral resuscitation is controversial.

ETOMIDATE

Etomidate (R-(+)-l-(α-methylbenzyl)-imidazole-5-ethylcarboxylate sulphate) is an imidazole derivative and an ester (Fig. 6.1). Although the sulphate salt is freely soluble in water, proprietary preparations of the drug usually contain propylene glycol (35% v/v). This improves the stability of the solution and reduces its local irritant effects. Etomidate is usually prepared and administered as a 0.2% solution (2 mg ml^{-1}). Normal induction doses (0.3 mg kg^{-1}) produce immediate loss of consciousness; its duration of action is dose dependent and the drug shows little or no tendency to cumulate (even with repeated dosage). Its mode of action is uncertain; it is generally assumed to act in a similar manner to other intravenous anaesthetics.

The most significant advantage of etomidate is its relatively high safety margin. There is a 30-fold difference between the anaesthetic dose and the lethal dose, which compares favourably with the five to tenfold difference for the intravenous barbiturates. In particular, etomidate has little or no adverse effects on the cardiovascular system. It usually causes a slight fall in peripheral resistance and blood pressure; blood flow in most organs is generally unchanged or slightly increased. Myocardial contractility, oxygen consumption, and coronary blood flow are usually unaffected. Etomidate reduces cerebral blood flow and intracranial pressure, and hypnotic doses cause respiratory depression (as assessed by the changes in ventilation produced by alterations in inspired Pco$_2$).

Both anaphylactic and anaphylactoid reactions to etomidate are uncommon. Occasionally, histamine release from mast cells causes skin rashes during the induction of anaesthesia. Severe reactions (e.g. generalized erythema, hypotension, and bronchospasm) appear to be commoner when etomidate is used with other drugs. In these conditions, it is difficult or impossible to incriminate the causative drug.

After intravenous etomidate, there is usually a biexponential decline in the plasma concentration of the drug. The initial fall in concentration (half-life = 2–5 min) reflects the distribution of the drug to well-perfused tissues. The subsequent slower decline in plasma concentration is due to the elimination of etomidate from the body (terminal half-life = 68–75 min). The apparent volume of distribution of etomidate is slightly greater than total body water, and its clearance is approximately 50–80% of liver blood flow (Table 6.2). The relatively high extraction ratio is consistent with 'flow-limited' hepatic clearance (although it is uncertain whether the liver is the only organ concerned with the metabolism of etomidate). Etomidate is bound to plasma albumin to a significant extent (i.e. 70–80%), and the effects of the drug may be enhanced in the elderly and in hypoalbuminaemic states.

Etomidate is mainly eliminated from the body by metabolism, and only trace amounts (1–2% of the dose) are detected in urine and bile. The drug is mainly metabolized by ester hydrolysis to ethyl alcohol and its corresponding carboxylic acid (l-(α-methylbenzyl)-imidazole-5-carboxylic acid). The metabolism of etomidate appears to be mainly dependent on non-specific hepatic esterases, although the drug may also be hydrolysed by plasma cholinesterase. Etomidate can also inhibit plasma cholinesterase, since it may compete with other substrates for the enzyme.

In spite of its advantages, several undesirable effects have restricted the use of etomidate in anaesthetic practice. In the first place, etomidate may cause local pain on intravenous injection. This phenomenon occurs in 25–50% of patients, and is commoner when slow injections are given into small veins (e.g. on the back of the hand or the wrist). Its incidence can be reduced by premedication or pretreatment with benzodiazepines or opioid analgesics. Secondly, etomidate commonly causes excitatory effects, particularly spontaneous movements and hypertonicity of voluntary muscle. These phenomena can also be modified by suitable premedication, or the prior administration of alfentanil or fentanyl. Finally, postoperative nausea and vomiting are commoner after etomidate (when compared with other intravenous induction agents).

Prolonged intravenous infusions of etomidate cause suppression of adrenocortical function. In these conditions, etomidate impairs the synthesis of both glucocorticoids (cortisol) and mineralocorticoids (aldosterone) by the adrenal cortex. The characteristic adrenal response to stress and ACTH is also inhibited. Qualitatively similar biochemical effects probably occur when single doses of etomidate are used to induce anaesthesia. These effects probably reflect the suppressant effects of etomidate on adrenocortical enzymes concerned with steroid hydroxylation. Since etomidate is an imidazole derivative, it will suppress hydroxylation in the adrenal cortex, and thus impair the synthesis of hydrocortisone (cortisol) and aldosterone. For similar reasons, it may interfere with hepatic oxidative drug metabolism by cytochrome P-450. These considerations suggest that etomidate may indirectly induce ('derepress') the enzyme ALA synthetase, and thus increase the formation of porphobilinogen and other porphyrins. For these reasons, the use of etomidate should be avoided in patients with acute intermittent porphyria.

PROPOFOL

Propofol (2,6-diisopropylphenol; Fig. 6.1) is a chemically inert phenolic derivative with anaesthetic properties. It has a high lipid solubility, but is almost insoluble in water; the original preparation contained the solubilizing agent Cremophor EL (polyethoxylated castor oil). This formulation was assessed in a number of preliminary clinical studies, but was discarded due to the anaphylactoid potential of Cremophor EL. In the current preparation, propofol is available as a 1% (10 mg ml^{-1}) isotonic emulsion, which contains soybean oil and purified egg phosphatide.

The normal induction dose of propofol (1.5–2.5 mg kg^{-1}) produces rapid loss of consciousness, due to the immediate uptake of the lipid-soluble drug by the CNS. Within several minutes of intravenous administration, the plasma concentration of propofol decreases, due to the distribution of the drug throughout the body and its uptake by peripheral tissues. As the plasma concentration falls, propofol is rapidly removed from the CNS; consequently, when bolus doses of the drug are used to induce anaesthesia, there is a rapid recovery of full consciousness and awareness. Postoperative nausea and vomiting appear to be extremely uncommon. In general, its safety margin is less than etomidate but greater than the intravenous barbiturates. The rapid recovery from anaesthesia is one of the most significant clinical advantages of propofol, and makes it a suitable agent for short procedures and day-case surgery (Table 6.1).

The mode of action of propofol on the CNS is uncertain, although it is generally assumed to act in a similar manner to other intravenous anaesthetics. Recent experimental evidence suggests that propofol potentiates inhibitory transmission in the CNS by facilitating the postsynaptic actions of GABA (γ-aminobutyric acid). Thus it appears to act in a similar manner to barbiturates and certain other hypnotics and anaesthetics. In general, drugs that potentiate GABA-mediated inhibitory transmission act at the benzodiazepine binding site (e.g. the benzodiazepines) or directly interact with the GABA$_A$ receptor complex (e.g. barbiturates; Chapter 12). Propofol is unlikely to directly interact with benzodiazepine receptors, since its anaesthetic effects are not modified by the benzodiazepine antagonist flumazenil.

Similarly, propofol does not mimic the effects of GABA when it is directly applied to the cerebral cortex of experimental animals. These considerations suggest that propofol primarily and directly affects chloride ion channels in the CNS (presumably by increasing mean channel opening times in a similar manner to the intravenous barbiturates). Propofol has no effect on excitatory transmission mediated by amino acid neurotransmitters (e.g. aspartate and glutamate).

Propofol frequently causes a significant reduction in systolic and diastolic blood pressure, which may fall to 70–80% of its pre-injection level. Hypotension is related to the dose and the rapidity of intravenous injection, and is usually maximal within 5–10 min. The reduction in blood pressure is mainly due to decreased systemic vascular resistance, and is not usually accompanied by reflex tachycardia. Indeed, cardiac output may fall slightly (presumably due to the direct effects of propofol on the heart). In experimental studies, propofol increases the threshold to adrenaline-induced arrhythmias, when compared to halothane anaesthesia. When propofol is injected as a soybean oil–egg phosphatide emulsion, hypersensitivity and anaphylactoid responses appear to be uncommon, although local oedema, bronchospasm, laryngospasm, and hypotension are occasionally observed. These reactions are probably due to the release of histamine and other mediators from mast cells.

Propofol is extensively bound to plasma proteins; after anaesthetic doses, approximately 97–98% is bound to plasma albumin. After intravenous injection, the plasma concentration of propofol usually declines in a biexponential or a triexponential manner. The initial fall in concentration has an extremely rapid half-life (1–3 min), reflecting the almost immediate distribution of the lipid-soluble drug from plasma to tissues. Indeed, most of the drug removed from the blood in the first 2 hours is due to tissue uptake. Estimated values for pharma-cokinetic constants after injection of propofol are extremely variable. In early studies, it was suggested that the terminal half-life of propofol was 1–5 h, and that the total apparent volume of distribution of the drug was approximately ten times greater than total body water. The clearance of propofol was more than liver blood flow, suggesting that there might be significant extrahepatic meta-bolism of the drug. More recent studies have thrown some doubt on these con-cepts. Prolonged blood sampling suggests that the half-life of propofol is about 60 h, and that its clearance is usually less than hepatic blood flow (i.e. approxi-mately 1000 ml min^{-1}). These studies suggest that the elimination of propofol is entirely dependent on hepatic metabolism, and may be sensitive to changes in liver blood flow (but not to protein binding or enzyme activity). Propofol is mainly metabolized to the glucuronide conjugates of 2,6-diisopropylphenol and 2,6-diisopropylquinol. These conjugates are subsequently eliminated in urine. There is no evidence that propofol adversely affects renal or hepatic function, or induces enzymes involved in drug metabolism or porphyrin synthesis.

The main advantage of propofol in clinical practice is that rapid recovery of full consciousness and awareness occurs when bolus doses are used to induce anaesthesia; similarly, significant cumulation does not usually occur after infusion or repeated administration of the drug. Nevertheless, a number of studies suggest that the drug has a relatively long half-life, and prolonged infusions and multiple doses should be used with caution. Occasionally, the prolonged infusion of propofol is associated with delayed recovery from the effects of the drug (Table 6.1).

When injected into small veins on the dorsum of the hand or the wrist, propofol causes discomfort or pain in 30–40% of patients. This complication is less common when the drug is injected into veins in the antecubital fossa. Spontaneous movements, tremor, and hypotonus are occasionally observed, but are less common than with methohexitone or etomidate. There is no definitive evidence that propofol has significant effects on hepatic or renal function, or that the drug adversely affects steroid synthesis by the adrenal cortex.

The pharmacological properties and pharmacokinetics of propofol are summarized in Tables 6.1 and 6.2.

KETAMINE

Ketamine ((2-chlorophenyl)-2-(methylamino)-cyclohexanone hydrochloride) (Fig. 6.1) is chemically related to cyclohexamine and phencyclidine. Although it does not usually produce loss of consciousness in one arm–brain circulation time, it is commonly classified as an induction agent. Ketamine hydrochloride is freely soluble in water, forming an acidic solution (pH = 3.5–5.5). Three different concentrations (10 mg ml^{-1}, 50 mg ml^{-1}, and 100 mg ml^{-1}) are available for intravenous injection (dose = 1–2 mg kg^{-1}) or intramuscular administration (dose = 5–10 mg kg^{-1}). Ketamine is a racemic mixture of two enantiomers; the (+) enantiomer is 3.4 times more potent than the (−) isomer.

Ketamine differs from other intravenous agents (Table 6.1); it is almost devoid of hypnotic properties, but produces a state of 'dissociative anaesthesia', in which dose-related anterograde amnesia and profound analgesia are present. The drug has a relatively slow onset of action, when compared with other intravenous anaesthetics. After intravenous injection, up to 90 seconds may elapse before effects on the CNS are observed; after intramuscular administration, a delay of up to 8 min usually occurs. It can be difficult to determine the precise time of the onset of action, and patients may gaze into the distance for several minutes without closing their eyes. Hypertonus and spontaneous involuntary muscle movements, including tonic–clonic activity of the limbs, may occur during induction. Muscular relaxation is often poor, and the tone of the jaw muscles may be increased, causing obstruction of the airway. Respiratory activity is little affected (although respiratory rate may slightly increase), and the response to alterations in $Paco_2$ is normal. Coughing and laryngospasm are extremely rare; indeed, experimental studies suggest that ketamine antagonizes the effects of histamine, acetylcholine, and 5-hydroxytryptamine on bronchial smooth muscle. The drug can be safely used in asthmatic patients. Although most reflex responses are not affected by ketamine, some depression of laryngeal reflexes may occur. This usually precludes its use for operations on the upper airway.

In contrast to most other anaesthetic agents, ketamine invariably produces tachycardia, increases cardiac output, and raises plasma noradrenaline concentrations. Both systolic and diastolic blood pressures (as well as pulmonary vascular resistance and arterial pressure) are usually increased by 20–40%. These changes usually occur within 5 min, and last for 10–20 min. Nevertheless, cardiac arrhythmias are extremely uncommon, and ketamine may produce an increase in peripheral blood flow. The effects of ketamine on the cardiovascular system are probably secondary to its direct action on neuronal pathways in the CNS; they are not produced by peripheral effects at sites that are innervated by the sympathetic nervous system. Ketamine also affects the brain and the cerebral circulation, and cerebral blood flow, oxygen consumption, CSF tension, and intracranial pressure are all increased.

The duration of action of ketamine (like that of most other intravenous anaesthetic agents) is dependent on the dose of the drug. Normal intravenous doses (2 mg kg^{-1}) act for 10–20 min, although the precise duration of action may be difficult to assess. Nausea and vomiting are not infrequent during the postoperative period. In addition, there is a significant possibility of emergence phenomena, ranging from vivid dreams and visual images to hallucinations and delirium, which may continue for 24 h after administration (Table 6.1). Psychotomimetic sequelae may be extremely unpleasant, and it has been suggested that they are due to the misperception or misinterpretation of sensory information (particularly visual or auditory stimuli). Emergence phenomena may be considerably modified by the use of appropriate premedication with opiates, benzodiazepines, or droperidol (which itself may give rise to psychotomimetic side-effects). They tend to be commoner in women, but are relatively rare in children, particularly when their postoperative recovery is undisturbed.

The effect of ketamine on the CNS is associated with characteristic changes in the EEG. The α-rhythm is usually depressed, and is replaced by θ- and δ-wave activity. These changes may persist for the duration of analgesia. Electrophysiological studies suggest that ketamine mainly affects thalamocortical projection pathways, and has only minimal effects on the reticular activating system, the limbic system, and most thalamic nuclei. Analgesia may be due to effects on afferent pathways in the spinoreticular tracts that are concerned with the perception of pain, or to the binding of the drug by opioid receptors (particularly δ-receptors). More recent evidence suggests that ketamine and other phencyclidine analogues specifically antagonize glutamate (an excitatory neurotransmitter) at certain receptor sites in the CNS (i.e. at NMDA receptors). Antagonism between ketamine and NMDA (*N*-methyl-D-aspartate) is non-competitive, suggesting that the drug may produce indirect changes at receptor sites (e.g. it may produce conformational changes in ion channels that are normally activated by glutamate and other excitatory amino acids). In the CNS, glutamate is known to be released at corticostriate nerve endings, and plays an important role as a central neurotransmitter.

Ketamine is approximately 45% non-ionized (i.e. lipid-soluble) at pH 7.4. After intravenous administration, the drug is rapidly distributed in tissues and readily crosses the blood–brain barrier and the placental barrier. Plasma concentrations usually decrease in a biexponential manner; the initial rapid fall in plasma concentration (half-life $= 10-20\,\text{min}$) is followed by a slower decline (half-life $= 150-200\,\text{min}$), which is due to the elimination of ketamine (mainly by hepatic metabolism). The apparent distribution volume of ketamine is two to three times greater than total body water, and its clearance is approximately equal to liver blood flow. The relatively high extraction ratio is consistent with 'flow-limited' hepatic clearance, and drugs that reduce liver blood flow (e.g. inhalational anaesthetics, β-adrenoceptor antagonists, and cimetidine) can decrease ketamine clearance and prolong its terminal half-life. After intramuscular administration, ketamine is rapidly absorbed, and maximum plasma concentrations are invariably present within 30 min.

Ketamine is mainly eliminated from the body by hepatic metabolism; this is dependent on the mixed function oxidase system associated with the smooth endoplasmic reticulum (cytochrome P-450). Its main metabolite is norketamine (the demethylated analogue of ketamine). Norketamine has some hypnotic activity, but is generally less potent than ketamine. Both ketamine and norketamine may be further metabolized to hydroxylated derivatives, which are subsequently conjugated and eliminated as glucuronides (Table 6.2).

Ketamine has only a limited place in current anaesthetic practice, due to its undesirable effects on the CNS and the cardiovascular system. It is usually avoided in patients with cardiac impairment, hypertension, or a history of psychotic illness. Nevertheless, the drug has a definite role in certain situations. In paediatric practice, it is a useful agent when venepuncture is difficult or poorly tolerated, or when repeated anaesthesia is necessary. Thus, it may be used to provide anaesthesia for cardiac catheterization, burns dressings, and other minor procedures (e.g. radiotherapy and bone marrow biopsy). In adults, the indications for its use are more controversial and less well defined. It may be of value for repeated burns dressings, in the poor-risk elderly patient, and in certain emergency situations.

ADVERSE REACTIONS TO INTRAVENOUS ANAESTHETIC AGENTS

There has been a progressive increase in the apparent incidence of hypersensitivity reactions to intravenous anaesthetic agents since the first conclusive case associated with the use of thiopentone was reported in 1952. The increase has coincided with the introduction and use of many non-barbiturate agents; in recent years, two intravenous anaesthetics (i.e. propanidid and Althesin) have been withdrawn due to the adverse reactions associated with their use.

The incidence and severity of anaphylactoid and hypersensitivity reactions to intravenous anaesthetic agents is difficult to assess. In many instances, some undesirable effects (e.g. hypotension) may be due to the direct actions of anaesthetic agents on vascular smooth muscle, or an enhanced vasovagal response to venepuncture. In addition, mechanical problems with the airway related to kinked or misplaced endotracheal tubes may present as apparent bronchospasm. Anaesthetic techniques usually involve some polypharmacy, and the part played by other drugs (e.g. opiates, antimuscarinic drugs, and muscle relaxants) may be difficult to assess. On the other hand, it seems probable that many cases are unreported (particularly those in which serious sequelae do not occur).

Adverse reactions to thiopentone are relatively uncommon; when they occur, they usually have serious consequences, and a number of deaths have been associated with hypersensitivity reactions to thiopentone (Table 6.3). The incidence of adverse reactions to other intravenous anaesthetic agents is extremely variable. In recent years, two intravenous anaesthetics (propanidid and Althesin) have been withdrawn due to the relatively high incidence of anaphylactoid reactions associated with their use. In some surveys, these were as common as 1 in 100 to 1 in 1000. Both propanidid and Althesin contained the solubilizing agent Cremophor EL (polyethoxylated castor oil), which is a mixture of fatty acids with a molecular weight of approximately 3200. Cremophor EL is also present in some vitamin preparations and antifungal drugs. Although early studies suggested that Cremophor EL has little or no immunogenic or

Table 6.3 Incidence of hypersensitivity responses associated with intravenous anaesthetic agents.

Drug	Reported incidences	Number of deaths
Thiopentone	1 in 23 000 1 in 29 000 1 in 36 000	7
Methohexitone	1 in 7 000 1 in 22 000	0
Etomidate	3 in 1 400*	0
Propofol	0	0
Ketamine	0	0

* Skin manifestations only.

anaphylactoid potential, most of the recent evidence suggests that it plays a crucial role in the occurrence of adverse reactions to intravenous anaesthetics. Alternatively, its surfactant properties may enhance the immunogenic potential of propanidid and alphaxalone (the active steroid in Althesin).

The clinical features of hypersensitivity and anaphylactoid reactions to intravenous anaesthetics may include erythema, oedema, urticaria, bronchospasm, hypotension, peripheral vascular collapse, and occasionally abdominal pain. The clinical course of the reaction is variable; localized or generalized vasodilatation may occur within seconds of the injection, and can be rapidly followed by bronchospasm and cyanosis. The pulse may be impalpable and the blood pressure unrecordable (although the ECG shows an increase in heart rate). Localized or generalized oedema may subsequently develop. Occasionally, reactions to intravenous anaesthetics have a slower onset (over 10–90 min); their clinical features are usually relatively benign and their cause may not be recognized.

Many of the clinical features of anaphylactoid and hypersensitivity reactions resemble the pharmacological effects of histamine in man, or may be produced by other mediators of hypersensitivity reactions. After the induction of anaesthesia with intravenous agents, plasma concentrations of histamine are frequently raised, and may be related to the high local concentrations of the drug (which in turn is dependent on the dose and the rate of injection). When reactions to intravenous anaesthetics occur, there may be a close relation between the plasma concentration of histamine and the clinical severity of the reaction. Nevertheless, other mediators may also be involved (e.g. bradykinin, 5-hydroxytryptamine, leukotrienes and prostaglandins).

At least three mechanisms may be responsible for the increased plasma concentrations of histamine:

1 Histamine may be directly released from tissue mast cells and circulating basophil leucocytes. In these conditions, histamine release is usually dose related, and previous exposure or sensitization to the intravenous agent is usually unnecessary. These reactions are frequently referred to as 'anaphylactoid' or 'histamine-releasing' reactions, in order to distinguish them from hypersensitivity reactions involving immunoglobulins or complement activation ('anaphylactic' reactions). Anaphylactoid reactions usually account for the erythema and unexpected hypotension which is not infrequently observed after the induction of anaesthesia. A number of other agents used in anaesthetic practice (e.g. tubocurarine, morphine, pethidine, and polygeline) may also cause anaphylactoid reactions.

2 Type 1 hypersensitivity reactions may cause histamine release (Chapter 5). These reactions usually depend on previous exposure and sensitization to the intravenous agent, and the production of reaginic antibodies (usually IgE immunoglobulins). Occasionally IgG is involved in this type of reaction. The antibodies become bound to mast cells and basophils; subsequent exposure to the agent results in an antigen–antibody reaction on the mast cell membrane, and the disruption of its cytoplasmic granules. Subsequently, histamine and other mediators are released into the circulation (e.g. leukotrienes, prostaglandins, anaphylatoxin and chemotactic factors).

3 Complement activation (either by the classical pathway or the alternate pathway) may release histamine from mast cells. Activation of the classical pathway results in the consumption of C4 and C3 and the formation of C3a (anaphylatoxin). In the alternate pathway, a large proportion of C3 is converted to anaphylatoxins (C3a and C5a). Many of the reactions to Althesin involved the alternate pathway of complement activation.

Prevention of reactions

1 The rate of injection and the dose of the induction agent should be carefully considered. The severity of many reactions is reduced by the slow administration of moderate doses of intravenous agents.

2 Patients with a history of allergy or atopy may be especially prone to Type 1 hypersensitivity responses (particularly when there is evidence of increased IgE concentrations). The repeated exposure of these patients to induction agents known to produce reactions is particularly dangerous. Unfortunately, when two or more agents are given almost simultaneously, it may not be easy to identify the causative agent. Patients who have previously developed reactions to an identified agent can usually be safely anaesthetized with an alternative drug.

3 In certain circumstances, intradermal testing may be of value. It should be recognized that this procedure could provoke a systemic reaction, and facilities for resuscitation should always be available.

4 Patients who are considered to be at risk should probably be premedicated with a H_1-receptor antagonist and an H_2-receptor antagonist.

Treatment

The diagnosis should be firmly established and airway obstruction mimicking bronchospasm must be excluded.

Hypotension and peripheral circulatory collapse should be managed by tilting the patient in the head-down position and the infusion of colloid or crystalloid solutions as plasma expanders; 1–2 litres may be required, as a similar volume is rapidly lost by extravasation into tissues. In addition, intravenous adrenaline (1 in 10 000, i.e. $100\,\mu g\ ml^{-1}$) may be required in 50–100 µg increments. The drug should rapidly restore peripheral vascular tone, and may prevent the further release of histamine and other mediators from mast cells. Hydrocortisone hemisuccinate (100–200 mg) may also be of value, although the maximum response may be delayed for 1–3 h.

Bronchospasm is usually treated by the slow intravenous administration of aminophylline (250–500 mg) or salbutamol (250–500 μg). Hydrocortisone hemi-succinate (100–200 mg) may also be valuable. If not already instituted, endotra-cheal intubation and positive pressure ventilation with oxygen may be necessary. This is often of value in reactions in which bronchospasm and laryngeal oedema are minimal.

Antihistamines (i.e. H_1-receptor antagonists) are often useful in the treat-ment of urticaria, and in the prevention of glottic oedema. Chlorpheniramine (10–20 mg) is probably the drug of choice.

TOTAL INTRAVENOUS ANAESTHESIA

Total intravenous anaesthesia (or continuous infusion anaesthesia) is usually applied to techniques in which all anaesthetic agents are given intravenously during major surgical procedures. Thus, intravenous anaesthetics are used to induce hypnosis, opioids are given to prevent intraoperative pain, and neuro-muscular blockade is induced during controlled ventilation with air enriched with oxygen. In recent years, there has been considerable interest in total intravenous anaesthesia, due to environmental considerations and the introduction of drugs with suitable pharmacokinetic properties (e.g. propofol, alfentanil and atracur-ium). The use of continuous infusion techniques has considerable practical advantages, including minimal cardiovascular depression, rapid recovery, and the elimination of the hazards of exposure to inhalational agents. Unfortunately, they are relatively expensive, since they usually depend on the accurate and controlled infusion of drugs with a short duration of action and a rapid recovery. In addition, they require precise pharmacokinetic data that have been previously generated in a defined patient population, as well as the determination and assessment of the various factors that are liable to influence the behaviour of drugs in the body. Thus, the concurrent administration of other drugs as well as cardiovascular, renal, and hepatic impairment may affect the disposition and the activity of many intravenous agents. Present evidence suggests that there is considerable inter-individual variability in the metabolism and elimination of anaesthetic drugs; at least some of this variability may be determined by genetic factors. In recent years, there have also been problems with the accurate measurement of the plasma concentrations of certain drugs (e.g. opioid analgesics). For all these reasons, total intravenous anaesthesia is not a practical proposition at present; it remains a possible goal for the future.

FURTHER READING

Aveling W, Sear JW, Fitch W *et al*. Early clinical evaluation of minaxolone: a new intravenous steroid anaesthetic agent. *Lancet* 1979; **ii**: 71–73.

Avery AF, Evans A. Reactions to Althesin. *British Journal of Anaesthesia* 1973; **45**: 301–303.

Breimer DD. Pharmacokinetics of methohexitone following intravenous infusion in humans. *British Journal of Anaesthesia* 1976; **48**: 643–649.

Briggs LP, Clarke RSJ, Dundee JW, Wright PJ, Moore J, Bahar M, Wright PJ. Use of di-isopropylphenol as main agent for short procedures. *British Journal of Anaesthesia* 1981; **53**: 1197–1202.

Brown SS, Dundee JW. Clinical studies of induction agents. XXV: Diazepam. *British Journal of Anaesthesia* 1968; **40**: 108–112.

Christensen JH, Andreasen F, Janssen JA. Influence of age and sex on the pharmacokinetics of thiopentone. *British Journal of Anaesthesia* 1981; **53**: 1189–1196.

Christensen JH, Andreasen F, Janssen JA. Pharmacokinetics and pharmacodynamics of thiopentone — a comparison between young and elderly patients. *Anaesthesia* 1982; **37**: 398–404.

Christensen JH, Andreasen F, Janssen JA. Thiopentone sensitivity in young and elderly women. *British Journal of Anaesthesia* 1983; **55**: 33–39.

Clarke RSJ, Dundee JW, Barron DW, McArdle L, Howard PJ. Clinical studies of induction agents. XXVI: The relative potencies of thiopentone, methohexitone and propanidid. *British Journal of Anaesthesia* 1968; **40**: 593–601.

Clarke RSJ, Dundee JW, Carson IW. A new steroid anaesthetic — Althesin. *Proceedings of the Royal Society of Medicine* 1973; **66**: 1027–1029.

Collins GGS. Effects of the anaesthetic 2,6-diisopropylphenol on synaptic transmission in the rat olfactory cortex slice. *British Journal of Pharmacology* 1988; **95**: 939–949.

Doenicke A. Etomidate, a new intravenous hypnotic. *Acta Anaesthesiologica Belgica* 1974; **25**: 307–315.

Doenicke J, Kugler J, Penzel G *et al.* Hirnfunktion und Toleranzbreite nach Etomidate einem neuen barbituratfreien i.v. applizierbaren Hypnoticum. *Der Anaesthesist* 1973; **22**: 357–366.

Domino EF, Chodoff P, Corssen G. Pharmacologic effects of CI 581, a new dissociative anesthetic in man. *Clinical Pharmacology and Therapeutics* 1965; **6**: 279–290.

Dundee JW. Ketamine. *Proceedings of the Royal Society of Medicine* 1971; **64**: 39–40.

Dundee JW, Barron DW. The barbiturates. *British Journal of Anaesthesia* 1962; **34**: 240–246.

Dundee JW, Clarke RSJ. Propofol. *European Journal of Anaesthesiology* 1989; **6**: 5–22.

Dundee JW, Knox JWD, Black GW *et al.* Ketamine as an induction agent in anaesthetics. *Lancet* 1970; **i**: 1370–1371.

Dundee JW, McIlroy PDA. The history of the barbiturates. *Anaesthesia* 1982; **37**: 726–734.

Dundee JW, Moore J. Thiopentone and methohexital. A comparison as main anaesthetic agents for a standard operation. *Anaesthesia* 1961; **16**: 50–60.

Dundee JW, Price HL, Dripps RD. Acute tolerance to thiopentone in man. *British Journal of Anaesthesia* 1956; **28**: 344–352.

Dundee JW, Wyant GM. *Intravenous Anaesthesia*. Edinburgh: Churchill Livingstone, 1988; 1–358.

Edwards R, Ellis FR. Clinical significance of thiopentone binding to haemoglobin and plasma protein. *British Journal of Anaesthesia* 1973; **45**: 891–893.

Gjessing J. Ketamine (CI-581) in clinical anaesthesia. *Acta Anaesthesiologica Scandinavica* 1968; **12**: 15–21.

Healy TEJ, Hoffbrand BI, Kay B *et al.* Propofol ('Diprivan'). A new intravenous anaesthetic. *Postgraduate Medical Journal* 1985; **61** (Suppl. 3): 3–169.

Horton JN. Adverse reaction to Althesin. *Anaesthesia* 1973; **28**: 182–183.

Hudson RJ, Stanski DR. Burch PG. Pharmacokinetics of methohexital and thiopental in surgical patients. *Anesthesiology* 1983; **59**: 215–219.

Jarman R, Abel AL. Intravenous anaesthesia with pentothal sodium. *Lancet* 1936; **230 (i)**: 422–423.

Jessop E, Grounds RM, Morgan M, Lumley J. Comparison of infusions of propofol and methohexitone to provide light general anaesthesia during surgery with regional blockade. *British Journal of Anaesthesia* 1985; **57**: 1173–1177.

Johnston R, Noseworthy TW, Anderson B, Konopad E, Grace M. Propofol versus thiopentone for outpatient anaesthesia. *Anesthesiology* 1987; **67**: 431–433.

Kay B. A clinical assessment of the use of etomidate in children. *British Journal of Anaesthesia* 1976; **48**: 207–211.

Knell PJW. Total intravenous anaesthesia by an intermittent technique. Use of methohexitone, ketamine and a muscle relaxant. *Anaesthesia* 1983; **38**: 586–587.

Langrehr D. Dissoziative anästhesie durch Ketamine. *Actuelle Chirurgie* 1969; **4**: 71–78.

Lowenstein E, Hallowell P, Levine FH, Daggett WM, Austen WG, Laver MB. Cardiovascular response to large doses of intravenous morphine in man. *New England Journal of Medicine* 1969; **281**: 1389–1393.

Logan MR, Duggan JE, Levack ID, Spence AA. Single-shot i.v. anaesthesia for outpatient dental anaesthesia. Comparison of 2,6-diisopropylphenol and methohexitone. *British Journal of Anaesthesia* 1987; **59**: 179–183.

Lundy JS. Intravenous anesthesia: preliminary report of the use of two new thiobarbiturates. *Proceedings of Staff Meetings of the Mayo Clinic* 1935; **10**: 534–543.

Lundy JS, Tovell RM. Some of the newer local and general anesthetic agents. Methods of their administration. *Northwest Medicine* (Seattle) 1934; **33**: 308–311.

McCarthy DA, Chen G, Laump DH, Ensor C. General anesthetic and other pharmacological properties of 2-(O-chlorophenyl)-2-methylamino-cyclohexanone HCl (CI-581). *Journal of New Drugs* 1965; **5**: 21–33.

McClish A. Diazepam as an intravenous induction agent for general anaesthesia. *Canadian Anaesthetists' Society Journal* 1966; **13**: 562–575.

Mackenzie N, Grant IS. Comparison of the new emulsion formulation of propofol with methohexitone and thiopentone for induction of anaesthesia in day cases. *British Journal of Anaesthesia* 1985; **57**: 725–731.

Major E, Verniquet AJW, Waddell TK, Savege TM, Hoffler DE, Aveling W. A study of three doses of ICI 35868 for induction and maintenance of anaesthesia. *British Journal of Anaesthesia* 1981; **53**: 267–272.

Miller E, Munch JC, Crossley FS, Hartung WH. Thiobarbiturates. *Journal of the American Chemical Society* 1936; **58**: 1090–1091.

Morgan M. Total intravenous anaesthesia. Anaesthesia 1983; **38** (Supplement): 1–72.

Morgan M, Lunn JN. Experiences with propofol. *Anaesthesia* 1988; **43** (Supplement): 1–121.

Morton NS, Wee M, Christie G, Gray IG, Grant IS. Propofol for induction of anaesthesia in children. A comparison with thiopentone and halothane inhalational induction. *Anaesthesia* 1988; **43**: 350–355.

Pandit SK, Kothary SP, Kumar SM. Low dose intravenous infusion technique with ketamine. *Anaesthesia* 1980; **35**: 669–675.

Paul DL, Logan MR, Wildsmith JAW. Which intravenous induction agent for day case surgery? A comparison of propofol, thiopentone, methohexitone and etomidate. *Anaesthesia* 1988; **43**: 362–364.

Sanders LD, Isaac PA, Yeomans WA, Clyburn PA, Rosen M, Robinson JO. Propofol-induced anaesthesia. Double-blind comparison of recovery after anaesthesia induced by propofol or thiopentone. *Anaesthesia* 1989; **44**: 200–204.

Schuermans V, Dom J, Dony J, Scheijgrond H, Brugmans J. Multinational evaluation of etomidate for anesthesia induction. Conclusions and consequences. *Anaesthesist* 1978; **27**: 52–59.

Selye H. Studies concerning the correlation between anesthetic potency, hormonal activity and chemical structure among steroid compounds. *Anesthesia and Analgesia* 1942; **21**: 41–47.

Servin F, Desmonts JM, Haberer JP, Cockshott ID, Plummer GF, Farinotti R. Pharmacokinetics and protein-binding of propofol in patients with cirrhosis. *Anesthesiology* 1988; **69**: 887–891.

Stanski DR. Intravenous barbiturates. *Anaesthesia* 1981; **36**: 548–549.

Stoelting VK. Use of a new intravenous oxygen barbiturate 25398 for intravenous anesthesia. *Anesthesia and Analgesia* 1957; **36**: 49–51.

Valtonen M, Iisalo E, Kanto J, Rosenberg P. Propofol as an induction agent in children: pain on injection and pharmacokinetics. *Acta Anaesthesiologica Scandinavica* 1989; **33**: 152–155.

Weese H, Scharpff W. Evipan, ein neuartiges Einschlafmittel. *Deutsche Medizinische Wochenschrift* 1932; **58**: 1205–1207.

White PF, Ham J, Way WL, Trevor AJ. Pharmacology of ketamine isomers in surgical patients. *Anesthesiology* 1980; **52**: 231–239.

Whitwam JG. Methohexitone. *British Journal of Anaesthesia* 1976; **48**: 617–619.

Wyant GM, Barr JS. Further comparative studies of sodium methohexital. *Canadian Anaesthetists Society Journal* 1960; **7**: 127–135.

Wyant GM, Chang CA. Sodium methohexital: a clinical study. *Canadian Anaesthetists Society Journal* 1959; **6**: 40–50.

SEVEN

Inhalational Anaesthetic Agents

Although the introduction of inhalational anaesthetics revolutionised operative surgery, their general acceptance by the medical profession was relatively slow. The effects of nitrous oxide on sensation and voluntary power were described by Joseph Priestley as early as 1772; nevertheless, the gas was not generally used as an analgesic or an inhalational anaesthetic until well into the 19th Century. Diethylether and chloroform, which were initially used in the 1840s, were more rapidly accepted. There were few further significant advances until 1934, when trichlorethylene and cyclopropane were introduced into anaesthetic practice. Some 20 years later halothane was synthesized, and its general acceptance was followed by the introduction of other fluorinated anaesthetics, e.g. methoxyflurane, enflurane and isoflurane.

In the early days of anaesthesia, administration of a single anaesthetic agent was used to produce that state of reversible insensibility associated with the loss of consciousness, absence of pain and muscular relaxation known as general anaesthesia. By contrast, during the past 25 years 'balanced' techniques have become widely used, in which three different drugs are used to cause these effects. By this approach, the hazards of general anaesthesia are greatly reduced and postoperative recovery of vital functions is relatively rapid.

Drugs that are classified as inhalational anaesthetics primarily produce loss of consciousness; however, they may also produce significant analgesia (e.g. nitrous oxide, methoxyflurane, enflurane, isoflurane) or muscle relaxation (particularly enflurane and isoflurane). They are stored either as gases or volatile liquids at ambient temperatures, although in practice this distinction is unimportant.

MODE OF ACTION

Sites of action in the CNS

Study of evoked cortical responses in the anaesthetized state has revealed that the *primary* effect of anaesthetics is on transmission of information from the periphery to the cortex. The main site in the pathway that is affected is at the level of the ventrobasal thalamus. However, there are also effects on cortical level V, the reticular activating system, basal ganglia, cerebellum, sensory and motor pathways in the spinal cord and medullary centres concerned with control of respiration and vascular tone. It is probable that instead of being dependent solely on depression of reticular nuclei, the neurological manifestations of anaesthesia are due to actions at different sites within the CNS depending on the agent used. Furthermore, there is some experimental evidence that suggests that cortical cells are more sensitive to inhalational anaesthetics than the reticular activating system, in spite of the large number of synaptic relays in the latter. Indeed, polysynaptic transmission may be less sensitive to inhalational anaesthetic agents than monosynaptic transmission.

Basic physical principles underlying the action of inhalational agents

Due to the rapid onset and reversibility of most inhalational anaesthetics, it appears improbable that they act by means of the formation of stable covalent chemical bonds in the CNS. Their action is presumably dependent on their physical properties or on the presence of reversible, low-energy, intermolecular forces (e.g. Van der Waals forces, dipole–dipole interactions, or the formation of ionic and hydrogen bonds). Although the precise basis for their action has not been defined, it has been known for many years that they possess certain similar physicochemical properties. For example, all of the inhalational anaesthetics introduced into clinical practice since 1842 are either aliphatic hydrocarbons or ethers with less than four carbon atoms, and have boiling points less than 90°C (with the exception of methoxyflurane); all are lipid-soluble and the anaesthesia produced is reversed by the application of pressure. The number of agents that will behave as inhalational anaesthetics is very large and includes many gases, hydrocarbons, halogenated hydrocarbons, ethers, halogenated ethers and other organic solvents. Most are unacceptable for clinical usage because of side-effects such as convulsant activity. Interestingly, some agents only have an anaesthetic effect when given at sufficiently high partial pressures. Thus the anaesthetic effect of nitrogen gas only became evident in scuba diving; at 30 atm, nitrogen is a potent anaesthetic.

Inhalational anaesthetics vary greatly in potency (i.e. the alveolar concentration that is required to produce a given anaesthetic effect) and to some extent, this is related to molecular structure. For example, the anaesthetic potency of organic compounds increases as a given halogen is replaced with successively larger halogens. Nitrous oxide is a relatively non-potent anaesthetic and concentrations of 80% in oxygen are usually insufficient to maintain anaesthesia. By contrast, concentrations of 1–2% of halothane or enflurane will produce general

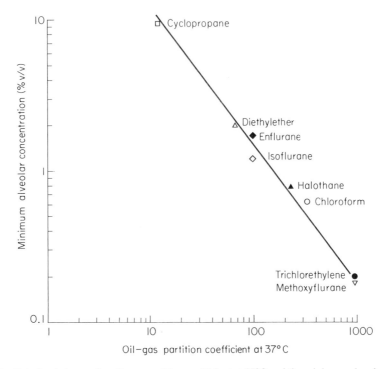

Fig. 7.1 Relation between the oil–gas partition coefficient at 37°C and the minimum alveolar concentration.

anaesthesia. When anaesthetic potency is expressed in terms of minimum alveolar concentration (MAC), i.e. the minimum concentration that produces no reaction to a surgical stimulus (skin incision) in 50% of subjects at atmospheric pressure, there is a particularly close correlation (correlation coefficient = 0.96) between potency and the oil : gas partition coefficient at 37°C when expressed on a logarithmic scale (Fig. 7.1). In general, with the exception of solubility in octanol (see below), the correlation between potency and alternative partition coefficients or other physical and chemical properties is not as marked.

An alternative to MAC is the anaesthetic dose for 95% of the population or 'AD95'. In practice, this is about 5–40% higher than the MAC of the agent and is a more useful guide to the amount of anaesthetic actually required.

The MAC of an inhalational agent is affected by many physiological and pharmacological factors, and these are summarized in Table 7.1. It should also be remembered that the effects of inhalational anaesthetic agents are additive so that, for example, 50% of the nitrous oxide MAC plus 50% of the MAC of a second drug is equal in anaesthetizing effect to that of 100% MAC of either agent alone.

Table 7.1 Some factors affecting MAC. (*Data from human studies unless otherwise stated.*)

Stimulus	Effect on MAC
General	
Type of stimulation	None
Duration of anaesthesia	None
Sex	None
Pregnancy	↓
Age	↓ in elderly; ↑ in newborns
Circadian rhythms[1]	↑ during period of greatest metabolic activity
Low body temperature[2]	↓ ↓ (for a 10°C decrease)
High body temperature[2]	Up to 42°C ↑ ; >42°C ↓
Acid–base and respiratory	
Hypocarbia (21 mmHg)	None
Hypercarbia (up to 95 mmHg)[2]	None (if CSF pH >7.10)
Hypercarbia (>95 mmHg)[2]	↓ (if CSF pH <7.10)
Metabolic acidosis[2]	↓ if end-tidal $Paco_2$ normal
Metabolic alkalosis[2]	None
Hypoxia (PaO_2 >38 mmHg)[2]	None
Hyperoxia[2]	None
Anaemia[2]	None (if haematocrit > 10%)
Cardiovascular	
Hypotension[2]	↓ (if MAP reduced by 50%)
Hypertension[2]	None
Neurotransmission	
Raised catecholamines/5HT[2]	↑ (α_2-agonists decrease MAC)
Reduced catecholamines/5HT[2]	↓
Opiate analgesics[1,2]	
acute administration	↓ (depends on dose of drug)
chronic administration	↑
Naloxone	None
Amphetamine[2]	
acute administration	↑ ↑ ↑
chronic administration	↓
Sedatives and tranquillizers	↓ ↓ (depends on dose of drug)
Ethyl alcohol	
acute administration[3,4]	↓
chronic administration[1,3]	↑ (may take many weeks to return to normal after cessation of intake)
Metabolic and biochemical	
Hypothyroid[2]	↓ (change from gross hypothyroidism to gross hyperthyroidism increases MAC by 20%)
Hyperthyroid[2]	↑
Hypermagnesaemia	↓
Hypercalcaemia[4]	↓
Hyperkalaemia[2]	None
Lithium	↓
Hypernatraemia[2]	↑ ↑
Hyponatraemia[2]	↓ (if accompanied by changes in brain sodium levels)

Single arrow, up to 30% change; two arrows, up to 60% change; and three arrows, >60% change.
[1] = rats; [2] = dogs; [3] = mice; and [4] = cats.

THEORIES OF ANAESTHESIA

Historical perspectives

Almost 90 years ago, Meyer and Overton independently showed that anaesthetic potency was closely related to the solubility of the agent in olive oil (relative to water solubility). Hence, olive oil was the first model of the CNS and it was suggested that the effects of inhalational agents were due to interaction with lipids in the CNS. The importance of the physical properties of inhalational anaesthetics was emphasized in the late 1930s by Ferguson who expressed their thermodynamic activity (or molal free energy) in terms of their effective vapour pressure. For a chemical to be usable as an anaesthetic agent, its 'activity' had to fall within a certain range regardless of the concentration.

The Overton–Meyer hypothesis has been recently re-examined by investigating the solubility of inhalational anaesthetics in a range of solvents with different properties. In particular, the partition of anaesthetics between octanol, a slightly polar solvent, and water provides a better correlation with anaesthetic potency than olive oil and water. This suggests that a pure lipid is not the best model of the CNS and that ideally, anaesthetic agents should be amphipathic, i.e. have both hydrophobic and hydrophilic properties.

Membrane structure

In the CNS and other tissues, the limiting membrane of most cells is approximately 10 nm wide and consists of a bimolecular layer of phospholipid with intercalated molecules of protein (Fig. 1.1). Some protein molecules are situated on the internal or external aspects of the membrane (extrinsic or peripheral proteins); others are contained within the lipid membrane (intrinsic or integral proteins) and may traverse the membrane. Some of them provide a ring surrounding fine pores or channels, approximately 0.5 nm in diameter (Fig. 1.1). The opening and closing of these channels leads to ionic changes that govern neuronal activity. The phospholipid components can migrate within the neuronal membrane, and are responsible for the permeability barrier that limits the diffusion of most polar compounds. The lipid immediately surrounding the membrane proteins (boundary lipid) is particularly important for modulating protein function and is in a loosely arranged state to provide room for the conformational changes that occur when proteins function.

In the past, it has been suggested that individual molecules of anaesthetic are enclosed within a cage of molecules in the brain as hydrates (or clathrates). If structural proteins formed part of the clathrate, conformational changes could occur that would interfere with the function of the cellular membrane. These concepts did not provide as good a correlation with potency as lipid solubility and are not now accepted.

Importance of lipid solubility for anaesthetic action

The correlation between oil : gas partition coefficient *in vitro* and pharmacological potency is one of the most consistent features of drugs that produce inhalational anaesthesia. This relationship has been the basis of many theories of anaesthetic action and suggests that inhalational anaesthetics mainly produce their effects by interacting at non-polar (hydrophobic) sites on the lipid or protein components of neuronal membranes in the CNS. These interactions, which then interfere with membrane function in some way such as reducing ion transport, have been thought to occur in three ways.

First, the inhalational agents may interact directly with membrane *proteins* possibly causing conformational changes in their structure. Experimental studies *in vitro* measuring optical rotation or using nuclear magnetic resonance (NMR) suggest that inhalational anaesthetics and similar molecules can cause reversible conformational changes in a number of model protein systems, e.g. albumin, haemoglobin, and acetylcholine receptor protein.

Second, inhalational anaesthetics may alter the physical conditions that determine the degree of order or disorder within the lipid membrane. The resultant increase in phospholipid mobility could indirectly modify the functional activity of membrane proteins in various ways. The membranes may be less able to accommodate the conformational changes in proteins that may be the basis for important membrane events such as transmitter release; the many interactions between protein molecules and the boundary lipids may be prevented or disrupted; or the volume and width of neuronal membranes may be increased, so that ion channels can no longer function properly. All of these possibilities have been supported by some experimental evidence. The theory that alterations in membrane disorder (or fluidity) are solely responsible for the action of inhalational anaesthetics has been discounted. The fluidity changes caused by anaesthetics in clinical concentrations are very small and equivalent to those produced in membranes by a temperature increase of about one degree. Furthermore, the suggestion that anaesthetics disorder the membrane in some way does not explain the anaesthetic action of low temperatures when a reduction in membrane fluidity should occur leading to an increase in MAC; in fact MAC decreases. Presumably the anaesthetic effect of low temperatures relates partly to a reduction in enzyme activity and partly to an increase in the hydrophobic solubility of an inhalational agent so that MAC decreases (by approximately 8% per °C) in order to maintain the same concentration at the site of action.

Third, inhalational anaesthetics may affect non-polar sites in the membrane in an inert manner and physically modify the relationship between pressure and volume within the neuronal membrane. This concept has arisen from studies on luminous bacteria, newts, and mice which showed that anaesthesia with a wide range of anaesthetic agents could be reversed when the environmental pressure is increased. The hypothesis put forward to explain this was called the 'critical volume hypothesis' which proposed that 'anaesthesia would occur when the volume of a hydrophobic region (in the cell membrane) is caused to expand beyond a certain critical amount by absorption of molecules of an inert substance'. If the volume could be restored by changes in pressure, then anaesthesia will be removed. A modification of this theory was the 'mean excess volume hypothesis' which postulated that it is not the volume of cell membrane plus anaesthetic agent that is important, but the extra increase in volume that occurs by virtue of the physical interaction between the drug and the membrane lipids. For example, if 50 ml of ethanol is mixed with 50 ml of decane (an apolar solvent), the final volume exceeds 100 ml because the molecules of the two substances do not interact. These theories have not been substantiated by further studies. In particular, non-anaesthetic molecules can also expand the membrane, and the change in membrane volume is of the same order as that caused by a temperature increase of about 1°C. Furthermore, it could be that reversibility of anaesthesia following the application of pressure is a manifestation of the high pressure neurological syndrome which occurs in humans and other mammalian species at >30 atm and is characterized by tremor, convulsions and periods of microsleep. Arousal might then be due to pressure causing a general increase in excitability counteracting the general decrease caused by anaesthetics rather than any effect on membrane volume. Undoubtedly, the phenomenon of pressure 'reversal' of anaesthesia represents an effect at multiple sites in the nervous system since analysis at a single synapse has shown pressure and anaesthesia to be additive rather than antagonistic. The observation that different agents have different pressure reversal characteristics gave rise to the 'multi-site expansion hypothesis' which proposed that anaesthesia is produced by an action at more than one molecular site. This has been supported by the fact that not all anaesthetics produce a similar state of anaesthesia, each agent producing its own pattern of CNS depression and activation.

Current theories

In the last 15 years, concepts of the molecular mechanisms of anaesthesia have changed considerably. The basis of the action of inhalational anaesthetics is now believed to be by an interference with neurotransmission, and this is probably achieved by effects at a number of sites at the cellular level rather than merely by the physical presence of an anaesthetic agent in the cell membrane. Current evidence favours action principally on membrane proteins either directly at the hydrophobic regions, indirectly via the 'boundary' lipids that immediately surround the proteins, or at the interface between the two. These proteins may form part of the ion channels in the cell membrane or part of the receptor systems that mediate the effects of synaptic transmitters. The effects of inhalational agents on intracellular processes are much less clearly defined.

Many *in vivo* studies have concentrated on looking at the effect of a variety of factors on MAC to indicate the possible cellular site(s) of action of inhalational anaesthetic agents. The usual technique has been to stimulate or block specific ion channels or receptors and then assess the subsequent effect, if any, on MAC. If the MAC alters, this suggests that the receptor or ion channel may play a role in the production of general anaesthesia. For example, α_2-adrenoreceptor agonists such as clonidine, azepexole and dexmedetomidine can reduce the MAC of inhalational agents to the point of completely replacing them. This effect can be reversed or prevented by the administration of an α-adrenoreceptor blocker such as tolazoline, idazoxan or yohimbine. This type of effect should be differentiated from the MAC reduction seen when narcotic analgesics are administered as this occurs by reducing afferent input and not by affecting the anaesthetic 'process'.

An alternative *in vivo* approach has been to administer drugs which stimulate or block a particular type of neurotransmission to see if these agents can induce anaesthesia. Recently, a γ-aminobutyric acid analogue has been shown to produce anaesthesia in rats and mice.

In vitro studies have investigated the interaction between inhalational anaesthetic agents and a particular aspect of normal cellular function. These drugs have been shown to:(1) affect the way in which endogenous ligands bind to their receptors, (2) disturb the opening and closing of ion channels, (3) impair neurotransmitter release, and (4) alter the activity of intracellular enzymes. One enzyme that may well have a role in the mechanism of anaesthesia is protein kinase C. It is found in all tissues, particularly in the synapses of mammalian brain from where it was first isolated. Protein kinase C is a calcium ion-activated phospholipid-dependent enzyme that phosphorylates a variety of cellular proteins involved in transmembrane signalling. Recently, concentration-dependent inhibitory effects on this enzyme by clinical concentrations of a variety of anaesthetic agents have been demonstrated.

The types of studies outlined above have indicated a number of possible sites at which inhalational anaesthetic agents may alter normal cellular function to produce general anaesthesia, and these are listed in Table 7.2.

The overall size of a molecule is important for anaesthetic effect and an abrupt loss of potency can be demonstrated among the higher molecular weight members of homologous families of anaesthetics such as the primary alcohols, regardless of lipid solubility. The mechanism of this phenomenon is unknown but may be related to changing the amounts of volatile agent present in different parts of the cell membrane as molecular size increases. It has been suggested that there might be a specific 'anaesthetic receptor', the cut-off phenomenon reflecting the

Table 7.2   Aspects of cellular function that may be involved in the production of general anaesthesia.

Ligand–receptor interaction
Acetylcholine
Glycine
γ-aminobutyric acid
5-Hydroxytryptamine
Catecholamines

Intracellular functions
Protein kinase C
Transmitter release from synaptic vesicles

Ion channels
Potassium
Calcium
Sodium
Magnesium
Chloride

presence of a membrane site of restricted size, although recent evidence would seem to refute this. For example stereoselectivity for inhalational agents has not been reported, and the range of anaesthetic substances is great, very often with no structural similarity.

It should be emphasized that most current views on the molecular basis of anaesthetic action are derived from experimental work carried out *in vitro*. Interpretation of the results of some of these studies are extremely controversial and changes observed *in vitro*, and/or experimental animals, do not necessarily reflect the effects of these agents during clinical anaesthesia. No one single theory adequately explains all of the diverse effects of anaesthetic action and it is not known which, if any, of the known effects on neuronal processes is responsible for anaesthesia. It has been suggested that this may mean that anaesthesia can be induced by a variety of mechanisms. Indeed, the fact that it can be caused by such a large range of substances from small molecules to complex steroids may be taken as strong evidence that anaesthesia is the end result of any number of possible disruptions to neuronal function.

ONSET OF ACTION

General anaesthesia occurs when the partial pressure (tension) and hence concentration of inhalational agents in the CNS is sufficiently great to induce loss of consciousness. The uptake and elimination of a volatile anaesthetic is a series of exponential processes. During the induction of anaesthesia by the inhalation of a constant concentration of an anaesthetic, a series of diffusion gradients are established. The diffusion gradients occur: (1) between the concentration of inspired gas or vapour and its tension in pulmonary alveoli, (2) between the alveolar and pulmonary capillary tensions, (3) between pulmonary capillary and cerebral blood tensions, and (4) between the cerebral blood tension and the concentration of the anaesthetic in the cells and tissues in the CNS. In practice, the rapidity of action is mainly dependent on the rate at which the alveolar, and hence brain tension of the agent increases and approaches the inspired gas or vapour tension. A rapid rise in alveolar tension produces a maximal diffusion gradient between the alveoli and pulmonary capillary blood. Once equilibrium is achieved, the partial pressure of anaesthetic in the alveoli will be approximately equal to the tension of the agent in the brain.

Similar but opposite changes occur during recovery from inhalational anaesthesia. The inspired gas tension falls to zero and a series of diffusion gradients are established between the partial pressure of the anaesthetic in the CNS and the exhaled vapour. The speed of recovery is mainly dependent on the rapidity with which the alveolar tension decreases and thus produces a large diffusion gradient between pulmonary blood and the alveoli. Thus factors that affect the onset of action of inhalational anaesthetics will also affect recovery in an equal and opposite manner.

Factors determining alveolar concentration

As stated above, the potency of inhalational anaesthetics (expressed as the minimum alveolar concentration) is closely related to their oil: gas partition coefficient. By contrast, the rate of onset of action is mainly dependent on a different physical property, i.e. their blood: gas partition coefficient. Clearly, if an anaesthetic is completely insoluble in blood, no uptake from the lungs will occur and the alveolar tension will rapidly increase and approach inspired tension. Anaesthetics that are poorly soluble in blood tend to behave in this manner; their partial pressure in the alveoli rapidly increases towards the inspired tension, diffusion into pulmonary capillaries causes a marked rise in their partial pressure in blood and the onset of anaesthesia is rapid. By contrast, agents which are more soluble are extensively removed from the alveoli due to rapid solution in pulmonary capillary blood. The partial pressure in the alveoli and the vascular system remains low and CNS tension only rises slowly. The onset of anaesthesia is correspondingly slow since the diffusion gradient between cerebral blood and the CNS is relatively low.

In addition to the solubility in the blood, differences in tissue solubility may also be important for determining the speed of action of each inhalational agent. For example, although uptake of isoflurane from the alveolar space into the blood is faster than for halothane due to its lower blood: gas partition coefficient (1.4 vs 2.3), movement from the blood to the brain is not. Consequently, there is clinically very little difference in the speed of induction of anaesthesia between isoflurane and halothane.

Recovery from anaesthesia obeys similar principles to those outlined above except that the substantial amount of halothane that is biotransformed can contribute considerably to postanaesthetic drowsiness, particularly after long procedures, and in such instances, recovery from isoflurane is very much faster.

The solubility of anaesthetics in blood is usually expressed in terms of the blood : gas partition coefficient, which can be defined as the ratio of the amounts of an anaesthetic in blood and gas, the two phases being of equal volume, in equilibrium and at 37°C. It is numerically equal to the Ostwald solubility coefficient of the agent. Table 7.3 shows the blood : gas partition coefficients of some common inhalational anaesthetics. Anaesthetics with a low coefficient are poorly soluble in blood and have a rapid onset of action; those with a higher value are more soluble in blood and have a slower onset of action. Changes in the composition of blood, such as alterations in the levels of free fatty acids, albumin and haemoglobin can affect the partition coefficient.

The alveolar tension of inhalational anaesthetics is also influenced by several other factors. In non-rebreathing circuits, the uptake of anaesthetic is primarily dependent upon pulmonary ventilation. Thus changes in ventilation and abnormal ventilation : perfusion ratios in the lung will significantly alter the alveolar partial pressure of anaesthetic agents. The functional residual capacity (FRC) acts as a buffer between the inspired concentration of a gas and the alveolar concentration. As a result, an increase in FRC significantly slows the rate at which the alveolar concentration rises. A reduced FRC has the opposite effect. Ventilation/perfusion inequality alters anaesthetic uptake by either increasing end-tidal anaesthetic concentration (dead-space effect) or by reducing the arterial uptake (shunting effect). Hyperventilation increases the alveolar tension of inhalational anaesthetics and leads to the more rapid onset of anaesthesia by indirectly enhancing the diffusion gradient between cerebral blood and the CNS. Conversely, any reduction in pulmonary ventilation, which may be due to pathological processes as well as intravenous anaesthetics, narcotic analgesics or

Table 7.3 Blood : gas partition coefficients of some common inhalational anaesthetics.

Desflurane	0.4
Cyclopropane	0.5
Nitrous oxide	0.5
Sevoflurane	0.7
Isoflurane	1.4
Enflurane	1.8
Halothane	2.3
Chloroform	8.4
Trichlorethylene	9.0
Diethylether	12.0
Methoxyflurane	12.0

muscle relaxants, decreases the rise in alveolar tension during inhalation of the anaesthetic. These effects of ventilation are most evident when anaesthesia is induced with a soluble agent, i.e. one with a high blood : gas partition coefficient because in these cases, all of the agent that enters the lung is taken up by the blood so that, for example, doubling ventilation will therefore double uptake.

Any increase in the inspired gas or vapour tension will obviously tend to raise the alveolar partial pressure and produce a more rapid onset of anaesthesia. Thus concentrations higher than those required for the maintenance of anaesthesia may be used during induction to accelerate the onset of anaesthesia. This principle is well demonstrated by the single-breath technique for the induction of anaesthesia. After maximum expiration, the subject takes a full breath of a gas mixture containing either 4% halothane or 2% isoflurane and holds it in the lungs for as long as comfortable. This is followed by normal tidal breathing until conscious-ness is lost within 1–2 minutes.

The relation between the inspired gas tension and its alveolar partial pressure is complex. It has been shown that when a constant concentration of halothane is inspired, the rise in alveolar concentration is accelerated by the concomitant administration of nitrous oxide. This was called the 'second gas effect' and was postulated to occur because the uptake of a large volume of nitrous oxide created a potential subatmospheric intrapulmonary pressure which in turn led to an increased inspiratory flow. In addition to this, however, there is also a 'concentration effect' which occurs because the nitrous oxide is taken up more quickly than the halothane which is then present in a smaller volume so that its concentration rises. For example, consider the situation in which 1% of a volatile agent is administered with 80% nitrous oxide in oxygen. The nitrous oxide is taken up quickly in large amounts and as a result, the concentration of the volatile agent increases to almost 2%, i.e. there has been an increase in the concentration of the volatile agent as a result of removing some of the nitrous oxide. The uptake of the volatile agent is then accelerated because of the increase in its alveolar partial pressure. In practice, these effects are only seen when nitrous oxide is the 'first' gas because this is the only agent in current use that is administered at high enough concentrations and is taken up in large enough amounts at a fast rate (in an adult subject at an inspired concentration of 60%, uptake in the first few minutes usually exceeds 1 litre min^{-1}).

Changes in cardiac output and regional blood flow may alter the diffusion gradient between the alveoli, pulmonary capillary blood and the tissues during the induction of anaesthesia. Raised cardiac output increases the gradient and the uptake of anaesthetic from the lungs; opposite effects are produced by a reduction in pulmonary blood flow. This may be significant when anaesthesia is induced by agents with a high blood : gas partition coefficient. Similarly, the diffusion gradient across the pulmonary epithelium is reduced as the partial pressure of anaesthetic in systemic venous blood rises. When complete equilibration occurs (i.e. when the tension in the alveoli and pulmonary capillary blood are equal), diffusion ceases and no uptake of anaesthetic occurs. In practice, complete equilibration never occurs because of the time required and because some anaesthetic is always being removed from the body by metabolism and excretion. Thus inhalational anaesthesia is a state of partial equilibrium.

Both the inspired gas or vapour tension and hence its alveolar partial pressure may be modified by absorption of the agent into components of the anaesthetic circuit. All halogenated anaesthetics are soluble in rubber (some extremely so); they are also taken up by soda lime, especially when dry. As a result, the concentration leaving the vaporizer may not be the same as the inspired concentration. This is particularly evident when low flows are used. Furthermore, release of the agent from the rubber may significantly affect a subsequent anaesthetic. Although saturation of the anaesthetic agent in components of the circuit never occurs (even after several weeks), significant gradients may be present at the beginning and end of anaesthesia. The problem can be minimized by using less soluble agents.

Another effect of anaesthetic circuitry relates to the differences between non-rebreathing and circle systems. In the former, uptake of anaesthetic is primarily dependent upon ventilation because the inspired concentration is fixed to the amount set at the vaporizer. By contrast, in a circle system, the inspired concentration depends upon the expired concentration as well as the amount in the fresh gas supply. Thus if uptake is low, for example because of breath holding, more anaesthetic is left in the expired gas. However, 'fresh' anaesthetic is still added and the inspiratory concentration is therefore raised, the alveolar–arterial gradient is increased and hence so is uptake. Consequently, ventilation variables do not seriously affect rate of uptake in circle system anaesthesia. The effect of altering cardiac output on alveolar concentration is greater with a circle system than a non-rebreathing system because removal of a given amount of agent by the blood will have a greater effect upon the residual concentration in the circuit.

The ways in which inhaled anaesthetics are taken up and distributed around the body, and the effects of changes in inspired tensions, ventilation and anaesthetic circuitry, as well as some patient variables, have been well described by Mapleson using a water analogue.

HAZARDS OF TRACE CONCENTRATIONS

In recent years, there has been increasing interest in the adverse effects of chronic exposure to inhalational anaesthetics. Hospital staff who work in operating theatres are continually exposed to trace amounts of inhalational agents and small concentrations of the agents or their breakdown products have been detected in plasma, breast milk and exhaled air for up to several days after exposure. The long-term effects of occupational exposure are unknown but are of great potential importance. Many animal studies have been carried out to address these questions. However, uncertainties about extrapolating the findings to man, insufficient attention to detail (for example, the suggestion that isoflurane can cause liver cancer in mice was disproved when it was demonstrated that the animals in the first experiment had been exposed (inadvertently) to known carcinogens) and the non-representative nature of many of the studies (many experiments have used inappropriate amounts of anaesthetic to demonstrate an effect) preclude any conclusive interpretation of the results. The consensus of data from such experiments has yielded no convincing evidence of fetotoxicity or carcinogenicity.

A number of epidemiological investigations have therefore been carried out with particular emphasis on the possible risk to female anaesthetists. All but one of these studies were done retrospectively and many have suffered from serious inaccuracies such as a poorly selected control group, difficulty in collecting data, and difficulty in demonstrating cause and effect. The only finding was that there *may* be an increased incidence of spontaneous abortion among exposed women. There is little or no evidence that the concentrations present in an operating theatre have any other toxic effects or impair performance.

In an effort to get round the methodological problems encountered with previous studies, a ten year *prospective* study of all women doctors aged 40 years or less was carried out between 1977 and 1986. This has yielded a vast amount of data and as yet (spring 1991), the results have not been formally reported. The interim conclusions, however, are that 'there is no obvious association between medical specialty, hours in the operating theatre, the use or non-use of scavenging, and the miscarriage rate'. The study has confirmed the already known effects on the fetus of maternal smoking and alcohol consumption.

There are a few reports of abnormal liver function in anaesthetists chronically exposed to low concentrations of halothane, and this has occasionally led to hepatitis which resolved when exposure to the drug ceased.

Although the hazards of trace concentrations of inhalational anaesthetics appear to be small or non-existent, the number of hospital staff exposed is relatively large. In consequence, there has been recent interest in the development and application of monitoring and scavenging systems in the operating theatre. Despite their high cost, the use of these systems is probably justifiable since they will minimize any occupational hazards of inhalational anaesthetics. The only remaining hazard will then be to the environment as nitrous oxide, along with carbon dioxide, is an important 'greenhouse' gas; the halogenated inhalational anaesthetics are, however, thought to present a minimal threat to the ozone layer.

Biotransformation of inhalational anaesthetics

It was not until the mid-1960s that it was recognized that volatile anaesthetics are metabolized in the body and that this has important implications for toxicity. All

Table 7.4 Extent of metabolism of volatile anaesthetics in humans.

Methoxyflurane	75%
Chloroform	50%
Halothane	25%
Diethyl ether	6%
Enflurane	3%
Isoflurane	0.2%

of the agents in current use are either halogenated alkanes or ethers. It is difficult to directly break a single carbon–halogen bond; the C–F bond is the most stable, followed by C–Cl, C–Br and C–I in that order. Additional stability is generally conferred by the presence of two or more halogen atoms on the same carbon atom. For example, the trifluoromethyl group found in halothane, isoflurane, sevoflurane and desflurane is very stable. A configuration that is very susceptible to enzymatic dehalogenation is when there are one or two chlorine atoms on the *terminal* carbon, as found in trichloroethylene and methoxyflurane, the two most extensively metabolized of the volatile agents (Table 7.4).

Halogen atoms attract electrons from the atoms adjacent to the carbon atom to which they are attached leading to an unequal distribution of charges on the molecule. This renders those adjacent atoms more susceptible to attack by an electron-donating group such as oxygen. Thus *oxidative dehalogenation*, the most common reaction that the volatile anaesthetics undergo, does not occur as a result of direct attack on a carbon–halogen bond but as a result of addition of oxygen to the electron-depleted carbon. This destabilizes the molecule which subsequently breaks down to release halogen, with possible toxic consequences. The biotransformation of anaesthetics to toxic metabolites or reactive intermediates can cause renal or hepatic injury. For example, methoxyflurane is metabolized extensively to release fluoride ions which can cause a reversible nephropathy at plasma levels greater than $40 \mu mol$ litre^{-1}.

The metabolic route along which volatile anaesthetics are biotransformed depends to some extent on oxygen availability in the liver. The main enzymes responsible for the (oxidative) biotransformation are the cytochrome P-450 system, however, an alternative (reductive) cytochrome P-450 pathway exists and this will alter the type of metabolites formed. Thus under normal circumstances, little or no defluorination of halothane takes place; however, in the presence of hepatic hypoxia, significant amounts of fluoride may be produced.

Many drugs, such as phenytoin, barbiturates and ethanol, as well as physiological variables such as diet, can induce the cytochrome P-450 enzymes although not all of these factors produce the same pattern of induction. As a result, the biotransformation of a given substance will be affected differently by different enzyme inducers. There is also some evidence to suggest that when inhaled in trace amounts over a period of time, volatile agents themselves can induce hepatic enzymes. The situation after a single anaesthetic is less clear but the consensus view is that hepatic microsomal enzymes are induced following minor surgery in man, but this is related more to the stress of surgery than to general anaesthesia. In practice, the maintenance and recovery from general anaesthesia is not affected by any preexisting enzyme induction because the 'anaesthetic' effects of the volatile agents depend upon exhalation rather than metabolism.

Toxicity, however, is a different matter because biotransformation commences as soon as exposure to the drug occurs. In this situation, the tissue solubility of the anaesthetic may be an important factor. For example, hepatic microsomes have been shown to metabolize methoxyflurane and sevoflurane at the same rate *in vitro*, although the *in vivo* inorganic fluoride levels are much lower with the latter. This probably reflects the very low tissue solubility of sevoflurane so that not only are adequate brain levels achieved after inhalation of only small amounts of the agent but also that it is completely exhaled more rapidly. By contrast, the greater solubility of methoxyflurane creates a large tissue reservoir which slows the elimination of the drug from the body and allows more time for its biotransformation.

If a volatile agent can be metabolised to a toxic product, then enzyme induction may enhance this effect. For example, phenobarbitone has been shown to considerably increase the biotransformation of methoxyflurane; conversely, enzyme inhibitors would be expected to have the opposite effect. Enflurane, sevoflurane, isoflurane and desflurane are not metabolized to any great extent so that enzyme inducers have little clinically significant effect on the biotransformation of these substances. Thus, the risk to patients from the accumulation of drug metabolites would seem to be declining as newer, less biotransformed volatile anaesthetics are introduced into clinical practice. Although most research has been carried out on laboratory animals, it is important to realize that accurate and meaningful extrapolation of the results to humans is not possible. Further details of the metabolism of individual volatile anaesthetics will be given in the following sections.

The effects of inhalational anaesthetics on drug disposition

In view of the ability of some volatile anaesthetics to induce hepatic enzymes, it is reasonable to ask whether this will affect the handling of concomitantly administered drugs. The investigation of this problem is difficult because many factors in the perioperative period can affect drug clearance. Using antipyrine clearance as an index of hepatic drug metabolism, some studies have shown an increase in the clearance of the drug after surgery performed under general anaesthesia with volatile anaesthetics. Antipyrine clearance, however, may not be representative of the real situation and many perioperative events such as starvation can change its value. Other work suggests that if anything, there is a decrease in drug clearance intraoperatively and postoperatively and has been demonstrated to occur with many drugs including fentanyl, lignocaine, propranolol, and verapamil. This is due to a depressant effect on the cytochrome P-450 system and a reduction in hepatic blood flow. There may also be an effect on drug distribution leading to greater uptake in the tissues. Thus the exact nature of the perioperative changes in drug disposition remains unclear at present but generally, these appear not to be great enough to be of major practical significance.

Hepatotoxicity of inhalational anaesthetics

Halothane. One of the first reports of postoperative jaundice and death after exposure to halothane appeared in the literature in 1958 and was likened to the effects of chloroform poisoning. In the wake of such reports, several large retrospective studies were carried out, including the National Halothane Study in the USA in 1963. Although many of these epidemiological and pathological studies were of limited value (particularly because the problem in question occurs rarely and could not always be clearly differentiated from viral hepatitis), certain risk factors emerged as being associated with this condition. These are multiple exposures with a maximum susceptibility of 28 days between exposures, middle age (although more cases are now being reported in children), obesity, and it is twice as common in females.

Clinically, halothane can affect the liver in two different ways. The first is quite common, occurring in 8–40% of patients 1–3 days after receiving the drug, and is characterized by a transient rise in aminotransferases and absence of clinical abnormalities. The second is severe hepatic necrosis typically occurring 5 days (but can be up to 4 weeks) after the last exposure to the drug and accompanied by large rises in aminotransferases. The duration of exposure is not critical with many cases occurring after only short operative procedures. The overall incidence of this condition is 1 in 10 000 halothane administrations (the range quoted in different studies is 1 in 7000 to 1 in 35 000). It occurs in 1 in 3500 *multiple* administrations and has a mortality rate of 50–80%.

Following the observation that halothane is biotransformed in the body, various animal models were developed in an attempt to define the mechanism of halothane hepatotoxicity, the premise being that the condition is caused by a metabolite. These were the *PCB–halothane model* (rats were given polychlorinated biphenyls (PCBs) to induce liver enzymes and then exposed to halothane); the *halothane–hypoxia* model (halothane can be metabolized along a reductive pathway capable of producing reactive species which can covalently bind to liver macromolecules and cause damage); and the *tri-iodothyronine model* (rats were pretreated with tri-iodothyronine and then exposed to halothane under normal or hypoxic conditions to produce hepatic necrosis, possibly by an effect on carbo-hydrate metabolism). The validity of all of these models has been questioned as they are very poorly representative of the human situation. For example, hypoxia alone can cause liver damage, but this differs pathologically and temporally from that seen clinically. A better animal model has been developed in the guinea pig which produces a lesion similar to that seen clinically without the need for hypoxia or enzyme induction with phenobarbitone.

Recent investigation has focused on immunological mechanisms as the cause of halothane hepatotoxicity. One of the metabolites of the oxidative biotrans-formation of halothane, the trifluoroacetyl group (TFA), covalently binds to lysine residues on hepatic proteins (including cytochrome P-450 itself). This altered protein acts as an antigen in certain individuals so that antibodies are produced. Cleavage of the TFA groups from the proteins *in vitro* abolishes the antigenicity. Using a technique called ELISA (enzyme linked immunosorbent assay), it is now possible to demonstrate the presence of the circulating anti-TFA antibodies in about 70% of patients with fulminant hepatic failure following halothane but not in the serum of patients with other forms of liver disease or in those who have had a recent halothane anaesthetic without resultant liver necrosis. Titres may persist for 1–5 years. Thus this assay can be used to establish the diagnosis of halothane-induced hepatitis; it does not prove cause and effect. Why only a minority of individuals are sensitive to this immunogen is at present unknown.

If a metabolite of halothane is the first step towards halothane hepatotoxicity, it is reasonable to ask whether inhibition of this biotransformation would be protective. Cimetidine, an inhibitor of cytochrome P-450, has been shown to offer some protection against halothane hepatotoxicity in rats when given in large dosage but not in humans when given as a single preanaesthetic dose.

There is no doubt that the most important thing that the anaesthetist can do to protect his patient from the possibility of liver damage is to be aware of the problem. The recommendations by the Committee on Safety of Medicines in 1986 to address this problem were to take a careful anaesthetic history, 'avoid repeated exposure to halothane within a period of at least 3 months' and that 'a history of unexplained jaundice or pyrexia in a patient following exposure to halothane is an absolute contraindication to its future use in that patient'. However, if halothane hepatotoxicity does turn out to be immunologically mediated, albeit idiosyncrati-cally, then there would be no such thing as a safe period. The antibody titres are long lasting and there are cases on record of hepatotoxicity occurring after a 5 year gap between exposures to halothane.

Enflurane has been incriminated in the production of postoperative hepatic dysfunction although it is an extremely rare event estimated at about one in 2 million enflurane anaesthetics; *isoflurane* has not yet been conclusively linked with this problem. It had been hoped that these agents would be free of hepatotoxic effects because they undergo less hepatic biotransformation. Certainly the incidence of liver damage is much greater after halothane, suggesting that the amount of biotransformation is indeed an important factor. However, one of the metabolites of isoflurane is TFA, although as yet, there are no published case reports of antibodies to isoflurane metabolism.

Recent evidence suggests that there might be a common mechanism underlying the hepatotoxicity of all volatile agents as antibodies from patients with halothane hepatitis recognize hepatically bound intermediates from enflurane metabolism. All three volatile anaesthetics can produce metabolites which covalently bind to hepatic proteins and can then serve as antigens. The only difference is that halothane produces much greater quantities of immunoreactive protein than enflurane and isoflurane, the quantities correlating directly with the relative extents of metabolism of these agents. If cross sensitization does occur, it will no longer be acceptable to substitute one volatile agent for another.

PROPERTIES OF THE INDIVIDUAL AGENTS

Although the general effects of all inhalational anaesthetics on the brain are similar, they often have unique properties or toxic hazards that may limit their use and applicability. For this reason, the properties of different inhalational anaesthetics are described separately. A summary of the main properties and effects of the agents in current use in the UK is shown in Table 7.5 and the formulae are shown in Fig. 7.2.

Nitrous oxide

Nitrous oxide was discovered by Joseph Priestley in 1772 and the subjective and objective effects of the gas were first described by him. Subsequently, Humphrey Davy suggested that its analgesic properties might be useful in the management of pain during operative surgery. Its obvious potential as an analgesic and anaesthetic was ignored for many years. In 1844, Horace Wells, an American dentist, first used nitrous oxide to facilitate dental extraction. Unfortunately, his clinical demonstration of its effects was unsuccessful and its use fell into disrepute. The low potency of nitrous oxide, and the necessity for adequate oxygenation during anaesthesia, were only recognized in the 1870s. Since then, the gas has been frequently used as an adjuvant, and as a vehicle for the administration of more potent agents during inhalational anaesthesia. Nitrous oxide is also widely used as an analgesic, particularly in obstetric practice where it was first used as an 80% mixture in oxygen in 1881.

In some respects, nitrous oxide has the properties of the ideal inhalational

Table 7.5 Main properties of the inhalational anaesthetics in current use in the UK.

	Nitrous oxide N–N → O	Halothane CF₃.CHClBr	Enflurane CHF₂.O.CF₂.CHCl	Isoflurane CHF₂.O.CHCl.CF₃
Structure				
Boiling point at atmospheric pressure (°C)	−88	50	57	49
Vapour pressure at 20°C (kPa)	5200	32	23	33
MAC (% v/v)	105	0.8	1.7	1.2
Blood : gas partition coefficient	0–0.5	2.3	1.8	1.4
Analgesic properties	Marked	Poor	Moderate	Moderate
Effect of respiration	Non-irritant Enters air spaces Increased resp. rate maintains CO₂ levels	Non-irritant Increased rate Decreased tidal volume (least depressant)	Non-irritant Increased rate Decreased tidal volume (most depressant)	Slightly irritant Increased rate Decreased tidal volume
Effects on cardiovascular system	Little or no effect; no increased cardiac sensitivity to catecholamines	Bradycardia; hypotension Decreased cardiac output Peripheral resistance slightly reduced Increased cardiac sensitivity to catecholamines	Tachycardia; hypotension Decreased cardiac output Decreased peripheral resistance; slightly increased cardiac sensitivity to catecholamines	Slight tachycardia and hypotension Little myocardial depression Coronary steal possible Biggest decrease in peripheral resistance. Slightly increased sensitivity to catecholamines
Effects on electroencephalogram	None	Cortical depression	Changes resembling grand mal or focal seizure activity; may be associated with twitching or tonic–clonic movements	Cortical depression
Cerebral blood flow	Moderate increase	Big increase	Moderate increase	No change if <1 MAC
Potentiation of nondepolarizing neuromuscular blockade	None	Moderate	Marked	Marked
Effects on uterus	None	Slight relaxation	Slight relaxation	Slight relaxation
Metabolism	Minimal	20–45%	2.5–8.5%	0.2%
Toxic and hypersensitivity reactions	Inactivation of vitamin B₁₂ Neutropenia	Hepatic damage (rare)	Hepatic damage (very rare)	None

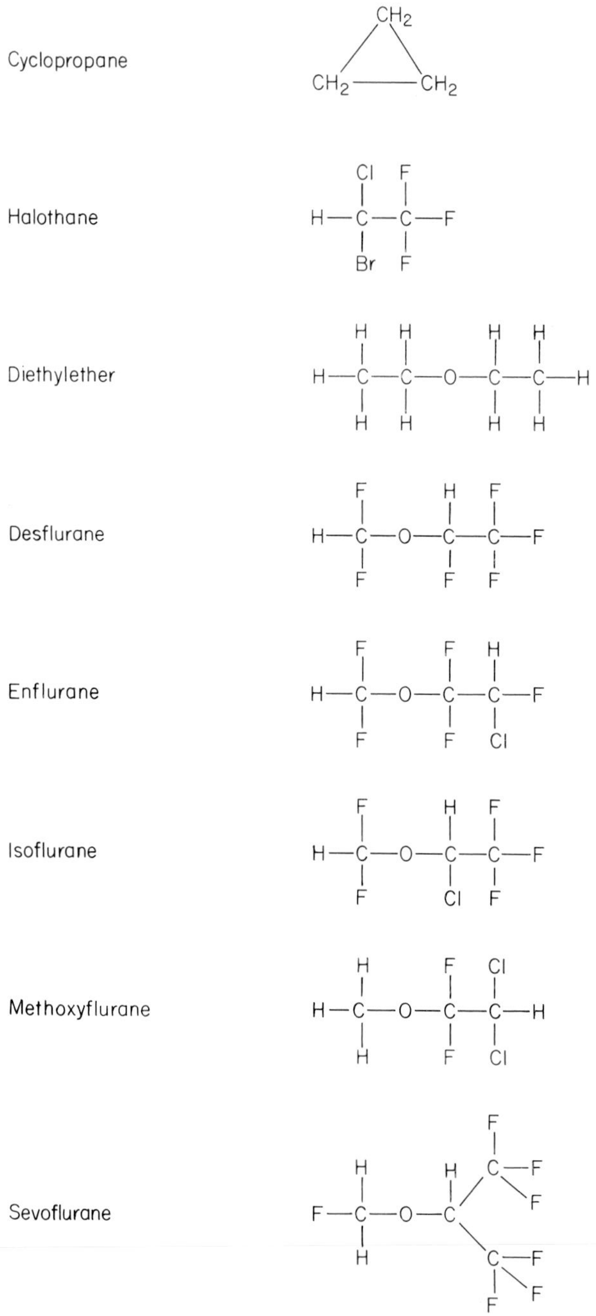

Fig. 7.2 Structural formulae of the inhalational anaesthetic agents.

anaesthetic. At room temperature, it is a colourless, odourless, non-flammable gas that is heavier than air; it is usually stored as a liquid under pressure in steel cylinders.

Nitrous oxide has one of the lowest blood : gas partition coefficients of all of the inhalational agents (0.5) so that during its administration, the partial pressure of the gas in arterial blood rapidly approaches its alveolar concentration. Consequently, both induction and recovery from anaesthesia are extremely rapid. It diffuses across the alveolar epithelium into pulmonary capillaries more rapidly than oxygen and the alveolar oxygen tension may therefore temporarily increase (see concentration effect above). Reverse changes may occur during recovery from anaesthesia as it diffuses rapidly from pulmonary capillary blood into the alveoli and may cause temporary hypoxia ('diffusion hypoxia'). The low solubility of nitrous oxide enables it to move more readily through the tissues than other anaesthetics; the diffusion rate through the skin is about 10 ml min^{-1} in the average adult. Nitrous oxide rapidly enters any enclosed air-containing spaces, such as the cuff of an endotracheal tube, intestinal gas, a pneumothorax and air emboli, and will increase their volume by an amount related to the concentration of nitrous oxide in the alveoli. For example, administration of 75% nitrous oxide doubles the size of a pneumothorax in 10 min and triples it in 30–45 min.

Uses

The use of nitrous oxide as an inhalational anaesthetic is restricted by its low potency and this is its main disadvantage in clinical practice. Its MAC of 104% makes it the least potent of the currently available inhaled agents. When the inspired concentration of nitrous oxide in oxygen is more than about 70%, this may result in arterial and tissue hypoxia. Since this proportion is usually insufficient to induce surgical anaesthesia, it is necessary to concurrently administer other depressant drugs which will have an additive effect to the nitrous oxide. Thus a 50–70% mixture of nitrous oxide and oxygen is widely used as a carrier gas for more potent inhalational agents, or in combination with other drugs (e.g. intravenous anaesthetics and narcotic analgesics).

Nitrous oxide is a potent analgesic and inhalation of a 10–20% mixture in oxygen may have an effect equivalent to 15 mg morphine or 100 mg of pethidine for certain types of pain. Consequently, a mixture of nitrous oxide and oxygen containing equal volumes of both gases (Entonox) is widely used in obstetric practice to relieve pain during childbirth. It may also be used in minor surgical procedures (e.g. the dressing of small burns and superficial wounds). The mechanism by which nitrous oxide produces this effect is unknown but may involve an action at opiate receptors as the analgesia is partially antagonized by naloxone.

Other effects

During the induction of anaesthesia, nitrous oxide may cause exhilaration and euphoria and has been used since the early 19th Century as an intoxicant, when it became known as 'laughing gas' because those who inhaled it became jovial and boisterous. However, unpremedicated patients anaesthetized only with nitrous oxide and oxygen may experience unpleasant dreams during surgery or even be wide awake.

Nitrous oxide inhibits the uptake of noradrenaline by the lungs and also causes sympathetic stimulation by a central effect. Although it has a direct myocardial depressant effect *in vitro*, the increase in sympathetic activity that occurs *in vivo* is sufficient to counteract any depressant effects and may also offset the cardiovascular depressant effects of the other inhalational agents. Experiments on dogs with critical coronary artery stenosis has suggested that nitrous oxide further reduces myocardial performance. This has not been supported by evidence from human studies and it seems that 70% nitrous oxide has no significant effect on haemodynamic performance even in patients undergoing coronary artery surgery. Heart rate is unaffected by nitrous oxide (in the absence of excitement) but systemic vascular resistance may rise slightly due to the sympathetic stimulation. Extrasystoles or ectopic rhythms are rarely induced and there is no evidence that sensitivity to endogenous or exogenous catecholamines is modified. Thus at present, nitrous oxide is not contraindicated in patients with serious cardiac disease.

Research on the effect of nitrous oxide on cerebral blood flow has produced some inconsistent results due to interspecies and methodological differences between studies. However, there is overall agreement that nitrous oxide not only increases cerebral blood flow on its own but also exaggerates the effect of the halogenated volatile agents. Consequently, some workers now recommend that it should be avoided in patients with serious intracranial pathology. In other patients, these effects are minor and of little practical importance.

In anaesthetic concentrations, nitrous oxide causes an increase in respiratory rate and a decrease in tidal volume so that $Paco_2$ is maintained at normal levels. Thus, substituting it for a portion of the anaesthetic requirement of one of the potent agents will minimize the increase in $Paco_2$ produced by the agent. The responses to an increase in carbon dioxide or to hypoxia are depressed as much as for the other volatile agents. There is some evidence that there is a greater incidence of atelectasis and a lower Pao_2 in the postoperative period when nitrous oxide has been used. It also has an inhibitory effect on neutrophils not seen with halothane but no depressant effect on mucociliary function.

Nitrous oxide has no effect on neuromuscular blockade and there is no evidence that any significant amounts are metabolized in man. In this respect, it may be unique among the currently used inhalational agents. Small amounts are converted to nitrogen in the course of the oxidation of vitamin B_{12} (see below) and some may be biotransformed (also to nitrogen) by intestinal bacteria.

The toxic effects of nitrous oxide are a result of its interference with the syntheses of methionine and deoxyribonucleic acid (DNA), as shown in Fig. 7.3. Nitrous oxide causes the oxidation of the cobalt ion at the centre of the B_{12} molecule from the monovalent to the bivalent form so that the vitamin is then no longer usable as a cofactor for methionine synthase (MSyn). In addition, this enzyme is inactivated by nitrous oxide, possibly due to the production of free radicals.

These effects can occur quite quickly. Thymidine synthesis is impaired within 1 hour in rats exposed to 50% nitrous oxide, and within 2 hours in some seriously ill patients after anaesthesia with nitrous oxide. There is some evidence from studies in animals that the degree of interference is related to the duration of anaesthesia. However, rat MSyn is considerably more sensitive to nitrous oxide than man's, an important factor in the evaluation of these effects.

Clinically, the problems that arise reflect the impairment of DNA synthesis. Exposure to anaesthetic concentrations of nitrous oxide for more than 5–6 days results in agranulocytosis but megaloblastic changes can appear in the bone marrow of any patient exposed to anaesthetic concentrations of the gas for more than 2 hours. The time scale is very variable and some patients may remain unaffected for several hours. These changes are accompanied by a rise in serum folate and a fall in serum methionine levels. After exposure has ceased, the marrow gradually returns to normal within 1 week. Recovery can be speeded up by the administration of folinic acid which acts as an alternative source of tetrahydrofolate and will restore normal thymidine synthesis within a few hours (Fig. 7.3). However, administration of methionine, even in large dosage, may

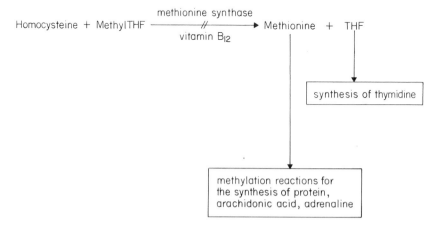

Fig. 7.3 Key metabolic pathways affected by nitrous oxide. $\nrightarrow$ pathway blocked by nitrous oxide.

only partially alleviate the shortage of it. Administration of vitamin B_{12} may speed up the recovery of methionine synthesis in some patients after exposure to nitrous oxide has ceased, but the main factor appears to be the time taken to synthesize new MSyn. There is little data regarding the actual recovery of MSyn activity in humans but circumstantial evidence suggests that it is slow (i.e. 2–3 days). Intermittent exposure to nitrous oxide within short periods therefore compounds the problem by not allowing time for the enzyme activity to recover.

The inactivation of vitamin B_{12} or MSyn by nitrous oxide in rats cannot be demonstrated below an inhaled concentration of 450 p.p.m. regardless of the duration of exposure and staff working in unscavenged theatres exposed to concentrations between 200 and 400 p.p.m. have normal serum methionine levels; the levels in a properly scavenged operating theatre are in the order of 50 p.p.m. By contrast, prolonged exposure to nitrous oxide in heavily contaminated unscavenged environments, such as a dental surgery, can produce a neurological disorder similar to that of subacute combined degeneration of the cord, presumably reflecting the chronic vitamin B_{12} deficiency induced by the nitrous oxide.

There are also implications for fetotoxicity since nitrous oxide is a weak teratogen in the rat if administered at concentrations over 50% for several days. This effect can largely be prevented by pretreatment with folinic acid, showing that the fetotoxic effect is due to inhibition of DNA synthesis. There is currently no published evidence of fetal abnormalities attributable to the administration of nitrous oxide to pregnant women during the period of organogenesis in spite of the large numbers that must have been exposed over the years. Nevertheless, one author has recommended that 'it would seem wise to avoid nitrous oxide during the first 4 weeks of pregnancy or to cover the anaesthetic with folinic acid' although he admits that 'the likelihood of actually discovering a pregnancy this early is very small indeed'.

In summary, nitrous oxide is a very safe inhalational agent. There have been suggestions that it should no longer have a place in modern anaesthesia but it continues to be used for several reasons. Firstly, it has the longest and best safety record of any inhalational anaesthetic in use today and billions of people have breathed it without apparent harm. Secondly, there is very little evidence to suggest that its potential hazards are actually seen in the clinical situation. Thirdly, there is nothing acceptable to replace it.

Halothane

Halothane (2-bromo-2-chloro-1,1,1-trifluoroethane) is one of a series of fluorinated hydrocarbons synthesized by Suckling between 1950 and 1955. Its pharmacology was subsequently investigated by Raventós and its anaesthetic effects in man and guidance for use with a Boyle's bottle were described by Johnstone. At present, halothane is still probably the most commonly used inhalational anaesthetic in the world although its use has declined considerably in recent years, especially in North America, following problems with hepatotoxicity and the subsequent development of alternative agents which are less potentially toxic. Halothane is a volatile, colourless liquid which is unstable in the presence of light and its decomposition is usually prevented by storage in amber bottles and with the addition of thymol (0.01%) to prevent the liberation of free bromine. In the conditions and concentrations used in anaesthesia, it is non-flammable and non-explosive. Halothane is administered by means of a calibrated vaporizer; concentrations of 2–4% are routinely required for induction and 0.5%–1.5% for the maintenance of anaesthesia. The blood : gas partition coefficient of halothane is quite low (2.3) so that both induction and recovery are relatively rapid and the level of anaesthesia is quite easily controlled. It has been shown to have little if any analgesic properties and may even have an 'antanalgesic' effect and lower the pain threshold.

Significant amounts (20–45%) of halothane are oxidatively biotransformed in the liver to trifluoroacetic acid and chloride and bromide ions. These are excreted slowly in the urine, and bromide in particular may be detected in the body for several weeks after prolonged anaesthesia with levels high enough to cause significant postoperative sedation. Reductive halothane metabolism only occurs to a small extent in man although this will be enhanced in the presence of hepatic hypoxia. This pathway produces fluoride ions and three halogenated 2-carbon molecules which are excreted as conjugated metabolites in the urine. The implications of halothane biotransformation for hepatic toxicity have been discussed above.

Halothane does not irritate the respiratory tract or increase salivary, laryngeal or bronchial secretions. As with all of the halogenated agents, it causes a reversible increase in mucus production and a decrease in mucociliary flow rates. Concentrations used to induce anaesthesia depress pharyngeal and laryngeal reflexes. Halothane also causes a reduction in bronchiolar muscle tone by a combination of β-adrenergic stimulation and a direct effect on the smooth muscle; it is therefore particularly useful in asthmatics. The ventilatory response to hypercarbia is depressed by 50% by 1 MAC of halothane and is almost completely absent at 2 MAC. The ventilatory response to hypoxia is abolished by 1 MAC of halothane, as with all of the inhalational agents. Halothane causes an increase in respiratory rate associated with a small decrease in tidal volume so that overall ventilation is virtually unchanged up to 1 MAC but decreases at greater concentrations.

During halothane anaesthesia, there are marked effects on the heart and circulation. It increases vagal tone, depresses the SA node and its response to sympathetic stimulation, and depresses AV conduction to produce a sinus bradycardia or an AV junctional escape rhythm. Myocardial contractility is also decreased (by about 30% at 1.5 MAC) resulting in a similar reduction in cardiac output, although values tend to return towards normal if anaesthesia is prolonged. The myocardial depression, which is potentiated by β-adrenoceptor and some calcium channel blocking drugs, is the main mechanism by which halothane reduces the blood pressure. The interaction between halothane and calcium channel blocker drugs is discussed further in the section on isoflurane (p. 219).

Halothane causes a small change in overall peripheral vascular resistance (7% reduction at 1.5 MAC), although this increases to 25% with progressive duration of anaesthesia. The change is small due to a combination of a decrease in resistance in some vascular beds, particularly in the cutaneous (at lighter an-aesthetic levels) and cerebral circulations, and an increase in others, notably splanchnic and muscle. The mechanism of these effects is unknown and has been variously attributed to the effects of halothane on central sympathetic pathways and baroreceptors, blockade of nicotinic receptors in autonomic ganglia, or to a direct action on vascular smooth muscle. During halothane anaesthesia, there is a fall in the plasma concentration of most endogenous catecholamines, including dopamine, noradrenaline and adrenaline and this could play a part in mediating some of the effects of halothane on the circulation. Autoregulation is also lost so that organ perfusion, such as in the brain, will reflect changes in cardiac output and therefore may alter in a detrimental fashion. For example, at about 2 MAC, there is up to a fourfold increase in cerebral blood flow but a 25% fall in hepatic blood flow, although these flow figures will depend to some extent on the arterial blood pressure. In addition, halothane abolishes the CO_2 responsiveness of the cerebral circulation so that hypocapnia will not offset the increase in cerebral blood flow.

Halothane inhibits hypoxic pulmonary vasoconstriction. Although it reduces coronary blood flow, it can have a beneficial effect on the myocardium by slightly reducing afterload and increasing the myocardial oxygen supply-to-demand ratio and myocardial tolerance of ischaemia. There is therefore a lower incidence of intraoperative ST depression than with other inhalational agents.

The overall result of these cardiovascular effects is a fall in blood pressure by an amount directly related to the inhaled concentration of the drug and this may therefore be used to produce controlled hypotension.

Cardiac arrhythmias sometimes occur during halothane anaesthesia. The most frequent and important cause of these is the level of circulating catecholamines although there are many other precipitating factors such as hypokalaemia, hypo-calcaemia, acidosis, alkalosis and sudden hypertensive episodes. It is well known that halothane sensitizes the myocardium to catecholamines although the exact mechanism of this effect is not clear. Recent work has demonstrated that simultaneous α_1 and β stimulation are necessary for sensitization to occur. An elevated blood pressure plays an important role but the chronotropic effect of β-adrenoceptor agonists contributes little to the arrhythmogenic action. Factors

that increase the physiological secretion of adrenaline (e.g. endotracheal intubation, hypoxia, hypercarbia, the presence of a phaeochromocytoma) and drugs
with either direct β-adrenergic effects (e.g. adrenaline and isoprenaline) or
indirect β-adrenergic effects (e.g. tricyclic antidepressants) can precipitate dangerous arrhythmias during halothane anaesthesia. Also, some other drugs such as
aminophylline and thiopentone lower the threshold for arrhythmias. A bigeminal
rhythm or multifocal ventricular extrasystoles are commonly seen and these may
progress to ventricular tachycardia or fibrillation. A particular hazard is presented
by injected or infused adrenaline and the use of this substance should ideally be
avoided completely during halothane anaesthesia. Other inhalational agents are
considerably safer from this point of view; for example, animal studies have
shown that the dose of intravenous adrenaline required to produce ventricular
extrasystoles at 1.2 MAC is about five times greater with enflurane than halothane.
If it is necessary to use adrenaline during halothane anaesthesia to effect local
haemostasis, then its use should be restricted. Concentrations of 1:100 000
($10\,\mu g\ ml^{-1}$) or less should be used and in an adult, no more than $100\,\mu g$ should
be given within a 10 min period. This dose can be doubled if administered in
combination with 0.5% lignocaine. By contrast, vasoconstrictor polypeptides
such as felypressin do not affect the excitability of the heart or increase the risk of
arrhythmias during halothane anaesthesia.

Arrhythmias induced during halothane anaesthesia usually cease spontaneously within a short period of time if aggravating factors, such as hypercarbia,
are treated. Specific therapy is only indicated to terminate life-threatening arrhythmias and the efficacy of such treatment will be greatly enhanced by the prior
institution of general corrective measures. Adrenaline-induced ventricular
arrhythmias may be treated with intravenous lignocaine or a β-receptor antagonist
such as propranolol. Metoprolol, a more cardioselective β-blocker, is an alternative for patients in whom the use of propranolol may be inadvisable, e.g.
asthmatics.

Halothane, like all of the volatile agents, has a depressant effect on all types
of smooth muscle (vascular, gastrointestinal, bladder and uterus) and skeletal
muscle, as well as cardiac muscle. Evidence regarding uterine muscle relaxation
suggests that equipotent concentrations (0.5 MAC) of halothane, enflurane and
isoflurane produce about the same degree of muscle relaxation, 1.5 MAC reducing
contractility by about 20%.

Halothane augments the effects of non-depolarizing muscle relaxants in a
dose-dependent manner although not to the same extent as enflurane and
isoflurane. The mechanism of this effect is unknown but is believed to be due to a
combination of factors. As well as depression of the central nervous system and
presynaptic inhibition of acetylcholine release, halogenated anaesthetics also
cause postsynaptic receptor desensitization (possibly by interfering with the
binding of acetylcholine to its receptor and the opening of the associated ion

channel). Clinically, smaller amounts of nondepolarizing agents will be required to produce a given amount of relaxation and their duration of action will be prolonged. This effect is greatest with *d*-tubocurarine and pancuronium, and is less marked with atracurium and vecuronium. When the volatile anaesthetic drugs are eliminated, there is a rapid reversal of the potentiated neuromuscular blockade.

In summary, halothane is a non-flammable and potent inhalational anaesthetic. Induction and recovery of anaesthesia are quite rapid and the level is easily controlled. Halothane does not irritate the respiratory tract, but it does depress the cardiovascular system causing bradycardia and a fall in cardiac output and blood pressure. It potentiates the effects of non-depolarizing muscle relaxants and causes relaxation of uterine smooth muscle. The main disadvantages of halothane are its ability to sensitize the heart to the arrhythmogenic effects of catecholamines and its propensity to induce hepatic damage, although in severe form this is very rare.

Enflurane

Enflurane (2-chloro-1,1,2-trifluoroethyl difluoromethyl ether) has been extensively used in the USA and in Europe during the past 20 years. It is currently the most popular volatile agent in the UK, having taken over from halothane in the wake of the problems of hepatic toxicity with that agent. Enflurane is a volatile colourless liquid with as pleasant a smell as any of the inhalational agents. It is only flammable at concentrations above 5.75%. Enflurane has a low blood : gas partition coefficient (1.8), so induction and recovery are rapid and the level of anaesthesia is easily controlled. It is less potent than halothane and concentrations of up to 5% are required for induction and 1–2% for the maintenance of anaesthesia. Enflurane is invariably administered by means of a calibrated vaporizer. It has been shown to have analgesic properties when administered in subanaesthetic concentrations (about 0.8%) and may be used effectively during labour and for burns dressings. However, it is not as convenient as Entonox and continuous administration, even of subanaesthetic doses, can cause excessive drowsiness.

Unlike halothane, enflurane is not extensively metabolized and over 90% of the amount absorbed is eliminated unchanged. The remainder is oxidatively metabolized to carbon dioxide, difluoromethoxy difluoroacetic acid, and inorganic fluoride and chloride ions. In both experimental animals and in man, the breakdown of enflurane is not affected by inducers or inhibitors of hepatic drug metabolism, with the possible exception of isoniazid. Toxic or hypersensitivity reactions affecting the liver are very rare and even prolonged enflurane anaesthesia only causes slight changes in hepatic function in normal subjects. Hepatotoxicity associated with enflurane has been discussed above.

Inorganic fluoride is of particular importance as plasma levels greater than

$40\,\mu$mol litre^{-1} can give rise to an ADH-resistant polyuria; this is the main reason why methoxyflurane is no longer in use today. Peak plasma fluoride levels occur at 4–8 h after enflurane anaesthesia in contrast to anaesthesia with methoxyflurane, when the peak levels are found at about 24 h postoperatively and may persist for a further 24–48 h. This is because methoxyflurane is about ten times more fat-soluble than enflurane and there is therefore a large reservoir of the drug left in the body after anaesthesia that is available for metabolism in the postoperative period. After enflurane anaesthesia, the levels of fluoride in the plasma and urine only rise to a limited extent although they may not return to baseline for several days. Nevertheless, the likelihood of renal damage is very small and even after prolonged anaesthesia, there may only be a small reduction in ADH sensitivity lasting for a few days.

Enflurane is non-irritant to the respiratory tract and produces some bronchodilation, although less than halothane. It does not usually induce bronchospasm or laryngospasm, but does cause a reversible increase in mucus production. During spontaneous ventilation, enflurane causes an increase in respiratory rate but a decrease in tidal volume. It depresses the ventilatory response to carbon dioxide to a greater extent than halothane and is in fact, the most respiratory depressant of all of the volatile agents in current use. Ventilatory response to hypoxia and hypoxic pulmonary vasoconstriction are depressed in a dose-related manner to about the same extent with all of the inhalational agents.

Enflurane depresses all cardiovascular parameters with the exception of heart rate, and has a more profound effect than halothane except at the lightest levels of anaesthesia (0.5 MAC). Furthermore, for a given change in inhaled concentration, there is a greater change in effect than for any other agent, so that enflurane has the narrowest margin of safety of all the volatile agents in current use. During light anaesthesia (0.5 MAC), stroke volume and cardiac output are well maintained, but the blood pressure decreases slightly due to a decrease in systemic vascular resistance. Higher concentrations significantly depress cardiac contractility and at 1.5 MAC, stroke volume falls to about 50% of the awake value. This negative inotropic effect may be enhanced if the patient is on β-adrenoceptor or some calcium-channel blocking drugs. The mechanism of how inhalational anaesthetics modify myocardial performance is not known but is probably related to their interference with calcium ion movement across cell membranes. Heart rate is unaffected by 0.5 MAC enflurane but tends to rise thereafter more than with any other agent, and this helps to reduce the fall in cardiac output that would otherwise occur at higher inspired concentrations. Even so at 1.5 MAC, cardiac output is only 65% of the awake value. Peripheral vascular resistance is reduced by about 25%, regardless of the depth of anaesthesia, and the combination of this and the myocardial depression causes a more marked fall in arterial blood pressure than is seen with halothane. Paradoxically, this may make enflurane potentially safer than halothane for controlled hypotension since less myocardial depression is required to achieve a given blood pressure. The coronary circulation is either unaffected or slightly vasodilated by enflurane.

All halogenated anaesthetics may potentially induce cardiac arrhythmias during the induction of anaesthesia and can sensitize the heart to the effects of adrenaline and other sympathomimetic amines, although the secretion of endogenous catecholamines is in fact decreased during enflurane anaesthesia. It is much less likely than halothane to induce these complications and the plasma concentration of adrenaline associated with ventricular arrhythmias is about five to ten times greater during enflurane anaesthesia than during halothane anaesthesia, although there is a wide variation in individual response. The explanation for these differences between halothane and enflurane is uncertain; halothane is a fluorinated hydrocarbon while enflurane is a fluorinated ether, and the administration of ethers is generally associated with cardiovascular stability. Unlike halothane, enflurane causes little change in AV conduction time except in the presence of the calcium-channel blockers verapamil and diltiazem, when there is an increase in the conduction time which may lead to arrhythmias, particularly an AV junctional escape rhythm. This interaction is discussed further in the section on isoflurane. In practice, arrhythmias during enflurane anaesthesia are unlikely after subcutaneous injection or local application of adrenaline and it is therefore preferable to halothane in situations associated with the presence of excessive amounts of catecholamines.

Inhalation of 0.5 MAC of enflurane impairs the autoregulation of cerebral blood flow, and 1 MAC abolishes it completely so that blood flow increases or decreases in proportion to the systemic blood pressure. These changes are potentiated by hypercarbia and antagonized by hypocarbia. Inhalation of enflurane, particularly at concentrations of about 3%, produces abnormal EEG activity, especially when $Paco_2$ tensions are decreased by hyperventilation and in children, paroxysms of generalized electrical activity that resemble grand mal epilepsy may be induced. In adults, changes indicative of focal seizure activity are more commonly observed. The abnormal EEG activity may be reduced or even abolished by decreasing the concentration of enflurane and increasing $Paco_2$ tension but may persist for between 6 and 30 days after anaesthesia. There have been no cases of permanent neurological disturbance resulting from the seizure activity produced by enflurane. Occasionally, these EEG changes may be associated with peripheral effects such as fasciculation, twitching, or tonic–clonic movements of the face and limbs. There is no evidence that these phenomena are more common in epileptic patients; however, it is probably best to avoid the use of enflurane in subjects with convulsive disorders.

Enflurane, like other halogenated anaesthetics, has indirect muscle relaxant properties and tends to enhance the effects of non-depolarizing muscle relaxants, being more potent in this respect than halothane or isoflurane when used with vecuronium and atracurium. It is generally recommended that the dosage of non-depolarizing agents should be reduced, particularly when higher concentrations of enflurane are used. In practice, the potentiation of muscle relaxation diminishes rapidly once the volatile agent is discontinued. Similar effects are produced on the ocular muscles and there is often a significant fall (about 30–40%) in intraocular tension. This is not quite as great as that seen with halothane and isoflurane (about 50%) when administered at the same MAC concentration and in the presence of the same blood pressure. Enflurane also causes relaxation of uterine smooth muscle by the same amount as halothane.

In summary, enflurane is an inhalational agent with similar properties to other fluorinated anaesthetics. When compared with halothane, it is approximately half as potent although induction times are not significantly different. It is less likely to sensitize the heart to the arrhythmic effects of catecholamines and is a more potent muscle relaxant than halothane. It may induce EEG abnormalities and muscle twitching although in practice, these are of little consequence in most patients. Enflurane is only metabolized to a limited extent, and is unlikely to induce hepatic or renal damage.

Isoflurane

Isoflurane (1-chloro-2,2,2-trifluoroethyl difluoromethyl ether) is an isomer of enflurane but with several quite different properties. It is the most commonly used inhalational agent in the USA and is fast gaining popularity in the UK. It does not decompose in light or at room temperature and requires no preservatives, having a shelf-life of at least 5 years. Isoflurane is not flammable at anaesthetic concentrations and is the most stable of the inhalational agents in current use in soda lime. It has a low blood : gas partition coefficient (1.4) so that induction of anaesthesia is quick and the level of anaesthesia is easily controlled. The potency of isoflurane (MAC 1.2) is intermediate between halothane and enflurane and concentrations of up to 4% are required for induction and 1–1.5% for the maintenance of anaesthesia. Like enflurane, isoflurane has analgesic properties when administered in subanaesthetic concentrations (about 0.5%) and has been used during labour and for burns dressings. However, it is not as convenient as entonox and may produce excessive drowsiness if used continuously.

Of all the halogenated inhalational agents in current use, isoflurane is the least metabolized and only 0.2% of an absorbed dose is biotransformed. The principal metabolites are trifluoroacetic acid, fluoride ions and small quantities of other organic fluoride compounds, none of which have to date been linked with anaesthetic toxicity. Peak inorganic fluoride levels reach only about 5 µmol litre^{-1} and are never likely to be high enough to cause renal damage even in the presence of hepatic enzyme-inducing agents. Furthermore, unlike enflurane, the peak levels of fluoride occur at the time of anaesthesia, reflecting the lower tissue solubility of isoflurane.

Isoflurane is slightly irritating to the upper airway but does not cause bronchoconstriction in normal man and is not associated with any greater incidence of postoperative pulmonary complications than halothane. If it does have any bronchodilatory effects, these are only mild and like enflurane and halothane, it causes a reversible depression in mucus production. During spontaneous ventilation, isoflurane causes a dose-dependent respiratory depression that is intermediate between halothane and enflurane; it depresses hypoxic pulmonary vasoconstriction to about the same extent as halothane.

The main differences between isoflurane, and enflurane and halothane lie in its effects on the cardiovascular system. All inhalational anaesthetics cause a dose-dependent depression of myocardial contractility resulting in a reduction in stroke volume and a fall in cardiac output. The fall in cardiac output can be offset to some extent by increases in heart rate. Anaesthetic concentrations (1–1.5 MAC) of isoflurane cause only a small fall (10–20%) in myocardial contractility and stroke volume and hence cardiac output alters very little. Heart rate tends to rise slightly as isoflurane has little depressant effect on baroreceptor reflexes. The tachycardia, which is by an amount intermediate between halothane and enflurane, is mainly seen in people under 40 years old and can actually raise the cardiac output to above normal awake levels. In older people, in whom baroreflex activity is normally reduced, the pulse rate tends to stay at preanaesthetic levels.

Isoflurane does not disturb cardiac rhythm and causes even less sensitization of the myocardium to adrenaline than enflurane, although induction of anaesthesia with thiopentone has been shown to reduce the arrhythmic threshold to almost half for both of these agents. Isoflurane does not affect conduction through the AV node, but like halothane and enflurane, it further prolongs the increase in conduction time caused by the calcium channel blockers diltiazem and verapamil. This is discussed further below.

Isoflurane is a potent vasodilator, particularly at higher concentrations. It maintains or even increases blood flow through some vascular beds, notably the hepatic arterial circulation and in the myocardium, and therefore allows better tissue oxygenation. In the cerebral circulation, significant vasodilation is only seen at concentrations greater than 1 MAC and up to that level, isoflurane causes no increase in cerebral blood flow or intracranial pressure. Furthermore, there is little impairment of cerebral autoregulation or carbon dioxide responsiveness, so that isoflurane is currently the inhalational agent of choice for neurosurgical anaesthesia.

The safety of isoflurane when used in patients with coronary arterial disease has been called into question. Following the demonstration that isoflurane is a potent coronary vasodilator, it was suggested that the drug might provoke myocardial ischaemia on the basis of coronary 'steal', in which blood is diverted away from stenosed segments of the coronary circulation by dilation of the normal parts. Investigation in patients about to undergo coronary artery bypass grafting has shown that isoflurane, but not halothane, decreases blood flow through the great cardiac vein, indicating reduced regional perfusion, and this is good evidence in favour of the 'steal' theory. This work has been supported by studies in dogs with stenosis of the left anterior descending (LAD) coronary artery. In this experimental model, substitution of halothane for isoflurane caused a 20% increase in flow through the stenosed LAD and a corresponding decrease through the unconstricted left circumflex coronary artery, with resultant improvement in myocardial function. However, a recent study of over 1000 patients undergoing coronary bypass operations revealed no difference in the incidence of ischaemic episodes and mortality between halothane, enflurane and isoflurane.

The overall picture is confusing but it would seem that some patients are at risk from isoflurane whereas others may not be. It is important to remember that there are other important factors which determine myocardial blood flow and therefore may affect the incidence of intraoperative ischaemia. Hypotension, particularly in the presence of a tachycardia, can also induce myocardial ischaemia particularly if the ratio of mean blood pressure to heart rate falls to one or less. These circumstances may be more likely to arise during isoflurane anaesthesia due to its tendency to cause peripheral vasodilation and raise the heart rate. Thus it would be advisable to be cautious when using isoflurane in patients with severe coronary artery disease until more evidence is available, and to pay meticulous attention to ensure that blood pressure is maintained and tachycardia is avoided.

There is some evidence that isoflurane and halothane are beneficial in the presence of a 'stunned' myocardium. This is a condition characterized by temporary (hours–days) deficits in contractile function accompanied by a depression of myocardial biochemical processes and follows brief periods (seconds) of coronary artery occlusion. It has been shown that both isoflurane and halothane speed up recovery of the affected myocardium and the return to baseline contractility.

There is considerable potential for significant interactions to occur between the calcium channel blocking drugs (CCBs) and the halogenated inhalational anaesthetic agents, principally in relation to the cardiovascular system. There is a similarity between the modes of action of the two groups of drugs. Halothane and enflurane have calcium channel blocking activity resembling verapamil and diltiazem respectively, and predominantly affect the myocardium. By contrast, isoflurane mainly affects intracellular calcium kinetics and more closely resembles nifedipine and nicardipine, acting predominantly on the peripheral vasculature. The clinical effects of any interaction between these groups of drugs depends on the pattern of administration. In the closed chest situation in patients with reasonable ventricular function, significant haemodynamic effects are only likely to occur when high doses of the inhalational agents are used (>1.5 MAC) in the presence of high plasma levels of CCB, whether given in acute or chronic dosage. Typically, there will be hypotension due to reductions in systemic vascular resistance and myocardial contractility, but AV block or sinus arrest may also occur, particularly with verapamil. Cardiovascular depression is more pronounced with enflurane than isoflurane or halothane. By contrast, in the open chest situation and in patients with poor ventricular function, there is considerable myocardial depression even with small dosages of CCB, except when agents with mainly peripheral actions are used (i.e. nifedipine and nicardipine). The presence of a β-adrenoceptor blocking drug will further enhance cardiac depression.

There is also a pharmacokinetic interaction between CCBs and inhalational anaesthetic agents. The latter reduce hepatic blood flow and inhibit drug metabolism so that higher blood levels of the CCB may be expected.

The management of severe cardiovascular depression occurring as a result of the interaction between CCBs and inhalational anaesthetic agents may be difficult. Apart from reducing the inspired concentration of the inhalational agent, intravenous fluids may help to elevate the blood pressure. Catecholamines are not always effective probably because calcium flux is too heavily blocked. An intravenous bolus dose of calcium has a short-lived positive inotropic action, and the polypeptide hormone glucagon and phosphodiesterase inhibitors have been shown experimentally to improve cardiac function. However, all of these agents are ineffective against AV conduction disorders.

Other effects

In contrast to enflurane, isoflurane depresses cortical EEG activity and does not induce convulsions. It is more potent than halothane in augmenting the effects of non-depolarizing muscle relaxants and has approximately the same potency as enflurane in this respect, although this depends on the relaxant used. Isoflurane causes the same degree of uterine muscle relaxation as halothane and enflurane.

In summary, isoflurane differs in many ways from halothane and enflurane. Although it also causes a fall in blood pressure, it does this predominantly by vasodilation whereas halothane reduces blood pressure by myocardial depression and enflurane by a mixture of vasodilation and myocardial depression. In some patients with coronary artery disease, however, differential vasodilation of the coronary artery bed can provoke myocardial ischaemia by directing blood away from stenosed areas and this will be aggravated by the tendency of isoflurane to reduce the blood pressure by peripheral vasodilation and raise the heart rate. Isoflurane is chemically very stable; it does not undergo a significant amount of hepatic biotransformation and as yet, no definite cases of hepatic damage attributable to it have been reported.

NEW INHALATIONAL ANAESTHETIC AGENTS

Sevoflurane

Research with sevoflurane has been continuing since 1975 and although not yet approved for general use, it is undergoing clinical trials in Japan. It is another fluorinated ether (methyl-isopropyl) and is less potent than other volatile agents with an oil:gas partition coefficient of 47 and a MAC in humans of about 1.7%. With low blood:gas (0.68) and tissue:blood partition coefficients, induction of and recovery from anaesthesia would be expected to be faster than with any agent in current use. It is less soluble than isoflurane in the plastic and rubber components of anaesthetic circuitry which would be an advantage when used in low flow systems. Sevoflurane is not flammable at concentrations used for anaesthesia. However, significant amounts are taken up by soda lime and broken down to produce toxic substances including formaldehyde, hydrofluoric acid and methanol.

About 2.5% of sevoflurane undergoes biotransformation *in vivo*, but this is increased in the presence of hepatic enzyme induction, and one of the metabolites is inorganic fluoride. The peak levels of fluoride are not high enough to be nephrotoxic and plateau after about 1 h, falling quickly after the cessation of anaesthesia due to the rapid exhalation of the drug. Evidence from animal studies and initial trials in humans suggests that there is no difference in the degree of hepatic and pulmonary injury compared with isoflurane.

The cardiovascular system is not greatly disturbed by sevoflurane with organ blood flow being well maintained. It causes only a small fall in blood pressure, virtually no change in pulse rate and is as safe as isoflurane in the presence of adrenaline. Sevoflurane is a respiratory depressant like all volatile agents and causes a moderate rise in $Paco_2$ of about 2 kPa. It potentiates the effects of non-depolarizing muscle relaxants and has similar effects on the CNS as isoflurane, causing only a slight increase in cerebral blood flow at 1 MAC.

Desflurane (I-653)

Desflurane was synthesized in the late 1960s. Its structure differs from isoflurane by the substitution of fluorine for chlorine at the 1-carbon position. The vapour pressure of desflurane is 89 kPa at 20°C (in comparison with 32 kPa for isoflurane) so that a pressurized vapourizer is required. Initially, little interest was shown in this agent as it is difficult and expensive to synthesize, and investigation of its suitability as an anaesthetic agent did not begin until 1987. It is less potent than other modern inhalational anaesthetic agents with an oil:gas partition coefficient of 18.7 and a MAC in humans of about 6%. The blood:gas partition coefficient of 0.42 is the lowest of all of the inhalational agents, including nitrous oxide, as are its other tissue : blood partition coefficients. This suggests that induction of and recovery from anaesthesia should be more rapid than with any other agent including sevoflurane, and this has been shown to be the case in studies in humans and in rats. It is non-flammable at clinical concentrations and is highly stable in soda lime, with almost no degradation occurring regardless of the temperature.

Desflurane is minimally biotransformed in the body and current evidence suggests that it is very safe. In rats it causes small increases in the serum inorganic fluoride levels but these are considerably less than with isoflurane, and occur only when hepatic enzymes have been induced with phenobarbitone. Repeated anaesthesia over a short period of time and prolonged anaesthesia (up to 9.7 MAC h) have not been shown to cause tissue damage. In hypoxic rats, it causes no evidence of hepatic or renal damage in contrast to halothane, isoflurane or sevoflurane when administered in similar conditions.

To date, there is very little clinical experience with the drug and most of the work on it has been done in animals. One study in human volunteers has shown a dose-dependent fall in systemic vascular resistance and an initial fall in cardiac output and heart rate. However, at deeper levels (>1.5 MAC), the cardiac output rises and can exceed baseline levels at 2.5 MAC. This has been attributed to β-adrenergic activity as seen with diethyl ether and fluoroxene. Desflurane does not sensitize the myocardium to catecholamines to any greater extent than isoflurane. The margin of safety (the ratio of the fatal concentration, i.e. that which causes total cardiovascular collapse, to MAC) is greater than for enflurane and halothane but slightly less than that for isoflurane. As with other inhaled anaesthetics, the concentration causing cardiovascular collapse exceeds that which produces apnoea making such an event very unlikely during spontaneous ventilation.

Desflurane is a respiratory depressant and increases the resting $Pa\text{co}_2$ in humans and decreases the ventilatory response to carbon dioxide at $1-2$ MAC. The effects on the electroencephalogram of pigs are indistinguishable from those of isoflurane and hypocarbia has a minimal effect.

Thus it would appear that of the two new inhalational agents, desflurane has more to offer than sevoflurane in terms of cardiovascular stability, pharmacokinetics, lower potential toxicity and a greater overall improvement over existing agents.

Cyclopropane

Cyclopropane is a colourless and odourless gas introduced into anaesthetic practice in 1934, although it had been synthesized in 1882. It is stored as a liquid under pressure, in metal cylinders. Like nitrous oxide, it has a low blood : gas partition coefficient (0.5), and both induction and recovery are very rapid. A few breaths of 50% cyclopropane are sufficient to render a patient unconscious. Respiratory depression may be more marked than with other inhalational agents and hypercarbia is likely to occur in the absence of controlled ventilation. Cyclopropane does not irritate the respiratory tract, although laryngospasm or bronchospasm may occur (particularly in asthmatic subjects), due to an increase in the tone of bronchial muscle. During anaesthesia, there is usually a slight but generalized increase in sympathetic tone, producing a small rise in blood pressure. Cyclopropane is a potent muscle relaxant, and may potentiate the effects of non-depolarizing agents. Little is known of its metabolism in man although experimental evidence suggests that it is partly metabolized to carbon dioxide; no significant toxic effects are produced by its use.

Unfortunately, cyclopropane anaesthesia is associated with two significant hazards. Firstly, cardiac excitability is increased and a variety of arrhythmias may occur, particularly during the induction of anaesthesia. In these conditions, ventricular ectopic beats or ventricular tachycardia may precipitate ventricular fibrillation. Similar arrhythmias are more likely to be induced by β-adrenergic agonists, by factors that increase endogenous adrenaline levels (such as hypercarbia), or by anticholinergic drugs. During cyclopropane anaesthesia, the use of sympathomimetic amines is therefore extremely hazardous. Secondly, cyclopropane is explosive and inflammable in the concentrations required to produce anaesthesia. For this reason, it is invariably administered in a closed circuit. These two disadvantages have restricted the use of cyclopropane and it is now not commonly used.

Diethylether

Diethylether was introduced by William Morton in 1846 and was the first inhalational anaesthetic to be used successfully during surgical operations. It is a volatile, inflammable liquid, with a high blood : gas partition coefficient (12). Thus, both induction and recovery are relatively slow, and it may take many hours to be entirely eliminated from the body. Diethylether tends to increase sympathetic tone so that respiratory rate, blood pressure, and heart rate are usually maintained or slightly increased during anaesthesia. There is marked irritation of the respiratory tract, with an increase in secretions, and premedication with atropine or a similar drug is usually essential. Diethylether enhances the action of non-depolarizing agents and causes some relaxation of uterine muscle.

Little is known of the metabolism of diethylether in man, although its administration is not associated with any significant toxicity. In experimental animals, about 6% of an administered dose is metabolized to a number of compounds including ethanol, acetaldehyde, and acetic acid. One of the main advantages of diethylether is the absence of any deleterious effects on the cardiovascular system. There is no tendency to arrhythmias or increased sensitivity to catecholamines. However, postoperative nausea and vomiting are frequent side-effects.

The main disadvantages of diethylether are its slow onset and recovery, its irritant effect on the respiratory tract, and its inflammability. Nevertheless, the drug was widely used until the advent of halothane in 1958. In recent years, its use has greatly declined and it is rarely if ever employed in anaesthetic practice. Diethylether may still be used occasionally in the intensive care situation in the management of severe asthma. The bronchorrhoea which it causes increases the effectiveness of bronchial lavage performed in these patients.

FURTHER READING

Albrecht RF, Miletich DJ. Speculations on the molecular nature of anesthesia. *General Pharmacology* 1988; **19**: 339–346.

Atlee JL III, Hamann SR, Brownlee SW, Kreigh C. Conscious state comparisons of the effects of the inhalational anesthetics and diltiazem, nifedipine, or verapamil on specialized atrioventricular conduction times in spontaneously beating dog hearts. *Anesthesiology* 1988; **68**: 519–528.

Benjamin SB, Goodman ZD, Ishak KG, Zimmerman HJ, Irey NS. The morphologic spectrum of halothane-induced hepatic injury: analysis of 77 cases. *Hepatology* 1985; **5**: 1163–1171.

Brett RS, Dilger JP, Yland KF. Isoflurane causes 'flickering' of the acetylcholine receptor channel: observations using the patch clamp. *Anesthesiology* 1988; **69**: 161–170.

Brown BR Jr, Gandolfi AJ. Adverse effects of volatile anaesthetics. *British Journal of Anaesthesia* 1987; **59**: 14–23.

Buffington CW. Hemodynamic determinants of ischemic myocardial dysfunction in the presence of coronary stenosis in dogs. *Anesthesiology* 1985; **63**: 651–662.

Carpenter RL, Eger EI II, Johnson BH, Unadkat JD, Sheiner LB. Pharmacokinetics of inhaled anesthetics in humans: measurements during and after the simultaneous administraton of enflurane, halothane, isoflurane, methoxyflurane, and nitrous oxide. *Anesthesia and Analgesics* 1986; **65**: 575–582.

Cheng-S-Z, Brunner EA. A hypothetical model on the mechanism of anesthesia. *Medical Hypotheses* 1987; **23**: 1–9.

Christ DD, Kenna JG, Kammerer W, Satoh H, Pohl LR. Enflurane metabolism produces covalently bound liver adducts recognized by antibodies from patients with halothane hepatitis. *Anesthesiology* 1988; **69**: 833–838.

Conway CM. Gaseous homeostasis and the circle system. Factors influencing anaesthetic gas exchange. *British Journal of Anaesthesia* 1986; **58**: 1167–1180.

Eger EI II (ed.) *Anesthetic Uptake and Action*. Baltimore: Williams & Wilkins, 1974.

Eger EI II (ed.) *Nitrous Oxide*. London: Arnold, 1985.

Eger EI II, Saidman LJ, Bandstater B. Minimum alveolar concentration: a standard of anesthetic potency. *Anesthesiology* 1965; **26**: 756–763.

Eger EI II, Smith NT, Stoelting RK, Cullen DJ, Kadis LB, Whitcher CE. Cardiovascular effects of halothane in man. *Anesthesiology* 1970; **32**: 396–409.

Eger EI II, Smuckler EA, Ferrell LD, Goldsmith CH, Johnson BH. Is enflurane hepatotoxic? *Anesthesia and Analgesia* 1986; **65**: 21–30.

Epstein RM, Rackow H, Salanitre E, Wolf GL. Influence of the concentration effect on the uptake of anesthetic mixtures: the second gas effect. *Anesthesiology* 1964; **25**: 364–371.

Firestone L. General anaesthetics. *International Anesthesiology Clinics* 1988; **26**: 248–253.

Fogdall RP, Miller RD. Neuromuscular effects of enflurane, alone and combined with *d*-tubocurarine, pancuronium, and succinylcholine in man. *Anesthesiology* 1975; **42**: 173–178.

Forrest JB, Chambers C. Effects of volatile anaesthetics on tracheal mucociliary transport. *Canadian Anaesthetists Society Journal* 1983; **30**: S76–77.

Franks NP, Lieb WR. What is the molecular nature of the general anaesthetic target sites? *Trends in Pharmacological Sciences* 1987; **8**: 169–174.

Frost EAM. Inhalation anaesthetic agents in neurosurgery. *British Journal of Anaesthesia* 1984; **56**: 47S–56S.

Gelman S, Fowler KC, Smith LR. Regional blood flow during isoflurane and halothane anesthesia. *Anesthesia and Analgesia* 1984; **63**: 557–565.

Gillman MA. Analgesic (sub anesthetic) nitrous oxide interacts with the endogenous opioid system: a review of the evidence. *Life Sciences* 1986; **39**: 1209–1221.

Halsey MJ. A reassessment of the molecular structure–functional relationships of the inhaled general anaesthetics. *British Journal of Anaesthesia* 1984; **56**: 9S–25S.

Halsey MJ. Anaesthetic mechanisms. *British Journal of Hospital Medicine* 1986; **36**: 445–447.

Halsey MJ. Drug interactions in anaesthesia. *British Journal of Anaesthesia* 1987; **59**: 112–123.

Halsey MJ, Wardley-Smith B, Green CJ. Pressure reversal of general anaesthesia—a multisite expansion hypothesis. *British Journal of Anaesthesia* 1978; **50**: 1091–1096.

Hansen TD, Warner DS, Todd MM, Vust LJ. Effects of nitrous oxide and volatile anaesthetics on cerebral blood flow. *British Journal of Anaesthesia* 1989; **63**: 290–295.

Hayashi Y, Sumikawa K, Tashiro C, Yamatodani A, Yoshiya I. Arrhythmogenic threshold of epinephrine during sevoflurane, enflurane, and isoflurane anesthesia in dogs. *Anesthesiology* 1988; **69**: 145–147.

Haydon DA, Hendry BM, Levinson SR. The molecular mechanisms of anaesthesia. *Nature* 1977; **268**: 356–358.

Jones RM. Clinical comparison of inhalation anaesthetic agents. *British Journal of Anaesthesia* 1984; **56**: 57S–69S.

Jones RM, Cashman JN, Eger EI II, Damask MC, Johnson BH. Kinetics and potency of desflurane (I-653) in volunteers. *Anesthesia and Analgesia* 1990; **70**: 3–7.

Kapur PA, Matarazzo DA, Fung DM, Sullivan KB. The cardiovascular and adrenergic actions of verapamil or diltiazem in combination with propranolol during halothane anesthesia in the dog. *Anesthesiology* 1987; **66**: 122–129.

Keane PE, Biziere K. Minireview. The effects of general anaesthetics on GABAergic synaptic transmission. *Life Sciences* 1987; **41**: 1437–1448.

Kenna JG, Neuberger J, Williams R. An enzyme-linked immunosorbent assay for detection of antibodies against halothane-altered hepatocyte antigens. *Journal of Immunological Methods* 1984; **75**: 3–14.

Kenna JG, Neuberger J, Williams R. Specific antibodies to halothane-induced liver antigens in halothane-associated hepatitis. *British Journal of Anaesthesia* 1987; **59**: 1286–1290.

Kenna JG, Satoh H, Christ DD, Pohl LR. Metabolic basis for a drug hypersensitivity: antibodies in sera from patients with halothane hepatitis recognize liver neoantigens that contain the trifluoroacetyl group derived from halothane. *Journal of Pharmacology and Experimental Therapeutics* 1988; **245**: 1103–1109.

Khambatta HJ, Sonntag H, Larsen R, Stephan H, Stone G, Kettler D. Global and regional myocardial blood flow and metabolism during equipotent halothane and isoflurane anesthesia in patients with coronary artery disease. *Anesthesia and Analgesia* 1988; **67**: 936–942.

Landers DF, Becker GL, Wong KC. Calcium, calmodulin, and anesthesiology. *Anesthesia and Analgesia* 1989; **69**: 110–112.

Mapleson WW. Pharmacokinetics of inhalational anaesthetics. In: Nunn JF, Utting JE, Brown BR (eds) *General Anaesthesia*, 5th edn. London: Butterworths, 1989; 44–59.

Maze M, Mason Jr DM. Aetiology and treatment of halothane-induced arrhythmias. In: Mazze RI (ed.) *Clinics in Anaesthesiology—Inhalation Anaesthesiology*. Philadelphia: WB Saunders, 1983; **1**: 301–321.

Mazze RI. Nephrotoxicity of fluorinated anaesthetic agents. In: Mazze RI (ed.) *Clinics in*

Anaesthesiology—Inhalation Anaesthesiology. Philadelphia: WB Saunders. 1983; **1**: 469–483.

Mazze RI. Metabolism of the inhaled anaesthetics: implications of enzyme induction. *British Journal of Anaesthesia* 1984; **56**: 27S–41S.

Merin RG. Calcium channel blocking drugs and anesthetics: is the drug interaction beneficial or detrimental? *Anesthesiology* 1987; **66**: 111–112.

Merin RG, Chelly JE, Hysing ES *et al*. Cardiovascular effects of and interaction between calcium blocking drugs and anesthetics in chronically instrumented dogs. IV: chronically administered oral verapamil and halothane, enflurane, and isoflurane. *Anesthesiology* 1987; **66**: 140–146.

Merrell WJ, Gordon L, Wood AJJ, Shay S, Jackson EK, Wood M. The effect of halothane on morphine disposition: relative contributions of the liver and kidney to morphine glucuronidation in the dog. *Anesthesiology* 1990; **72**: 308–314.

Miletich DJ, Ivankovich AD, Albrecht RF, Reimann CR, Rosenberg R, McKissic ED. Absence of autoregulation of cerebral blood flow during halothane and enflurane anaesthesia. *Anesthesia and Analgesia* 1976; **55**: 100–105.

Mitchell MM, Prakash O, Rulf ENR, van Daele MERM, Cahalan MK, Roelandt JRTC. Nitrous oxide does not induce myocardial ischemia in patients with ischemic heart disease and poor ventricular function. *Anesthesiology* 1989; **71**: 526–534.

Moody EJ, Suzdak PD, Paul SM, Skolnick P. Modulation of the benzodiazepine/gamma-aminobutyric acid receptor chloride channel complex by inhalation anesthetics. *Journal of Neurochemistry* 1988; **51**: 1386–1393.

Munson ES, Embro WJ. Enflurane, isoflurane, and halothane and isolated human uterine muscle. *Anesthesiology* 1977; **46**: 11–14.

Neigh JL, Garman JK, Harp JR. The electroencephalographic pattern during anesthesia with enflurane. *Anesthesiology* 1971; **35**: 482–487.

Neuberger J, Williams R. Halothane anaesthesia and liver damage. *British Medical Journal* 1984; **289**: 1136–1139.

Nunn JF. Clinical aspects of the interaction between nitrous oxide and vitamin B_{12}. *British Journal of Anaesthesia* 1987; **59**: 3–13.

Nunn JF, Chanarin I, Tanner AG, Owen ERTC. Megaloblastic bone marrow changes after repeated nitrous oxide anaesthesia. *British Journal of Anaesthesia* 1986; **58**: 1469–1470.

Plummer JL, Wanwimolruk S, Jenner MA, Hall P de la M, Cousins MJ. Effects of cimetidine and ranitidine on halothane metabolism and hepatotoxicity in an animal model. *Drug Metabolism and Disposition* 1984; **12**: 106–110.

Pollard JB, Hill RF, Lowe JE *et al*. Myocardial tolerance to total ischemia in the dog anesthetized with halothane or isoflurane. *Anesthesiology* 1988; **69**: 17–23.

Priebe HJ. Isoflurane and coronary hemodynamics. *Anesthesiology* 1989; **71**: 960–976.

Priebe HJ, Skarvan K. Cardiovascular and electrophysiologic interactions between diltiazem and isoflurane in the dog. *Anesthesiology* 1987; **66**: 114–121.

Quasha AL, Eger EI ii, Tinker JH. Determination and applications of MAC. *Anesthesiology* 1980; **53**: 315–334.

Rasmussen H. The calcium messenger system—Part 1. *New England Journal of Medicine* 1986; **314**: 1094–1101.

Rasmussen H. The calcium messenger system —Part 2. *New England Journal of Medicine* 1986; **314**: 1164–1170.

Reilly CS, Wood AJJ, Koshakji RP, Wood M. The effect of halothane on drug disposition: contribution of changes in intrinsic drug metabolising capacity and hepatic blood flow. *Anesthesiology* 1985; **63**: 70–76.

Reiz S, Bålfors E, Sørensen MG, Ariola S Jr, Friedman A, Truedsson H. Isoflurane—a powerful coronary vasodilator in patients with coronary artery disease. *Anesthesiology* 1983; **59**: 91–97.

Righi DF, Lowenstein E. Volatile anaesthetics and the ischaemic myocardium. In: Foëx P (ed.) *Anaesthesia for the Compromised Heart. Clinical Anaesthesiology*. Edinburgh: Baillière Tindall, 1989; **3**: 185–204.

Roth SH. Mechanisms of anaesthesia: a mystery. *Canadian Journal of Anaesthesia* 1988; **35**: S1–3.

Roth SH, Miller KW (eds) *Molecular and Cellular Mechanisms of Anesthetics*. New York: Plenum, 1986.

Rudo FG, Krantz Jr JC. Anaesthetic molecules. *British Journal of Anaesthesia* 1974; **46**: 181–189.

Ruffle JM, Snider MT, Rosenberger JL, Latta WB. Rapid induction of halothane anaesthesia in man. *British Journal of Anaesthesia* 1985; **57**: 607–611.

Rupp SM, Miller RD, Gencarelli PJ. Vecuronium-induced neuromuscular blockade during enflurane, isoflurane, and halothane anesthesia in humans. *Anesthesiology* 1984; **60**: 102–105.

Sahlman L, Henriksson B-Å, Martner J, Ricksten S-E. Effects of halothane, enflurane, and isoflurane on coronary vascular tone, myocardial performance, and oxygen consumption during controlled changes in aortic and left atrial pressure. *Anesthesiology* 1988; **68**: 1–10.

Segal I, Vickery RG, Walton JK, Doze VA, Maze M. Dexmedetomidine diminishes halothane anesthetic requirements in rats through a postsynaptic alpha$_2$ adrenergic receptor. *Anesthesiology* 1988; **69**: 818–823.

Shackleton S, Harrington JM. The pollution controversy. In: Lunn JN (ed.) *Epidemiology in Anaesthesia*. London: Arnold, 1986; 93–122.

Slogoff S, Keats AS. Randomized trial of primary anesthetic agents on outcome of coronary artery bypass operations. *Anesthesiology* 1989; **70**: 179–188.

Stoelting RK, Blitt CD, Cohen PJ, Merin RG. Hepatic dysfunction after isoflurane anesthesia. *Anesthesia and Analgesia* 1987; **66**: 147–153.

Stoelting RK, Eger EI II. An additional explanation for the second gas effect: a concentrating effect. *Anesthesiology* 1969; **30**: 273–277.

Targ AG, Yasuda N, Eger EI II, Huang G, Vernice GG, Terrell RC. Halogenation and anesthetic potency. *Anesthesia and Analgesia* 1989; **68**: 599–602.

Targ AG, Yasuda N, Eger EI II. Solubility of I-653, sevoflurane, isoflurane, and halothane in plastics and rubber composing a conventional anesthetic circuit. *Anesthesia and Analgesia* 1989; **69**: 218–225.

Terrell RC. Physical and chemical properties of anaesthetic agents. *British Journal of Anaesthesia* 1984; **56**: 3S–7S.

Trudell JR. A unitary theory of anesthesia based on lateral phase separations in nerve membranes. *Anesthesiology* 1977: **46**: 5–10.

Ueda I, Kamaya H. Molecular mechanisms of anesthesia. *Anesthesia and Analgesia* 1984; **63**: 929–945.

Warltier DC, Al-Wathiqui MH, Kampine JP, Schmeling WT. Recovery of contractile function of stunned myocardium in chronically instrumented dogs is enhanced by halothane and isoflurane. *Anesthesiology* 1988; **69**: 552–565.

Webster NR, White DC. Study of the uptake of inhalational agents by modelling. In: Kaufman L. (ed.) *Anaesthesia Review* Volume 6. Edinburgh: Churchill Livingstone, 1989; 267–285.

Weiskopf RB, Eger EI II, Homes MA *et al.* Epinephrine-induced premature ventricular contractions and changes in arterial blood pressure and heart rate during I-653, isoflurane, and halothane anesthesia in swine. *Anesthesiology* 1989; **70**: 293–298.

Weiskopf RB. New inhaled anesthetics. *Current Opinion in Anesthesiology. Current Science*; 1989; **2**: 421–424.

White DC. A review of nitrous oxide. In: Atkinson RS, Adams AP (eds) *Recent Advances in Anaesthesia and Analgesia* Volume 16. Edinburgh: Churchill Livingstone, 1989; 19–42.

Williams R. Halothane and the liver—a medical review. In: Halothane and the liver: the problem revisited, pp. 12–21. *Proceedings of a Symposium, 1986*. Bristol: Sir Humphrey Davy Department of Anaesthesia, 1986.

EIGHT

Local Anaesthetic Agents

Local anaesthetic agents can be defined as drugs which are used clinically to produce the reversible loss of sensation in a circumscribed area of the body. Their action depends on the reversible inhibition of the conduction of impulses in peripheral nerve fibres and nerve endings. At high concentrations, many drugs that are used for other purposes possess local anaesthetic or membrane stabilizing properties. These drugs include:

1 Anticonvulsants (e.g. phenytoin, carbamazepine).
2 Phenothiazines (e.g. chlorpromazine).
3 Antihistamines (H_1-histamine antagonists) (e.g. cyclizine).
4 Barbiturates (e.g. pentobarbitone).
5 Opioid analgesics (e.g. pethidine).
6 Antiarrhythmic drugs (e.g. quinidine, disopyramide).
7 β-adrenoceptor antagonists (e.g. propranolol, acebutalol).

Similarly, local anaesthetic drugs are commonly used as antiarrhythmic agents, and are occasionally used as anticonvulsants.

In addition, a number of naturally occurring biotoxins reversibly inhibit the conduction of impulses in peripheral nerves and nerve endings. Thus, one variety of the Japanese 'puffer fish' (*Spheroides spengleri*) contains the poison tetrodotoxin; it is also present in the octopus, salamanders, newts and amphibia, and is probably derived from micro-organisms that synthesize the toxin. (During his voyages of discovery in the South Seas, Captain James Cook tasted 'puffer fish' and subsequently suffered from tetrodotoxin poisoning.) An unrelated series of toxins (the saxitoxins) are produced by the dinoflagellates (i.e. flagellated unicellular organisms which contaminate shellfish). Both tetrodotoxin and saxitoxin are extremely potent local anaesthetics; unfortunately, they are relatively polar compounds and do not readily penetrate perineuronal tissues.

STRUCTURE AND FUNCTION OF NERVE FIBRES

Peripheral nerves consist of the dendrites and axons of sensory and/or motor nerves, which are bound together and surrounded by connective tissue. Layers of longtitudinally arranged collagen surround individual nerve fibres (the en-

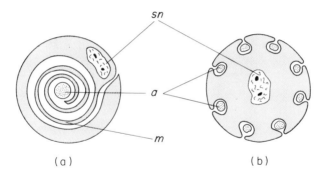

Fig. 8.1 Diagram showing transverse section of (a) myelinated, and (b) unmyelinated nerve fibre, *sn*: Schwann cell nucleus, *a*: axon, *m*: myelin sheath.

doneurium) or groups of nerve fibres (the perineurium); an outer connective tissue sheath (the epineurium) surrounds the nerve trunk and carries its blood vessels, nerve supply, and lymphatics. Each nerve fibre is connected with a central cell body or perikaryon from which it receives its nutritional requirements, and is surrounded by a sheath of Schwann cell cytoplasm. Unmyelinated fibres are usually enclosed in groups by the sheath of a single Schwann cell (which may be up to 0.5 mm long); at junctions, the cytoplasm of adjacent Schwann cells is in contact. In contrast, each myelinated fibre is enclosed by the cytoplasm of a single Schwann cell, with its phospholipid cell membrane wound spirally around the axon (Fig. 8.1). The double phospholipid cell membrane of the Schwann cell (the myelin sheath) does not extend continuously along the axon; between individual Schwann cells the myelin sheath is absent. The junctions between Schwann cells are known as the nodes of Ranvier. The internodal distance is related to the size of the Schwann cells and the diameter of the nerve fibres. In large myelinated nerves, the internodal distance may be 1–2 mm.

Nerve fibres consist of a central core (the axoplasm) which is enclosed by a limiting cell membrane (the axolemma or axonal membrane). The axoplasm contains mitochondria, microtubules, and neurofilaments, which are required for normal neuronal metabolism. In contrast, the axonal membrane is a characteristic phospholipid membrane (p. 1), containing integral proteins which play an important functional role as ion channels.

Various techniques have been used to study the electrophysiology of neuronal conduction and its modification by drugs. These methods include measurement of changes in potential by intracellular microelectrodes, the use of fluorescent probes, and the analysis of voltage clamp recordings, in which the membrane potential is changed in small steps, and separate phases of ionic flow are studied.

In the inactive state, there is a difference in potential of approximately 80 mV across the neuronal membrane (i.e. the inside is electronegative relative to the

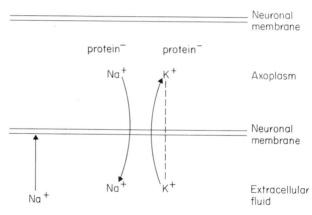

Fig. 8.2 The origin of the resting membrane potential. The ionic pump (the enzyme Na$^+$/K$^+$ ATPase) maintains a high internal potassium concentration and a high external sodium concentration. In the resting state, the membrane is effectively impermeable to sodium ions, although potassium ions can diffuse from the axoplasm to extracellular fluid. The tendency for potassium ions to leave the fibre is opposed by the anionic charges on intracellular protein, giving rise to the resting membrane potential.

outside). This potential difference (the resting potential) mainly reflects the selective permeability of the neuronal membrane to potassium ions, and can be regarded as a 'potassium diffusion potential'. In nerve fibres, as in many other cells, an ionic pump (the enzyme Na$^+$/K$^+$ ATPase) maintains a high internal potassium concentration and a high external sodium concentration. The intracellular concentration of potassium (K$_i^+$) is normally 25–30 times greater than in extracellular fluid (K$_o^+$). In the resting state, the neuronal membrane is effectively impermeable to sodium ions (Fig. 8.2); consequently sodium ions play little or no part in the production of the resting membrane potential. In contrast, the membrane is relatively permeable to potassium ions, and there is a tendency for potassium ions to diffuse from the axon. This tendency is opposed by the anionic charge on intracellular proteins, which tends to prevent outward potassium ion diffusion, and the balance between these two forces represents the resting membrane potential (-80 mV). Consequently, the resting membrane potential is closely related to the intracellular/extracellular concentration ratio of potassium ions (K$_i^+$/K$_o^+$). In these conditions, the neurone acts as a potassium electrode, and the resting potential can be modified by alterations in extracellular potassium concentration. On electrical stimulation, characteristic changes occur in the transmembrane potential. Initially, there is a slow phase of depolarization as the cell becomes progressively less negative. When the threshold potential is reached, there is rapid and transient depolarization to approximately $+30$ mV, followed by a return to the resting value (repolarization). These changes in transmembrane potential are referred to as the action potential, and occur within

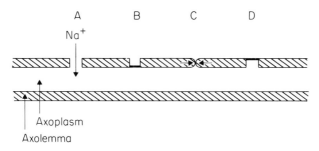

Fig. 8.3 Site of action of local anaesthetic agents. A, influx of Na$^+$ via unblocked channels to produce depolarization. B, Na$^+$ channels blocked by cationic form of local anaesthetic esters or amides. C, Na$^+$ channels blocked by uncharged base ('membrane expansion'). D, Na$^+$ channels blocked by tetrodotoxin.

1–2 ms; they are due to changes in the ionic permeability of axonal membranes. The property of electrical excitability (i.e. the ability to generate an action potential) depends on the presence of voltage-sensitive sodium channels in the axonal membrane. During excitation, the neurone slowly depolarizes, and the transmembrane potential decreases until the threshold potential is reached (at approximately −50 mV). At this point, sodium permeability rapidly increases due to the opening of voltage-dependent ion channels, and sodium ions rapidly diffuse across the axonal membrane (Fig. 8.3). This causes a transient reversal of the membrane potential to approximately +30 mV. Sodium ion diffusion ceases (since the transmembrane potential equals the Na$^+$ equilibrium potential), and the channels close spontaneously (inactivation). At the same time, potassium permeability increases due to the opening of different specific ion channels in the axonal membrane. Potassium ions diffuse across the axonal membrane into extracellular fluid, resulting in repolarization and the restoration of the resting membrane potential. During the refractory period these changes are reversed (i.e. sodium ions are transferred from the axoplasm to extracellular fluid, and potassium ions are concentrated by the neurone). Re-establishment of the ionic gradient depends on active transport by the enzyme Na$^+$/K$^+$ ATPase (the sodium pump), and requires the expenditure of cellular energy.

Calcium ions are present in the neuronal membrane (and other cellular membranes), and can interact with negatively charged phosphate groups associated with the heads of phospholipids. These hydrophilic groups are present at the internal and external aspects of the membrane (Chapter 1); interaction with calcium ions alters the charge distribution in the membrane, impedes sodium conductance, and may modify the action of local anaesthetics.

In experimental conditions, the threshold potential required for sodium channel opening is reduced when the local concentration of Ca^{2+} is increased (although the resting potential is unaltered).

In unmyelinated fibres, depolarization produces a local flow of current in the neuronal membrane which decreases the transmembrane potential of the adjacent nerve. Voltage-sensitive sodium channels are activated and impulses are propagated along the nerve fibre. Retrograde conduction cannot occur, due to the inactivation of sodium channels in the wake of the impulse.

In myelinated fibres, current flows from one node of Ranvier to another; since the internodal distance may be 1–2 mm, conduction in myelinated fibres (saltatory conduction) is much more rapid (approximately $120\,\mathrm{m\ s^{-1}}$).

HISTORY OF LOCAL ANAESTHETICS

The alkaloid cocaine is the only naturally occurring local anaesthetic, and was the first of these drugs to be used clinically. It is derived from a shrub (*Erythroxylon coca*) that grows in the foothills of the Andes, and for many centuries its leaves have been chewed by the Peruvian Indians, in order to obtain cocaine. The drug was particularly valued for its mood-elevating and stimulant properties, and its numbing effects on the buccal mucosa were well-known. Pure cocaine was first isolated by Niemann in 1860, who confirmed its effects on sensation; its pharmacological actions were studied by Von Anrep between 1870 and 1880. The drug was first introduced into clinical practice by Freud and Köller in 1884. Sigmund Freud used cocaine in an attempt to treat a morphine-dependent colleague, but converted him into a cocaine addict; he also took cocaine himself for a period of 10 years (while he was writing *The Interpretation of Dreams*). Karl Köller initially used cocaine to provide corneal anaesthesia in experimental animals. He rapidly appreciated its potential advantages, and introduced it in ophthalmological practice as a surface anaesthetic; its use for infiltration, conduction and spinal anaesthesia soon followed. Unfortunately, its potential for producing drug dependence was not fully appreciated at this time. Nevertheless, by 1890 the dangers of cocaine were well-recognized, and a search began for newer and safer drugs. The first synthetic local anaesthetic, the *para*-aminobenzoate ester procaine, was synthesized by Einhorn about 1905. Many other synthetic local anaesthetic esters were subsequently investigated; most of them have now been discarded, and are now solely of historical interest. However chloroprocaine, which was introduced in 1952, is still used clinically in the USA; it is the least toxic local anaesthetic ester.

An important milestone occurred in 1943 when lignocaine, the first aminoacyl-amide local anaesthetic, was synthesized by Lofgren. This compound was the prototype of a new group of local anaesthetics with significant clinical advantages. Since the advent of lignocaine, many other amide anaesthetics have been introduced (e.g. mepivacaine, bupivacaine, and prilocaine). Etidocaine is also an extremely potent amide anaesthetic; it is not available for clinical use in the UK.

LOCAL ANAESTHETIC PREPARATIONS

Most local anaesthetics are bases that are almost insoluble in water. Consequently, their hydrochloride salts, which are extremely water-soluble, are usually dissolved in modified isotonic Ringer solution. Dilute preparations of local anaesthetics are usually acid (pH range = 4.0–5.5), and contain a reducing agent (e.g. sodium metabisulphite) to enhance the stability of added vasoconstrictors (which may oxidize in solution). They also usually contain a preservative and a fungicide. The preservative helps to maintain the stability of the local anaesthetic solution, while the fungicide (usually a small concentration of thymol) prevents the growth of contaminating fungi. Solutions of local anaesthetics are extremely stable and usually have an effective shelf-life of more than 2 years.

Most local anaesthetics also produce some degree of vasodilatation, and they may be rapidly absorbed after local injection. Consequently, vasoconstrictors are frequently added to local anaesthetic solutions, in order to enhance their potency and prolong their duration of action by localizing them in tissues. In addition, vasoconstrictors decrease the systemic toxicity and increase the safety margin of local anaesthetics by reducing their rate of absorption (which is mainly dependent on local blood flow). In these conditions, the effectiveness of vasoconstrictors is extremely variable. In most infiltration procedures and in conduction blockade, vasoconstrictors usually prolong and enhance local anaesthesia; on the other hand, they may have little effect on the duration of extradural or intrathecal blockade (particularly when induced by etidocaine or bupivacaine).

Adrenaline is the most commonly used vasoconstrictor; it is added to local anaesthetic solutions in concentrations ranging from 1 in 80 000 (12.5 µg ml^{-1}) to 1 in 300 000 (3.3 µg ml^{-1}). Preparations containing noradrenaline (1 in 80 000) are also available, but are usually avoided due to their pressor effects (which are particularly hazardous in patients with ischaemic heart disease or who are on tricyclic antidepressant drugs). The vasoconstrictor felypressin is added to some local anaesthetics (i.e. prilocaine) in a concentration of 0.03 i.u.ml^{-1}. Felypressin is a non-catecholamine vasoconstrictor that is chemically related to vasopressin, the posterior pituitary hormone. It is a synthetic octapeptide that only affects peripheral blood vessels; it has no action on the heart. Although it produces less marked vasoconstriction than adrenaline, it may be useful in patients with ischaemic heart disease, or when the use of catecholamines is undesirable. Other vasoconstrictors (e.g. phenylephrine) have also been studied; however, adrenaline is more effective than phenylephrine (or noradrenaline) in reducing the rate of absorption of most local anaesthetics.

Chemical and physicochemical properties

All local anaesthetics have certain chemical and physicochemical properties in common. Chemically, they consist of a lipophilic aromatic group (R_1), an

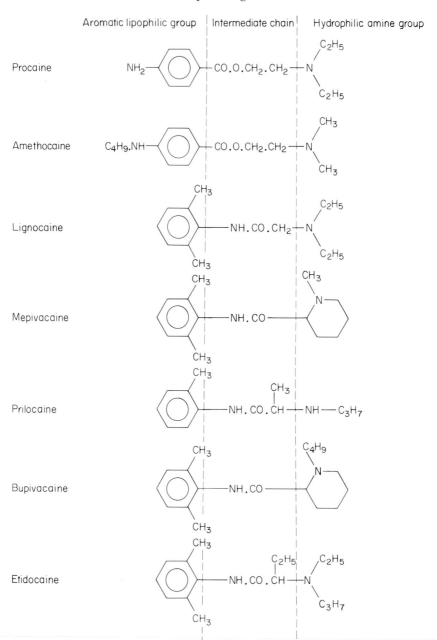

Fig. 8.4   Chemical structure of local anaesthetic agents.

intermediate ester $(-CO.O-)$ or amide $(-NH.CO-)$ chain, and a hydrophilic secondary or tertiary amine group (R_2). The intermediate chain is an important determinant of the duration of action; it also allows the classification of local anaesthetics as esters or amides (Fig. 8.4).

Ester local anaesthetics include:

1 Procaine.
2 Chloroprocaine.
3 Amethocaine.

Amide local anaesthetics are:

1 Lignocaine.
2 Prilocaine.
3 Mepivacaine.
4 Bupivacaine.
5 Etidocaine.

There are important practical differences between these two groups of local anaesthetics. Esters are relatively unstable in solution, and are rapidly hydrolysed in the body by plasma cholinesterase (and some other esterases). *Para*-aminobenzoate (PABA) is usually one of the main hydrolytic products; this metabolite may be associated with the presence of allergic reactions and other hypersensitivity phenomena. By contrast, amides are relatively stable in solution, and are slowly broken down by amidases in the liver. In addition, hypersensitivity reactions to amide local anaesthetics are almost unknown. In current practice, esters are only rarely used to produce local anaesthesia; they have been largely superseded by the amides.

Modification of the chemical structure of local anaesthetics may have a profound effect on their physicochemical characteristics. In particular, anaesthetic properties may be modified by changes in (1) lipid-solubility, (2) plasma and tissue protein binding, and (3) the dissociation constant (i.e. the pK_a value). Values for these constants in ester and amide local anaesthetics are shown in Table 8.1.

In general, there is a close correlation between lipid-solubility and anaesthetic potency (particularly in *in vitro* conditions). This relationship presumably reflects the ability of different anaesthetics to penetrate the perineuronal tissues and the neuronal membrane, and reach their site of action in the axoplasm.

Plasma and tissue protein binding primarily affect the duration of action of local anaesthetics. For example, procaine (which is not extensively bound to plasma or tissue proteins) has a short duration of action in most clinical situations; by contrast, amethocaine, bupivacaine, and etidocaine are extensively bound and have prolonged effects. Lignocaine, mepivacaine and prilocaine are moderately bound to plasma and tissue proteins, and have an intermediate duration of action (Table 8.1).

Table 8.1 Physicochemical properties and pharmacological effects of local anaesthetic agents.

	pK_a value (25°C)	Relative lipid solubility	Relative potency	Protein binding (%)	Onset of action	Duration of action	Clinical use	Properties
Esters								
Procaine	8.9	1	1	6	Slow	Short	Limited Vascular spasm Diagnostic procedures	Vasodilatation Allergenic
Amethocaine	8.5	200	8	76	Slow	Long	Topical anaesthesia Spinal anaesthesia	Systemic toxicity
Amides								
Lignocaine	7.7	150	2	64	Fast	Moderate	Infiltration anaesthesia Peripheral nerve blockade Extradural blockade IVRA	Versatile Moderate vasodilatation
Mepivacaine	7.6	50	2	78	Fast	Moderate	Infiltration anaesthesia Peripheral nerve blockade	Similar to lignocaine
Prilocaine	7.7	50	2	55	Fast	Moderate	Infiltration anaesthesia Peripheral nerve blockade IVRA	Methaemoglobinaemia Low systemic toxicity
Bupivacaine	8.1	1000	8	96	Moderate	Long	Infiltration anaesthesia Peripheral nerve blockade Extradural and spinal anaesthesia	Separation of sensory and motor blockade
Etidocaine	7.7	5000	6	96	Fast	Long	Infiltration anaesthesia Peripheral nerve blockade Extradural blockade	Profound motor blockade

IVRA, intravenous regional anaesthesia.

The dissociation constant (pK_a value) of local anaesthetics is the most important factor affecting their rapidity and onset of action. In order to produce their effects, local anaesthetics must diffuse across the nerve sheath and the neuronal membrane in the form of the unionized, uncharged free base. The dissociation constant (pK_a value) represents the pH at which the concentration of the non-ionized base (B) and the ionized base (BH^+) are equal; it can be used to calculate the proportion of the free base present in solution at different pH values. For example, lignocaine and prilocaine have a pK_a value of approximately 7.7; at pH 7.4, 33% is present in solution as the free base B, and is available to diffuse across the nerve sheath. High pK_a values are associated with a slower onset of blockade, since less of the drug is present as the free base B. Conversely, lower pK_a values are reflected by the more rapid onset of anaesthesia, since more of the drug is present as the unionized base at physiological pH values. These considerations may explain the slower onset of action of procaine, amethocaine, and bupivacaine, and the more rapid effects of mepivacaine and etidocaine, in relation to lignocaine and prilocaine (Table 8.1). Nevertheless, the rapidity of onset and latency of action of local anaesthetics can also be modified by unrelated factors (e.g. the dose and the resultant concentration of the drug in tissues).

Mode of action

Most local anaesthetic agents are tertiary amine bases (B) that are administered as water-soluble hydrochlorides (B.HCl). After injection, the tertiary amine base is liberated by the relatively alkaline pH of tissue fluid:

$$B.HCl + HCO_3^- = B + H_2CO_3 + Cl^-.$$

In tissue fluid, the local anaesthetic will be present in both an ionised (BH^+) and a non-ionized form (B); their relative proportions will depend on the pH of the solution and the pK_a of the individual compound, as determined by the Henderson–Hasselbalch equation:

$$pK_a - pH = \log [BH^+]/[B].$$

The non-ionized base B then diffuses through the nerve sheath, perineuronal tissues, and the neuronal membrane to reach the axoplasm, where it partially ionizes again:

$$B + H^+ \rightleftharpoons BH^+.$$

In the ionized form BH^+, the local anaesthetic enters the sodium channel from the axoplasm (i.e. from the interior of the nerve fibre); it either occludes the channel, or combines with a receptor that results in channel closure (Fig. 8.3). Indeed, the sodium channel itself may be the receptor for local anaesthetics, or there may be multiple binding sites for drugs in the sodium channel. The binding of drugs to open ion channels is required for local anaesthetics to reach their site of action; consequently, in experimental conditions the degree of nerve blockade is proportional to the rate of stimulation.

Thus, although the presence of the diffusable base is essential to reach its site of action in the axoplasm, the anaesthetic acts in an ionized, cationic form. The most convincing evidence to support this explanation has been obtained from experiments in which lignocaine and its N-ethylated quaternary derivative have been applied to the inside and the outside of the neuronal membrane. Lignocaine produces local anaesthesia when applied to the inside or the outside of the axonal membrane; in contrast, its quaternary derivative is only effective when applied to the axoplasmic aspect of the membrane, implying the presence of a site of action that is only accessible from the axoplasm.

Although local anaesthetics primarily prevent sodium entry and thus prevent depolarization, they may also affect other ionic channels (e.g. potassium channels). Nevertheless, they do not modify the resting potential of the neurone (except in extremely high concentrations). Similarly, they do not alter the threshold potential required for impulse propagation; although the rates of depolarization and repolarization are decreased, the refractory period is prolonged, and conduction velocity is diminished. Similar effects may be produced in other excitable tissues; for instance, in cardiac muscle, the rate of depolarization of ventricular muscle (phase 0) is reduced (Chapter 15). In addition, local anaesthetics may modify the effects of calcium ions on the charge distribution and excitability of neuronal membranes.

All local anaesthetics do not act in the manner described above. Certain agents (e.g. benzocaine, benzyl alcohol, and n-butanol) are only present as an uncharged, tertiary base, and must therefore act by a different mechanism. They may cause conduction blockade by 'membrane expansion' (i.e. by causing swelling of the lipoprotein matrix of the sodium channel). To some extent, other local anaesthetics (which are partly present in the axolemma and the axoplasm as the uncharged, tertiary base) may act in this way.

In clinical practice, local anaesthesia may be influenced by the local availability of the free base (B), since this is the form of the drug that readily diffuses through connective tissue and crosses the neuronal membrane. Thus, local anaesthetics are relatively inactive when injected into tissues with an acid pH (e.g. pyogenic abscesses). This is presumably due to the reduced availability of the free base for diffusion, and to the more rapid removal of the drug due to increased vascularity. Conversely, carbonated solutions have also been used to improve the speed of onset and the quality of conduction blockade. In isolated preparations, carbon dioxide rapidly diffuses across the neuronal membrane and decreases the axoplasmic pH. This enhances the conversion of the local anaesthetic to the active, cationic form, and the gradient for the diffusion of the free base from the extracellular fluid to the axoplasm is also increased. In these conditions, the speed of onset and the depth of local anaesthesia should be enhanced (due to the presence of a greater proportion of the free base at its site of action). It is debatable whether these advantages are present in clinical practice, since injected carbonic acid and carbon dioxide may be rapidly buffered by intracellular proteins. In addition, carbonated solutions are unstable, the local anaesthetic may be precipitated, and any added vasoconstrictor is more easily hydrolysed. Other agents (e.g. sodium bicarbonate and various dextrans) have also been added to local anaesthetic solutions, in an attempt to increase the intensity and duration of action (presumably by modifying the proportion of the free base that is present in solution).

During conduction blockade, different sensations may be affected to an unequal extent by local anaesthetics. The sensation of pain usually disappears before touch and pressure, while motor fibres may remain functional although sensory pathways are blocked. These differences may be related to the diameter of the nerve fibres mediating different sensations; smaller diameter fibres may differ in their susceptibility to the effects of local anaesthetics. Non-myelinated fibres have a relatively large surface area (due to the absence of a myelin sheath). In contrast, myelinated fibres have a relatively small surface area, and are only susceptible to nerve blockade at the nodes of Ranvier. In addition, sequential blockade of two to three nodes of Ranvier may be required to interrupt neuronal transmission. Since the internodal distance is related to nerve fibre diameter, the larger diameter myelinated fibres are less susceptible than smaller fibres, which in turn are less susceptible than non-myelinated fibres. Consequently pain (which is partly mediated by non-myelinated C fibres) is commonly blocked before touch and pressure (mediated by $A\beta$ and $A\gamma$ fibres) which in turn are blocked before proprioception and motor fibres (which are dependent on $A\alpha$ fibres). Nevertheless, these considerations do not adequately explain several clinical observations. For instance, myelinated fibres of the $A\delta$ group (which conduct the sensation of fast or 'first' pain) may be blocked before some non-myelinated C fibres. This phenomenon may reflect the anatomical distribution of nerve fibres, and their accessibility to drugs.

Physicochemical factors may also account for the differential effects of local anaesthetics on sensory and motor function. For instance, low concentrations of bupivacaine may readily affect unmyelinated C fibres, due to its high lipid-solubility; in contrast, it may not rapidly diffuse across myelinated $A\alpha$ fibres and cause motor blockade (due to its high pK_a value). Consequently, bupivacaine may possess the optimal physicochemical characteristics required to cause differential sensory and motor blockade.

Pharmacokinetics

Significant absorption of local anaesthetics occurs from their site of injection. For each individual drug, the amount of local anaesthetic absorbed and the peak plasma concentration will be dependent on the dose, and may also be modified by the presence or the absence of a vasoconstrictor (particularly during infiltration or conduction anaesthesia). The site of injection is also important; for example, higher blood levels are attained after intercostal and caudal blockade than with lumbar epidural or brachial plexus blockade. Thus, for every 100 mg lignocaine injected in an adult, the peak venous plasma concentration ranges from 1.5 μg ml^{-1} (intercostal blockade), 1.2 μg ml^{-1} (caudal and paracervical blockade), 1.0 μg ml^{-1} (epidural blockade), 0.6 μg ml^{-1} (brachial plexus blockade) to 0.4 μg ml^{-1} (intrathecal blockade). This range of concentrations is mainly due to differences in vascularity, although other factors (e.g. uptake by tissue lipids) may also be involved. In these conditions, adherence to dose limits for local anaesthetics (e.g. 200–500 mg for lignocaine and 150 mg for bupivacaine) may obscure potential differences in systemic toxicity, depending on the site of injection. Clearly, identical doses of local anaesthetics may be more toxic in certain injection sites than in others.

Many local anaesthetics are also well absorbed from mucous membranes. The rate of uptake is closely related to the surface area available for absorption (e.g. it is extremely rapid when topical local anaesthetic sprays are applied to the tracheobronchial tract). In addition, the inherent effects of drugs on vascular tone may affect their rate of absorption. Thus, cocaine prevents the neuronal uptake of catecholamines (Uptake$_1$) and inhibits the enzyme monoamine oxidase; this produces vasoconstriction and delays drug absorption. All other local anaesthetics may have a biphasic action on vascular smooth muscle; in the concentrations present clinically they all tend to produce some degree of vasodilatation (usually in the order procaine > prilocaine > lignocaine > mepivacaine > bupivacaine). This may affect the rate of absorption of the individual drugs. Procaine, chloroprocaine and related esters are potent vasodilators, and are readily absorbed after injection; they are also rapidly broken down in tissues and plasma by esterase enzymes. The inactivation of procaine by vascular mucous membranes accounts for its relative lack of surface anaesthetic activity.

After absorption from the site of injection, the plasma concentration of local anaesthetics depends on their rate of distribution in tissues and their elimination from the body. The prolonged absorption of local anaesthetics may preclude or obscure the accurate determination of their pharmacokinetics. After intravenous injection, the plasma concentration of all local anaesthetics invariably declines in a biexponential or triexponential manner. There is an initial rapid distribution phase (half-life = 1–3 min), associated with the rapid uptake of the drugs by highly perfused organs (e.g. lung, liver, and kidney). Local anaesthetics are also distributed to skeletal muscle. One (or more than one) initial distribution phase is followed by a slower decline in the plasma concentration of the drug. This final phase represents the removal of the local anaesthetic by metabolism and excretion. The terminal half-life of most ester anaesthetics is relatively short (appro-

Table 8.2 Pharmacokinetics and metabolism of local anaesthetics.

	Terminal half-life (min)	Clearance (litre min^{-1})	Apparent volume of distribution (litres)	Metabolites
Esters				
Cocaine	Uncertain	Uncertain	Uncertain	Norcocaine Ecgonine Benzoylated derivatives
Procaine	Uncertain	Uncertain	Uncertain	*para*-aminobenzoic acid Diethylaminoethanol
Amethocaine	Uncertain	Uncertain	Uncertain	Butylaminobenzoic acid Dimethylaminoethanol
Amides				
Lignocaine	100	1.0	91	Monoethylglycinexylidide *N*-ethylglycine; 2,6-xylidine 4-hydroxy-2,6-xylidine
Mepivacaine	115	0.8	84	3-hydroxymepivacaine 4-hydroxymepivacaine
Prilocaine	100	2.4	191	*O*-toluidine *N*-propylamine
Bupivacaine	160	0.6	73	Pipecolic acid Pipecolylxylidide
Etidocaine	160	1.1	134	Numerous unidentified metabolites

ximately 10 min), due to their rapid hydrolysis by plasma cholinesterase. In contrast, the elimination half-life of amides ranges from 100 min (lignocaine) to 180 min (bupivacaine). Their volume of distribution is rather greater than total body water, while their plasma clearance is comparable with liver blood flow (Table 8.2). Pathological conditions may alter the pharmacokinetics of local anaesthetics. In particular, cardiovascular disease and hepatic cirrhosis may decrease the clearance and volume of distribution of local anaesthetics, with variable effects on the terminal half-life. In neonatal life, clearance of local anaesthetics is decreased and the half-life is prolonged. In addition, a number of drugs (e.g. halothane and propranolol) can decrease the clearance of amide local anaesthetics.

The binding of local anaesthetics by plasma proteins may also affect their pharmacokinetic behaviour and pharmacodynamic effects. In general, ester local anaesthetics are not significantly bound by plasma proteins (i.e. 5–10%). In contrast, amide local anaesthetics are mainly bound by α_1-acid glycoprotein, in the order bupivacaine > mepivacaine > lignocaine > prilocaine. The extent of protein-binding usually ranges from 50–80%; it is usually readily reversible, and does not appear to limit or restrict the uptake of local anaesthetics by most tissues and organs. Plasma protein binding is significantly influenced by physiological and pathological changes in the concentration of α_1-acid glycoprotein (which may occur in infancy, pregnancy, old age, myocardial infarction, renal failure, malignant disease, and after operative surgery). In these conditions, protein-binding is increased, the free (unbound) concentration of drugs is reduced, and the total plasma concentration of local anaesthetics may not be related to their effective concentration. The protein-binding of local anaesthetics may also affect placental transfer. In general, highly protein-bound drugs have a low umbilical vein:maternal blood (UV:M) concentration ratio. Thus, the UV:M ratio for bupivacaine is approximately 0.2; for lignocaine and prilocaine, the UV:M ratio is 0.5. These values do not necessarily reflect the relative safety of the local anaesthetics in pregnancy and labour (since they do not take account of differential α_1-acid glycoprotein binding in maternal and fetal blood). Nevertheless, it is generally accepted that the placental transfer of bupivacaine is less than lignocaine and prilocaine, and that this may have possible implications in pregnancy and labour.

Metabolism and elimination

The metabolism of local anaesthetics is determined by their chemical structure. Esters and amides are metabolized in different ways by different tissues.

Ester local anaesthetics are broken down by plasma cholinesterase (and, to some extent, by other esterase enzymes in certain tissues). Only small amounts are eliminated unchanged in urine. For example, procaine is hydrolysed to *para*-aminobenzoic acid (which is excreted unchanged in urine) and diethylaminoethanol (which is mainly further metabolized by alcohol dehydrogenase to diethylglycine). Most other ester local anaesthetics (e.g. chloroprocaine and amethocaine) are metabolized in an essentially similar manner. In contrast, cocaine is relatively resistant to hydrolysis by plasma cholinesterase. It is extensively metabolized in the liver, and only trace amounts (approximately 1% of the dose) are excreted unchanged. Studies using radiolabelled cocaine suggest that the drug is converted to several metabolites (i.e. norcocaine, ecgonine, and their benzoylated analogues). Some of these metabolites may be responsible for the stimulant effects of cocaine on the CNS.

In contrast to most ester anaesthetics, the amides are extensively metabolized by hepatic enzymes (mainly by amidases that are associated with the cytoplasm and the smooth endoplasmic reticulum). Lignocaine is almost entirely metabolized by the liver; its clearance is approximately 70–80% of normal liver blood flow, and after oral administration only trace amounts gain access to the systemic circulation (i.e. it has an extremely high 'first pass effect'). It is initially de-alkylated to monoethylglycinexylidide and acetaldehyde. Monoethylglycine-xylidine is mainly hydrolysed to *N*-ethylglycine and 2,6-xylidine. The latter compound is hydroxylated to 4-hydroxy-2,6-xylidine, which is the main metabo-lite of lignocaine eliminated in urine (accounting for approximately 70% of the dose). Some of the metabolites of lignocaine have local anaesthetic activity, while others appear to have convulsive properties. Monoethylglycinexylidide has antiemetic and antiarrhythmic properties, and may potentiate convulsions produced by lignocaine. Glycinexylidide (a minor metabolite of lignocaine) has local anaesthetic effects and may depress the CNS; it has a relatively long half-life and may take several days to be eliminated from the body.

Prilocaine is more rapidly metabolized than other amide anaesthetics; although it is mainly metabolized by the liver, it may also be broken down by the kidney and the lung. Its principal metabolites are *O*-toluidine and *N*-propylamine. *O*-toluidine is probably responsible for the methaemoglobinaemia and cyanosis which sometimes occurs approximately 6 h after large doses of prilocaine. It usually resolves spontaneously, but may be treated with reducing agents (e.g. ascorbic acid or methylene blue).

Mepivacaine is rapidly metabolized in the liver. At least three hydroxylated metabolites are formed; most of the drug is excreted in urine as 3-hydroxymepivacaine or 4-hydroxymepivacaine.

Bupivacaine has a relatively low hepatic clearance, and is only slowly metabolized by the liver. In man, the main metabolite is probably pipecolic acid (a product of hydrolysis of bupivacaine); only 5% of the dose is eliminated in urine as a dealkylated metabolite (pipecolylxylidide).

Pharmacological effects of local anaesthetics

Cardiovascular effects

Cocaine causes tachycardia and arrhythmias by both central and peripheral effects. In the CNS, it increases neuronal activity in sympathetic centres in the hypothalamus and the medulla; peripherally, it enhances the effects of endoge-nous catecholamines and produces sympathomimetic effects. Both these actions are due to its effects on Uptake$_1$ ('the amine pump'), which is responsible for the removal of catecholamines from extracellular fluid by central and peripheral nerve endings. Thus inhibition of Uptake$_1$ by cocaine increases the central and peripheral effects of adrenaline and noradrenaline. In contrast, the membrane stabilizing effects of other local anaesthetics has led to their development and use as anti-arrhythmic agents. Most local anaesthetics affect sodium channels in myocardial and junctional tissues (as well as in peripheral nerves). Bupivacaine may also affect calcium channels in cardiac muscle. Consequently, local anaesthetics decrease the maximum rate of increase of phase 0 of the cardiac action potential (V_{max}) in a dose-dependent manner. The slowing of conduction of the cardiac action potential prolongs the PR and the QRS intervals of the electrocardiogram. The excitability of atrial and ventricular muscle cells is decreased, and the refractory period of conducting tissue is prolonged. In the past, procaine was used as an antiarrhythmic agent. Its short duration of action led to the development of its analogue procainamide (which is not significantly broken down by plasma cholinesterase); this drug was widely used in the management of ventricular arrhythmias and in the treatment of supraventricular tachycardias (Chapter 14).

In recent years, lignocaine has become the standard agent for the suppression of ventricular arrhythmias associated with myocardial infarction or cardiac surgery. In general, lignocaine does not affect atrial muscle fibres; it may act preferentially on ischaemic myocardium, prolong the effective refractory period of junctional tissues, and be more effective when the extracellular potassium concentration is high. Lignocaine has a terminal half-life of approximately 1.6 hours; thus, constant intravenous infusion of the drug requires some time (approximately 7–8 h) to approach a steady state. Consequently lignocaine is usually administered as a loading dose (75–100 mg i.v. or 300 mg i.m.), and a constant infusion of 2–4 mg min^{-1} is then maintained. Drowsiness and numbness are frequently observed at high rates of infusion, and the metabolism of the drug is reduced in heart failure.

High doses of local anaesthetics are associated with significant cardiotoxicity. Myocardial contractility and conduction in junctional tissues is depressed, with widening of the QRS complex and distortion of the ST segment. High concentrations of local anaesthetics (particularly bupivacaine) may predispose to the development of re-entrant arrhythmias, which may be potentiated by hypoxia, acidosis and hyperkalaemia.

Peripheral vascular effects

Cocaine possesses inherent vasoconstrictor activity, since it inhibits the uptake of adrenaline and noradrenaline by peripheral sympathetic nerve endings. Other commonly used local anaesthetics may produce variable effects on vascular smooth muscle. Exposure of isolated blood vessels to local anaesthetics frequently produces an increase in tone. Intravascular injection of most amides produces a biphasic effect on vascular smooth muscle; extremely low concentrations enhance its activity and increase peripheral resistance, while higher concentrations cause vasodilatation. This may be due to changes in the Ca^{2+} concentration of the vessel wall. In the doses commonly used to produce local anaesthesia, vasodilatation usually occurs in the order procaine > chloroprocaine > prilocaine > lignocaine > mepivacaine > bupivacaine.

The vasodilatation produced by procaine has been used to advantage in the management of vascular spasm associated with inadvertent intra-arterial injections, trauma, or surgery.

Central nervous system

Local anaesthetics and their metabolites are weak bases, and cross the blood–brain barrier relatively easily. They may produce biphasic effects on the CNS. Although small doses of lignocaine ($2-4\,mg\ kg^{-1}$) have anticonvulsant effects, and have been used in the treatment of status epilepticus, signs of CNS excitation usually follow the absorption of significant amounts of the drug. Increasing plasma concentrations of local anaesthetics are associated with numbness of the tongue and mouth, lightheadedness, visual disturbances, slurring of speech, muscular twitching and tremors, restlessness, and irrational conversation. At concentrations of $2\,\mu g\ ml^{-1}$ (bupivacaine) or $9\,\mu g\ ml^{-1}$ (lignocaine), grand mal convulsions may occur. The threshold for convulsions is influenced by the presence of other drugs that affect the CNS, and by acidosis and hypoxia. Some local anaesthetics (e.g. procaine) are relatively free from convulsant activity. The excitatory effects of local anaesthetics are probably due to the selective depression of inhibitory cortical neurones, and may be followed by signs of cortical and medullary depression (e.g. unconsciousness, coma and apnoea).

Unwanted effects

Due to absolute or relative overdosage

Severe and occasionally fatal CNS and CVS toxicity may occur with gross overdosage of local anaesthetic agents (or when large doses inadvertently reach the vascular system). As long as the injection is not too rapid, the early signs of CNS toxicity described above may be recognized before more serious effects occur.

Convulsions should be treated by maintaining adequate ventilation and controlled by anticonvulsant drugs. Thiopentone ($150-250\,mg$ i.v.) has an immediate onset of action and a relatively short duration of action. Alternatively, diazepam ($10-20\,mg$ i.v., repeated if necessary) may be used. It has a slower onset of action, but is unlikely to potentiate the phase of CNS depression. If convulsions are prolonged, the use of a muscle relaxant and mechanical ventilation may be required.

Profound hypotension and bradyarrhythmias may occur due to depression of the cardiovascular system. Intravenous atropine ($1.2-1.8\,mg$) and colloid or crystalloid infusions as plasma expanders may be necessary. Fetal bradycardia and other signs of fetal distress may occur after paracervical block for analgesia in labour. As mentioned above, absorption of local anaesthetics from this site is extremely rapid.

Accidental injection of large volumes of local anaesthetic into the CSF during epidural or paravertebral block can produce 'total spinal' anaesthesia. This presents as complete respiratory paralysis (due to motor and medullary involvement) and hypotension (due to autonomic blockade). Treatment includes mechanical ventilation and circulatory support, and the use of a vasopressor may be indicated.

As part of the therapeutic effect

If multiple intercostal blocks are performed, respiratory insufficiency may occur, due to unavoidable paralysis of some motor fibres. During spinal anaesthesia, a variable degree of hypotension is not uncommon, due to autonomic blockade; epidural analgesia during labour may potentiate the effects of hypotension due to inferior vena caval compression. Prophylactic measures usually minimize these complications, but symptomatic treatment may be required.

Due to the added vasoconstrictor

Most of these effects are undoubtedly due to accidental intravascular injection. Cardiac arrhythmias and hypertensive responses are predictable side-effects when sympathomimetic amines are used, although the local anaesthetic itself may exert some protective effect on the heart. In general, the use of sympathomimetic vasoconstrictors should be restricted in susceptible patients, e.g. those with a known history of cardiovascular disease, or who are taking drugs that inhibit Uptake$_1$, such as tricyclic antidepressants. It has been shown that concentrations of adrenaline greater than 1 in 200 000 do not further enhance local anaesthetic effects when most amide-type drugs are used to produce conduction blockade.

Sympathomimetic amines with predominant α-adrenoceptor effects, such as noradrenaline and phenylephrine, have theoretical advantages as vasoconstrictors; in practice they appear to be less effective than adrenaline. Felypressin does not cause arrhythmias, although some elevation of blood pressure may occur.

Vasoconstrictor agents must not be given with local anaesthetics when anaesthesia is produced in digital extremities or in areas with a terminal vascular supply, as the intense ischaemia produced may lead to gangrene. Similarly, these solutions must never be given intravenously.

Specific effects

Allergic responses to most currently used local anaesthetics are extremely rare. Skin reactions following repeated handling of ester-type drugs have been most frequently reported; occasionally, anaphylactic responses have occurred. The metabolite *para*-aminobenzoic acid (PABA) probably acts as a hapten and induces the antibody response. Allergic reactions associated with the amide group are even less common; cross-sensitization between amide and ester local anaesthetics is almost unknown. Some reactions may occur when multi-dose ampoules are used (possibly due to the added preservative).

Sulphonamides produce bacteriostatic effects by preventing the incorporation of PABA into the folic acid nucleus, thus inhibiting the growth and multiplication of bacteria. Procaine and related esters are hydrolysed to PABA, and thus may antagonize the effects of sulphonamides; the concurrent use of ester local anaesthetics and sulphonamides or preparations containing sulphonamides (e.g. co-trimoxazole) is therefore undesirable.

Methaemoglobinaemia formation may occur when high doses of prilocaine are given (e.g. more than 600 mg extradurally), probably due to the accumulation of its main metabolite O-toluidine (and various hydroxylated derivatives). The fetus is at special risk, since its erythrocytes are deficient in methaemoglobin reductase (the enzyme that reduces methaemoglobin to haemoglobin). When necessary, methylene blue ($5\,\text{mg kg}^{-1}$) is an immediate and effective antidote in the mother and the child.

Clinical uses

Topical anaesthesia

Local anaesthetics may be applied to the skin, the eye, the ear, the nose, and the mouth, as well as other mucous membranes (particularly in the tracheobronchial tree and the genitourinary tract). In general, cocaine, amethocaine, lignocaine, lignocaine and prilocaine are the most useful and effective local anaesthetics for this purpose. When used to produce topical anaesthesia, they usually have a rapid onset of action (5–10 min) and a moderate duration of action (30–60 min). The powerful vasoconstrictor properties of cocaine make it a useful agent when both the reduction of bleeding and local anaesthesia is required. Its main indication in current practice is to provide surface anaesthesia for intranasal procedures; for this purpose, aqueous solutions containing 10 or 20% cocaine (with adrenaline 1 in 1000) are available. Cocaine is occasionally used to produce corneal anaesthesia; its desiccating effect is a marked disadvantage and may lead to corneal ulceration. It has largely been replaced in this field by other drugs (e.g. amethocaine, which is an excellent topical anaesthetic).

Various preparations of lignocaine are available as aqueous solutions (4%) or in water-miscible bases as gels, ointments, and sprays (2–10%). These may be variously used as eye drops, or to provide anaesthesia of the tracheobronchial tract prior to endotracheal intubation or bronchoscopic examination. They may also be used to produce anaesthesia of the urethra during diagnostic urological procedures, in order to eliminate the need for general anaesthesia. Sprays may be applied to mucosal surfaces to provide anaesthesia for suturing of episiotomy wounds or minor lacerations. Significant absorption may occur from the more vascular areas, and fatalities have occurred after the topical application of local anaesthetics to mucosal surfaces.

Benzocaine (a non-ionized ester) is incorporated into ear-drops used for the relief of pain in otitis media, and into various ointments and creams used for the symptomatic relief of muscle strains, pruritis, and painful fissures.

Absorption of local anaesthetics through intact skin is usually slow and unreliable, and high concentrations (e.g. 20% benzocaine or 40% lignocaine) are required. In recent years, a eutectic mixture of local anaesthetics (EMLA) has been widely used to produce surface anaesthesia of the skin (particularly in paediatric practice). In this preparation, the crystalline tertiary bases of lignocaine and prilocaine are present in equal proportions, forming an oil at temperatures greater than 16°C. The eutectic mixture is present in an emulsion which can be applied as a cream to the skin. An occlusive dressing is usually necessary to ensure cutaneous contact and at least 60 min is required to demonstrate significant surface analgesia.

Infiltration anaesthesia

Infiltration techniques are frequently employed in dentistry and to provide anaesthesia for minor surgical procedures. Amide anaesthetics with a moderate duration of action (lignocaine, prilocaine and mepivacaine) are commonly used. The site of action is at the unmyelinated nerve endings; with all these agents, the onset of action is almost immediate after submucosal or subcutaneous injection, and provides satisfactory operating conditions in over 90% of cases. The duration of local anaesthesia is variable. Procaine has a short duration of action (15–30 min), while lignocaine, mepivacaine and prilocaine have a moderate duration of action (usually 70–140 min). Bupivacaine has the longest duration of action (approximately 200 min). The addition of adrenaline (1 in 200 000) will increase the quality and prolong the duration of anaesthesia. Nevertheless, there is no significant difference in the duration of effect when lignocaine (1%) and bupivacaine (0.25%) containing adrenaline are used to produce infiltration anaesthesia. Residual anaesthesia persists longer after intradermal injection (4–7 h) than after submucosal injection (1–3 h), presumably due to differences in vascular absorption.

Conduction anaesthesia

Conduction anaesthesia is usually arbitrarily divided into minor nerve blockade of a moderately accessible single nerve entity (e.g. ulnar, radial, or intercostal nerve blockade); and major blockade of deeper nerves or nerve trunks with a wide dermatomal distribution (e.g. sciatic nerve or brachial plexus blockade).

In current practice, amides are almost invariably used to produce conduction anaesthesia. Lignocaine, mepivacaine and prilocaine have a moderate duration of action, while etidocaine and bupivacaine have a prolonged effect. Solutions containing vasoconstrictors are usually administered in these techniques, and for each individual agent the duration of anaesthesia will be chiefly determined by the total dose of the drug, rather than the volume or the concentration used.

When amide local anaesthetics are used to produce minor nerve blockade, they have a relatively rapid onset of action (3–6 min). The duration of local anaesthesia is more variable; lignocaine, mepivacaine and prilocaine have a moderate duration of action (1–2 h), while bupivacaine and etidocaine produce local anaesthesia for 2–6 h. The duration of action is prolonged by increasing the dose of the local anaesthetic, or by the addition of a vasoconstrictor. Thus, the duration of action of lignocaine during minor nerve blockade is usually increased from 1–2 h to 4–5 h by the addition of adrenaline (1 in 200 000). Drugs with a moderate duration of action produce anaesthesia for 1–2 h; etidocaine and bupivacaine act for 2–6 h.

In major nerve blockade, the onset of action is more variable, mainly due to anatomical factors which can delay or restrict the access of the local anaesthetic to its site of action. During brachial plexus or sciatic nerve blockade, solutions of local anaesthetics may be placed outside the fascial planes or connective tissues that surround the nerve trunks. Consequently, local anaesthetic bases must diffuse across extensive connective tissue barriers as well as the myelin sheaths of nerve trunks; they may be also taken up by the surrounding adipose tissue and by muscle. Thus, their onset of action is more variable. In general, lignocaine, mepivacaine and prilocaine have a more rapid onset of action (approximately 14 min) than bupivacaine (23 min). Analgesia persists for 3–4 h with lignocaine, prilocaine and mepivacaine, but up to 10 h with bupivacaine. Etidocaine has a shorter onset time (9 min) but a similar duration of action to bupivacaine; however, the differential blockade of motor fibres may tend to limit its use. Persistent paraesthesia after nerve blockade is probably due to mechanical trauma, rather than a pharmacological effect.

Procaine is an ideal diagnostic agent, due to its relatively short duration of action (15–45 min) and its localizing effects (which are due to poor diffusion properties). In the treatment of chronic pain it can be used to block somatic or autonomic fibres; the efficiency of permanent neurolytic blockade can then be more easily assessed.

Extradural anaesthesia

The deposition of local anaesthetic solutions in the area between the dura mater and the periosteum lining the vertebral canal is widely used to provide surgical anaesthesia and for analgesia during labour. Extradural anaesthetics are commonly administered in the thoracolumbar region of the spinal cord. The epidural space is filled with adipose tissue, lymphatics and blood vessels (mainly the peridural venous plexus). After injection, local anaesthetic solutions spread widely in all directions, and produce analgesia by blocking conduction at the intradural spinal nerve roots; the local anaesthetic diffuses through the thin dural sleeve and the numerous arachnoid villi that are present in this region. After extradural injection, high concentrations of local anaesthetics are invariably present in intradural nerve roots, and the dermatomal spread of analgesia is consistent with conduction blockade at this site. Spread into the paravertebral spaces may also occur in younger subjects, and there may be some uptake of local anaesthetics by the spinal cord. Indeed, the pattern of recovery from extradural anaesthesia suggests that transverse blockade of the spinal cord may eventually occur.

In general terms, extradural anaesthesia may be considered as multiple minor nerve blockade. The onset of action is slightly longer (10–20 min), presumably due to the greater distance for diffusion, but the duration of action is equal to ulnar or intercostal nerve blockade. The quality and extent of the blockade produced by each agent is determined by the volume as well as the total dose of the drug. Other important factors are the site of injection, the speed of administration, and the position of the patient. The spread of local anaesthetic solution may be more extensive in parturient women, when the peridural venous plexus is distended due to inferior vena caval compression, and the volume of the potential space is reduced. Consequently, the dose of local anaesthetic required to produce extradural blockade in pregnancy is usually reduced. Similarly, enhanced effects may be seen in arteriosclerotic patients and the elderly, due to the impairment of vascular absorption from the epidural space.

Bupivacaine (0.5%) is usually used to produce extradural anaesthesia. Its duration of action is usually suitable, its protein-binding capacity and high lipid-solubility delay its absorption into the systemic circulation, and a relatively low concentration of the drug reaches the fetal circulation. Bupivacaine (0.75%) has recently been introduced, and may be preferred when some degree of motor blockade is desired (e.g. for caesarean section under epidural anaesthesia). Dose requirements vary between 1–3 ml for each segment blocked. The ester chloroprocaine (1–3%) has a shorter duration of action (30–90 min) and may be even safer in certain circumstances, although there have been occasional reports of permanent neurological sequelae after accidental dural puncture.

Caudal block is a form of extradural anaesthesia; the nerves of the cauda equina descending in the sacral canal are blocked by local anaesthetics inserted through a needle in the sacral hiatus, to produce sacral or perineal anaesthesia. The anaesthetic agent does not need to traverse a dural sleeve; the slow onset of action and the significant failure rate are probably due to considerable vascular absorption and the wide distribution of the drug through the various sacral foramina.

Tachyphylaxis (i.e. the development of rapid drug tolerance) may occur after the repeated administration of lignocaine or mepivacaine into the epidural space. This phenomenon may be related to the local changes in pH produced by the introduction of relatively acid local anaesthetic solutions (pH = 4–5). The decrease in pH reduces the relative concentration of the free base that is available for diffusion across the neuronal membrane. In these conditions, there is a progressive decrease in the degree of analgesia produced by local anaesthetic solutions.

Spinal anaesthesia

The introduction of local anaesthetic solutions directly into the CSF produces spinal anaesthesia. The central attachments of ventral and dorsal nerve roots are unmyelinated; when local anaesthetic solutions are introduced into the subarachnoid space, their tertiary bases are rapidly taken up by the nerve roots and the spinal cord. Consequently, their potency is approximately ten times greater than after extradural administration, and motor blockade is more pronounced. In addition, the onset of anaesthesia is more rapid after subarachnoid (intrathecal) administration, since local anaesthetics do not need to penetrate extensive tissue or diffusion barriers in order to reach their site of action. Due to the smaller doses of local anaesthetics that are used, the duration of spinal anaesthesia is usually shorter than extradural anaesthesia.

The quality and extent of blockade is related to the dose of local anaesthetic administered, the speed of injection, the position of the patient, and the specific gravity of the solution injected (when compared with CSF). Hyperbaric solutions of local anaesthetics are frequently used to produce subarachnoid blockade. The spread of these solutions in the CSF is affected by gravity and by posture. Hyperbaric solutions of amethocaine (0.2%), lignocaine (5%), prilocaine (5%), bupivacaine (0.5%) and mepivacaine (4%) are commonly used to produce spinal analgesia. Prilocaine and mepivacaine have a slightly longer duration of action than lignocaine; bupivacaine has the longest duration of action. Isobaric solutions of local anaesthetics are also used to produce spinal anaesthesia. These solutions are more physiological and their spread in the CSF does not depend on the position of the patient; unfortunately, their effects are less predictable.

Spinal analgesia may be affected by the volume and capacity of the subarachnoid space. Thus, compression of the inferior vena cava (e.g. in pregnancy) distends the vertebral venous plexus and decreases the volume of the subarachnoid space. Consequently, the degree of analgesia is increased.

Neurological complications of spinal anaesthesia are usually related to CSF leakage, mechanical trauma, the introduction of infection, or pre-existing pathology. However, the incidence of arachnoiditis and cauda equina syndromes is probably commoner when high concentrations of local anaesthetics are used.

Intravenous local anaesthesia

Procaine (1% in saline) has been used by intravenous infusion as a supplement to general anaesthesia, to produce analgesia for burns dressings, and to relieve postoperative pain. Its action is rather unpredictable and side-effects are not uncommon. It is rarely if ever used for this purpose in current anaesthetic practice.

In contrast, intravenous regional anaesthesia (IVRA) is a useful method of providing analgesia for minor surgical procedures. In this technique, a local anaesthetic agent is injected into the vein of a limb that has been previously exsanguinated and occluded by a tourniquet. The site of action is probably the unmyelinated nerve terminals, which drugs must reach by retrograde spread in the vascular bed. Nerve conduction is not usually affected, although motor paralysis may occur due to presynaptic and postsynaptic effects at the neuro-muscular junction. The onset of analgesia is almost immediate; its quality and duration are dependent on the dose of local anaesthetic administered, the effic-iency of exsanguination, the period of ischaemia prior to injection, and the site of injection. It may also be influenced by the effects of local acidosis, and vaso-dilatation due to CO_2 accumulation.

Most of the commonly used agents are effective, and the period of residual anaesthesia (30–350 min) is related to the drug that is used. Local anaesthetics that are significantly bound to plasma or tissue protein (e.g. bupivacaine and etidocaine) should not be used to produce intravenous regional anaesthesia; the use of bupivacaine, in particular, has been associated with several deaths during IVRA, due to cardiac complications.

Lignocaine or prilocaine (200 mg, i.e. 40 ml of a 0.5% solution) are commonly used for regional anaesthesia in the arm. Larger doses are required for the lower limb, and the results are less satisfactory. Systemic blood levels of these local anaesthetics are unlikely to be significant if the tourniquet is released more than 15 min after injection.

Other uses

Cocaine is sometimes used in analgesic mixtures that are administered orally (e.g. for the relief of intractable pain associated with terminal malignant disease). Gastric sedation may be related to its local anaesthetic effects, and euphoria may be produced. However, the occurrence of excitatory side-effects (as well as the world shortage of cocaine) has tended to restrict its use for this purpose.

Procaine forms less soluble conjugates with some other drugs (e.g. penicillin), producing slow-release preparations; procaine may also reduce the pain of injection. Similarly, lignocaine is sometimes used with intramuscular injections of irritant drugs (e.g. amoxycillin) in order to decrease the pain of injection.

Finally dibucaine (cinchocaine, nupercaine) selectively inhibits the normal (typical) plasma cholinesterase enzyme, and is used to study the genetic variants in this condition.

FURTHER READING

Adriani J, Campbell B. Fatalities following topical application of local anaesthetics to mucous membranes. *Journal of the American Medical Association* 1956; **162**: 1527–1530.

Adriani J, Dalili H. Penetration of local anesthetic through epithelial barriers. *Anesthesia and Analgesia* 1971; **50**: 834–841.

Adriani J, Zepernick R, Arens J, Authement E. The comparative potency and effectiveness of topical anesthetics in man. *Clinical Pharmacology and Therapeutics* 1964; **5**: 49–62.

Albert J, Lofström B. Bilateral ulnar nerve blocks for the evaluation of local anesthetic agents. III: Tests with a new agent, prilocaine, and with lidocaine in solutions with and without epinephrine. *Acta Anaesthesiologica Scandinavica* 1965; **9**: 203–211.

Atkinson DI, Modell J, Moya F. Intravenous regional analgesia. *Anesthesia and Analgesia* 1965; **44**: 313–317.

Bassett AL, Wit AL. Recent advances in electrophysiology of antiarrhythmic drugs. *Progress in Drug Research* 1973; **17**: 33–58.

Bell HM, Slater EM, Harris WH. Regional anesthesia with intravenous lidocaine. *Journal of the American Medical Association* 1963; **186**: 544–549.

Bigger JT. Jr. Arrhythmias and antiarrhythmic drugs. *Advances in Internal Medicine* 1972; **18**: 251–281.

Blair MR. Cardiovascular pharmacology of local anaesthetics. *British Journal of Anaesthesia* 1975; **47**: 247–252.

Blaschke TF. Protein binding and kinetics of drugs in liver diseases. *Clinical Pharmacokinetics* 1977; **2**: 32–44.

Boakes AJ, Laurence DR, Lovel KW, O'Neil R, Verrill PJ. Adverse reactions to local anaesthetic vasoconstrictor preparations: a study of the cardiovascular responses to xylestesin and hostacain-with-noradrenaline. *British Dental Journal* 1972; **133**: 137–140.

Boyes RN. A review of the metabolism of amide local anaesthetic agents. *British Journal of Anaesthesia* 1975; **47**: 225–230.

Braid DP, Scott DB. The systemic absorption of local analgesic drugs. *British Journal of Anaesthesia* 1965; **37**: 394–404.

Braun H. Ueber einige neue örtliche Anaesthetica (Stovain, Alypin, Novocain). *Deutsche Medizinische Wochenschrift* 1905; **31**: 1667–1671.

Bromage PR. Physiology and pharmacology of epidural analgesia. *Anesthesiology* 1967; **28**: 592–622.

Bromage PR. Mechanism of action of extradural analgesia. *British Journal of Anaesthesia* 1975; **47**: 199–212.

Bromage PR, Gertel M. An evaluation of two new local anaesthetics for major conduction blockade. *Canadian Anaesthetists Society Journal* 1970; **17**: 557–564.

Cahalan MD, Almers W. Interactions between quaternary lidocaine, the sodium channel gates and tetrodotoxin. *Biophysical Journal* 1979; **27**: 57–74.

Calvey TN. Drugs affecting administration of anaesthetics. *British Dental Journal* 1980; **149**: 185–186.

Catchlove RFH. The influence of CO_2 and pH on local anesthetic action. *Journal of Pharmacology and Experimental Therapeutics* 1972; **181**: 298–309.

Chambers WA, Littlewood DG, Logan MR, Scott DB. Effect of added epinephrine on spinal anesthesia with lidocaine. *Anesthesia and Analgesia* 1981; **60**: 417–420.

Covino BG. Pharmacokinetics of local anaesthetic drugs. In: Prys-Roberts C, Hug CC (eds) *Pharmacokinetics of Anaesthesia*. Oxford: Blackwell Scientific Publications, 1984; 270–292.

Covino BG. Pharmacology of local anaesthetic agents. *British Journal of Anaesthesia* 1986; **58**: 701–716.

Crawford OB. Comparative evaluation in peridural anaesthesia of lidocaine, mepivacaine and L-67, a new local anesthetic agent. *Anesthesiology* 1964; **25**: 321–329.

Eccles JC. *The Understanding of the Brain*. New York: McGraw-Hill, 1973.

Ehrenström Reiz GM, Reiz SL. EMLA — a eutectic mixture of local anaesthetics for topical anaesthesia. *Acta Anaesthesiologica Scandinavica* 1982; **26**: 596–598.

Foldes FF, Davidson GM, Duncalf D, Kunabara S. The intravenous toxicity of local anesthetic agents in man. *Clinical Pharmacology and Therapeutics* 1965; **6**: 328–335.

Franz DN, Perry RS. Mechanisms for differential block among single myelinated and non-myelinated axons by procaine. *Journal of Physiology* 1974; **236**: 193–201.

Frazier DT, Narahashi T, Yamada M. The site of action and active form of local anesthetics. II. Experiments with quaternary compounds. *Journal of Pharmacology and Experimental Therapeutics* 1970; **171**: 45–51.

Gissen AJ, Covino BG, Gregus J. Differential sensitivity of mammalian nerves to local anesthetic drugs. *Anesthesiology* 1980; **53**: 467–474.

Hallén B, Carlsson P, Uppfeldt A. Clinical study of a lignocaine–prilocaine cream to relieve the pain of venepuncture. *British Journal of Anaesthesia* 1985; **57**: 326–328.

Heath M. Deaths after intravenous regional anaesthesia. *British Medical Journal* 1982; **285**: 913.

Hille B. The common mode of action of three agents that decrease the transient charge in sodium permeability in nerves. *Nature* 1966; **210**: 1220–1222.

Hille B. *Ionic Channels of Excitable Membranes*. Sunderland, Massachusetts: Sinauer Associates, 1984.

Hodgkin AL. *The Conduction of the Nervous Impulse*. Liverpool: Liverpool University Press, 1964.

Huxley AF. Ion movements during nerve activity. *Annals of the New York Academy of Sciences* 1959; **81**: 221–246.

Huxley AF, Stämpfli R. Evidence for saltatory conduction in peripheral myelinated nerve fibres. *Journal of Physiology* 1949; **108**: 315–339.

Knapp RB. Drug distribution following intravenous regional analgesia. *Journal of the American Medical Association* 1967; **199**: 760–762.

Lubens HM, Ausdenmoore RW, Shafer AD, Reece RM. Anesthetic patch for painful procedures such as minor operations. *American Journal of Diseases of Children* 1974; **128**: 192–194.

Maunuksela E-L, Korpela R. Double-blind evaluation of a lignocaine–prilocaine cream (EMLA) in children. *British Journal of Anaesthesia* 1986; **58**: 1242–1245.

Mihaly GW, Moore RG, Thomas J, Triggs EJ, Thomas D, Shanks CH. The pharmacokinetics of the anilide type local anesthetics in neonates: I. Lignocaine. *European Journal of Clinical Pharmacology* 1978; **13**: 143–152.

Moore DC. Local anesthetic drugs: tissue and systemic toxicity. *Acta Anaesthesiologica Scandinavica* 1981; **4**: 283–300.

Moore DC, Bridenbaugh LD, Bagdi PA, Bridenbaugh PO, Stander H. The present status of spinal (subarachnoid) and epidural (peridural) block: A comparison of the two technics. *Anesthesia and Analgesia* 1968; **47**: 40–49.

Moore DC, Bridenbaugh LD, Bridenbaugh PO, Tucker GT. Bupivacaine hydrochloride: laboratory and clinical studies. *Anesthesiology* 1970; **32**: 78–83.

Narahashi T, Yamada M, Frazier DT. Cationic forms of local anesthetics block action potentials from inside the nerve membrane. *Nature* 1969; **223**: 748–749.

Nation RL, Triggs EJ, Selig M. Lignocaine kinetics in cardiac patients and aged subjects. *British Journal of Clinical Pharmacology* 1977; **4**: 439–448.

Nishimura N, Morioka T, Sato S, Kuba T. Effects of local anesthetic agents on the peripheral vascular system. *Anesthesia and Analgesia* 1965; **44**: 135–139.

Ochs HR, Carstens G, Greenblatt DJ. Reduction in lidocaine clearance during continuous infusion and by co-administration of propranolol. *New England Journal of Medicine* 1980; **303**: 373–377.

Piafsky KM. Disease-induced changes in the plasma binding of basic drugs. *Clinical Pharmacokinetics* 1980; **5**: 246–262.

Piafsky KM, Knoppert D. Binding of local anesthetics to α_1-acid glycoprotein. *Clinical Research* 1978; **26**: 836A.

Reisner LS, Hochman BN, Plumer MH. Persistent neurologic deficit and adhesive arachnoiditis following intrathecal 2-chloroprocaine injection. *Anesthesia and Analgesia* 1980; **59**: 452–454.

Reiz S, Nath S. Cardiotoxicity of local anaesthetic agents. *British Journal of Anaesthesia* 1986; **58**: 736–746.

Reynolds F. Adverse effects of local anaesthetics. *British Journal of Anaesthesia* 1987; **59**: 78–95.

Ritchie JM. Mechanism of action of local anesthetic agents and biotoxins. *British Journal of Anaesthesia* 1975; **47**: 191–198.

Ritchie JM, Ritchie B, Greengard P. The active structure of local anesthetics. *Journal of Pharmacology and Experimental Therapeutics* 1965; **150**: 152–159.

Ritchie JM, Ritchie B, Greengard P. The effect of the nerve sheath on the action of local anesthetics. *Journal of Pharmacology and Experimental Therapeutics* 1965; **150**: 160–164.

Scott DB. Toxic effects of local anaesthetic agents on the central nervous system. *British Journal of Anaesthesia* 1986; **58**: 732–735.

Scott DB, Jebson PJR, Braid DP, Örtengren B, Frisch P. Factors affecting plasma levels of lignocaine and prilocaine. *British Journal of Anaesthesia* 1972; **44**: 1040–1049.

Scott DB, McClure JH, Giasi RM, Seo J, Covino BG. Effect of concentration of local anaesthetic drugs in extradural block. *British Journal of Anaesthesia* 1980; **52**: 1033–1037.

Strichartz GR (ed.) *Local Anesthetics. Handbook of Experimental Pharmacology* 81: 1–292. Heidelberg: Springer-Verlag, 1987.

Strong JM, Mayfield DE, Atkinson AJ, Burris BC, Raymon F, Webster LT. Pharmacological activity, metabolism, and pharmacokinetics of glycinexylidide. *Clinical Pharmacology and Therapeutics* 1975; **17**: 184–194.

Swerdlow M, Jones R. The duration of action of bupivacaine, prilocaine and lignocaine. *British Journal of Anaesthesia* 1970; **42**: 335–339.

Thorn-Alquist A-M. Intravenous regional anesthesia. *Acta Anaesthesiologica Scandinavica* 1971; **40** (Supplement) 1–35.

Tillement JP, Lhoste F, Giudicelli JF. Diseases and drug protein binding. *Clinical Pharmacokinetics* 1978; **3**: 144–154.

Tucker GT. Pharmacokinetics of local anaesthetics. *British Journal of Anaesthesia* 1986; **58**: 717–731.

Tucker GT, Boyes RN, Bridenbaugh PO, Moore DC. Binding of anilide-type local anesthetics in human plasma. I. Relationships between binding, physicochemical properties, and anesthetic activity. *Anesthesiology* 1970; **33**: 287–303.

Tucker GT, Mather LE. Clinical pharmacokinetics of local anaesthetic agents. *Clinical Pharmacokinetics* 1979; **4**: 241–278.

Tucker GT, Wiklund L, Berlin-Wahlen A, Mather LE. Hepatic clearance of local anesthetics in man. *Journal of Pharmacokinetics and Biopharmaceutics* 1977; **5**: 111–122.

Von Anrep B. Ueber die physiologische Wirkung des Cocain. *Archiv für die gesammte Physiologie des Menschen und der Tiere* (Pflügers) 1880; **21**: 38–77.

Wildsmith JAW. Peripheral nerve and local anaesthetic drugs. *British Journal of Anaesthesia* 1986; **58**: 692–700.

Wildsmith JAW, Gissen AJ, Gregus J, Covino BG. Differential nerve blocking activity of amino-ester local anaesthetics. *British Journal of Anaesthesia* 1985; **57**: 612–620.

Wood M, Wood AJ. Changes in plasma drug binding and alpha-1 acid glycoprotein in mother and newborn infant. *Clinical Pharmacology and Therapeutics* 1981; **29**: 522–526.

NINE

Drugs that Act on the Neuromuscular Junction

STRUCTURE OF THE NEUROMUSCULAR JUNCTION

Motor nerve fibres branch extensively within skeletal muscle, and each anterior horn cell normally innervates 10–150 muscle fibres (the motor unit). As the motor nerve terminal approaches skeletal muscle it loses its myelin sheath; the neuromuscular junction commences at the non-myelinated nerve ending that is distal to the last node of Ranvier. Each axonal terminal lies in a junctional fold or gutter on the surface of the muscle fibre (the motor endplate). In most mammalian muscles, each muscle fibre has a single motor endplate, i.e. it is innervated near its midpoint by one axonal terminal ('focal innervation'). This usually forms an elevation on the surface of the fibre, which is called an 'en plaque' neuromuscular junction. These focally innervated fibres are supplied by fast conducting Aα axons, and have rapid rates of contraction and relaxation. Conversely, some other muscle fibres are densely innervated at numerous sites by slower conducting Aγ axons. This type of innervation (known as 'multiple innervation') occurs in extra-ocular muscles, intrinsic laryngeal muscles, and some facial muscles. The termination of motor nerves in multiply innervated fibres in these muscles resembles a bunch of grapes (an 'en grappe' neuromuscular junction).

The subcellular features of the motor endplate can be demonstrated by electron microscopy (Fig. 9.1). The axonal terminal lies in a cleft in the sarcolemmal membrane, and contains numerous mitochondria and synaptic vesicles. Many of the synaptic vesicles are associated with specialized zones in the axonal membrane that correspond to sites of neurotransmitter release. The synaptic vesicles are synthesized in the anterior horn cells of the spinal cord, and are transported to the motor nerve terminal through the intraneuronal microtubular system. The external surface of the axonal membrane is covered by processes of Schwann cell cytoplasm, which surround the motor nerve terminal (Fig. 9.1). The axolemmal membrane is separated from the postsynaptic membrane by a gap of approximately 50 nm; this includes a basement lamina approximately 20 nm

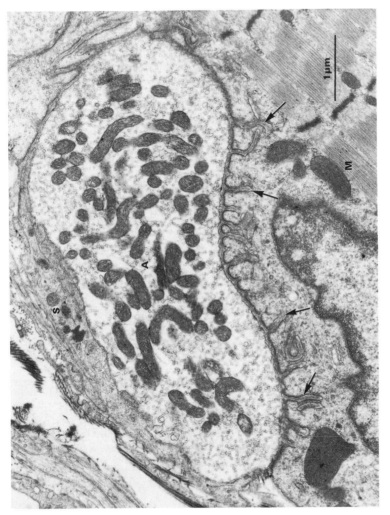

Fig. 9.1 Electron micrograph of part of a normal neuromuscular junction. The axonal terminal (A) lies in a deep indentation of the sarcolemmal membrane and contains abundant mitochondria and synaptic vesicles. The external surface of the axon is covered by processes of Schwann cell cytoplasm (S). There are numerous infoldings (arrowed) of the sarcolemma beneath the axon and basal lamina material lies between nerve and muscle (M) and fills these subneural folds (×30 000). (Courtesy of Professor L. W. Duchen.)

wide, and mainly consists of mucopolysaccharides. The sarcolemmal postsynaptic membrane is convoluted, forming junctional folds (Fig. 9.1). Acetylcholine receptors are primarily present in discrete groups on the shoulders of the junctional folds; the distal valleys are mainly associated with the hydrolytic enzyme acetylcholinesterase. Both acetylcholine receptors and acetylcholinesterase are also present at presynaptic sites on the motor nerve terminal.

THE SYNTHESIS AND STORAGE OF ACETYLCHOLINE

Neuromuscular transmission depends on the synthesis, storage and release of acetylcholine by the motor nerve terminal. At the motor endplate, extracellular

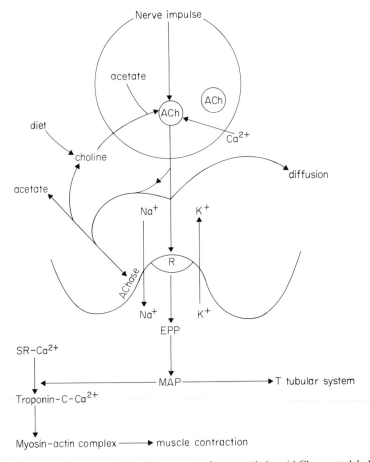

Fig. 9.2 A diagrammatic representation of neuromuscular transmission. (ACh = acetylcholine; R = acetylcholine receptor; AChase = acetylcholinesterase; EPP = endplate potential; MAP = muscle action potential; SR = sarcoplasmic reticulum.)

choline is partly derived from dietary and plasma choline, and partly produced by the hydrolysis of acetylcholine. It is transported from extracellular fluid into the axoplasm by a high affinity carrier system that is present in all cholinergic nerves (Fig. 9.2). Choline transport is usually the rate-limiting step in the synthesis of acetylcholine in the axoplasm by the enzyme choline acetyltransferase, according to the reaction:

$$\text{Choline} + \text{acetyl-coenzyme A} \rightarrow \text{acetylcholine} + \text{coenzyme A}$$

In general, the synthesis of acetylcholine is increased by the release of the neurotransmitter; it is not usually possible to deplete the nerve ending of acetylcholine by choline deficiency, or by rapid and unphysiological rates of nerve stimulation.

Most of the synthesized acetylcholine is then transferred from the axoplasm to the synaptic vesicles, where it is stored as molecular packages or quanta. Some acetylcholine remains in the axoplasm, and leaks across the axonal membrane. Each synaptic vesicle contains approximately 10 000 molecules of acetylcholine. In the motor nerve terminal, there are at least two separate pools of synaptic vesicles; one of these represents reserve acetylcholine, while the smaller fraction is available for immediate release ('readily releasable acetylcholine'). In the synaptic vesicles, acetylcholine is probably bound as an ATP–mucopolysaccharide complex, and purine nucleotides (particularly adenosine) are probably released with acetylcholine at the neuromuscular junction.

Acetylcholine receptors

At the neuromuscular junction, acetylcholine receptors are mainly present in discrete groups on the shoulders of the junctional folds of the postsynaptic membrane. They are also present at presynaptic sites on the motor nerve terminal. During the past 20 years, there has been considerable progress in their isolation and purification; more recently, their precise structure has been determined by molecular biological techniques. Similar acetylcholine receptors are present in abundance in the electroplaque organs of certain fishes (e.g. the South American freshwater eel and the giant electric ray). These receptors are irreversibly bound by the toxins of certain snakes (e.g. α-bungarotoxin derived from the Taiwan banded krait, and α-cobra toxin from the cobra). Consequently, nicotinic acetylcholine receptors in electroplaque tissues and mammalian muscle can be irreversibly bound by radiolabelled α-bungarotoxin, and the receptors can then be isolated and purified by affinity chromatography. In addition, acetylcholine receptors have been sequenced and inserted into artificial and amphibian oocyte membranes by molecular biological techniques.

These studies have shown that the acetylcholine receptor at the neuromuscular junction is an integral membrane protein with a molecular weight of approximately 250 kDa (250 000). In adult man, it consists of five subunits (α, α, β, δ and ε) which cross the postsynaptic membrane and surround the ion channel or ionophore. The structure of the receptor is slightly different in fetal life; the ε-subunit is replaced by a partly homologous but distinct entity (the γ-subunit). In the adult, the ε-subunit appears to be responsible for the short channel opening time and higher ionic conductance. Two of the receptor subunits (the α-subunits) have a molecular weight of approximately 40 kDa (40 000) and contain acetylcholine binding sites at the amino acid residues Cys 192–Cys 193. Combination of the neurotransmitter with the binding sites on the α-subunits results in conformational changes that open the ion channel; the probability of this occurring is considerably increased when both the sites are occupied by acetylcholine ('positive cooperativity'). The diameter of the acetylcholine receptor complex is approximately 10 nm, and causes a slight elevation of the postsynaptic membrane. Acetylcholine receptors on the motor nerve terminal (presynaptic receptors) have a slightly different molecular structure, since they are not bound by α-bungarotoxin or cobra toxin, and are differentially affected by neuromuscular blockade.

Neuromuscular transmission

Acetylcholine is released from the motor nerve terminal as distinct packets or quanta (each containing approximately 10 000 molecules of the neurotransmitter) (Fig. 9.2). Each quanta of acetylcholine probably corresponds to the release of a single synaptic vesicle. In the absence of nerve impulses, synaptic vesicles randomly collide with the limiting axonal membrane, releasing acetylcholine which diffuses across the synaptic cleft and combines with receptors on the postsynaptic membrane. This causes spontaneous electrical activity at the motor endplate, in the form of discrete, randomly distributed miniature endplate potentials (mepps) with an amplitude of 0.5–1.5 mV. Thus, miniature endplate potentials correspond to the release of a single quantum of acetylcholine, which represents the minimum unit of neurotransmitter release.

In contrast, when a nerve action potential reaches the axonal terminal, approximately 200 quanta of acetylcholine are released (i.e. about 200 synaptic vesicles fuse with the presynaptic membrane and release their contents of acetylcholine into the synaptic cleft). The adenylate cyclase–cAMP system and calcium ions may play an important part in the release of acetylcholine. On arrival of the nerve impulse at the motor nerve terminal, cAMP is formed from ATP (Chapter 3); this intermediate messenger may then activate protein kinases that are coupled to calcium channels in the neuronal membrane (N channels). The increased synthesis of the nucleotide may account for the improvement in neuromuscular transmission which can occur in myasthenic patients when sympathomimetic drugs (e.g. ephedrine) are administered.

An alternative view suggests that depolarization of the motor nerve terminal directly opens voltage-sensitive calcium channels, and that the changes in cyclic nucleotides are secondary phenomena. The entry of calcium ions into the axoplasm, and its subsequent binding by intraneuronal calmodulin, causes the fusion of synaptic vesicles with the limiting axonal membrane, resulting in the release of acetylcholine. The quantal release of acetylcholine can be described in statistical terms by the Poisson distribution; the average number of quanta released by each nerve impulse (m) is given by m = np (where n is the number of quanta of acetylcholine immediately available for release, and p is the probability of quantal release when the nerve terminal is depolarized). The amount of acetylcholine released is greater than that required to produce endplate depolarization (i.e. there is a considerable 'safety margin' in neuromuscular transmission).

Released acetylcholine diffuses across the synaptic cleft and combines with the α-subunits of acetylcholine receptors which surround the ion channel on the postsynaptic membrane. Combination of the neurotransmitter with these binding sites results in conformational changes that open the ion channel; the probability of this occurring is considerably increased when both binding sites on the α-subunits are occupied by acetylcholine. Ion channel opening is an extremely rapid all or none phenomenon that lasts for 5–10 ms, and causes a non-specific increase in permeability to small ions (mainly sodium, potassium, and calcium ions). In experimental conditions, it has been estimated that acetylcholine causes the transfer of 10 000 ions per ionophore during each millisecond that the channel is open. These ionic changes result in multiple single channel currents; each of these has an amplitude of approximately 4 pA (i.e. 4×10^{-12} A). The single channel currents summate to produce the endplate current, which tends to depolarize the postsynaptic membrane. A small and localized endplate potential is produced; if this reaches a critical amplitude (which normally requires a change of 10–15 mV), voltage-sensitive sodium channels open, the muscle fibre is depolarized, and a propagated muscle action potential is conducted along its surface (Fig. 9.2). (The quantal content of the endplate potential (m) can be calculated from the equation: m = amplitude of endplate potential/amplitude of miniature endplate potentials.) The propagated muscle action potential is conducted along the electrically excitable muscle membrane and enters the transverse tubular system (T-tubular system) at the end of the sarcomere (Fig. 9.2). Depolarization of the T-tubular system causes the release of calcium ions from the sarcoplasmic reticulum (possibly by increasing the synthesis of the intermediate messenger inositol trisphosphate). Released calcium ions are bound by Troponin C, producing conformational changes in other troponins and tropomyosin. Simultaneously, myosin ATPase is activated and ATP is hydrolysed to ADP; this provides an abundant supply of intracellular energy. In these conditions, cross-bridges are formed between actin and myosin, resulting in the phenomenon of muscle contraction (Fig. 9.2). The sequence of physiological and biochemical changes be-

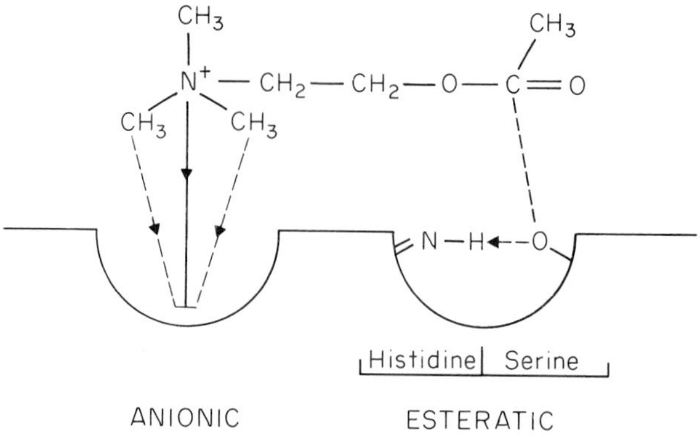

Fig. 9.3 Binding sites of acetylcholinesterase (AChE).

tween depolarization of the T-tubular system and muscle contraction are known as excitation–contraction coupling (EC coupling).

The action of acetylcholine at receptors on the postsynaptic membrane is rapidly terminated by the enzyme acetylcholinesterase. Normally, each molecule of acetylcholine only activates a single receptor before its hydrolysis to choline and acetate ions (or its removal by diffusion). The enzyme is primarily present on the junctional clefts of the postsynaptic membrane, although some is also present at presynaptic sites (i.e. on the motor nerve terminal and in the axoplasm). Acetylcholinesterase has two binding sites for acetylcholine (the anionic site and the esteratic site), which are approximately 0.5 nm apart (Fig. 9.3). The anionic site is negatively charged, and probably consists of aspartate or glutamate groups; consequently, it forms an electrostatic (ionic) bond with the quaternary nitrogen atom of acetylcholine, which is supplemented by London–Van der Waals dispersion forces. In contrast, the esteratic site consists of the hydroxyl group of serine and the imidazole group of histidine. Hydrogen bonding between these groups enhances the nucleophilic properties of serine, and allows it to react with the ester group in acetylcholine (Fig. 9.3). A covalent bond is formed and choline is released, resulting in the production of the acetylated enzyme; this is rapidly hydrolysed, causing the regeneration of the enzyme and the formation of acetic acid. The reactions involved are extremely rapid, and the half-life of the acetylated enzyme is approximately 40 µs (4×10^{-5} s). The rapid destruction of the neurotransmitter is essential, in order to prevent the repetitive firing of the motor endplate.

When acetylcholine is released from the motor nerve terminal, it mainly produces its effects at nicotinic receptors on the postsynaptic membrane. Nevertheless, there is some evidence that acetylcholine receptors are also present on the motor nerve terminal, and at the most distal node of Ranvier. Acetylcholine receptors on the motor nerve terminal may play an important part in maintaining transmitter output at high rates of nerve stimulation; their blockade by non-depolarizing neuromuscular blocking agents may be responsible for the phenomenon of decrement or fade (p. 269). In contrast, acetylcholine receptors at the last node of Ranvier may induce retrograde or antidromic firing of the motor nerve. Thus, the injection of acetylcholine into the popliteal artery of experimental animals not only produces activity of the appropriate muscle groups, but also gives rise to action potentials in the motor nerve which are conducted in a retrograde manner. These antidromic potentials can be recorded from the ventral nerve roots by appropriate electrophysiological techniques. Similar effects can be produced by repetitive nerve stimulation, anticholinesterase drugs, or suxamethonium. These results suggest that drugs that act at the neuromuscular junction may also affect the motor nerve terminal. Nevertheless, the functional importance of these effects is a matter of conjecture, and most of the evidence suggests that the main effects of acetylcholine occur at postsynaptic sites.

DRUGS THAT AFFECT NEUROMUSCULAR FUNCTION

In general, drugs that modify neuromuscular transmission may affect:
1   Acetylcholine release.
2   Acetylcholine action.
3   Acetylcholine breakdown.
4   EC coupling.

Drugs that affect the release of acetylcholine

The release of acetylcholine from the motor nerve terminal may be affected by:
1   Calcium ions and calcium ion antagonists.
2   Local and general anaesthetics.
3   Neurotoxins.
4   Guanidine and aminopyridine.
5   Other drugs.

Calcium ions and calcium ion antagonists

The release of acetylcholine from the motor nerve terminal is dependent on the entry of calcium ions from extracellular fluid to the axoplasm (p. 261). Consequently, alterations in extracellular calcium might be expected to affect neurotransmitter release from the motor nerve terminal. In practice, although hypocalcaemia and hypercalcaemia have important effects on the excitability of tissues and cardiac contraction, they do not usually modify acetylcholine release (except in experimental conditions).

Nevertheless, drugs that prevent the entry of calcium ions into the motor nerve terminal may decrease acetylcholine release (and thus prolong non-depolarizing neuromuscular blockade). Thus, calcium channel antagonists (e.g. verapamil, diltiazem and nifedipine) occasionally prevent the entry of calcium ions into the axoplasm; in these conditions they may impair neurotransmitter release and interact with muscle relaxants. Similarly, certain antibiotics may impair neuromuscular transmission and prolong non-depolarizing blockade by decreasing the entry of calcium ions into the motor nerve terminal. Although this phenomenon has been mainly reported with the aminoglycosides and the polymyxins, it may also occur with other antibiotics (e.g. colistin, tetracyclines and lincomycin). Although the primary action of these antibiotics is presynaptic, effects on the motor endplate and voluntary muscle may also occur. Classically, neuromuscular function was impaired in tuberculous patients on long-term streptomycin; alternatively, neostigmine-resistant curarization occurred after abdominal surgery in which large doses of intraperitoneal aminoglycoside antibiotics were used. Calcium salts (e.g. calcium gluconate) may cause the reversal of antibiotic-induced neuromuscular blockade; less commonly, anticholinesterase drugs are useful. The problem is not frequently encountered in current anaesthetic practice. A similar phenomenon may occur when antibiotics are given to patients with myasthenia gravis.

Magnesium ions compete with calcium ions for transport into the motor nerve terminal, and thus decrease the release of acetylcholine. Consequently, parenteral magnesium sulphate, or magnesium-containing antacids, may reduce neurotransmitter release and interact with muscle relaxants (particularly in patients with renal failure).

Local and general anaesthetics

Most local anaesthetics can decrease the release of acetylcholine from the motor nerve terminal. After systemic administration or absorption, they may affect conduction in unmyelinated nerve endings; alternatively, conduction blockade of major or minor nerve trunks may prevent the transmission of nerve impulses from anterior horn cells.

General anaesthetics (particularly inhalational agents) may also decrease the release of acetylcholine from the motor nerve terminal. They produce depression of the CNS and thus decrease the generation of nerve impulses by anterior horn cells. In addition, some fluorinated anaesthetics may have direct effects on the muscle cell membrane. Consequently, many volatile anaesthetic agents may profoundly affect the degree of non-depolarizing neuromuscular blockade. Diethylether classically potentiates the effects of muscle relaxants; similar effects are produced by the fluorinated ethers, enflurane and isoflurane. Halothane is a fluorinated hydrocarbon, and has less potent effects on neuromuscular transmission. Nevertheless, it can still prolong the effects of non-depolarizing drugs. The cardiovascular effects of inhalational anaesthetics may also modify the pharmacokinetics of muscle relaxants.

Neurotoxins

Certain neurotoxins also prevent the release of acetylcholine by the motor nerve terminal. Black widow spider venom contains α-latrotoxin which affects transmitter release in all cholinergic nerves. At the neuromuscular junction, α-latrotoxin initially produces the irreversible fusion of synaptic vesicles with the terminal axonal membrane. Subsequently, the synaptic vesicles become disorganized, and lose their ability to concentrate newly synthesized acetylcholine. Botulinus toxin also affects all cholinergic nerves. It prevents the release of acetylcholine from synaptic vesicles, but has little or no effect on the ultrastructure or the neurotransmitter content of the motor nerve terminal.

Guanidine and aminopyridine

Both guanidine and aminopyridine prolong the duration of the neuronal action potential, increase calcium ion entry, and thus facilitate the release of acetylcholine from the motor nerve terminal (and other cholinergic nerve endings). Their mode of action is slightly different; guanidine delays the inactivation of sodium channels, while aminopyridine tends to inactivate potassium channels (and thus prevents repolarization). Both drugs have been used to increase the release of acetylcholine from the motor nerve terminal in botulinism and the Eaton–Lambert syndrome. (This condition is a rare disorder of neuromuscular transmission which is usually associated with a small cell carcinoma of the bronchus.) In Bulgaria, aminopyridine has been used to reverse non-depolarizing neuromuscular blockade. Unfortunately, both guanidine and aminopyridine readily cross the blood–brain barrier, and may cause convulsions; this has severely restricted their clinical use.

Other drugs

Many other drugs can affect acetylcholine release in experimental conditions (e.g. dendrotoxin, catechol, phenol, tetraethylammonium, and adenosine). Theophylline and other xanthine derivatives can enhance the release of acetylcholine (either by adenosine receptor blockade, or by phosphodiesterase inhibition and accumulation of cAMP). This phenomenon may also explain the improvement which occurs in myasthenia gravis when sympathomimetic drugs (e.g. ephedrine) are administered.

Drugs that affect the action of acetylcholine

Drugs can modify the action of acetylcholine by combining with nicotinic receptors on the postsynaptic membrane. These compounds are traditionally referred to as neuromuscular blocking agents (or 'muscle relaxants').

They are commonly divided into two groups:

1 Depolarizing agents (e.g. suxamethonium and decamethonium).
2 Non-depolarizing agents (e.g. tubocurarine, gallamine, alcuronium, pancuronium, vecuronium and atracurium).

As their name implies, depolarizing agents produce depolarization of the motor endplate immediately before the onset of neuromuscular blockade. In contrast, non-depolarizing agents do not produce depolarization (except in experimental conditions in embryonic and cultured muscle cells).

Mode of action

Both depolarizing and non-depolarizing agents have non-specific effects, and may affect neuromuscular transmission at different sites. Consequently, the interpretation of their actions on neuromuscular function in terms of their molecular and electrophysiological effects is imprecise and controversial.

Depolarization blockade is probably due to the rapid inactivation of voltage-sensitive sodium channels in the muscle cell membrane, immediately adjacent to the motor endplate. The intra-arterial injection of small doses of acetylcholine near the motor endplate normally produces a brief contraction of voluntary muscle. In these conditions, the hydrolysis of acetylcholine is extremely rapid, and subsequent stimulation of the motor nerve produces little change in the twitch response. When larger doses of acetylcholine are injected (or its activity is prolonged by anticholinesterase drugs), the initial muscle contraction is followed by neuromuscular blockade, resulting in the depression of the maximal twitch response to nerve stimulation. Similar effects can be produced by other drugs that are structurally related to acetylcholine, but are less rapidly removed from the motor endplate (e.g. suxamethonium and decamethonium).

In normal conditions, depolarization of the motor endplate by acetylcholine activates voltage-sensitive sodium channels in the adjacent muscle fibre, resulting in the generation and propagation of a muscle action potential. If depolarization is maintained, several action potentials may be produced. However, persistent depolarization is rapidly followed by the generation of local current circuits and the inactivation of voltage-sensitive sodium channels in the adjacent muscle fibre, immediately peripheral to the motor endplate. In the inactivated state, these channels are closed, and cannot be opened by the persistent depolarization of the motor endplate. This phenomenon occurs within several milliseconds, and produces a zone of electrical inexcitability surrounding the motor endplate, which extends for 1–2 mm along the muscle fibre membrane. This zone will not transmit or propagate impulses, although the remainder of the muscle fibre is normally excitable. Consequently neuromuscular blockade is a direct consequence of persistent depolarization of the motor endplate.

In contrast, non-depolarizing neuromuscular blockade is primarily due to competition of drugs with acetylcholine for receptor sites on the postsynaptic membrane. Consequently, these drugs are frequently referred to as 'competitive' neuromuscular blocking agents (although it is difficult to be certain that all of their effects are due to the competitive antagonism of acetylcholine). The reversible combination of non-depolarizing agents with postsynaptic receptors does not produce any change in membrane conductance or ionic permeability, so that depolarization by acetylcholine is progressively diminished (due to a reduction in the available receptors). Since the formation of an effective agonist–receptor complex is prevented, the amplitude of the endplate potential gradually decreases. Eventually, it fails to generate a propagated muscle action potential, resulting in neuromuscular blockade. Normal neuromuscular function is restored when adequate redistribution and/or elimination of the muscle relaxant occurs, or when sufficient acetylcholine accumulates to displace the non-depolarizing agent from postsynaptic receptors.

In normal conditions, the amount of acetylcholine released by nerve stimulation exceeds that required to produce an endplate potential and its subsequent muscle action potential. Similarly, there is an excessive number of receptors on the postsynaptic membrane, in comparison with the number of molecules of acetylcholine released to combine with them. Consequently, there must be considerable receptor occupation by the antagonist before there is evidence of neuromuscular blockade. Experimental evidence suggests that approximately 80% of receptors must be occupied by non-depolarizing agents before any reduction in neuromuscular transmission occurs; 90–95% receptor occupation is required for complete neuromuscular blockade.

In addition to their effects on acetylcholine receptors on the postsynaptic membrane, non-depolarizing agents affect neuromuscular transmission in at least two additional ways. In the first place, they may combine with receptors on the motor nerve terminal which are normally responsible for the maintenance of transmitter output at high rates of stimulation. Consequently, during partial neuromuscular blockade, acetylcholine release decreases during repetitive nerve stimulation, resulting in decrement or fade. Secondly, non-depolarizing relaxants (and some other drugs) may physically occlude ion channels on the postsynaptic membrane (and possibly at presynaptic sites as well). This type of blockade is most likely to occur when ion channel opening is most frequent (i.e. when acetylcholine, other agonists, or anticholinesterase drugs are also used). Its contribution to non-depolarizing blockade in current clinical practice is uncertain.

Characteristic features of neuromuscular blockade

Depolarizing and non-depolarizing blockade have characteristic and distinctive features, which may be of clinical significance. These differences are classically seen after the administration of suxamethonium and tubocurarine in man (Table 9.1).

1 Depolarization blockade is preceded by muscle fasciculations; in non-depolarizing blockade, muscle activity does not occur.

Muscle fasciculations are incoordinated contractions due to the repetitive firing of muscle fibres, and are associated with increased electromyographic activity in voluntary muscle. It is unlikely that muscle fasciculations simply reflect the depolarization of the motor endplate. Acetylcholine receptors are present at presynaptic sites on the motor nerve ending, and their depolarization may initiate a local antidromic axon reflex within the terminals of an entire motor unit. Consequently, fasciculations are probably due to the synchronous release of acetylcholine from a number of motor nerve terminals, and thus reflect the pre-synaptic actions of depolarizing drugs. Reflex effects mediated by acetylcholine receptors in muscle spindles may play a secondary role.

In contrast, during non-depolarizing blockade muscle fasciculations are absent, since presynaptic receptors are occupied by acetylcholine antagonists. Indeed, non-depolarizing drugs may decrease suxamethonium-induced fasciculations by preventing prejunctional depolarization and the occurrence of local axon reflexes, thus reducing the rate of motor unit firing. Consequently, pretreatment with non-depolarizing relaxants may prevent suxamethonium-induced fasciculations and muscle pain.

2 In depolarization blockade, there is a decrease in potential amplitude during repetitive indirect stimulation, but no evidence of fade (i.e. the progressive decrease in the electrical or the mechanical response to continuous nerve stimula-

Table 9.1 Differences between depolarizing and non-depolarizing neuromuscular blockade.

	Depolarizing blockade	Non-depolarizing blockade
Preceded by muscle fasciculations	Yes	No
Neuromuscular decrement ('fade')	Absent	Present
Post-tetanic potentiation	Absent (usually)	Present
Effect of anticholinesterase drugs	Increased	Antagonized
Effect of non-depolarizing drugs	Antagonized	Increased
Tachyphylaxis and dual blockade	May occur	Absent

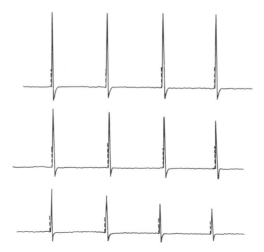

Fig. 9.4 Muscle action potentials evoked by indirect nerve stimulation during the induction of neuromuscular block. A 'train-of-four' was used in each instance.

tion). In contrast, in non-depolarizing blockade there is a gradual decrease in the amplitude of the muscle action potential or the twitch height during repetitive indirect stimulation ('decrement' or 'fade'; Fig. 9.4).

In depolarization blockade, acetylcholine output is probably maintained during subtetanic or tetanic stimulation, due to the effects of depolarization on pre-synaptic receptors that preserve transmitter output at high rates of impulse con-duction. In any case, variations in acetylcholine release are unlikely to affect the degree of neuromuscular blockade, since this is due to persistent depolarization of the motor endplate. During partial recovery from depolarization blockade, there is a decrease in potential amplitude during repetitive indirect stimulation, but no evidence of fade.

By contrast, in non-depolarizing blockade there is a significant decrease in the quantal release of acetylcholine during rapid indirect stimulation. It is not entirely clear whether this is a pharmacological phenomenon; it may be related to blockade of presynaptic receptors on the motor nerve terminal. Since post-synaptic receptors are also affected (i.e. the safety factor of neuromuscular transmission is compromised), the progressive decrease in transmitter release with repetitive stimulation is reflected in the amplitude of the muscle action potential or the twitch height. This phenomenon of decrement (fade) is character-istically seen during the onset or recovery from non-depolarizing blockade. It is widely used to monitor the effects of drugs on neuromuscular transmission (e.g. by the train-of-four, which compares the amplitude of the first and the fourth response to a train-of-four stimuli (Fig. 9.4)). It may or may not reflect the effects of muscle relaxants on neurotransmitter release from the motor nerve ending.

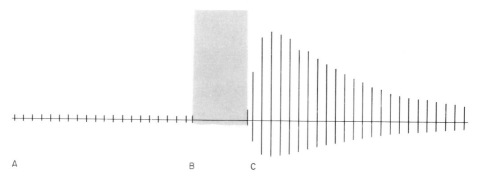

A   B   C

Fig. 9.5 Post-tetanic potentiation during partial recovery from non-depolarizing neuromuscular blockade. A, compound muscle action potentials evoked by repetitive indirect stimulation. B, conditioning tetanus; its amplitude is due to the presence of a stimulus artefact. C, post-tetanic potentiation after reversion to original rate of stimulation.

3   During the onset or partial recovery from depolarization blockade, significant post-tetanic potentiation does not occur. In contrast, in non-depolarizing blockade post-tetanic potentiation can usually be demonstrated (in both the electromyogram and the mechanical response to indirect stimulation; Fig. 9.5).

Subtetanic or tetanic stimulation of motor nerves results in the decreased release of acetylcholine per stimulus; this is rapidly followed by enhanced synthesis and transmitter mobilization. Consequently, when the tetanus ends, acetylcholine output per stimulus is increased. In normal circumstances, this does not affect neuromuscular function, due to the presence of the 'safety margin' for synaptic transmission (p. 267); consequently, post-tetanic potentiation is not observed on the electromyogram. Nevertheless, some post-tetanic potentiation may be present in the twitch response; this probably reflects increased muscle contractility, possibly due to the enhanced entry of calcium ions into muscle cells during tetanic stimulation. The phenomenon is sometimes referred to as 'augmentation of muscle contraction'.

During depolarization blockade, the enhanced transmitter release per stimulus produced by a conditioning tetanus does not significantly affect the degree of depolarization or the depth of neuromuscular blockade. Consequently, significant post-tetanic potentiation does not usually occur (although some 'augmentation of contraction' may be seen in the twitch response, as in normal circumstances).

In contrast, post-tetanic potentiation is an established feature of non-depolarizing blockade; the increase in transmitter output produced by the conditioning tetanus increases endplate depolarization above the threshold level in a proportion of partially blocked muscle fibres. In this instance, post-tetanic potentiation is due to 'facilitation of transmission', i.e. a temporary increase in acetylcholine output which displaces non-depolarizing relaxants from their postsynaptic sites. During profound neuromuscular blockade, the 'post-tetanic count' can be used to monitor the effects of muscle relaxants on the motor endplate.

4 Anticholinesterase drugs may increase the depth and duration of depolarization blockade. In contrast, they reverse or antagonize non-depolarizing blockade.

Anticholinesterase drugs increase the depth and duration of depolarization blockade for two main reasons. In the first place, they may prolong depolarization at the motor endplate by preventing the breakdown of released acetylcholine. Secondly, they may prevent the metabolism of depolarizing drugs that are esters (i.e. suxamethonium). Drugs that inhibit cholinesterase (i.e. tetrahydroamin-acrine and hexafluorenium) were at one time used to extend the duration of action of suxamethonium. In general, their action is unreliable and unpredictable.

In non-depolarizing blockade, anticholinesterase drugs cause the accumulation of acetylcholine at the motor endplate; the neurotransmitter progressively displaces non-depolarizing muscle relaxants from postsynaptic and presynaptic sites, resulting in the antagonism of neuromuscular blockade.

5 Non-depolarizing drugs reverse or antagonize depolarization blockade; in contrast, they invariably potentiate non-depolarizing blockade produced by other drugs.

Non-depolarizing drugs compete for and combine with acetylcholine receptors on the postsynaptic membrane. Consequently, in depolarization blockade they tend to reduce endplate depolarization, and may restore normal neuromuscular transmission. In practice, they are not used clinically for this purpose since their effects are rather unpredictable.

In contrast, non-depolarizing drugs invariably increase the depth and duration of non-depolarizing blockade produced by other drugs. In some instances, supra-additive or potentiating effects may be observed.

6 Depolarization blockade may be associated with the development of tachy-phylaxis and dual block. These complications do not occur in non-depolarizing blockade.

In depolarization blockade, tachyphylaxis is usually recognized by a decreased response to successive doses of the drug. This phenomenon may precede the gradual development of a second phase of neuromuscular blockade. Changes consistent with non-depolarizing blockade occur, and are usually referred to as dual block or phase II block. In man, this is most commonly seen when large doses or prolonged infusions of suxamethonium are used, or when drug elimination is compromised by enzyme abnormalities or other drugs.

The explanation for the development of dual block is not entirely clear. It may reflect the continual presence of depolarizing drugs at the motor endplate, resulting in receptor desensitization or ion channel blockade. Receptor desensitization effectively reduces the number of functional receptors on the postsynaptic membrane. If this reduction is profound, neuromuscular blockade occurs, which is potentiated by non-depolarizing drugs and antagonized by anticholinesterase agents. Similar features might be present if depolarizing drugs progressively blocked open ion channels at the motor endplate. Unfortunately, there is no definite evidence that either receptor desensitization or ion channel blockade can occur in man, and the cause of dual block is unclear.

Nevertheless, tachyphylaxis and dual block are only associated with depolarization blockade; they do not occur when neuromuscular blockade is produced by non-depolarizing drugs (Table 9.1).

Depolarizing agents

In general, all depolarizing agents have a similar chemical structure (Fig. 9.6). They are slender, elongated, and flexible molecules ('leptocurares') with methyl or ethyl groups attached to their quaternary heads, which are separated by a distance of 1.2–1.4 nm. In the past, decamethonium and suxamethonium have been used to produce neuromuscular blockade; in current practice, only suxamethonium is used for this purpose.

Acetylcholine

Suxamethonium

Decamethonium

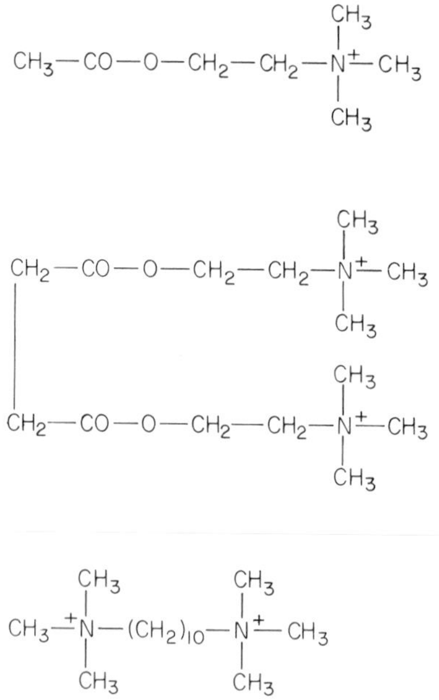

Fig. 9.6 The chemical structure of acetylcholine, suxamethonium, and decamethonium.

Table 9.2 Undesirable effects of suxamethonium.

Muscle fasciculations
Postoperative myalgia
Hyperkalaemia
Tachyphylaxis and dual blockade
Increased intra-ocular pressure
Malignant hyperthermia
Parasympathomimetic effects
bradycardia
increased respiratory secretions
increased intragastric pressure
increased uterine tone
Prolonged paralysis due to delayed metabolism

Suxamethonium

Suxamethonium is a quaternary amine ester (Fig. 9.6); chemically, it consists of two molecules of acetylcholine, joined together at their non-quaternary ends (i.e. through their acetyl groups). Its ability to produce depolarization blockade in man was first recognized in 1949–1951 (although its pharmacological properties were first investigated in curarized animals in 1906).

After the intravenous injection of suxamethonium, profound muscle relaxation preceded by observable muscle fasciculations normally occurs within 1 min. The duration of neuromuscular blockade after normal doses of suxamethonium ($1.0–1.5\,mg\,kg^{-1}$) is usually 4–6 min; during this time there is a rapid fall in the plasma concentration of the drug. Neuromuscular blockade is due to the persistent depolarization of the motor endplate, which rapidly inactivates voltage-sensitive sodium channels in the adjacent muscle fibre (p. 266). Unfortunately, suxamethonium produces a number of additional undesirable effects (Table 9.2).

1 Muscle fasciculations. Muscle fasciculations may be slight (usually involving the small muscles of the hand and the facial muscles), moderate (involving larger muscle groups in the limbs), or severe (involving most muscle groups in the body). Moderate and severe fasciculations can facilitate venous return and cause an increase in cardiac output; arterial blood pressure may rise and an increase in intracranial tension can occur. Fasciculations that involve the abdominal muscles may cause an increase in intragastric pressure.

2 Myalgia. Postoperative muscle pains are a frequent complication of the administration of suxamethonium, and occur chiefly in the subcostal region, the trunk, and the shoulder girdle. Women are more susceptible than men, and symptoms are more frequently encountered in patients who have been mobilized soon after surgery, and in subjects unaccustomed to muscular exercise. The frequency of postoperative myalgia after suxamethonium varies between 6 and 60%; creatine kinase levels are significantly raised, and myoglobinuria occasionally occurs. These findings suggest that suxamethonium myalgia may be related to muscle damage caused by drug-induced fasciculations. Nevertheless, in many studies the incidence of muscle fasciculations is not directly related to the occurrence of postoperative pain (although pretreatment with a small dose of non-depolarizing drugs modifies the fasciculations and reduces the incidence of pain).

3 *Hyperkalaemia.* Depolarization of the motor endplate, and the resulting muscle contraction, causes the efflux of intracellular potassium ions into the extracellular fluid. In normal conditions, plasma potassium rises by approximately 0.5 mmol litre^{-1}; this increase is rarely of clinical significance (although it may accentuate the cardiac effects of subsequent doses of suxamethonium).

In contrast, in patients with severe burns, peripheral nerve injuries, or neurological conditions, much greater increases in serum potassium concentrations may occur. Rises of $4-9$ mmol litre^{-1} have been reported; in neurological conditions, the major hyperkalaemic response can be demonstrated in the venous blood draining the paralysed or injured limbs. A latent period may be required between the time of injury and the development of an excessive hyperkalaemic response. This suggests that the rise in serum potassium may be related to receptor upregulation after muscle damage or peripheral denervation (i.e. 'denervation supersensitivity'). In peripheral denervation (and during fetal life), acetylcholine receptors on the postsynaptic membrane are not just localized to the motor endplate, but extend along the entire surface of the muscle fibre. In these conditions, the increased loss of potassium from muscle is related to the extensive area of the muscle membrane depolarized by suxamethonium.

There have been numerous reports of cardiac arrest after the use of suxamethonium in patients with severe burns and neurological conditions (particularly between 20 and 60 days after the initial injury). Although clear evidence of muscle damage or denervation may not be present, hyperkalaemia is probably the main causal factor. Hypovolaemia, acidosis, and autonomic imbalance may also be involved.

When pre-existing hyperkalaemia is present (e.g. in renal failure or severe acidosis), undesirable cardiac effects should be anticipated if suxamethonium is used.

4 *Tachyphylaxis and dual blockade* (phase II blockade). Suxamethonium, like other drugs that produce depolarization blockade, may cause tachyphylaxis (a decreased response to successive doses of the drug). This may precede the gradual development of dual blockade (phase II blockade), in which changes consistent with non-depolarizing blockade may occur. This phenomenon is most

commonly seen when large doses or prolonged infusions of suxamethonium are used, or when the elimination of the drug is compromised (e.g. by enzyme abnormalities or other drugs). The cause of tachyphylaxis and phase II blockade is uncertain (p. 272).

5 *Increased intra-ocular pressure.* Suxamethonium causes a rise in intra-ocular tension, which may last for several minutes. Consequently, the drug should be used with caution in patients with penetrating eye injuries, and during open ocular surgery.

In man, the extrinsic muscles of the eye are multiply innervated by relatively slowly conducting Aγ axons (i.e. each muscle fibre is innervated by more than one axonal terminal). In this respect, their innervation is similar to avian muscle. In many birds, suxamethonium characteristically produces a slow and sustained contraction (contracture) of voluntary muscle. Similar effects are probably produced in human extra-ocular muscles, causing a transient rise in intra-ocular pressure.

6 *Malignant hyperpyrexia* (malignant hyperthermia). In susceptible individuals, malignant hyperpyrexia may be triggered by suxamethonium. The initial dose of suxamethonium may fail to produce muscle relaxation; there may be generalized muscle rigidity, associated with a rapidly rising temperature, which may develop within a few minutes. Suxamethonium probably precipitates the release of calcium ions from the sarcoplasmic reticulum of susceptible individuals, causing sustained muscle contraction.

7 *Parasympathetic effects.* Suxamethonium is chemically related to acetylcholine, and has some activity at muscarinic receptors. Thus, bradycardia or AV nodal rhythm may occur after a large single dose, or with repeated administration (especially in children). Potentiation of these muscarinic effects on the heart may occur with digoxin, or with other drugs that alter autonomic balance in favour of parasympathetic activity (e.g. β-adrenoceptor antagonists). Other muscarinic effects are not uncommon. Increased production of bronchial and salivary secretions are frequently observed, especially with repeated dosage. Gastric tone is increased, and a rise in intragastric pressure occurs (although this is partly related to fasciculations involving the abdominal muscles). Repeated doses of suxamethonium may cause a marked increase in uterine tone during caesarean section. All these parasympathetic effects can be prevented or attenuated by premedication with atropine, or other antimuscarinic drugs.

8 *Metabolism of suxamethonium.* Occasionally, prolonged paralysis and apnoea are related to the delayed metabolism of suxamethonium. In general, problems

may be due to the presence of genetic variants of plasma cholinesterase, or to the concurrent use of other drugs that can inhibit the enzyme.

The transient effects of a single dose of suxamethonium are due to its rapid hydrolysis by plasma cholinesterase ('pseudocholinesterase'). The breakdown of the drug occurs in two stages. Initially, succinylmonocholine is formed, which has weak neuromuscular blocking activity (approximately 5% of the potency of suxamethonium). Subsequently, succinylmonocholine is broken down to succinic acid and choline. Prolongation of the effects of suxamethonium may be due to genetic polymorphism, decreased availability, or inhibition of cholinesterase.

Plasma cholinesterase is synthesized by the liver; severe hepatic dysfunction, usually associated with marked hypoalbuminaemia, may cause abnormally low cholinesterase levels, and some prolongation of the action of suxamethonium is likely. More significant problems can arise from genetically determined abnormalities of the enzyme. Genetic polymorphism is present, and at least four allelomorphic genes have been identified at a single locus of chromosome 3. These genes are called E_1^u, E_1^a, E_1^f, and E_1^s; they produce the normal (usual) enzyme, the atypical enzyme, the fluoride-resistant enzyme, and the absent (silent) enzyme respectively. The commonest genetic variant (the atypical enzyme) can

Table 9.3 The classical genetic variants of plasma cholinesterase.*

Genotype	Approximate incidence per 1000 population	Dibucaine number	Prolonged response to suxamethonium
$E_1^u E_1^u$	950	80	No
$E_1^u E_1^a$	40	60	Occasionally
$E_1^u E_1^f$	4	75	Occasionally
$E_1^u E_1^s$	6	80	Occasionally
$E_1^a E_1^a$	<1	20	Yes
$E_1^a E_1^f$	<1	50	Occasionally
$E_1^a E_1^s$	<1	20	Yes
$E_1^f E_1^f$	<1	65	Occasionally
$E_1^f E_1^s$	<1	65	Occasionally
$E_1^s E_1^s$	<1	–	Yes

*During the past decade, this system of classification has been extended by the use of DNA-cloning techniques. At least ten allelomorphic genes (and a possible 28 phenotypes) have been identified; some genetic variants (e.g. the K-variant, the J-variant, and the H-variant) are quantitative variants in which reduced enzyme activity is associated with normal kinetic properties. The amino acid sequence of the normal and the atypical enzyme have also been determined. The atypical (dibucaine-resistant) enzyme is associated with a single mutation at nucleotide 209 (GAT to GGT), which changes amino acid 70 from aspartate to glycine. This substitution at the active site of the acidic (anionic) amino acid aspartate by neutral glycine accounts for the resistance to dibucaine inhibition and the reduced affinity for the quaternary amine suxamethonium.

be distinguished from the usual enzyme by its resistance to inhibition by the local anaesthetic cinchocaine (dibucaine). The 'dibucaine number' is defined as the enzyme inhibition (%) produced by dibucaine (10^{-5}M), using benzoylcholine as the substrate. Normal homozygotes ($E_1^u E_1^u$) have dibucaine numbers of 80; heterozygotes for the atypical enzyme ($E_1^u E_1^a$) have dibucaine numbers of 60, while homozygotes for the atypical enzyme ($E_1^a E_1^a$) have dibucaine numbers of 20 (Table 9.3). Since four allelomorphic genes are present, ten genotypes have been identified; three of these genotypes will show a greatly prolonged response to suxamethonium (Table 9.3). Their total incidence in the general population is about 1 in 2000. In recent years, at least six additional allelomorphic genes have been identified (Table 9.3). In addition, a second distinct locus is associated with two further genetic variants ($E_{Cynthiana}$ and C_5) which may be responsible for increased cholinesterase activity.

Drugs that inhibit plasma cholinesterase may extend the duration of action of suxamethonium. Some agents (i.e. tetrahydroaminacrine and hexafluorenium) have been intentionally used for this purpose. More serious drug interactions (e.g. prolongation of neuromuscular blockade, tachyphylaxis and the increased likelihood of phase II block) may be due to the concurrent use of drugs that are substrates or inhibitors of plasma cholinesterase. These include edrophonium, neostigmine, pyridostigmine, ecothiopate, other organophosphorus compounds, alkylating agents, trimetaphan, pitocin, and ester local anaesthetics.

Decamethonium

Decamethonium was first used clinically in 1949, after the investigation of several bisquaternary compounds for curare-like activity. It was originally considered to cause less depression of respiration because of a diaphragm sparing activity; however, it soon became apparent that the production of effective relaxation also produced respiratory paralysis. After the administration of a single dose (usually 4–6 mg), there is a relatively slow onset of action (3–5 min) and a moderate duration of action (10–20 min); its effects are potentiated by passive hyperventilation. The drug is almost entirely excreted in urine unchanged. The effects of decamethonium may be antagonized by other methonium compounds (e.g. pentamethonium and hexamethonium); these drugs may cause considerable hypotension due to ganglion blockade. Decamethonium has been extensively used in experimental studies, but has not been generally available in the UK since 1958. Nevertheless, it may be imported, or a suitable preparation may be made up by a hospital pharmacist from decamethonium powder, and the drug is still occasionally used in clinical anaesthesia. Some of the advantages claimed for decamethonium include a marked degree of cardiovascular stability, little or no histamine release, and a lower incidence of muscle fasciculation and postoperative myalgia than with other depolarizing relaxants.

Non-depolarizing agents

The classical non-depolarizing muscle relaxant, 'curare', is a generic term for various South American arrow poisons; it is used correctly to describe the crude extracts obtained from certain species of the plants *Chondrodendron* and *Strychnos*. The impure extracts, containing several different alkaloids, have been used for many centuries by South American Indians as an 'arrow' or 'blow-dart' poison, in order to kill wild animals for food. Their preparation of curare was shrouded in mystery and ritual, and the samples of the drug which first reached civilization were classified by the containers in which they had been transported; pot curare was carried in earthenware jars, tube curare in bamboo tubes, and calabash curare in gourds. Scientific interest in curare dates from the classical observations of Claude Bernard in 1856; he correctly localized the paralytic effects of curare to the neuromuscular junction, since the drug did not affect nervous conduction or the response of voluntary muscle to direct stimulation. Its clinical use dates from 1932, when purified fractions were used in the treatment of tetanus and spastic disorders. Subsequently, the *d*-isomer of tubocurarine was isolated, and its provisional chemical formula (which was later revised) was established by King in 1932. The drug was later used to control pentylenetetra-zole-induced convulsions during the treatment of psychiatric disorders. It was finally introduced into anaesthetic practice in 1942.

Since then, other drugs have been widely used to produce neuromuscular blockade. The first synthetic relaxant, gallamine triethiodide, was introduced by Bovet in 1947, and alcuronium (a semi-synthetic derivative of a curare alkaloid) has been used in the UK since 1962. The bisquaternary aminosteroid pancur-onium has been widely employed for 20 years, while two newer drugs with significant advantages (i.e. vecuronium and atracurium) have been introduced during the past decade. Vecuronium is the monoquaternary analogue of pancuronium, while atracurium is a bisquaternary ester with a novel molecular structure, which is spontaneously broken down in the body. At least three other drugs are currently under development for clinical use. All of these compounds contain quaternary amine groups, and many of them have a bulky molecular structure (i.e. they are 'pachycurares'; Fig. 9.7).

Although all these drugs have similar effects on the neuromuscular junction, they differ in certain other respects (Table 9.4). In general, these differences are related to:

1 Effects of extracellular pH on their activity.
2 Histamine release.
3 Effects on the cardiovascular system.
4 Distribution and pharmacokinetics.
5 Metabolism and elimination.

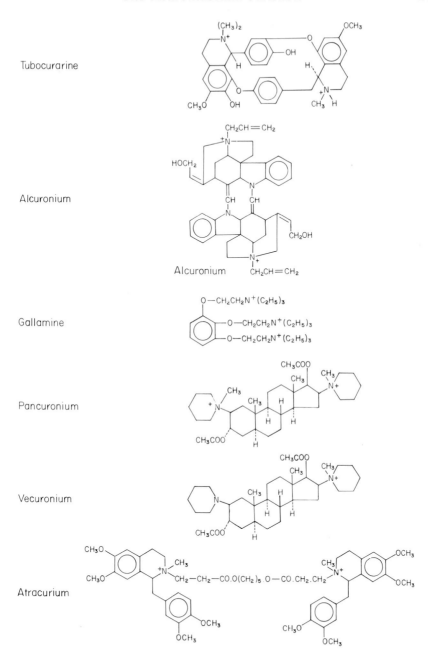

Fig. 9.7 The chemical structure of non-depolarizing muscle relaxants in current clinical use. (The associated anions have been omitted).

Table 9.4 Pharmacological differences between non-depolarizing relaxants.

	Onset of action	Histamine release	Cardiovascular effects	Duration of action	Plasma protein binding (%)	Volume of distribution (ml kg^{-1})	Clearance (ml min^{-1} kg^{-1})	$t_{\frac{1}{2}}$ (min)	Elimination
Tubocurarine	Slow	Common	Hypotension	Long	30–50	290	1.5	190	Not metabolized; eliminated in urine (70%) and bile (30%)
Alcuronium	Moderate	?Rare	Hypotension	Long	<20	300	1.5	200	Not metabolized; eliminated in urine (70%) and bile (30%)
Gallamine	Rapid	Rare	Tachycardia	Medium	<20	230	1.2	150	Not metabolized; eliminated in urine (100%)
Pancuronium	Moderate	Rare	Tachycardia	Medium	20–60	270	1.5	130	Metabolized (30%) to 3 deacetylated metabolites; 70% eliminated unchanged (mainly in urine)
Vecuronium	Moderate	Rare	None	Short	<20	230	4.0	60	Metabolized (20%) to deacetylated metabolites; 80% eliminated unchanged (mainly in bile)
Atracurium	Moderate	Rare	None	Short	<20	160	5.5	20	Metabolized (95%) to laudanosine, a quaternary acrylate, acid and alcohol; 5% eliminated unchanged.

Values for the volume of distribution, clearance and $t_{\frac{1}{2}}$ (terminal half-life) are median values obtained in patients without hepatic or renal impairment.

Extracellular pH

The potency and duration of action of individual muscle relaxants may be modified in different ways by changes in plasma and extracellular pH. In particular, the potency and duration of action of tubocurarine is prolonged by respiratory acidosis, and decreased by respiratory alkalosis. This phenomenon may be related to the effects of pH on the physicochemical properties of tubocurarine, which has one tertiary and one quaternary amine group (Fig. 9.7). In acidic conditions, the ionization of the tertiary amine group ($pK_a = 8$) is increased due to protonation; the ionization of the two hydroxyl groups ($pK_a = 8$ and 9.3) may also be modified. These changes increase the potency of tubocurarine. Similar effects on ionization may occur in metabolic acidosis and metabolic alkalosis. However, in these conditions the shift of K^+ between cells and extracellular fluid may be a complicating factor. Hypokalaemia tends to prolong non-depolarizing blockade, since it tends to increase the resting membrane potential and prevent depolarization.

The effects of gallamine may be potentiated by alkalosis and antagonized by acidosis; the action of other muscle relaxants is not usually affected by pH changes within the physiological range. Any alterations that do occur are probably related to the effects of pH on electrolyte balance, rather than to an inherent effect on the activity of the drugs.

Histamine release

Many drugs that contain amine groups can release histamine and other autocoids from mast cells, either by displacement or by exocytosis. Some muscle relaxants (e.g. tubocurarine, atracurium, and possibly suxamethonium) are particularly likely to cause histamine release from mast cells. This may be evident in 20–25% of patients after intravenous injection of tubocurarine (as seen by the 'weal and flare' response, i.e. local oedema and arteriolar vasodilatation). Histamine release by tubocurarine and atracurium may be dependent on several factors, e.g. the initial high local concentration of the drugs, and their injection into relatively small veins. Intra-arterial injection can produce a marked rise in histamine concentration in venous blood. Both tubocurarine and atracurium may cause systemic effects after intravenous administration. Cutaneous flushing is frequently seen, and histamine release may be implicated in the transient hypotension which is often observed. An increase in airway resistance occasionally occurs, but is usually slight and of short duration. Rarely, both tubocurarine and atracurium cause severe anaphylactoid or anaphylactic reactions, with widespread oedema, severe bronchospasm, bradycardia, and peripheral vascular collapse.

Significant histamine release is less commonly seen with other muscle relaxants; it is occasionally observed with gallamine and alcuronium. A number of other drugs used in anaesthesia are potent histamine-releasing agents (e.g. morphine, pethidine and some plasma substitutes).

Effects on the cardiovascular system

Most non-depolarizing agents may cause a fall in blood pressure immediately after their administration. This may be related to histamine release, a decrease in venous return caused by loss of muscle tone, or other effects.

Tubocurarine commonly causes a fall in blood pressure of 20–30 mmHg or more. Reflex tachycardia is rare; indeed, a slight decrease in pulse rate (less than 10 beats per min) is usually present. The fall in blood pressure is partly due to histamine release, and partly to blockade of sympathetic ganglia; the absence of reflex tachycardia suggests that ganglion blockade is the most important factor. In general, alcuronium has similar effects to tubocurarine, although significant histamine release is uncommon. A slight fall in blood pressure may occur, probably due to blockade of sympathetic ganglia.

In contrast, both gallamine and pancuronium commonly produce tachycardia. Gallamine usually increases pulse rate by 20–30 beats per min; blood pressure is usually unaltered or raised. After injection of atropine, a further rise in pulse rate may occur. Gallamine produces selective antagonism of muscarinic receptors in the heart (M_2-receptors), by causing conformational changes that reduce their affinity for acetylcholine. Muscarinic receptors in other tissues are not affected. In addition, the release of noradrenaline by cardiac sympathetic nerves is increased; this may be due to antagonism of presynaptic muscarinic receptors on sympathetic nerves (which normally mediate the decreased release of noradrenaline). Similarly, pancuronium commonly increases pulse rate, blood pressure, and venous return, although these effects are usually less marked than with gallamine. Pancuronium has complex effects on cardiac autonomic nerves; it inhibits Uptake$_1$ (i.e. the uptake of noradrenaline by sympathetic nerve endings), and may also have antimuscarinic effects which indirectly increase noradrenaline release. Both these actions tend to increase pulse rate and blood pressure.

Vecuronium and atracurium do not usually affect the cardiovascular system. They may apparently induce bradycardia and hypotension, but this is probably due to the unopposed effects of other drugs on cardiac vagal tone. Occasionally atracurium causes profound bradycardia during halothane anaesthesia.

Distribution and pharmacokinetics

Since all non-depolarizing relaxants are quaternary amines, they are not significantly absorbed from the gut. After intravenous administration, they are mainly distributed in extracellular fluid, and may be partly bound to plasma proteins. *In vitro* techniques (e.g plasmapheresis, equilibrium dialysis, and ultrafiltration) have been widely used to assess the protein binding of individual relaxants. Most of the results suggest that 30–50% of tubocurarine and 20–60% of pancuronium are bound by IgG and by albumin, but that only minor amounts of other relaxants are bound to plasma proteins. Changes in the binding of muscle relaxants to plasma proteins are probably of little practical significance. Patients in whom IgG concentrations are raised (e.g. those with severe burns and liver disease) may be resistant to tubocurarine and pancuronium; it is unclear whether this phenomenon is related to altered plasma protein binding or not. In the past, attempts have been made to correlate the individual dosage requirements of different relaxants with the concentration of different plasma proteins. In general, there is a positive correlation between tubocurarine dosage and IgG levels and between alcuronium dosage and albumin. The requirements of pancuronium were not related to any fraction of plasma proteins.

Due to their chemical structure, non-depolarizing relaxants do not cross the blood–brain barrier or the placental barrier in appreciable amounts. Nevertheless, small concentrations of muscle relaxants (usually less than 5% of the maternal level) can be detected in the fetal circulation or cord blood after administration to the mother. However, fetal apnoea is only rarely associated with the use of these drugs during anaesthesia for caesarean section (although paralysis has occurred following repeated dosage during long-term ventilation in pregnancy). Gallamine is more liable to cross the placenta than other relaxants, and its use in anaesthesia for caesarean section is usually avoided.

After intravenous administration of non-depolarizing agents, there is a rapid fall in plasma concentration during the first 2–10 min, mainly due to the uptake of the drug by renal and hepatic cells. Small concentrations are localized at the motor endplate and are non-specifically bound at anionic sites in the junctional cleft and at the basement membrane of muscle fibres. Subsequently, there is a further slower phase of exponential decline, which reflects the removal of the muscle relaxant by renal or biliary excretion, or by metabolism. Consequently, the disposition of most muscle relaxants has usually been represented in terms of models containing two compartments. Constants derived from these models can be used to calculate pharmacokinetic parameters; alternatively they may be derived by model-independent methods (Chapter 2). The total apparent volume of distribution of most muscle relaxants is similar to, or slightly greater than, extracellular fluid volume (i.e. 200–400 ml kg^{-1}). Their clearance is more variable, ranging from 1–2 ml min^{-1} kg^{-1} (tubocurarine, alcuronium, gallamine, and pancuronium) to 5–6 ml min^{-1} kg^{-1} (vecuronium and atracurium). These differences in clearance are reflected in the terminal half-lives of different relaxants, which in general are ranked in the order tubocurarine = alcuronium > pancuronium > gallamine > vecuronium > atracurium (Chapter 2; Table 9.4). This order also corresponds to the relative duration of neuromuscular blockade after the administration of equipotent doses. Indeed, with many relaxants (e.g.

tubocurarine) there is a close relation between their steady-state plasma concentration and the degree of neuromuscular blockade. In the past, it has been suggested that the main factor determining the duration of action of muscle relaxants is the rate of dissociation of the drug–receptor complex at the neuromuscular junction. These views are not now generally accepted.

The pharmacokinetics of muscle relaxants may be modified in renal and hepatic disease. In renal failure, the half-life of most non-depolarizing relaxants is increased, due to a reduction in their clearance. However, the half-life and the clearance of atracurium and vecuronium are not significantly affected. In hepatic disease, the pharmacokinetics of muscle relaxants that are mainly eliminated by the liver (e.g. vecuronium) may be modified.

Metabolism and elimination

Most muscle relaxants are partly excreted unchanged in urine, and are not readily metabolized by hepatic enzyme systems. Nevertheless, they all appear to enter liver cells, and some may be significantly secreted in bile (depending on the number of quaternary centres and their molecular weight).

Tubocurarine is not significantly metabolized by the liver or by other tissues. Normally, it is eliminated unchanged in urine (although small amounts are also present in bile, since it is a monoquaternary compound with a molecular weight of more than 400 Da). In renal failure, the amount of tubocurarine eliminated in bile is greatly increased. Similarly, the related drug alcuronium is probably not metabolized, but is mainly eliminated from the body in urine and in bile.

Gallamine is also not significantly metabolized by the body, but is almost entirely eliminated unchanged in urine. Only trace amounts are excreted in bile, since gallamine is a low molecular weight compound with more than one quaternary group. Consequently, in renal failure its clearance is greatly decreased and its half-life prolonged 10–20 times.

Pancuronium is mainly eliminated unchanged in urine, although 15–40% may be metabolized by the liver to three de-acetylated compounds (3-hydroxy-pancuronium, 17-hydroxypancuronium and 3,17-dihydroxypancuronium). At least one of these metabolites (3-hydroxypancuronium) has non-depolarizing actions, and is half as potent as pancuronium; it was at one time used as a muscle relaxant (dacuronium). Only trace amounts of pancuronium are eliminated in bile. In contrast, the related aminosteroid vecuronium is mainly eliminated from the body by active secretion in bile, since it is a monoquaternary compound. Vecuronium is also eliminated in urine, and small amounts are deacetylated by the liver.

Finally, atracurium is a unique muscle relaxant, since its chemical structure allows the partial termination of its action by spontaneous degradation *in vivo*. Atracurium is stable in solution in acid conditions (pH 4) at 4°C; in contrast, at pH 7.4 and 37°C, it is rapidly broken down to a tertiary amine (laudanosine) by a spontaneous chemical reaction (Hoffman elimination). Since atracurium is a bisquaternary ester, it is also metabolized by lung and plasma esterases to a monoquaternary alcohol and a monoquaternary acid. Although laudanosine has effects of its own (e.g. it is a glycine antagonist), its accumulation in renal or hepatic disease is unlikely. The spontaneous recovery from the effects of atracurium is a marked advantage, and the drug is the relaxant of choice in patients with renal or liver disease.

Drugs that affect the breakdown of acetylcholine

Anticholinesterase drugs prevent the hydrolysis of acetylcholine by combining with the enzyme acetylcholinesterase. Consequently, they cause the accumulation of acetylcholine at all cholinergic synapses to which they gain access. All anticholinesterase drugs produce effects on neuromuscular transmission and the autonomic nervous system; in addition, some of them (i.e. physostigmine and most organophosphorus compounds) produce central effects. Anticholinesterase drugs also inhibit plasma cholinesterase, and may prolong the effects of drugs that are esters, e.g. suxamethonium.

Drugs that inhibit acetylcholinesterase can be classified into three main groups:
1   Edrophonium.
2   Carbamate esters, e.g. neostigmine, pyridostigmine, distigmine and physostigmine (eserine).
3   Organophosphorus compounds.

Edrophonium

Edrophonium is a phenolic quaternary amine with a simple chemical structure (Fig. 9.8), which combines reversibly with acetylcholinesterase. Its quaternary group is attracted to the anionic site on acetylcholinesterase (Fig. 9.3); hydrogen bonding also occurs at the esteratic site, producing a drug–enzyme complex which is reversible and rapidly dissociable. Thus, edrophonium inhibits enzyme activity by preventing the access of acetylcholine to the active site. At the neuromuscular junction, edrophonium also has direct effects on the motor nerve terminal, resulting in increased acetylcholine release.

After intravenous injection, edrophonium characteristically causes muscle fasciculations which are frequently associated with autonomic effects (e.g. bradycardia, increased secretions and an increase in smooth muscle tone). Since it is a quaternary amine, it does not cross the blood–brain barrier or the placental barrier. After intravenous administration, it is rapidly distributed in extracellular fluid but may also enter hepatic and renal cells. The plasma concentration of the

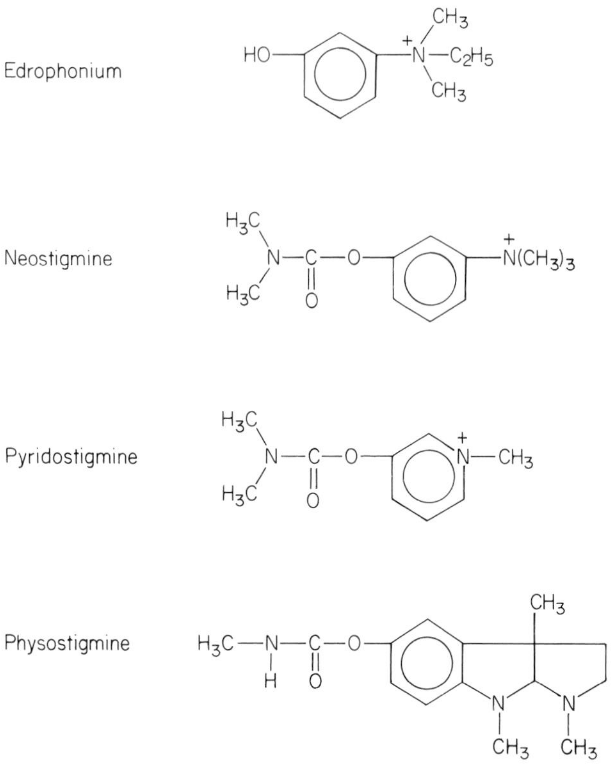

Edrophonium

Neostigmine

Pyridostigmine

Physostigmine

Fig. 9.8   The chemical structure of some anticholinesterase drugs. (The associated anion has been omitted.)

drug declines in a biexponential manner, with a distribution half-life of less than 2 min, followed by a slower decline (terminal half-life = 25–45 minutes). As the plasma concentration falls, acetylcholinesterase inhibition is rapidly reversed, and the effects of the drug are usually transient. It is mainly eliminated by glucuronide conjugation, and by renal excretion of the unchanged drug.

Edrophonium (in doses of 2–10 mg) has been widely used as a diagnostic test in suspected cases of myasthenia gravis; it may also be used to distinguish between 'myasthenic' and 'cholinergic' crises in the established disease. In anaesthetic practice, it has been occasionally used to confirm the development of phase II blockade (dual blockade) after the administration of suxamethonium or decamethonium.

More recently, the drug has been used in the reversal of non-depolarizing blockade produced by vecuronium or atracurium, since its duration of action is shorter than other anticholinesterase drugs. In these conditions, relatively large doses of edrophonium are required (e.g. 0.5–1.0 mg kg^{-1}) in order to ensure that plasma concentrations and enzyme inhibition persist for long enough to prevent recurarization.

Carbamate esters

All carbamate inhibitors of acetylcholinesterase affect the enzyme in a similar manner. They are attracted to the anionic site by an ionized group, which may be a tertiary amine (physostigmine) or a quaternary amine (neostigmine, pyridostigmine and distigmine). Subsequently, the methylcarbamyl group (Fig. 9.8) combines with the serine residue at the esteratic site, and the esters are simultaneously hydrolysed to phenolic derivatives which are released from the enzyme. Thus, the combination of carbamate inhibitors with acetylcholinesterase is essentially similar to the physiological substrate acetylcholine (Fig. 9.3). However, the hydrolysis of the methylcarbamylated enzyme (half-time = approximately 30 min) is 10^7–10^8 times slower than the acetylated enzyme (half-time = $42\,\mu s$). The slow hydrolysis of the carbamylated enzyme is mainly responsible for enzyme inhibition (although reversible enzyme inhibition also occurs). Carbamates are sometimes known as 'time-dependent', 'acid-transferring', or 'oxydiaphoretic' inhibitors of acetylcholinesterase, since they mainly act by transferring a methylcarbamic acid to the enzyme. Carbamates, particularly neostigmine, may also have a direct effect on neuromuscular transmission and autonomic function, probably due to their chemical similarity to acetylcholine. They also inhibit plasma cholinesterase and may prolong the effects of suxamethonium.

In general, neostigmine and pyridostigmine produce similar effects on neuromuscular transmission and the autonomic nervous system. Since both drugs are quaternary amines, they do not significantly cross the blood–brain barrier or the placental barrier. Neostigmine is four to five times more potent than pyridostigmine, since its quaternary group is outside the aromatic ring (Fig. 9.8). The absorption of both drugs from the gut is relatively poor, and their potency after oral administration is only 10–20% of their parenteral potency. Neostigmine is more rapidly absorbed than pyridostigmine, and has a greater first pass metabolism. It also has the more rapid onset of action after intravenous administration (usually 5–7 min). Its duration of action is less prolonged, since it has a shorter terminal half-life (approximately 30–45 min). Nevertheless, the relatively long duration of action of both neostigmine and pyridostigmine, which far exceeds their removal from plasma and usually prevents recurarization, probably reflects the slow hydrolysis of inhibited acetylcholinesterase in the synaptic gap. Both drugs are partly metabolized by the liver, and partly eliminated unchanged in urine. Pyridostigmine may produce less marked autonomic side-effects than neostigmine; it is occasionally used to reverse non-depolarizing blockade. Neostigmine, pyridostigmine, and the related compound ambenonium are sometimes used orally in the long-term management of myasthenia gravis. Tolerance to their muscarinic side-effects may develop, so that concurrent therapy with anti-cholinergic drugs is not always necessary. Neostigmine has also been used in the management of supraventricular tachycardias, and to improve smooth muscle activity in the bladder and the bowel, particularly in the postoperative period.

Distigmine is a combination of two molecules of pyridostigmine, which are joined by a methylene chain at their non-quaternary ends. Distigmine has a relatively long duration of action, and may be used to improve smooth muscle activity during the postoperative period. It may also be used in the management of the neurogenic bladder.

Physostigmine (eserine) is a naturally occurring anticholinesterase drug derived from the Calabar bean, and was once used by native tribes in West Africa in 'trial by ordeal'. Unlike edrophonium, neostigmine and pyridostigmine, it is a mono-methylcarbamate ester and a tertiary amine (Fig. 9.8). Consequently, it is well absorbed from the gastrointestinal tract, penetrates cellular membranes, and crosses the blood–brain barrier and the placental barrier. It has been used in the treatment of poisoning with anticholinergic drugs (e.g. atropine and the tricyclic antidepressants). Physostigmine eye-drops are a popular miotic agent, and are sometimes used in the treatment of narrow angle glaucoma.

Organophosphorus compounds

Organophosphorus compounds inhibit acetylcholinesterase by phosphorylation of the esteratic site of the enzyme (Fig. 9.3), forming an extremely stable complex which is resistant to hydrolysis or reactivation. In some instances, chemical changes take place after phosphorylation which prevent the reactivation of the enzyme ('ageing'). Consequently, recovery from the effects of inhibition is mainly dependent on the synthesis of new enzyme, and organophosphorus compounds are often considered to be irreversible inhibitors of acetylcholinesterase. Most of these drugs are also potent inhibitors of plasma cholinesterase. The classical organophosphorus compounds are diisopropylfluorophosphonate (DFP; dyflos) and tetraethylpyrophosphate (TEPP). Many of their analogues have been widely used as insecticides, and a number of volatile and lipid-soluble agents were syn-thesized during World War II as chemical warfare agents. These compounds are readily absorbed by the lungs and through the skin. Exposure leads to numerous toxic manifestations, including nicotinic effects (muscle weakness, paralysis and hypotension) and muscarinic effects (increased smooth muscle tone and salivary and respiratory secretions). In addition, excitation of the central nervous system occurs (causing tremors and convulsions), which may be followed by subsequent depression, with coma and respiratory paralysis. Organophosphorus poisoning is treated with reactivators of acetylcholinesterase (e.g. pralidoxime and obidoxime), which promote the hydrolysis of the phosphorylated enzyme. Repeated administration of atropine (2–4 mg) and anticonvulsant drugs, and mechanical ventilation of the lungs, may also be necessary. Pretreatment with carbamates has a protective effect against organophosphorus poisoning. Chronic exposure to these agents may lead to the development of a severe polyneuritis.

Ecothiopate is an organophosphorus compound which also has a quaternary amine group. Consequently, it is attracted to the anionic site on acetylcholinesterase, but subsequently phosphorylates the esteratic site, resulting in stable and prolonged inhibition. Proprietary preparations of ecothiopate are no longer available in the UK; an ophthalmic preparation was sometimes used as a miotic in narrow angle glaucoma, and its chronic administration was associated with prolonged apnoea after suxamethonium.

Drugs that interfere with EC coupling

Normal voluntary muscle contraction depends on the release of calcium ions from the sarcoplasmic reticulum, and their subsequent binding by Troponin C. The binding of calcium ions causes conformational changes in the Troponin–Tropomyosin complex, resulting in activation of myosin ATPase and muscle contraction (EC coupling; p. 262).

Dantrolene prevents the release of calcium ions from the sarcoplasmic reticulum, and thus indirectly prevents the activation of myosin ATPase and muscle contraction. Muscle action potentials are not affected, although the amplitude of the subsequent muscle contraction is reduced. Dantrolene does not usually impair the contractility of cardiac muscle or vascular smooth muscle; in these tissues, muscle contractility is not primarily dependent on the release of calcium ions from the sarcoplasmic reticulum.

Dantrolene sodium is used in the prevention and treatment of malignant hyperpyrexia (p. 294). In this rare genetic disease, calcium release from the sarcoplasmic reticulum may be precipitated by certain 'triggering agents'. The increase in intracellular calcium may then precipitate a sequence of physiological, biochemical and metabolic effects, producing the clinical signs of the disease. Dantrolene prevents EC coupling, controls muscle spasticity, and reduces abnormal heat production; thus it can reverse or attenuate the clinical effects of malignant hyperpyrexia.

Dantrolene is also used orally for the treatment of spasticity associated with chronic neurological disorders (e.g. cerebrovascular accidents, multiple sclerosis, spinal cord injury, and cerebral palsy). Central effects (e.g. dizziness, weakness, and fatigue) are not uncommon, and occasional hepatotoxicity can occur. In general, the drug should be administered in gradually increasing doses until the optimum effect is attained.

PRACTICAL CONSIDERATIONS

Choice of relaxant

Suxamethonium is indicated for short procedures (e.g. electroconvulsive therapy, and the reduction of fracture–dislocations), and to provide optimal conditions for rapid endotracheal intubation. During longer procedures, suxamethonium may be administered by intermittent or continuous infusion. This technique is not commonly used, since the development of phase II blockade may occur when the total dose infused is more than $7-8\,\text{mg kg}^{-1}$ during nitrous oxide–narcotic anaesthesia (or with considerably smaller doses during halothane, enflurane, or isoflurane anaesthesia).

An anticholinergic drug may be given prior to suxamethonium, at the discretion of the anaesthetist. However, atropine should always be administered if repeated dosage is contemplated, or in the presence of β-adrenoceptor blockade. Small doses of a non-depolarizing relaxant (e.g. tubocurarine 5 mg, gallamine 20 mg) are frequently given prior to suxamethonium in order to reduce the muscle fasciculations and subsequent muscle pains, or to modify the sustained activity in the extra-ocular muscles in cases of penetrating eye injury. In these circumstances, the dose of suxamethonium should be increased by 50%.

Contraindications to the use of suxamethonium include:
1   Major burns and neurological injuries.
2   Hyperkalaemic states (e.g. renal failure).
3   Myasthenic and myotonic diseases.
4   Major qualitative abnormalities of plasma cholinesterase.
5   A family history suggesting susceptibility to malignant hyperpyrexia.

The choice of a non-depolarizing drug is governed by the expected duration of the surgical procedure as well as the condition of the patient. The onset of sufficient muscle paralysis to provide adequate conditions for endotracheal intubation is more rapid with gallamine than with other non-depolarizing relaxants.

Other drugs may have different advantages. Tubocurarine is commonly used when hypotension is required to reduce bleeding during surgery. It is probably best avoided in patients with a history of asthma, or when its hypotensive effects could be dangerous (e.g. in hypovolaemic states and fixed output cardiac disease). Alcuronium is an acceptable alternative to tubocurarine, and has a shorter duration of action. It has some histamine-releasing and ganglion-blocking activity, but does not usually decrease blood pressure as much as tubocurarine. It is claimed to be more rapidly and completely reversible than tubocurarine, but this is doubtful. Pancuronium produces muscle relaxation of rapid onset and medium duration. Hypotension and histamine release are uncommon, and the drug may have advantages in asthmatic patients, as well as in cardiac surgery and cardiovascular disease. Gallamine has a more rapid onset and a shorter duration of action than pancuronium, and may be useful during short surgical procedures. Unfortunately, its use is limited by the problems of elimination in renal impairment, and the undesirable tachycardia that it commonly induces. Vecuronium is a newer muscle relaxant with a short duration of action, which is mainly eliminated in bile, and does not cumulate in patients with renal failure. Atracurium has the shortest duration of action, and is rapidly eliminated from the body by Hoffman degradation, a chemical reaction that is dependent on pH and temperature. Consequently, it is probably the drug of choice in renal disease, hepatic impairment, and in frail and elderly subjects. Unfortunately, it sometimes releases histamine, and should probably be avoided in patients with a history of asthma. Both vecuronium and atracurium have been used to provide neuromuscular blockade in patients with myasthenia gravis; in this condition other muscle relaxants may produce prolonged apnoea.

Non-depolarizing blocking drugs may be required to assist long-term ventilatory control (for example, in the management of tetanus, status epilepticus, or chest injuries). It is sometimes considered that the ganglion-blocking activity of tubocurarine may contribute to the development of paralytic ileus during artificial ventilation. Pancuronium is a logical alternative, although some tachycardia may be expected. In recent years, both atracurium and vecuronium have been widely used to assist the control of ventilation; these drugs do not cumulate and offer the advantage of flexibility.

Reversal of neuromuscular blockade

Neostigmine (usually $0.07\,\text{mg kg}^{-1}$, with a maximum dose of 5 mg) is commonly used to antagonize non-depolarizing neuromuscular blockade. Atropine ($0.02\,\text{mg kg}^{-1}$, with a maximum dose of 1.2 mg) is usually administered simultaneously, in order to control the muscarinic effects of neostigmine (although secretomotor activity appears to be more favourably modified if atropine is given 5 min previously). Full oxygenation and efficient pulmonary ventilation should be maintained during the administration of these drugs, as hypoxia and hypercarbia increase the risk of cardiac arrhythmias. Pyridostigmine ($0.3\,\text{mg kg}^{-1}$, with a maximum dose of 20 mg) may also be used, and is sometimes a useful alternative to neostigmine. It has a longer latency and duration of action than neostigmine, and appears to produce less muscarinic activity; consequently the dose of atropine may be reduced as appropriate. In recent years, edrophonium ($0.5-1.0\,\text{mg kg}^{-1}$) has also been used to antagonize neuromuscular blockade with the newer muscle relaxants (i.e. vecuronium and atracurium). It has a more rapid onset of action than neostigmine, and its duration of action is sufficiently long to prevent residual curarization (when used with short-acting relaxants).

In order to minimize the possibility of recurarization, anticholinesterase drugs should not be administered less than half an hour after full doses of the commonly used non-depolarizing muscle relaxants, and preferably when there is some evidence of return of muscle tone. Clinical evaluation of ventilatory activity and muscle strength have been classically used to measure recovery form neuromuscular blockade. Signs of adequate reversal include: an efficient tidal volume with some return of the cough reflex and absence of tracheal tug, a return of jaw tone and ability to protrude the tongue, and a head lift which can be sustained for at least 5 s. These clinical signs of reversal are closely correlated with the electrical or mechanical activity in voluntary muscles induced by indirect stimulation. When clinical signs of adequate reversal are present, there is a least 75% recovery from neuromuscular blockade (i.e. the amplitude of the final response to a train-of-four supramaximal stimuli is at least 75% of the amplitude of the first response). It should be recognized that clinical signs of reversal may be difficult to elicit in patients recovering from 'general anaesthesia without the risk of awareness; undoubtedly, the use of a nerve stimulator is the method of choice in the assessment of residual neuromuscular blockade.

The development of bradycardia during the postoperative period is often attributed to the muscarinic effects of neostigmine, since the drug has a longer duration of action than atropine. In these conditions, an antimuscarinic drug with a longer duration of action (e.g. glycopyrrolate) may be useful.

In some cases of neostigmine-resistant curarization or other disorders (e.g. the Eaton–Lambert syndrome and botulinism), drugs may be administered to increase neurotransmitter release from the motor nerve terminal. Guanidine delays inactivation of sodium channels in the motor nerve terminal, and thus prolongs depolarization (although it may produce unpleasant side-effects). The aminopyridines also act presynaptically, and delay repolarization by blockade of potassium channels; they may also increase contractility by a direct action on muscle fibres. Moderate doses ($0.35\,\text{mg kg}^{-1}$) can prolong the duration of action of neostigmine, while higher doses ($1\,\text{mg kg}^{-1}$) may reverse non-depolarizing neuromuscular blockade. At these doses, CNS stimulation with postoperative restlessness and convulsions can occur.

Drug interactions

Clinically significant interactions involving the use of non-depolarizing relaxants in patients on other drugs are uncommon. Many drugs may modify acid–base balance, or influence the plasma concentration of certain cations (e.g. antacids, steroids, chelating agents, diuretics and lithium); in these instances, prolongation of the effects of relaxants, although anticipated, is infrequently present.

Similarly, calcium transport at presynaptic sites may be influenced by many other drugs, e.g. aminoglycoside antibiotics, calcium antagonists and drugs with local anaesthetic properties, including quinidine, propranolol, chlorpromazine and phenytoin; again, the practical implications are usually minimal.

On the other hand, interactions with other drugs administered as part of the anaesthetic technique are usually much more important. Many volatile anaesthetic agents may profoundly influence the degree of non-depolarizing neuromuscular blockade. Diethylether has long been known to potentiate this type of blockade, and similar dose-related effects are produced by halothane, enflurane, and isoflurane. The chief mode of action is probably depression of somatic reflexes in the central nervous system, which consequently reduces transmitter release at the motor nerve terminal. However, there is some evidence that direct depression at presynaptic sites may also be involved; the effect of inhalational agents on muscle blood flow may also play a part. Diazepam may slightly prolong non-depolarizing blockade by a combination of prejunctional and central effects.

Drugs that block autonomic ganglia such as trimetaphan, which may be used to produce hypotension during anaesthesia, can complicate neuromuscular blockade. These drugs have some affinity for both acetylcholine receptors and acetylcholinesterase, and in high doses they may prolong non-depolarizing blockade. As mentioned previously, neostigmine-resistant curarization has been observed when large doses of certain antibiotics (particularly streptomycin and neomycin) have been instilled into the peritoneal cavity; calcium salts may partially reverse this type of blockade.

More serious drug interactions are associated with the use of suxamethonium. Prolongation of neuromuscular blockade, and an increased tendency to develop dual blockade, may be due to inhibition of plasma cholinesterase activity (e.g. by anticholinesterase drugs, alkylating agents, trimetaphan and pitocin). Drugs which use plasma cholinesterase for their own metabolism may also prolong the action of suxamethonium (e.g. procaine and possibly other local anaesthetics). Potentiation of the muscarinic effects of suxamethonium (particularly with respect to the cardiac vagus) may also occur with digoxin, or other drugs which alter autonomic balance in favour of parasympathetic activity (e.g. β-adrenoceptor antagonists).

Neurological and muscle diseases

Patients with myasthenia gravis are extremely sensitive to non-depolarizing blockade, but are usually resistant to decamethonium and suxamethonium. Both phenomena have been used as diagnostic tests in myasthenic patients. The differential effects of depolarizing and non-depolarizing drugs in myasthenia are due to the presence of antibodies to acetylcholine receptors at the motor endplate; in these conditions, the endplate potential induced by acetylcholine release is decreased, so that the effects of non-depolarizing agents are enhanced. In myasthenia gravis, different muscle groups are affected to a variable extent, and the reaction to muscle relaxants is unpredictable. The use of most muscle relaxants should be avoided in myasthenic patients undergoing major surgery (including thymectomy), since they may induce prolonged postoperative curarization. However, low doses of vecuronium and atracurium have been successfully used to produce neuromuscular blockade in myasthenia gravis. Suxamethonium has also been used; large doses may be required to produce muscle relaxation, and the elimination of the drug may be retarded by concurrent anticholinesterase therapy.

In the Eaton–Lambert (myasthenic) syndrome, muscle weakness improves with exercise, and an increase in twitch amplitude is observed during tetanic stimulation. The condition may accompany malignant disease, particularly bronchogenic carcinoma. In general, there is a marked sensitivity to non-depolarizing blockade, and resistance to anticholinesterase drugs is present.

In myotonic syndromes (myotonia dystrophia, myotonia congenita, and paramyotonia), generalized muscle spasm may occur with depolarizing agents, and is not responsive to tubocurarine. In other genetically determined myopathies (e.g. muscular dystrophy and familial periodic paralysis) the response to muscle relaxants is unpredictable, and their use is best avoided. A similar response may occur in other types of myopathy. In diseases and trauma associated with lower motor neurone lesions, and in burn patients, suxamethonium may cause significant and dangerous hyperkalaemia; increased sensitivity to non-depolarizing drugs can also occur.

In malignant hyperpyrexia, there is an inherited susceptibility to the development of fulminating hyperpyrexia, often associated with muscle rigidity and convulsions. In the established syndrome, there is a mortality rate of 60–70% associated with anaesthesia. The condition has a high familial incidence and is linked to an autosomal dominant gene. Patients at risk may exhibit minor myopathies, and an elevated creatine kinase and qualitative variants of plasma cholinesterase may be present. They may also be identified by muscle biopsy, as they may show an abnormal contractile response to caffeine or halothane in *in vitro* conditions. A similar condition may be induced in Landrace and Pietrain pigs. Malignant hyperpyrexia may be induced in susceptible individuals by the administration of suxamethonium, although most inhalational anaesthetics have also been incriminated as triggering agents. Typically, the initial dose of suxamethonium fails to produce adequate relaxation, and generalized muscle rigidity, in association with a rapidly rising temperature develops within several minutes. These effects are considered to be related to the fulminating release of calcium ions into the myoplasm of susceptible individuals, leading to sustained contraction and a rise in body temperature.

Treatment should commence as soon as the diagnosis is suspected. Administration of the suspected triggering agent must be stopped, and surgery discontinued as soon as possible. Active cooling and generalized supportive measures to the cardiovascular and respiratory system should be instituted; blood gases should be estimated and any metabolic acidosis corrected by an infusion of sodium bicarbonate. Previous drug therapy has included the administration of large doses of procaine and steroids, but it is doubtful if they are of any real value. Present evidence suggests that the drug of choice is dantrolene sodium. Dantrolene acts by inhibiting the release of Ca^{2+} from the sarcoplasmic reticulum of striated muscle, thus preventing EC coupling and the abnormal heat production. An intravenous preparation of the drug (sodium dantrolene with mannitol and sodium hydroxide) is available as a powder for reconstitution with water. The initial dose ($1 \, mg \, kg^{-1}$) may be repeated at 5–10 min intervals to a maximum dose of $10 \, mg \, kg^{-1}$. Dantrolene sodium is also available as an oral preparation for the treatment of various spastic disorders (p. 289); its prophylactic use has been proposed in patients with a susceptibility to malignant hyperpyrexia who require general anaesthesia.

Monitoring of neuromuscular blockade

Individual responses to muscle relaxants vary widely, and may be modified by age, body temperature, plasma and extracellular pH, electrolyte changes, the presence of other drugs, and pathological conditions. Consequently, in individual patients the response to muscle relaxants or their antagonists may be unpredictable, and the effects of some drugs (particularly vecuronium and atracurium) may change rapidly during recovery from neuromuscular blockade. Methods of monitoring the effects of muscle relaxants are therefore desirable; in certain circumstances, they may be essential. The most commonly used methods depend on indirect supramaximal stimulation of the ulnar nerve, and the recording of the compound muscle action potential or the mechanical twitch response of adductor pollicis. A square wave stimulus of short duration (0.1–0.2 ms) is commonly used in order to prevent repetitive muscle firing. In anaesthetized patients, tetanic rates of stimulation (>50 Hz) may be used; more frequently a 'train-of-four' stimulus (2 Hz for 2 s) is employed. Neuromuscular blockade may be monitored by comparing the amplitude of the first response in the train (T1) with the control response before the administration of the relaxant (T0). This ratio (T1:T0) is probably the most accurate measurement of postsynaptic neuromuscular blockade. More commonly, transmission is monitored by observing the amplitude (or presence, absence, or reappearance) of the fourth response (T4) compared to the first response (T1) within train-of-four stimuli (i.e. the ratio T4:T1). This method avoids the necessity for a control response, although it may reflect the presynaptic effects of muscle relaxants, rather than their postsynaptic actions. In practice, the difference is probably unimportant, since there is usually a close relation between the ratios T1:T0 and T4:T1.

FURTHER READING

Ali HH. Monitoring of neuromuscular function. *Seminars in Anesthesia* 1984; **3**: 284–292.

Ali HH, Savarese JJ. Monitoring of neuromuscular function. *Anesthesiology* 1976; **45**: 216–249.

Ali HH, Savarese JJ, Embree PB, Basta SJ, Stout RG, Bottros LH, Weakly JN. Clinical pharmacology of mivacurium chloride (BW B1090U) infusion: comparison with vecuronium and atracurium. *British Journal of Anaesthesia* 1988; **61**: 541–546.

Azar I. The response of patients with neuromuscular disorders to muscle relaxants: a review. *Anesthesiology* 1984; **61**: 173–187.

Beemer GH, Cass NM, Monitoring the neuromuscular junction. *Anaesthesia and Intensive Care* 1988; **16**: 62–65.

Bell CF, Florence AM, Hunter JM, Jones RS, Utting JE. Atracurium in the myasthenic patient. *Anaesthesia* 1984; **39**: 961–968.

Bowman WC. *Pharmacology of Neuromuscular Function*. Bristol: John Wright and Sons, 1980; 1–186.

Bowman WC. Prejunctional and postjunctional cholinoceptors at the neuromuscular junction. *Anesthesia and Analgesia* 1980; **59**: 935–943.

Buckett WR. Steroidal neuromuscular blocking agents. *Advances in Drug Research* 1975; **10**: 53–92.

Budd A, Scott RFP, Blogg CE, Goat VA. Adverse effects of suxamethonium. *Anaesthesia* 1985; **40**: 642–646.

Calvey TN. Assessment of neuromuscular blockade by electromyography: a review. *Journal of the Royal Society of Medicine* 1984; **77**: 56–59.

Calvey TN, Wareing M, Williams NE, Chan K. Pharmacokinetics and pharmacological effects of neostigmine in man. *British Journal of Clinical Pharmacology* 1979; **7**: 149–155.

Calvey TN, Williams NE, Muir KT, Barber HE. Plasma concentration of edrophonium in man. *Clinical Pharmacology and Therapeutics* 1976; **19**: 813–820.

Calvey TN, Wilson H. Muscle relaxant drugs and their antagonists. In: Gray TC, Nunn JF, Utting JE (eds) *General Anaesthesia*, 4th edn. London: Butterworths, 1980; 319–335.

Ceccarelli B, Hurlbut WP. The vesicle hypothesis of the release of quanta of acetylcholine. *Physiological Reviews* 1980; **60**: 351–396.

Changeux J-P, Giraudat J, Dennis M. The nicotinic acetylcholine receptor: molecular architecture of a ligand-regulated ion channel. *Trends in Pharmacological Sciences* 1987; **8**: 459–465.

Collier C. Suxamethonium pains and fasciculations. *Proceedings of the Royal Society of Medicine* 1975; **68**: 105–108.

Cullen DJ. The effect of pretreatment with nondepolarizing muscle relaxants on the neuromuscular blocking action of succinylcholine. *Anesthesiology* 1971; **35**: 572–578.

Desaki J, Uehara Y. The overall morphology of neuromuscular junctions as revealed by scanning electronmicroscopy. *Journal of Neurocytology* 1981; **10**: 101–110.

Drachman DB, Adams RN, Josifek LF, Pestronk A, Stanley EF. Antibody-mediated mechanisms of ACh receptor loss in myasthenia gravis: clinical relevance. *Annals of the New York Academy of Sciences* 1981; **377**: 175–188.

Dundee JW, Gray TC. Resistance to *d*-tubocurarine chloride in the presence of liver damage. *Lancet* 1953; **2**: 16–17.

Durant NN, Katz RL. Suxamethonium. *British Journal of Anaesthesia* 1982; **54**: 195–208.

Ebashi S. Muscle contraction and pharmacology. *Trends in Pharmacological Sciences* 1979; **1**: 29–31.

Eccles JC. *The Understanding of the Brain*. New York: McGraw-Hill, 1973; 1–238.

Endo M. Calcium release from the sarcoplasmic reticulum. *Physiological Reviews* 1977; **57**: 71–108.

Fambrough DM. Control of acetylcholine receptors in skeletal muscle. *Physiological Reviews* 1979; **59**: 165–216.

Ghonheim MM, Long JP. The interaction between magnesium and other neuromuscular blocking agents. *Anesthesiology* 1970; **32**: 23–27.

Gronert GA, Mott J, Lee J. Aetiology of malignant hyperthermia. *British Journal of Anaesthesia* 1988; **60**: 253–267.

Gwinutt CL, Meakin G. Use of the post-tetanic count to monitor recovery from intense neuromuscular blockade in children. *British Journal of Anaesthesia* 1988; **61**: 547–550.

Harrison GG. Dantrolene — dynamics and kinetics. *British Journal of Anaesthesia* 1988; **60**: 279–286.

Hilgenberg JC. Comparison of the pharmacology of vecuronium and atracurium with that of other currently available muscle relaxants. *Anesthesia and Analgesia* 1983; **62**: 524–531.

Hohlfeld R, Sterz R, Peper K. Prejunctional effects of anticholinesterase drugs at the endplate mediated by presynaptic acetylcholine receptors or by postsynaptic potassium efflux. *Pflügers Archiv für die gesamte Physiologie* 1981; **391**: 213–218.

Holmstedt B. Pharmacology of organophosphorus cholinesterase inhibitors. *Pharmacological Reviews* 1959; **11**: 567–688.

Holst-Larsen H. The hydrolysis of suxamethonium in human blood. *British Journal of Anaesthesia* 1976; **48**: 887–892.

Hunter JM. Adverse effects of neuromuscular blocking drugs. *British Journal of Anaesthesia* 1987; **59**: 46–60.

Hunter JM, Jones RS, Utting JE. Use of atracurium in patients with no renal function. *British Journal of Anaesthesia* 1982; **54**: 1251–1258.

Karlin A, Kao PN, DiPaola M. Molecular pharmacology of the nicotinic acetylcholine receptor. *Trends in Pharmacological Sciences* 1986; **7**: 304–308.

Katz B, Thesleff S. A study of the 'desensitization' produced by acetylcholine at the motor endplate. *Journal of Physiology* 1957; **138**: 63–80.

Kharkevich DA (ed.) *New Neuromuscular Blocking Agents. Handbook of Experimental Pharmacology* Berlin: Springer-Verlag, 1986; **79**: 1–717.

La Du BN. Identification of human serum cholinesterase variants using the polymerase chain reaction amplification technique. *Trends in Pharmacological Sciences* 1989; **10**: 309–313.

Lambert JJ, Durant NN, Henderson EG. Drug-induced modification of ionic conductance at the neuromuscular junction. *Annual Review of Pharmacology and Toxicology* 1983; **23**: 505–539.

Lee C, Chen D, Katz RL. Characteristics of non-depolarising neuromuscular block. (1) Post-junctional block by alpha-bungarotoxin. *Canadian Anaesthetists Society Journal* 1977; **24**: 212–219.

Lee C, Katz RL. Neuromuscular pharmacology. *British Journal of Anaesthesia* 1980; **52**: 173–188.

Meistelman C, Lienhart A, Leveque C, Bitker MO, Pigot B, Viars P. Pharmacology of vecuronium in patients with end-stage renal failure. *European Journal of Anaesthesiology* 1986; **3**: 153–158.

Mortier E, Moulaert P, De Somer A, Rolly G. Comparison of evoked electromyography and mechanical activity during vecuronium-induced neuromuscular blockade. *European Journal of Anaesthesiology* 1988; **5**: 131–142.

Newton DEF. Measurement of neuromuscular function. *Baillière's Clinical Anaesthesiology* 1988; **2**: 133–156.

O'Sullivan EP, Williams NE, Calvey TN. Differential effects of neuromuscular blocking agents on suxamethonium-induced fasciculations and myalgia. *British Journal of Anaesthesia* 1988; **60**: 367–371.

Parker CJR, Jones JE, Hunter JM. Disposition of infusions of atracurium and its metabolite, laudanosine, in patients in renal and respiratory failure in an ITU. *British Journal of Anaesthesia* 1988; **61**: 531–540.

Paton WDM. The effects of muscle relaxants other than muscular relaxation. *Anesthesiology* 1959; **20**: 453–463.

Paton WDM, Waud DR. The margin of safety of neuromuscular transmission. *Journal of Physiology* 1967; **191**: 59–90.

Payne JP, Hughes R. Evaluation of atracurium in anaesthetized man. *British Journal of Anaesthesia* 1981; **53**: 45–54.

Payne JP, Utting JE (eds) Atracurium. *British Journal of Anaesthesia* 1983; **55** (Suppl. 1): 1S–139S.

Ridley SA, Hatch DJ. Post-tetanic count and profound neuromuscular blockade with atracurium infusion in paediatric patients. *British Journal of Anaesthesia* 1988; **60**: 31–35.

Robertson EN, Booij LHDJ, Fragen RJ, Crul JF. Clinical comparison of atracurium and vecuronium (Org NC 45). *British Journal of Anaesthesia* 1983; **55**: 125–129.

Scott RPF, Norman J. Newer agents. *Current Opinion in Anaesthesiology* 1989; **2**: 493–496.

Shanks CA. Pharmacokinetics of the nondepolarizing neuromuscular relaxants applied to calculation of bolus and infusion dosage regimens. *Anesthesiology* 1986; **64**: 72–86.

Spence AA, Payne JP (eds) Proceedings of a symposium on atracurium. *British Journal of Anaesthesia* 1986; **58** (Suppl. 1): 1S–113S.

Stanski DR, Sheiner LB. Pharmacokinetics and dynamics of muscle relaxants. *Anesthesiology* 1979; **51**: 103–105.

Tammisto T, Wirtavuori K, Linko K. Assessment of neuromuscular block: comparison of three clinical methods and evoked electromyography. *European Journal of Anaesthesiology* 1988; **5**: 1–8.

Tobey RE, Jacobsen PM, Kahle CT, Clubb RJ, Dean MA. The serum potassium response to muscle relaxants in neural injury. *Anesthesiology* 1972; **37**: 332–337.

Tolmie JD, Joyce TH, Mitchell GD. Succinylcholine danger in the burned patient. *Anesthesiology* 1967; **28**: 467–470.

Torda TA. The 'new' relaxants. A review of the clinical pharmacology of atracurium and vecuronium. *Anaesthesia and Intensive Care* 1987; **15**: 72–82.

Viby-Mogensen J, Howardy-Hansen P, Chraemmer-Jorgensen B, Ording H, Engback J, Nielsen A. Post-tetanic count (PTC): a new method of evaluating an intense nondepolarising neuromuscular blockade. *Anesthesiology* 1981; **55**: 458–461.

Weber S, Brandom BW, Powers DM *et al.* Mivacurium chloride (BW B1090U)-induced neuromuscular blockade during nitrous oxide–isoflurane and nitrous oxide–narcotic anesthesia in adult surgical patients. *Anesthesia and Analgesia* 1988; **67**: 495–499.

Whittaker VP. The storage and release of acetylcholine. *Trends in Pharmacological Sciences* 1986; **7**: 312–315.

Williams NE, Webb SN, Calvey TN. Differential effects of myoneural blocking drugs on neuromuscular transmission. *British Journal of Anaesthesia* 1980; **52**: 1111–1115.

Wilson IB, Harrison MA. Turnover number of acetylcholinesterase. *Journal of Biological Chemistry* 1961; **236**: 2292–2295.

Wilson IB, Hatch MA, Ginsburg S. Carbamylation of acetylcholinesterase. *Journal of Biological Chemistry* 1960; **235**: 2312–2315.

Zaimis E (ed.) *Neuromuscular Junction. Handbook of Experimental Pharmacology* Berlin: Springer-Verlag, 1976; **42**: 1–746.

TEN

Analgesic Drugs

ANATOMY AND PHYSIOLOGY OF PAIN TRANSMISSION

Pain pathways

Two types of pain have been described. Fast pain allows the injury to be identified in time and space, initiates the rapid reflex withdrawal from the painful stimulus, and is of short duration. Slow pain occurs after fast pain, is less localized, and more persistent. Peripheral nociceptive receptors do not have a distinct histological structure, but are interwoven plexiform arrangements of free nerve endings which are widely distributed in interstitial tissues and around blood vessels; they respond specifically to painful stimuli of chemical, mechanical or thermal origin.

Afferent pain fibres can be divided into two groups:

1 Small myelinated Aδ fibres, 2–5 μm in diameter, which conduct 'first' or 'fast' pain and enter the deeper part of the dorsal horn (Rexed laminae IV and V).

2 Unmyelinated C fibres, less than 2 μm in diameter, which have a higher threshold and a lower conduction velocity. Unmyelinated C fibres conduct 'second' or 'slow' pain and synapse in the superficial area of the dorsal horn (Rexed laminae I and II).

Integration of the impulses in these two types of fibres takes place in laminae II of the dorsal horn (the substantia gelatinosa) and this may influence the quality and intensity of pain that is experienced. The input of nociceptive impulses may be further modified by collateral branches from the larger A fibres which ascend in the posterior columns; these conduct other sensory impulses, and have a lower threshold of activity and a greater conduction velocity than Aδ or C fibres.

Descending tracts from central grey matter (via the reticular formation) may also inhibit activity in the cells of the substantia gelatinosa (Fig. 10.1). Thus, a form of 'gate control' of nociceptive input appears to exist; this may explain why counter-irritation by heat or touch, or distraction of the individual, can reduce the intensity of the pain.

Second-order neurones relay in the dorsal horn, decussate in the spinal cord,

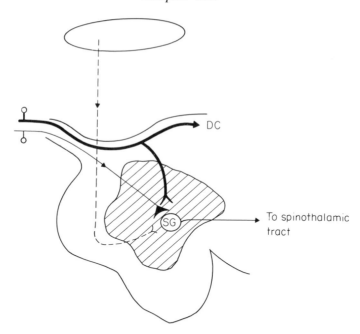

Fig. 10.1   Hemisection of spinal cord showing integration of pain impulses via the substantia gelatinosa. SG Substantia gelatinosa. DC Dorsal column. ⓩ A δ and C fibres conducting 'first' and 'second' pain impulses. ⓘ Large sensory A fibres sending collateral branch to inhibit (? presynaptically) pain transmission. - - Descending fibres via reticular formation inhibiting (? postsynaptically) pain transmission.

and ascend in the spinothalamic tract and the more diffuse spinoreticular pathways. They eventually terminate in the ventroposterior and medial nuclei of the thalamus, which is probably the main region associated with the appreciation of pain. However, further projections to the postcentral gyri are undoubtedly associated with the localization of nociceptive impulses, while connections with the prefrontal and temporal lobes and the limbic areas are related to the affective component and the memory of pain. Thus, it is not surprising that pain has been described as an unpleasant emotional state rather than as a simple sensory modality.

Pain production

Pain is produced by mechanical or thermal damage to superficial or deep tissues, ischaemia of somatic or visceral structures, spasm of smooth or striated muscle, and dilatation of blood vessels at the base of the brain. Many endogenous chemical substances are well-known excitants of peripheral nerve endings. These substances include H^+, K^+, acetylcholine, histamine, 5-hydroxytryptamine, cholecystokinin, and bradykinin; phosphate ions may also be implicated in the production of bone pain. It is thought that other substances (particularly the leukotrienes, prostaglandins, and their metabolites) are partly responsible for the increase in nociceptive sensitivity seen after tissue damage (both in the area of the injury and in surrounding uninjured tissues). This phenomenon not only leads to hyperalgesia in the affected areas, but also alters the local C fibre activity, increasing the sensitivity of the corresponding areas of the spinal cord. This hyperalgesic state can be attenuated both peripherally and centrally by the administration of opioids; these are much more effective if they are administered before the noxious stimulus is applied. In practical terms, this means that postoperative pain will be decreased if patients are given analgesics before surgical intervention.

Numerous studies have shown that there are many polypeptides in the dorsal horn that may influence the transmission of nociceptive impulses in the substantia gelatinosa (i.e. the 'gate' of Melzack and Wall). This interaction may lead to facilitation (so that the pain threshold is reduced) or inhibition (so that the threshold is increased). Over a dozen of these neurotransmitters have been identified, including γ-aminobutyric acid, cholecystokinin, bombesin, somatostatin, and several of the endogenous opioid peptides. Although some of these peptides are synthesized by the dorsal root ganglia, the activity of cells of the substantia gelatinosa is also modulated by other neurotransmitters (particularly catecholamines and 5-hydroxytryptamine), whether secreted by descending pathways or administered systemically. Thus, drugs that affect these pathways (e.g. 5-hydroxytryptamine and the α_2-agonist clonidine) can produce analgesia in a wide variety of patients when administered extradurally or intrathecally. These analgesic effects may be potentiated by the prior administration of agents that increase the local concentration of neurotransmitters (e.g. monoamine oxidase inhibitors). Part of the antinociceptive effect of clonidine may involve the activation of central opioid receptors; this action is antagonized by naloxone. Central pain occurs with ischaemic and other lesions of the thalamus; this may involve an imbalance of neurotransmitter activity.

In general, analgesics act by affecting processes of synthesis, release, receptor activation, degradation, and reuptake in different neurochemical systems. Their action involves the inhibition of systems that are nociceptive (e.g. the prostaglandins and bradykinin), and the facilitation of those that are antinociceptive (e.g. the endogenous opioids). However, since these systems have other physiological roles, analgesic drugs may have side-effects that reflect the widespread interruption of different neurochemical systems. It is therefore not surprising that the analgesic potential of some drugs was only discovered after their introduction into clinical practice for other indications. Thus, peripheral and central monoamines play a major role in the function of the cardiovascular system; although the centrally acting α_2-adrenergic agonist clonidine is an antihypertensive agent, it also has analgesic activity. Similarly, the benzodiazepines may have analgesic effects when injected extradurally or intrathecally, due to their interaction with the GABA receptor.

CLASSIFICATION OF ANALGESIC DRUGS

Analgesic drugs may be classified as:

1 Primary, general or non-specific analgesics. These drugs may be subdivided into:

(a) Opioid analgesics, e.g. morphine and its derivatives. This group includes all drugs with a chemical structure or pharmacological actions similar to morphine.

(b) Simple analgesics, e.g. aspirin and paracetamol. Many of these drugs also have anti-inflammatory and antipyretic effects (e.g. non-steroidal anti-inflammatory drugs or NSAIDs).

(c) Other analgesics, e.g. ketamine and nefopam. In some instances, the chemical structure of these drugs resembles the opioids sufficiently to allow the production of some analgesia. However, they may also be active at other sites in the CNS. Nitrous oxide may be included in this group; however, it is not clear whether its analgesic effects are mediated by the release of endogenous opioids or by a direct effect on opioid receptors.

2 Secondary, or specific analgesics. These drugs may be useful in specific painful conditions (e.g. antacids, vasodilators and carbamazepine).

3 Analgesic adjuncts. These non-analgesic drugs frequently enhance the effects of primary analgesics (e.g. caffeine and the tricyclic antidepressants).

OPIOID ANALGESICS

History

Opioid analgesics are classically known as narcotic analgesics (a name derived from the Greek word *narkoo*, to benumb). Opium (in Greek, *opion* or poppy juice) was first obtained from the capsules of the unripe Oriental poppy seed (*Papaver somniferum*) in the 4th Century BC. Early writings suggested that it was principally used for its antidiarrhoeal activity, but by the 16th Century the analgesic, sedative and antitussive properties of opium had become well recognized throughout Europe. The principal active ingredient, morphine, was isolated in 1806, and named after Morpheus, the Greek god of dreams.

Opium smoking became popular in the Orient in the 18th Century. The invention of the hypodermic syringe and needle in 1853, the ready availability of morphine and its increased usage in the treatment of battle injuries, and the migration of Chinese labourers all contributed to the development of the problem of compulsive drug usage and drug dependence in Western civilization. The semisynthetic opiate heroin (diamorphine or diacetylmorphine) was produced at St Mary's Hospital in 1874, with the aim of curing morphine dependence; it was many years before it was appreciated that it provided a cure by replacing morphine with a more powerful drug of addiction. The search for agents with the analgesic effects of morphine, but without its disadvantages of dependence and tolerance, has continued for many years; the introduction of drugs that appeared to be chemically dissimilar to morphine, e.g. pethidine (in 1939) and methadone (in 1942) was of little or no value in this respect.

The potential for drug abuse is undoubtedly present with all opioid analgesics. With some drugs, the tendency is relatively low, e.g. codeine and its derivatives; however, these agents are less effective analgesics than morphine, and increasing dosage is often associated with excitatory effects. In recent years, considerable promise has been shown by the development of analgesics with partial agonist activity, or with a mixed agonist–antagonist profile (although these drugs have their own particular disadvantages).

Nomenclature

The term 'opiate' has been generally used to refer to naturally occurring substances with properties similar to morphine. On the other hand, 'opioid' is a more specific term; it refers to all naturally occurring and synthetic drugs with an affinity for opioid receptors, and actions that can be stereospecifically antagonized by naloxone. In general, drugs that produce maximal responses at opioid receptors are called agonists (or more correctly, full agonists), e.g. morphine, pethidine and fentanyl. Their effects can be reversed by competitive reversible antagonists at opioid receptors (e.g. naloxone, naltrexone and nalmefene). Some drugs may produce submaximal responses at high doses, and are usually called partial agonists (e.g. buprenorphine). In theory, partial agonists may have antagonist properties; they may prevent the access of full agonists to receptor sites. Finally, mixed agonist–antagonists (or mixed antagonist–agonists) may be agonists at one type of opioid receptor (e.g. $\varkappa$-receptors) and antagonists at others (e.g. μ-receptors). The action of some analgesics at various opioid receptor sites is shown in Table 10.1.

Mode of action

Opioid analgesics modify the complex emotional experience of pain, as well as affecting its transmission as a sensory modality. Their influence on the reactive component of pain (i.e. anxiety, fear and suffering) can greatly influence the ability of patients to tolerate pain. In some experimental studies, the pain threshold (i.e. the intensity at which a stimulus is first appreciated as pain) is only slightly affected by opioid analgesics.

Table 10.1 Effects of opioids at receptors.

Receptor	Agonist	Partial agonist	Antagonist
μ	Morphine Fentanyl Pethidine Diamorphine Codeine β-endorphin	Buprenorphine* Meptazinol	Naloxone[†] Nalorphine Pentazocine Nalbuphine Butorphanol β-funaltrexamine SKF 10,047
ϰ	Pentazocine Butorphanol Ketocyclazocine Dynorphin Morphine[‡] Fentanyl	Nalorphine Nalbuphine Levallorphan	Naloxone
δ	Nalorphine Leu-enkephalin Met-enkephalin β-endorphin		Naloxone β-funaltrexamine
σ	Nalorphine Pentazocine SKF 10,047 Butorphanol Nalbuphine		Naloxone (weak)
ε	β-endorphin		Ketocyclazocine

*Buprenorphine may precipitate withdrawal symptoms in morphine-dependent subjects.
[†]Naloxone is 10 times more effective at the μ-receptor than at the other receptors.
[‡]Relative affinity of morphine for the ϰ-receptor is 200 times less than for the μ-receptor.

Various neurochemical changes (e.g. the increased utilization of brain amines, and cholinesterase inhibition) may be induced by opioid analgesics in experimental conditions. Nevertheless, approximately 20 years ago it was suggested that specific opioid receptors were present in the CNS. This suggestion was based on three main points:

1 Most opioid analgesics are stereospecific; almost invariably, analgesic activity is associated with the laevorotatory isomer.

2 Highly potent opioid analgesics had been developed (e.g. etorphine). Their development suggested that receptor mechanisms were involved.

3 The pure antagonist naloxone had been synthesized; most of its actions were consistent with the displacement of opioid analgesics from receptor sites.

Opioid receptors

It is generally accepted that opioid analgesics do not act at a single receptor site, but at several distinct but related receptor subtypes in the spinal cord and the brain (as well as in peripheral tissues). Evidence for the existence of different opioid receptors was initially based on clinical and experimental studies with nalorphine (*N*-allyl-normorphine), a classical opioid agonist–antagonist. Approximately 40 years ago, nalorphine was shown to antagonize the analgesic and the respiratory depressant effects of morphine, and was subsequently used in the management of morphine overdosage. It was also suggested that nalorphine might be a useful analgesic in clinical practice; unfortunately, doses of nalorphine that produced significant analgesia were associated with an unacceptable incidence of psychotomimetic side-effects.

At that time, the analgesic, respiratory depressant, and opioid antagonist profile of nalorphine was considered to reflect its activity on a single homogeneous population of receptors. Thus, nalorphine was envisaged as a classical partial agonist with relatively poor intrinsic activity. Subsequent studies were not entirely consistent with this view. It was shown that nalorphine did not antagonize the effects of morphine in a predictable or dose-related manner; high doses of nalorphine produced less antagonism than low doses, resulting in a biphasic dose–response relationship. This phenomenon was not consistent with the behaviour of a classical partial agonist on a homogeneous population of receptor sites. Subsequently, the concept of 'receptor dualism' was advanced, which postulated the existence of two distinct receptors for morphine and nalorphine. By acting as a classical competitive antagonist at the morphine receptor, nalorphine antagonized the analgesic and respiratory depressant effects of morphine; in addition, it acted as an agonist at the nalorphine receptor, producing analgesia. The concept of 'receptor dualism' adequately explained the dose–response relationship between morphine and nalorphine.

In subsequent studies, the pharmacology of various opioid analgesics was studied in the chronic spinal dog. Different syndromes were produced by morphine, ketocyclazocine and *N*-allyl-normetazocine (SKF 10047), and these syndromes were interpreted in terms of the actions of these drugs at three different receptor sites. In the first place, μ-receptors (prototype agonist morphine) mediated morphinomimetic effects such as a reduction in nociceptive responses, respiratory depression, miosis, bradycardia, hypothermia and a general indifference to environmental stimuli. They appeared to have an important role in producing physical dependence. Secondly, $\varkappa$-receptors (prototype agonist ketocyclazocine) were associated with analgesia, sedation, pupillary constriction, and a different syndrome of dependence; and finally, σ-receptors (prototype agonist *N*-allyl-normetazocine) produced mydriasis, tachypnoea, tachycardia, delirium, and mania.

Other work with naturally occurring opioid peptides showed that some peptides had a higher affinity than morphine for a different population of receptors, which were present in peripheral sites as well as the CNS (particularly the frontal cortex, the corpus striatum, and the amygdala). In man, the functional significance of these receptors (the ε-receptors) is unknown; they may or may not have an important role in mediating analgesia. Nevertheless, some peptides with δ-receptor selectivity have analgesic effects. Other opioid receptor subgroups (notably, ε-receptors) have also been identified.

More recently, the presence of different subtypes of opioid receptors has been demonstrated by receptor binding and autoradiographic techniques, in both isolated tissue preparations and in intact animals. These studies have been facilitated by the development of highly selective μ-agonists and ϰ-agonists (and by the selective deactivation of μ-receptors by the agent β-funaltrexamine). Most areas of the CNS contain more than one subtype of opioid receptor. In the spinal cord (particularly in the substantia gelatinosa) μ, ϰ and δ-receptors are present. In the brainstem, opioid receptors are localized to solitary nuclei which receive afferent vagal fibres, and are present in the area postrema (which is associated with the chemoreceptor trigger zone). Opioid receptors are also present in the periaqueductal grey matter, the amygdaloid nuclei, the cerebral cortex, and the thalamus. Experimental studies suggest that approximately equal numbers of μ, ϰ and δ-receptors are present in the CNS. Nevertheless, when opioids enter the CNS, only a small fraction is bound to specific opioid receptors; most of the drug is non-specifically bound at other sites. Thus, the administration of naloxone effectively antagonizes the effects of opioids without modifying the concentration of the drugs in the brain. The presence of opioid receptors outside the CNS may partially account for some other effects of analgesic drugs (e.g. constipation, and increased biliary tract pressure).

Many physiological functions, as well as analgesia, may be dependent on complex interactions between μ, ϰ and δ-receptors. However, interpretation and comparison of different studies is difficult, due to the varied experimental techniques that have been used. In addition, opioid receptors (like receptors at other sites) may be subject to upregulation and downregulation by alterations in agonist concentration (Chapter 3). Indeed, receptor downregulation may be an important cause of tolerance to opioids during their chronic administration.

In general, there is a significant correlation between the analgesic potency of opioids and their affinity for μ-receptors. Experimental evidence suggests that only a small degree of receptor occupation is required to produce significant analgesia. In recent years, the division of μ-receptors into two subtypes (μ_1 and μ_2) has been proposed. The μ_1-receptor mediates analgesia, has a high affinity for many μ-agonists, and is present in the substantia gelatinosa, the medial thalamus, and the periaqueductal grey matter. The μ_2-receptor mediates respiratory depression and intestinal motility, has a lower affinity for agonists, and is present in the brainstem and the gastrointestinal tract.

Some opioids (e.g. cyclazocine and *N*-allyl-normetazocine) bind preferentially to σ-receptors; these sites have a relatively low affinity for naloxone. The psychotomimetic and dysphoric effects of opioids appear to be mediated by σ-receptors. Similar effects may be produced by phencyclidine and ketamine, which may react with a stereospecific receptor, the PCP receptor. It is believed that the σ-receptor may be part of an opioid–PCP receptor complex, with a high-affinity site that is sensitive to opioids, and a low-affinity site which can be blocked by phencyclidine.

During the past 10 years, the molecular mechanisms underlying the action of opioids has been clarified. Opioid analgesics produce their effects by interfering with interneuronal communication, either by inhibiting depolarization or by modifying neurotransmitter release. At a cellular level, these effects are produced by modifying transmembrane ion currents, by affecting the synthesis or release of intermediate messengers, or by both these mechanisms. Thus opioid receptor activation may modify the synthesis of cyclic AMP (cAMP), or inhibit the release of intracellular calcium ions. Some opioid receptors are linked to G proteins (GTP binding proteins; Chapter 3) which are themselves coupled to transmembrane potassium channels.

Endogenous opioid peptides

Endogenous opioid peptides are usually classified as:
1 Enkephalins.
2 Endorphins (β-endorphins).
3 Dynorphins.

These endogenous peptides have differential potencies and are preferentially bound by different opioid receptors. Enkephalins are most active at δ-receptors; endorphins mainly act at μ-receptors; while dynorphins act on ϰ-receptors.

Although endogenous opioid peptides have been isolated from many sites in

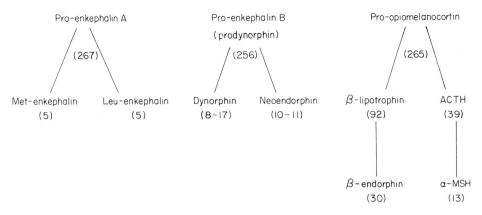

Fig. 10.2 Probable derivation of endogenous opioid peptides and related hormones. The number of amino acid residues in each polypeptide is shown in parentheses.

the body and have different molecular weights, they are all derived from three inactive precursors (pro-enkephalin A, pro-enkephalin B or prodynorphin, and pro-opiomelanocortin; Fig. 10.2). The peptides derived from these inactive precursors are widely distributed throughout the CNS, and are frequently found in the same region of the brain, but they do not occur in the same groups of neurones.

Enkephalins

The identification of opioid receptors naturally led to the search for endogenous opioids. In 1975, two similar pentapeptides (methionine (met-) enkephalin and leucine (leu-) enkephalin) were isolated from brain extracts. They were shown to produce analgesia, and to compete with the opioid antagonist naloxone for some brain receptor sites. The initial pentapeptide sequence of all endogenous opioids contains the structure of met-enkephalin or leu-enkephalin (Table 10.2).

Subsequent studies showed that regional variations in enkephalin levels reflected the distribution of opioid receptors. Enkephalins are widely distributed throughout the CNS, particularly in the spinal cord, the hypothalamus, the posterior pituitary, the globus pallidus, and the limbic system. They are also present in the gastrointestinal tract, sympathetic ganglia, the adrenal medulla, the eye, and the skin. Enkephalins have a selective affinity for δ-receptors, and are present in the CSF after some pain-relieving procedures (e.g. placebo analgesia, acupuncture and electrical stimulation of the periaqueductal grey matter). Naloxone antagonizes the analgesia produced by these procedures.

All enkephalins are derived from the inactive precursor pro-enkephalin A, and fulfil the accepted criteria for a classical neurotransmitter. They are rapidly hydrolysed in the body, partly by specific peptidases such as the enzyme enkephalinase. Their action may be prolonged by some enzyme inhibitors (e.g. D-phenylalanine). Due to the susceptibility of the natural peptides to proteolytic attack, many synthetic analogues with amino acid substitutions have been syn-

Table 10.2 Amino acid sequences of some endogenous opioid peptides.

14.4 Opioid peptide	Amino acid sequence
Leu-enkephalin	H-**Tyr-Gly-Gly-Phe-Leu**-OH
Met-enkephalin	H-**Tyr-Gly-Gly-Phe-Met**-OH
β-endorphin	H-**Tyr-Gly-Gly-Phe-Met**-Thr-Ser-Glu-Lys-Ser-Gln-Thr-Pro-Leu-Val-Thr-Leu-Phe-Lys-Asn-Ala-Ile-Ile-Lys-Asn-Ala-Tyr-Lys-Gly-Glu-OH
Dynorphin A	H-**Tyr-Gly-Gly-Phe-Leu**-Arg-Arg-Ile-Arg-Pro Lys-Leu-Lys-Trp-Asp-Asn-Gln-OH

thesized. Unfortunately, many of these analogues (as well as the endogenous pentapeptides) may produce tolerance and dependence.

Endorphins

The β-endorphins are derived from the inactive precursor pro-opiomelanocortin (Fig. 10.2). Each β-endorphin molecule contains about 30 amino acids and binds preferentially to μ-receptors. Their distribution in the CNS is more restricted than the enkephalins, and is mainly limited to the hypothalamus, the pituitary gland, and their connections. In general, the β-endorphins are far more potent and stable compounds than the enkephalins, and can produce profound and long-lasting analgesia (i.e. for several hours) when injected by the intraventricular or intrathecal routes. The endorphins appear to be independent of the enkephalins, since extirpation of the hypothalamopituitary axis in experimental animals does not lead to a decrease in enkephalin synthesis.

The inactive β-endorphin precursor pro-opiomelanocortin, which consists of 265 amino acid residues, is also the precursor of three non-opioids (i.e. ACTH, α-melanocyte stimulating hormone and β-lipotrophin). In response to acute pain and stress, both ACTH and β-endorphin are secreted in increased concentrations. Although β-endorphin contains the same amino acid sequence as met-enkephalin, it does not act as its precursor; all enkephalins are derived from pro-enkephalin A.

Dynorphins

The dynorphins (and the neo-endorphins) are derived from the inactive precursor pro-enkephalin B, which is mainly present in the posterior pituitary and the hypothalamus. The dynorphins are a group of peptides containing 8–17 amino acids, and are preferentially bound by ϰ-receptors (although they also interact with μ and δ-receptors). These peptides differ from other endogenous opioids, since they have no analgesic effects in the brain or the spinal cord. Their function appears to be the modulation of the effects of other opioids, such as analgesia, respiratory depression, and cardiovascular function. Some dynorphins may produce flaccid paralysis when injected intrathecally; it is possible that they have a role in the pathophysiology of spinal cord injuries. Thus, experimental studies have shown that dynorphin levels in the CNS are increased after spinal trauma. Administration of dynorphins may prolong survival and improve neurological deficits after cerebrovascular accidents.

Clinical significance of endogenous opioids

Current evidence suggests that endogenous opioids have important physiological roles in man. Opioid receptors may be involved in other physiological functions as well as nociception; these may include the regulation of body temperature, immunity, gastrointestinal motility, renal and hepatic function, behaviour patterns, extrapyramidal motor activity, cardiac and respiratory function, stress responses, appetite and thirst, and some endocrinological effects (e.g. those dependent on hypothalamic and pituitary function). There are high concentrations of μ and $\varkappa$-receptors in the vagal nuclei, and this may be related to the bradycardia frequently seen after opioid administration in anaesthetic practice.

Endogenous opioids have an important role in autonomic function, and there are similarities between the signs of opioid overdosage and those of circulatory shock. This has led to the hypothesis that endogenous opioid peptides are directly or indirectly linked to the manifestations of shock. Circulating levels of enkephalins and β-endorphin are elevated in experimental shock; in addition, opioids inhibit catecholamine-induced changes in myocardial contractility and heart rate in the intact heart. These effects may be related to interference with calcium influx across myocardial cell membranes. Although the administration of large doses of opioid antagonists (especially naloxone, $1-3 \, \text{mg kg}^{-1}$), may elevate blood pressure in experimental animals and human volunteers, clinical experience in shocked patients is unimpressive; in general, there has been little or no change in survival rates in patients with circulatory shock who have received naloxone. Furthermore, there are many potential disadvantages; reported complications of large doses of naloxone include grand mal seizure, pulmonary oedema and ventricular fibrillation. Some of these complications may be related to activation of the sympathetic nervous system. At present, there is insufficient clinical evidence to support the routine use of naloxone in patients with shock.

Spinally administered opioid analgesia

In 1976, the administration of morphine into the CSF was shown to have analgesic effects; in 1979, the procedure was introduced into modern clinical practice. Soon afterwards, the extradural route was found to be equally effective. Both methods are capable of producing prolonged analgesia, lasting for 15–20 h. Since then, perioperative regional analgesia using opioid drugs has become standard anaesthetic practice, providing effective analgesia with no accompanying motor or sympathetic blockade.

The initial hopes that opioids administered by these routes would provide analgesia without their usual side-effects were not fulfilled, and complications were soon reported. In addition, only certain types of pain can be managed in this way. Good results have been obtained in the management of selected cases of acute pain; for example, in patients with multiple rib fractures and acute myocardial infarction, and after some operations such as hip replacement, caesarean section and abdominal aortic surgery. The effectiveness of the analgesia is enhanced by the concurrent administration of small doses of a local anaesthetic agent, such as bupivacaine. Spinally administered opioids are not very effective in the management of labour pain, and carry the additional risk of respiratory depression in the fetus. Success with cancer pain has been mixed; the technique has some application in the management of continuous somatic or visceral pain, but is of little use in neurogenic and cutaneous pain.

There are few well-designed studies concerned with the place of intrathecal and extradural opioids in current clinical practice. Nevertheless, certain general conclusions can be drawn from these studies.

Intrathecal opioids

The mode of action of spinally administered opioids is unknown, but there is strong circumstantial evidence that drugs given intrathecally act directly on spinal opioid receptors (rather than at a higher, supraspinal level). This evidence is based on four main points:

1 Radiolabelled opioids (e.g. morphine and pethidine) can be detected in almost all laminae of the cord within minutes of administration (either autoradiographically or by liquid scintillation counting).

2 After intrathecal administration, the concentrations of morphine in plasma are extremely small (particularly with doses of 1 mg or less). In these conditions, a supraspinal action seems unlikely.

3 The duration of analgesia after intrathecal administration is several hours longer than when opioids are given by non-spinal routes. This is particularly true if large doses are used (e.g. 15–20 mg morphine), although the incidence of side-effects then becomes unacceptably high.

4 Undesirable systemic effects, such as respiratory depression, are easily antagonized by naloxone without affecting analgesia.

Morphine was the first opioid to be administered intrathecally, and continues to be the most popular drug in current use. Nevertheless, pethidine, diamorphine, and buprenorphine have also been used with equal success. The dosages used are typically about 10% of those used for intramuscular injection; doses as small as 1.25 mg of morphine or diamorphine, or 30–45 µg of buprenorphine, can produce long-lasting analgesia. Lower doses (0.1 mg morphine) may also be effective, and this probably reflects the direct delivery of the drug to its site of action. This may also affect the speed of onset of analgesia. Drugs with a relatively low lipid solubility (e.g. morphine) only pass slowly across the dura, so that the latency (i.e. the time to the onset of analgesia) is much longer after extradural administration.

Extradural opioids

Opioid analgesics that are given by extradural administration probably act by a combination of spinal and supraspinal mechanisms (in contrast to intrathecal opioids). Several studies have reported excellent analgesia at plasma concentrations that are well below the levels usually associated with analgesia. However, similar plasma concentrations may be present after intramuscular and extradural administration, suggesting considerable vascular uptake occurs from the extradural space. Absorption from the extradural venous plexus probably produces significant additional analgesia at a supraspinal level.

Most opioid analgesics have been delivered by the extradural route and all have been found to be effective (but only for certain types of pain). The shorter acting drugs (e.g. fentanyl and alfentanil) are best given by infusion, as single doses are only effective for a relatively short time (about 2–4 h). By contrast, long-acting drugs such as morphine and buprenorphine are usually administered as bolus injections, although infusions would be appropriate in certain circumstances (e.g. if a particularly long duration of action was desirable). In many early studies, the dosages used were comparable with those employed with other routes of administration (e.g. 100 mg pethidine, 0.1 mg kg^{-1} morphine). The current practice is to use much smaller doses of hydrophilic opioids (e.g. 1–2 mg morphine), since larger doses do not significantly enhance analgesia (although they do increase the incidence of side-effects). By contrast, more lipophilic drugs (e.g. fentanyl) are given in similar doses to those used parenterally, since there is significant uptake of the drug into adjacent areas such as extradural fat and vasculature. Thus a typical initial bolus dose of extradural fentanyl is 50–100 μg. The relative lipid solubilities of some opioid analgesics are shown in Table 10.3.

It was originally considered that opioids, like local anaesthetic agents, would only be effective if administered at the spinal level corresponding to the area of the pain. Since then, there have been several reports that administration by the lumbar route provides equally satisfactory analgesia after upper abdominal and thoracic surgery. In particular, morphine may produce satisfactory analgesia when given by the lumbar route, thus avoiding the need for a thoracic epidural. Even the caudal route has been used with good results in the treatment of postoperative pain in children following open heart surgery. The explanation for this effect is obscure. It has been suggested that morphine does not enter the spinal cord quickly, due to its relatively poor lipid solubility; consequently, it is able to diffuse throughout the CSF and produce widespread analgesia.

Table 10.3 The relative lipid solubility of some opioid analgesic bases.

Drug	Relative lipid solubility
Morphine	1
Pethidine	28
Alfentanil	90
Diamorphine	200
Fentanyl	580

Intrathecal administration has certain advantages over the extradural route. It is technically easier to perform, provides a longer duration of pain relief after a single dose, and avoids the problems of systemic absorption of drugs and possibility of localization in the extradural fat (which would limit the bioavailability of the drug). Nevertheless, most anaesthetists prefer the extradural route, because catheter techniques are routinely practised, so that the use of top-up doses or the institution of an infusion are possible.

Complications of spinal opioid analgesia

There are several adverse effects associated with spinal analgesia. Minor problems are relatively common; in some studies, they have occurred in almost every patient. They include nausea and vomiting, pruritus (usually over the head, neck and trunk), and urinary retention. Two major complications of spinally administered opioid analgesia can also occur. Firstly, neurological damage sometimes occurs; although this is rare, it may arise if preparations containing preservatives are used. Secondly, respiratory depression (which can proceed to respiratory arrest) occurs in 0.1–3% of patients, although the presence of certain risk factors may increase its incidence (Table 10.4). It is more common after intrathecal administration, and is dose-dependent. It typically occurs 6 h (range = 1–12 h) after administration of the opioid and can last as long as 24 h. Thus, close observation is recommended for 24 h after the last injection. Morphine is most commonly associated with this complication; its relatively low lipid solubility is thought to account for its tendency to spread rostrally in the CSF. Apart from the neurological sequelae, all of the complications described above are completely

Table 10.4 Factors predisposing to the development of respiratory depression after the spinal administration of opioids.

Patient factors	Drug factors
Elderly or disabled patients	Use of hydrophilic drugs (morphine)
Presence of coexisting respiratory disease	Large doses of opioids
Thoracic epidural administration	Repeated doses of opioids
Intrathecal administration	Concurrent administration of parenteral opioids
Presence of raised intrathoracic pressure (e.g. IPPV)	
Sensitivity to opioids (i.e. no previous exposure)	

antagonized by naloxone. This may need to be given repeatedly or by infusion, since these complications may persist for a considerable time. Naltrexone and nalmefene have a longer duration of action, and may be more suitable opioid antagonists.

PHARMACOKINETICS OF OPIOID ANALGESICS

After oral administration, most opioid analgesics are well absorbed from the small intestine. Since most opioids are weak bases and have high pK_a values (range = 6.5–9.3), they are mainly present in the stomach as ionized compounds; consequently, their absorption by the gastric mucosa is insignificant. By contrast, in the small intestine the pH is relatively alkaline, and opioid analgesics are mainly present in a non-ionized form; thus, they are rapidly and well absorbed in the upper small intestine. However, almost all opioid analgesics (with the single exception of methadone) undergo significant first pass metabolism in the gut wall and the liver so that their oral bioavailability is low (typically 20%; range = 15–30%). Consequently, this route of administration is only appropriate in situations where parenteral administration is undesirable or impractical. Opioid analgesics are more usually given by intramuscular administration. Their absorption from muscle is relatively rapid, and maximum plasma concentrations occur 15–60 min after administration. However, absorption will be prolonged by peripheral vasoconstriction (due to pain, hypovolaemia, hypotension, hypothermia, or any other cause). In this situation, a reservoir of drug may remain in the tissues for some time.

The distribution of opioid analgesics is affected by several factors including lipid solubility, ionization, and binding to plasma proteins and tissue components. Lipid solubility is the most important factor determining the rate of drug entry into, and exit from, the CNS. Highly lipid-soluble drugs such as fentanyl are able to equilibrate rapidly across the blood–brain barrier, and therefore have a rapid onset of action. By contrast, less lipophilic drugs such as morphine enter the CNS more slowly, leading to a delay in peak effect. The degree of ionization of opioid analgesics affects their lipid solubility, binding to plasma proteins, and their partitioning between tissues and plasma. This may be altered by changes in plasma pH. Finally, the uptake of lipid-soluble analgesics by tissues can be appreciable. If they are administered by repeated injections or infusions over a long period of time, they will accumulate and recovery will be prolonged. Changes in the amount of drug bound to plasma protein generally have little effect on the amount of drug entering the CNS, as the volumes of distribution of these drugs are very large; and small change in free drug concentration consequent to alterations in protein binding is of little or no significance.

The biotransformation of opioid analgesics mainly occurs in the liver; in general, drug metabolites are inactive, or are much less potent than the parent

Table 10.5 Typical pharmacokinetic and physicochemical parameters of some opioid analgesics.

	Terminal half-life (hours)	Clearance (ml min^{-1} kg^{-1})	Total volume of distribution (litres kg^{-1})	pK_a	% ionized at pH 7.4
Morphine	3	15	3.5	7.9	76
Pethidine	4	12	4.0	8.7	95
Fentanyl	3.5	13	4.0	8.4	91
Alfentanil	1.6	6	0.8	6.5	11

drug. Most pharmacokinetic studies of opioid analgesics have been based on intravenous drug administration, as this avoids the variability of drug absorption and simplifies the kinetic interpretation of the data. Nevertheless, there is a significant degree of inter-individual variability in the main pharmacokinetic constants; typical values for the terminal half-life of some commonly used analgesics are shown in Table 10.5. It should be recognized that the terminal plasma half-lives of opioid analgesics are not necessarily related to their duration of action; for example, morphine has a shorter terminal half-life than pethidine or fentanyl, but a longer duration of action. The volume of distribution of most opioids is several times greater than total body water, while their clearance is usually similar to liver blood flow (i.e. they are eliminated by flow-dependent hepatic clearance; Table 10.5).

CLASSIFICATION OF OPIOID ANALGESICS

Opioids may be classified into three main groups:
1 Drugs that are pure agonists.
2 Drugs that have mixed agonist/antagonist properties.
3 Drugs that are pure antagonists, and appear to have no intrinsic opioid activity in man.
  Further subdivisions are related to chemical structure.

Agonists

Agonists may be classified as:
1 Morphine.
2 Analogues or derivatives of morphine.
3 Phenylpiperidine derivatives.
4 Methadone and its congeners.
5 Benzomorphan derivatives.

1 Morphine

Morphine is the principal phenanthrene derivative in opium (which contains 9–17% by weight of morphine base), and is the standard agent with which all other opioids are compared. It has a complex chemical structure (Fig. 10.3); part

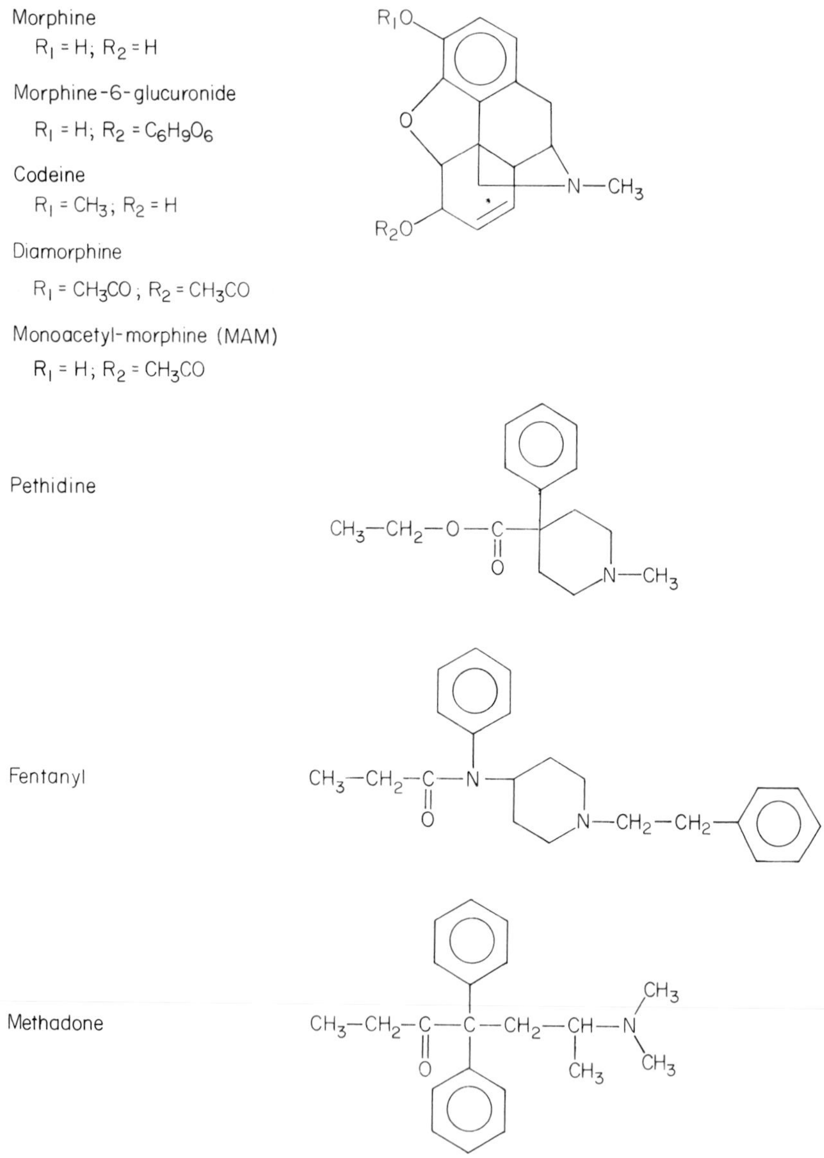
Morphine
R1 = H; R2 = H
Morphine-6-glucuronide
R1 = H; R2 = C6H9O6
Codeine
R1 = CH3; R2 = H
Diamorphine
R1 = CH3CO; R2 = CH3CO
Monoacetyl-morphine (MAM)
R1 = H; R2 = CH3CO
R1O
O
R2O
N—CH3
Pethidine
CH3—CH2—O—C
O
N—CH3
Fentanyl
CH3—CH2—C—N
O
N—CH2—CH2
Methadone
CH3—CH2—C—C—CH2—CH—N
O
CH3
CH3
CH3

Fig. 10.3 The chemical structure of some opioid analgesics.

of this structure (the 'chair' or piperidine ring) is a common feature of many other opioid analgesics.

Route of administration and pharmacokinetics

Morphine is usually administered (as a sulphate or hydrochloride salt) by intramuscular injection. Less commonly, it is given subcutaneously. It is well absorbed from these sites, and produces blood levels which are usually as high as after intravenous injection. The adult dose is normally 10–15 mg, but this should be reduced in frail and elderly subjects, or those with underlying respiratory disorders. A peak effect will be achieved after 30–60 min, and its duration of action is approximately 3–4 h. The onset of action is only slightly quicker after intravenous injection, as the main factor governing its latency is the permeability of the blood–brain barrier.

Morphine may also be administered orally. However, it undergoes extensive first pass effects so that only 20–30% of an orally administered dose reaches the systemic circulation; large doses have to be given to achieve adequate analgesia. Nevertheless, oral therapy with morphine solutions is commonly used in the long-term management of pain associated with malignancy. A slow release preparation and a suppository form of the drug are also available.

After the intravenous administration of a bolus dose of morphine, plasma concentrations decline in a triexponential manner. Distribution occurs rapidly at first, and then the plasma concentration declines more slowly. During this period, morphine enters the CNS; this occurs gradually, due to its low lipid solubility. These phases are followed by a slower phase of exponential decline, corresponding to the terminal half-life of the drug (approximately 3 h). Although the terminal half-life of morphine in plasma is shorter than that of pethidine or fentanyl, its duration of action is longer, because the decline in morphine concentrations in the brain is slower (due to the lower lipid solubility of the drug). Thus, there is no direct relationship between the plasma concentration of morphine and its clinical effects, such as respiratory depression (in contrast to lipid-soluble drugs such as fentanyl).

Morphine may also be given by intrathecal and extradural administration (p. 310).

Morphine is almost entirely metabolized by the gut wall or the liver to a number of active or inactive compounds; 90% of the dose is excreted within 24 h. The principal metabolite (accounting for 70% of the dose) is morphine-3-glucuronide. This metabolite is partly excreted in bile, but can be broken down by intestinal bacteria; morphine is released which may then be reabsorbed and metabolized by enterohepatic recirculation. Glucuronidation also takes place at the 6-carbon position, producing an active metabolite (morphine-6-glucuronide; Fig. 10.3).

Various factors may affect the pharmacokinetics of morphine. Neonates are more sensitive to the effects of morphine, because the conjugating capacity of the liver is not fully developed. In the elderly, the volume of distribution is about half that of younger subjects, so that peak plasma levels are higher. Morphine clearance is not altered in cirrhosis, since glucuronidation is largely unaffected. Any increased effects of the drug in hepatic cirrhosis are therefore likely to be due to increased sensitivity to morphine (i.e. a pharmacodynamic rather than a pharmacokinetic phenomenon). The accumulation of morphine-6-glucuronide in patients with renal failure may account for their increased sensitivity to morphine. The clearance of morphine administered parenterally appears to be reduced during halothane anaesthesia, due to a reduction in hepatic blood flow. This is unlikely to be of practical significance unless very large doses are administered.

Pharmacological effects

The principal pharmacological effects of morphine (Table 10.6) are almost entirely mediated by μ-receptors.

1 Analgesia. Morphine relieves most forms of pain. However, in clinical practice it is most valuable for the treatment of continuous, dull, poorly localized pain arising from deeper structures, and where there are associated symptoms of fear and anxiety. Patients frequently report that the pain is still present but that they feel more comfortable. Thus, it is most useful for the management of pain arising from acute abdominal catastrophes, postoperative pain, major trauma, myocardial infarction, and the management of pain associated with malignant disease.

Table 10.6 Principal pharmacological effects of morphine and related drugs.

Desirable effects	Undesirable effects
Effective analgesia	Tolerance
Relief of anxiety	Dependence
Sedation*	Dysphoria
Euphoria*	Nausea and vomiting
	Spasm of smooth muscle
	Constipation*
	Respiratory depression*
	Depression of cough reflex*
	Muscle rigidity

* These effects will vary according to circumstances. For example, respiratory depression will be an advantage during IPPV, whilst sedation and euphoria may be undesirable in the treatment of chronic pain in the ambulant patient.

It is less effective in experimentally induced pain, and in acute pain arising from superficial structures.

2 *Sedation*. Drowsiness usually occurs in man after the administration of morphine. Sleep is less commonly induced, although there is a shift of the electroencephalogram towards increased voltage and lower frequencies (a δ rhythm), and REM sleep is suppressed in animals. Some patients will experience euphoria (an unrealistic sense of well-being); however, dysphoria (an unpleasant sensation associated with mild anxiety or fear) may occur, especially when morphine is administered in the absence of pain. In anaesthetic practice, this may also be seen if the drug is administered a few minutes before the induction of anaesthesia.

3 *Respiratory depression*. Therapeutic doses of morphine will depress the depth (and more especially the rate) of respiration by a direct effect on the respiratory centres in the brainstem. Maximal respiratory depression is seen within 7 min of intravenous administration, but may occur up to 30 min after intramuscular administration. In both cases, it may last for 4–5 h. Responsiveness to carbon dioxide is decreased, as shown by a shift to the right and a flattening of the ventilation–response curve (although hypoxic stimulation may still be effective).

However, when the main stimulus to respiration is hypoxia, oxygen therapy may potentiate respiratory depression by suppressing reflex chemoreceptor stimulation. When other CNS depressants, particularly halogenated anaesthetic agents, are used concurrently, marked bradypnoea and periodic breathing may be anticipated. The fetal respiratory centre appears to be highly sensitive to morphine, which precludes the use of the drug as an analgesic during labour.

4 *Nausea and vomiting*. Nausea and vomiting are common and unpleasant side-effects of morphine. They are primarily due to stimulation of the dopamine and 5-HT$_3$ receptors associated with the chemoreceptor trigger zone in the area postrema of the medulla; the activity of the vomiting centre may actually be depressed (particularly after repeated doses of morphine). Effects on the vestibular apparatus and on the smooth muscle of the gut may also be involved.

5 *Cardiovascular effects*. After administration of morphine, a mild bradycardia often occurs. This may be due to the decreased sympathetic drive associated with sedation, or a direct effect on the vagal nuclei. However, a direct action on the SA node cannot be excluded, and halothane may potentiate this effect. Hypotension may occur, but is not usually significant in the normovolaemic supine patient; it is probably due to some reduction in sympathetic tone leading to peripheral vasodilatation, and the release of histamine from mast cells. Morphine causes no direct myocardial depression, and doses up to 3 mg kg^{-1} are well tolerated (for example, in patients with aortic valve disease undergoing open heart surgery).

Morphine has a particularly beneficial effect in the treatment of paroxysmal nocturnal dyspnoea, since it produces sedation, reduces preload, and depresses abnormal respiratory drive.

6 *Histamine release.* Morphine releases histamine from mast cells and may produce bronchospasm and hypotension in susceptible patients. Its use should be avoided, if possible, in patients with obstructive airways disease. Nasal pruritus (or even generalized pruritus) may occur; this phenomenon is probably also related to histamine release. Atropine may partially antagonize some of these effects.

7 *Effects on gastrointestinal function.* In general terms, morphine diminishes propulsive contractions and reduces secretory function throughout the gastro-intestinal tract. However, the resting tone in smooth muscle is increased (particularly in most gastrointestinal sphincters). This can result in a prolonged gastric emptying time, delayed passage through the intestine, and constipation. An important exception is lower oesophageal sphincter tone, which is decreased by morphine in patients with pre-existing reflux.

Spasm of the smooth muscle of the biliary tract and the sphincter of Oddi can also occur. The resulting rise of intraluminal pressure may lead to reflux of bile into the pancreatic duct; elevated levels of serum amylase and lipase are sometimes found following the administration of morphine. Therapeutic doses of the drug increase the tone and amplitude of contraction of the ureters.

8 *Miosis.* Miosis is due to stimulation of the Edinger–Westphal nucleus, depression of supranuclear pathways, or effects on central sympathetic activity. Pinpoint pupils are characteristic features of morphine overdosage.

9 *Hormonal effects.* The release of ACTH, prolactin, and gonadotrophic hormones is inhibited by morphine; by contrast, ADH secretion is increased. These effects may be mediated via dopamine receptors in the hypothalamus.

10 *Muscle rigidity.* Morphine (as well as all other opioids) may occasionally produce rigidity of the thoracic wall (or even generalized muscle rigidity). These effects are thought to be mediated via opioid receptors in the substantia nigra and striatum interacting with dopaminergic and GABA pathways, and can resemble convulsions. However, true convulsions only rarely occur, and are usually associated with gross overdosage of morphine.

11 *Tolerance and dependence.* Tolerance is characterized by decreased intensity and shortened duration of the usual effects of morphine, after repeated administration of the same dose of the drug. It may occur in subjects who have become socially habituated to the drug, or in patients who require continuous therapy for chronic pain. The pharmacokinetics of morphine are not altered by its repeated use; however, a negative feedback system may result in decreased production of endogenous opioids, and there may also be 'downregulation' of opioid receptors.

The development of morphine dependence can be demonstrated when the drug is suddenly withdrawn after repeated dosage. Various physical and psychological phenomena may develop, the severity of which are related to the total amount administered. Symptoms and signs include restlessness and irritability, frequent yawning, excessive sweating, lachrymation and salivation, painful muscle cramps, and intense and uncontrolled vomiting, diarrhoea and urination. Mild symptoms have been reported after only 48 h treatment.

2 Analogues and derivatives of morphine

Papaveretum (Omnopon)

Papaveretum is a semisynthetic mixture of the hydrochlorides of the opium alkaloids. The usual adult dose (20 mg) contains the equivalent of 10 mg anhydrous morphine (a dose equal to 12.5 mg morphine hydrochloride or 13.3 mg morphine sulphate). The drug also contains various other phenanthrene derivatives (e.g. codeine and thebaine) and the benzylisoquinoline derivatives papaverine and noscapine, which may antagonize some of the undesirable peripheral effects of morphine. Papaveretum may be given by intramuscular, intravenous or subcutaneous administration.

Diamorphine (diacetylmorphine; heroin)

Unchanged diamorphine has little or no affinity for opioid receptors. However, diamorphine is rapidly metabolized to monoacetylmorphine by esterases in plasma and tissues; both diamorphine and monoacetylmorphine are more lipid-soluble than morphine, and they consequently penetrate the blood–brain barrier more easily. In the CNS, both diamorphine and monoacetylmorphine are rapidly converted to morphine. Some clinicians consider that diamorphine has a greater euphoriant effect than morphine, and that it may cause less vomiting, although almost all of the drug is eventually hydrolysed to morphine (both *in vivo* and in prepared solutions). In many countries, the manufacture or importation of heroin, even for medical use, is illegal.

When patients with terminal malignant disease require large doses of morphine for pain relief, diamorphine can be administered (usually as the hydrochloride salt) by intramuscular injection in a smaller volume of solution than the equivalent dose of morphine. This is an important consideration in patients with muscle wasting and cachexia, and is the only significant advantage of diamorphine.

Codeine

Codeine (methylmorphine) and its derivatives have a higher oral bioavailability than morphine. This is presumably due to the presence of a methyl group in the C3 position, which protects the drug from the activity of conjugating enzymes. Codeine is less effective against severe pain than morphine, although about 10% is metabolized to the parent drug. Codeine has a low abuse potential, and large doses tend to produce excitement rather than central depression. Small doses of the drug (5–10 mg) are commonly incorporated with NSAIDs in analgesic compounds which are used in the treatment of pain of moderate intensity; it is also used in antitussive and antidiarrhoeal preparations. Dihydrocodeine, a related compound, is a valuable drug for the management of chronic pain; oxycodone is even more effective, but has a higher abuse potential.

Levorphanol

Levorphanol is about ten to 15 times as potent as morphine when used orally; it may also be given parenterally. Clinical reports suggest that nausea and vomiting are uncommon side-effects. The *d*-isomer (dextrorphan) is devoid of analgesic effects and possesses considerable antitussive activity.

Etorphine

Etorphine (an analogue of thebaine) is about 400 times more potent than morphine in man. It is frequently used in veterinary practice; it is a particularly valuable drug for immobilizing large animals in zoos and game reserves (due to its extremely high potency). It has undergone limited clinical trials in cancer patients, and tolerance and respiratory depression may be less pronounced than with equipotent doses of morphine. However, the development of etorphine has been discouraged by the World Health Organization; it is considered that its high potency conveys an increased risk of accidental overdosage and drug abuse.

3   Phenylpiperidines

Phenylpiperidine derivatives include pethidine, phenoperidine, fentanyl, alfentanil and diphenoxylate. They are structurally related to morphine and its derivatives (Fig. 10.3).

Pethidine

Although pethidine was originally developed as an anticholinergic agent, it was shown to have analgesic properties and was the first synthetic analgesic used in clinical practice (in 1939). Its apparent chemical dissimilarity to morphine suggested that it might not be associated with undesirable side-effects. However, there is little (if any) difference between the effects of equipotent doses of morphine and pethidine (e.g. analgesia, respiratory depression, nausea and vomiting, and tolerance and dependence). Pethidine is more lipid-soluble than morphine, and penetrates the blood–brain barrier more readily. Consequently, there is a clear relationship between the plasma concentration of pethidine and its effects (unlike morphine; p. 317). There are certain pharmacological differences between morphine and pethidine; these are summarized in Table 10.7. In particular, pethidine may produce serious adverse effects in patients receiving a monoamine oxidase inhibitor (MAOI), including coma, hypotension or hypertension, convulsions, and hyperpyrexia. The mechanism of this interaction is unknown; it may be mediated by 5-HT, although inhibition of pethidine metabolism by MAOIs has also been implicated. Pethidine should not be given if a MAOI has been taken in the preceding 2 weeks; although other opioids are probably safe, it may be preferable to withhold these drugs altogether. If this is not possible, a small

Table 10.7 Principal differences between morphine and pethidine.

	Morphine	Pethidine
Equipotent adult dosage	10 mg	100 mg
Cortical effects	Sedation: δ rhythm on EEG	Sedation less marked; no EEG change with single dosage; hallucinations
Pupillary effects	Miosis (see text)	Miosis less marked; ? atropine-like effect on sphincter pupillae
Cardiovascular effects	Bradycardia; slight fall in BP	Significant fall in BP may occur in elderly; tachycardia sometimes
Atropine-like effects	Nil	Dry mouth
Duration of action (i.m. or s.c.)	3–4 h	2–3 h
Use during labour	Generally contraindicated	Opioid of choice if administered >4 hours prior to delivery
Metabolism and excretion	Glucuronide conjugation; excretion in bile (enterohepatic circulation) and mainly via kidneys	Extensive metabolism in liver; two major pathways; one metabolite, norpethidine, may produce hallucinations and convulsions in toxic dosage or in combination with monoamine oxidase inhibitors

test dose (10% of the usual dose) should be given initially and titrated upwards.

The pharmacokinetics of pethidine show considerable inter-individual variability; typical findings are shown in Table 10.5. Pethidine is almost entirely metabolized by Phase I reactions in the liver; its main metabolites are norpethidine, pethidinic acid, and pethidine-*N*-oxide. Little or no unchanged pethidine is eliminated. About 70% of the dose is excreted in urine (as metabolites) within 24 hours, and this is enhanced by urinary acidification (and reduced by alkalinization). In patients with normal renal function, the elimination half-life of norpethidine is 14–21 h; the clearance of pethidine is reduced in liver disease, in the elderly, and in the perioperative period. In renal failure, both pethidine and norpethidine accumulate, and this may be associated with certain neurological sequelae including grand-mal seizures, particularly when the ratio of the metabolite to the parent compound is greater than one.

Pethidine is often used during labour. Since it is relatively lipid-soluble, it readily crosses the placenta and significant amounts reach the fetus over a period of several hours. By contrast, little norpethidine (or other metabolites) cross the placenta from the maternal circulation. The elimination of both pethidine and norpethidine is considerably prolonged in the neonate; their terminal half-lives are about three times longer than in adults (mainly due to a reduction in their clearance).

Phenoperidine

Phenoperidine is a potent analgesic and respiratory depressant, with a relatively short duration of action and considerable sedative effects. It is approximately five times more potent than morphine. It is invariably administered intravenously, and has been particularly popular in the management of patients requiring prolonged mechanical ventilation in the intensive care unit.

Its effects on respiratory function are maximal in 5–15 min, and the duration of action is usually less than 60 min. After intravenous administration, its plasma concentration shows a secondary peak after 30–40 min, which may be abolished by concurrent antacid therapy. This phenomenon is characteristic of other basic drugs (e.g. pethidine and fentanyl), and is due to their elimination into acidic gastric fluid, and their subsequent reabsorption from the small intestine. Phenoperidine is mainly metabolized to pethidine and norpethidine; both these metabolites (and traces of the unchanged drug) can be identified in urine.

Fentanyl

Fentanyl is the most potent analgesic used in the UK: it is approximately 100 times more potent than morphine. When given in small intravenous doses (1 μg kg^{-1}), it has a rapid onset and a short duration of action (about 30 min). Although it is structurally related to pethidine, it has little sedative activity at low doses; by contrast, in high doses ($50-150\,\mu g\ kg^{-1}$) sedation and unconsciousness are profound, and it may be used as the sole anaesthetic. However, awareness during surgery has been reported and this technique should be used with care. When given in high doses, muscular rigidity, particularly of the chest wall, may be a problem.

In many respects, fentanyl is similar to morphine. It depresses respiration in a dose-dependent manner. Cardiovascular stability is present even when the drug is administered in high dosage, and the position of fentanyl in cardiovascular anaesthesia is well established. During high-dose fentanyl anaesthesia, brady-cardia may occur; this may require treatment with atropine. High-dose fentanyl anaesthesia also reduces or eliminates the metabolic stress response to surgery.

Since fentanyl is highly lipid-soluble, it is rapidly and extensively distributed in tissues. Its duration of action is dose-dependent. In small doses ($1-2\,\mu g\ kg^{-1}$), its duration of action is short and there is rapid recovery; in these conditions, the plasma (and CNS) concentrations of the drug fall to below an effective level during the rapid distribution phase. However, after multiple or large doses of the drug, the duration of action is significantly prolonged. In these circumstances, the distribution phase is complete while the plasma concentration of fentanyl is still high. Recovery from the effects of the drug then depends on its relatively slow elimination from the body, and profound respiratory depression may be present for several hours during the postoperative period.

Many factors can affect the disposition of fentanyl, and many pharmacokinetic studies have shown considerable inter-individual variability. Typical pharmaco-kinetic parameters are shown in Table 10.5. After an intravenous bolus dose of fentanyl, plasma levels decline quickly (distribution half-life = approximately 13 min). The terminal half-life is 3–4 h in normal subjects, but may be as long as 7–8 h in some groups of patients. The volume of distribution is relatively large (approximately 4 litres kg^{-1}) indicating considerable tissue uptake, and the clearance is slightly less than hepatic blood flow. Fentanyl is predominantly metabolized in the liver; about two-thirds of the administered dose is excreted in the urine as inactive metabolites over 4 days. There is no evidence that fentanyl is any more likely to produce delayed respiratory depression than any other opioid analgesic.

Alfentanil

Alfentanil is a synthetic opioid structurally related to fentanyl; it has approximate-ly 10–20% of its potency, and has a shorter duration of action. Its effects on the respiratory and cardiovascular systems are similar to fentanyl, and it is used in similar situations. However, small doses of the drug can cause apnoea in some patients. Although this is usually very short-lasting, it is unpredictable; careful monitoring is essential, particularly in the elderly who are more sensitive to respiratory depression.

There are important pharmacokinetic differences between alfentanil and fentanyl (Table 10.5). Although it has a much lower lipid-solubility than fentanyl, more alfentanil in plasma is present in the unionized form (89% compared to 9% for fentanyl); consequently, its onset of action is more rapid than fentanyl. Alfentanil has a short distribution half-life (approximately 11 min), and a shorter terminal half-life than fentanyl (approximately 1.6 h); complete recovery is therefore more rapid, and alfentanil provides very little postoperative analgesia. Despite its shorter terminal half-life, its clearance is about half that of fentanyl, while its lower lipid solubility results in a much smaller volume of distribution. The shorter terminal half-life is mainly related to this factor.

Alfentanil is extensively metabolized in the liver, and less than 2% of the parent drug is excreted unchanged. Its clearance is unaffected by renal disease, but is prolonged in cirrhosis and in patients taking cimetidine.

Alfentanil may be administered in either bolus doses or as a continuous infusion. Bolus doses ($10\,\mu g\,kg^{-1}$) are useful to attenuate the cardiovascular responses to intubation and stimulation during surgery. However, its pharmacokinetics are consistent with administration by continuous intravenous infusion; it may be used as the sole anaesthetic agent, or for sedation in the intensive care unit in patients on mechanical ventilation. Typically, a loading dose of $25-50\,\mu g\,kg^{-1}$ is given, followed by an infusion of $0.5-2.0\,\mu g\,kg^{-1}\,min^{-1}$.

Sufentanil

Sufentanil is closely related to fentanyl in chemical structure, but has five to ten times its potency. It produces excellent cardiovascular stability and has a shorter duration of action than fentanyl. It has been widely used in the USA; it is particularly useful in patients undergoing cardiac surgery. More recently, it has been used in low dosage as a premedicant administered by intranasal spray.

Carfentanil

Carfentanil is approximately twice as potent as sufentanil; it has been mainly used in veterinary medicine to immobilize large animals. As little as 5 mg can immobilize an elephant (approximately 5000 kg). It is extremely potent, and a scratch from a loaded syringe dart in a human subject will quickly cause unconsciousness and apnoea.

Lofentanil

Lofentanil is about ten times as potent as fentanyl. A single dose has a prolonged duration of action and may cause respiratory depression for as long as 48 h. Its prolonged action is mainly due to the slow dissociation of the drug from the μ-receptor. Lofentanil might have an application in intensive care; at present, it is not available for clinical use.

Diphenoxylate

Diphenoxylate is chemically related to pethidine, and produces constipation in man. It has an extremely low abuse potential, since its salts are virtually insoluble in aqueous solution. It is commonly incorporated (with atropine salts) in an anti-diarrhoeal preparation (Lomotil).

Loperamide

Loperamide, like diphenoxylate, is a piperidine derivative that is poorly absorbed from the gastrointestinal tract and does not penetrate the blood–brain barrier. Its only use is in the treatment of diarrhoea.

4 Methadone and its congeners

Methadone

Methadone was synthesized by German chemists during World War II. It is active at μ-receptors, and has similar properties to morphine. Methadone and morphine are approximately equipotent.

Unlike most other opioid analgesics, methadone has a high oral bioavailability, and the oral and parenteral doses are usually equal (5–15 mg). Consequently, methadone is a particularly useful drug when oral dosage is preferred. Methadone has a long duration of action (terminal half-life = 15–20 h), and miosis and respiratory depression can be detected for more than 24 h. It is bound to tissue proteins, so that cumulative effects may be observed with repeated dosage, especially in elderly patients (who may experience marked sedation). Methadone is metabolized in the liver by the mixed-function oxidase system (cytochrome P-450). Drugs that induce this enzyme system (e.g. rifampicin) can produce withdrawal symptoms in patients on chronic methadone treatment.

Tolerance develops more slowly to methadone than to morphine; consequently, methadone is used in the treatment of morphine dependence. Thus, methadone may be substituted for morphine without precipitating an abstinence syndrome. However, the overall abuse potential of methadone is comparable to that of morphine, and this limits its use for this purpose.

Dextromoramide and dipipanone

Dextromoramide and dipipanone are analogues of methadone, and have similar properties and potency; however, they have a shorter duration of action than the parent drug. Dipipanone is usually used with the antiemetic drug cyclizine in a proprietary preparation (Diconal). Both dextromoramide and dipipanone may provide valuable oral therapy in the management of chronic pain associated with malignancy.

Dextropropoxyphene

Propoxyphene occurs as a racemic mixture (although only the dextrorotatory isomer possesses analgesic activity). It is about 50–65% as potent as oral codeine, and has been used alone or in compound preparations. A popular formulation in the UK has been coproxamol (Distalgesic); each tablet contains paracetamol (325 mg) and dextropropoxyphene (32.5 mg). Coproxamol has been prescribed for a wide variety of painful conditions. Unfortunately, the use of coproxamol is associated with several disadvantages; some degree of dependence to dextropro-poxyphene can occur, and a number of incidents of drug abuse, particularly in combination with alcohol, have been reported. In addition, overdosage or drug interaction involving coproxamol may lead to the rapid development of profound respiratory depression which precedes the manifestations of paracetamol hepato-toxicity. One of the metabolites of dextropropoxyphene (norpropoxyphene) has a longer half-life than the parent drug; it has some analgesic activity, but also has cardiotoxic properties.

5   Benzomorphan derivatives

Phenazocine

In the UK, phenazocine is the only available benzomorphan derivative that is a pure opioid agonist. It is approximately three times as potent as morphine, and is effective when administered orally or sublingually. There is some evidence that it may be useful in the treatment of biliary colic, since it has little or no spasmogenic effect on the sphincter of Oddi.

Analgesics with mixed agonist/antagonist properties

The characteristic feature of this group of drugs is that they act as agonists at one receptor and antagonists at another. Analgesic activity is mediated almost entirely at $\varkappa$-receptors, at which they are partial agonists or full agonists (rather than at μ-receptors). By contrast, most agonist/antagonist drugs have no agonist effects at μ-receptors, but are competitive antagonists at this site. The essential differences between pure agonist drugs and mixed agonist/antagonists are summarized in Table 10.8. In addition, the mixed agonist/antagonist drugs have more activity at σ-receptors than pure agonists, so that there is generally a higher incidence of dysphoria associated with these drugs. There are also important

Table 10.8 Comparison of pure agonists and mixed agonist/antagonists.

Effect	Pure agonist	Mixed agonist/antagonist
Dose–response relationship	Linear (except at extremes)	Plateau or bell-shaped
Effect vs dosage	Increasing dosage increases analgesia and respiratory depression	'Ceiling' effect at lower level of analgesia and respiratory depression than pure agonists
Effect at μ-receptor	Agonist	Antagonist above low dose
Effect at ϰ-receptor	Agonist	Full or partial agonist
Effect of naloxone	Antagonist	Antagonist
Effect of nalorphine	Antagonist	No effect

differences between the dose–response relationships of the two groups of drugs. In the case of pure agonists, increasing the dose causes an increase in analgesia and respiratory depression, and the maximum effect is only obtainable with doses well in excess of those used in routine clinical practice. By contrast, the dose–response curve of mixed agonist/antagonists generally shows a plateau or 'ceiling' effect, the top of the plateau representing the maximum effect possible for the agonist/antagonist (Fig. 10.4).

An additional dose - dependent effect may be possible at the same receptor for certain agonist/antagonist drugs. At low doses, the agonist action is most marked, but at higher concentrations, the antagonist action is predominant. If the transition between agonism and antagonism occurs within the clinical dose range, then the drug may be a less effective analgesic at higher dosages. This effect has been

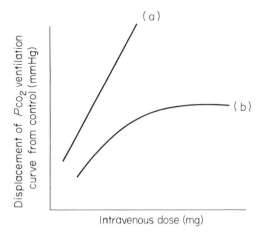

Fig. 10.4 Diagrammatic representation of the effects of (a) pure agonists, and (b) agonist/antagonists on the P_{CO_2} — ventilation response. In the case of agonist/antagonists, a plateau ('ceiling') effect occurs, so that further increases in dosage do not enhance respiratory depression.

demonstrated with nalbuphine which is actually less effective at high dosage than low to medium dosage, although the mechanism of this effect is not clearly understood.

The drugs in this group may be subdivided into those in which agonist (i.e. analgesic) activity predominates (e.g. pentazocine, butorphanol, nalbuphine and meptazinol), and those in which antagonist activity predominates (e.g. nalorphine, levallorphan and cyclazocine).

Pentazocine

Pentazocine was the first drug in this group developed for clinical use as an analgesic. It is a benzomorphan derivative, chemically related to phenazocine, and has approximately 25% of the analgesic potency of morphine. The principal differences between pentazocine and morphine (or similar analgesics that are pure agonists) are:

1 Pentazocine has a much lower abuse potential than most pure agonists. Nevertheless, there have been occasional reports of withdrawal symptoms occurring after prolonged use of the drug, particularly by parenteral administration. Consequently, it is now a controlled drug (Schedule 3) in the UK.

2 Pentazocine is a $\varkappa$-agonist, and is not very effective in relieving severe pain. This may be partly due to the absence of the euphoriant effects of morphine.

3 Psychotomimetic effects (e.g. bizarre dreams and hallucinations) occur in about 6% of patients after parenteral administration, due to its action at σ-receptors.

4 Intravenous pentazocine invariably produces an increase in both systemic blood pressure and heart rate, and an increase in circulating catecholamine levels. A rise in pulmonary vascular resistance and mean pulmonary artery pressure is not uncommon; the drug should not be used after myocardial infarction, in pulmonary or systemic hypertension, or in patients with heart failure.

5 The effects of an overdose of pentazocine will not be reversed by nalorphine.

6 Combined therapy with pentazocine and a μ-agonist in chronic pain states may produce unpredictable results. Pentazocine may antagonize the analgesic effects of the μ-agonist, while the full agonist may enhance the psychotomimetic side-effects of pentazocine. Since pentazocine has an antagonist action at the μ-receptor, the technique of 'sequential analgesia' was devised. Pentazocine was used at the end of surgery to antagonize the respiratory depression caused by large doses of intraoperative fentanyl without affecting the level of analgesia. This technique has not gained widespread acceptance.

The usefulness of pentazocine is limited by the high incidence of dysphoria, hallucinations and unpleasant dreams; the drug has been superseded by newer agonist/antagonist drugs that have a lower incidence of psychotomimetic side-effects.

Butorphanol

Butorphanol is approximately 20 times more potent than pentazocine, but has a similar profile of activity (particularly on the cardiovascular system). Therapeutic doses (1–2 mg) produce effective analgesia for 3–4 h. Butorphanol produces fewer dysphoric reactions than pentazocine (due to its reduced affinity for the σ-receptor). Butorphanol is no longer available in the UK (although it is still used in the USA).

Nalbuphine

Nalbuphine is structurally related to naloxone. It is a partial agonist at ϰ-receptors, but only has minimal effects on σ-receptors; in addition, it is a potent μ-antagonist and can precipitate withdrawal symptoms in patients who are physically dependent on opioid analgesics. It has also been used effectively in the technique of 'sequential analgesia'. Nalbuphine undergoes extensive first pass metabolism in the liver, and its oral bioavailability is low (about 10%). Consequently, it is only available as a parenteral preparation.

Nalbuphine and morphine are equipotent, and both drugs have a similar duration of action. It is similar to other agonist/antagonists, and has a plateau or 'ceiling' effect; increasing the dose has variable effects on the degree of analgesia. Unlike pentazocine, it causes no significant haemodynamic changes, and is a suitable analgesic for patients with heart disease.

Meptazinol

Meptazinol is only one-tenth as potent as morphine; unlike many opioids that are racemates, both of its enantiomers possess analgesic activity. Its mode of action is not clearly understood. It appears to be a relatively selective agonist at μ_1-receptors, although it also affects central cholinergic transmission. In opioid-dependent subjects, it has some opioid antagonist effects. Meptazinol may produce less respiratory depression than other opioids; although it rarely causes dysphoria, it may produce nausea and vomiting. This may be related to its effects on central cholinergic pathways in the cerebellum, labyrinth, and vestibular apparatus, which are known to be concerned with nausea and vomiting. The incidence of emetic complications can be reduced by anticholinergic drugs.

Buprenorphine

Buprenorphine is chemically related to thebaine, and is approximately 30 times more potent than morphine. Thus, 300 μg buprenorphine and 10 mg morphine produce the same degree of analgesia. It is a highly lipid-soluble drug, and is well absorbed sublingually.

Buprenorphine is not a classical agonist/antagonist drug, since it only acts at a single receptor subtype. It is a partial agonist at μ-receptors (i.e. it has a low intrinsic activity at this site). Thus, theoretical considerations suggest that if buprenorphine is given with morphine or similar drugs, the level of analgesia will decrease to the 'ceiling' level of buprenorphine. In practice, this interaction will only occur if all the available receptors are already occupied by the μ-agonist, or if extremely large doses of buprenorphine are given. These conditions are only present in subjects who receive large doses of morphine (e.g. cancer patients or drug addicts). In the more usual perioperative situation, the majority of opioid receptors are unoccupied and available for combination with other drugs; in these conditions, no significant interactions should occur. Buprenorphine may bind with low affinity to other opioid receptors (e.g. ϰ and σ-receptors), but it does not appear to produce pharmacological effects at these sites.

In general, buprenorphine and morphine produce similar effects and side-effects (e.g. drowsiness, nausea, vomiting, dizziness, and sweating). Since buprenorphine has an extremely high affinity for μ-receptors, its effects are not completely reversed by naloxone. Buprenorphine can produce respiratory depression; although a plateau or 'ceiling' for this effect has been described, this can still become clinically significant and should be managed with doxapram. Dysphoria is uncommon, and untoward haemodynamic effects mediated by CNS stimulation are rare (possibly due to its relatively low affinity for ϰ and σ-receptors). Although it was initially believed to have a low abuse potential, dependence may occur; in the UK, buprenorphine is now a controlled drug (Schedule 3).

Buprenorphine is extremely lipid-soluble, and is absorbed after sublingual administration; it has an extremely low oral bioavailability (due to its high first pass effect). Buprenorphine is metabolized by the liver, and 70% of a dose is eliminated in the faeces. Although its terminal half-life is similar to pethidine (3–4 h), it has a much longer duration of action (up to 8 h); this may be related to its slow dissociation from the μ-receptor. The clearance of buprenorphine is not affected by renal failure.

Nalorphine

In 1915, it was shown that *N*-allyl-norcodeine reversed or abolished the respiratory depression induced by morphine or heroin. Over 25 years later, the *N*-allyl derivative of morphine (*N*-allyl-normorphine; nalorphine) was found to have similar, but more pronounced, effects. In the following decade, nalorphine was used in the treatment of morphine overdosage, and was shown to produce withdrawal symptoms in morphine-dependent subjects. It was subsequently found to produce analgesia; it has approximately the same analgesic potency as morphine, but causes less respiratory depression. The development of nalorphine as an analgesic with a low abuse potential was limited by the occurrence of dysphoria and hallucinations (p. 305). However, it is now known that tolerance to these effects can occur in man. Nalorphine is now believed to act as an antagonist at one opioid receptor (μ), but as an agonist at others ($\varkappa$ and σ). The psychotomimetic and respiratory depressant effects of nalorphine can be antagonized by large doses of naloxone.

Levallorphan

Levallorphan is the *N*-allyl derivative of levorphanol; this drug also has mixed agonist/antagonist activity at the same opioid receptors as nalorphine. It is a more potent agonist at the $\varkappa$-receptor than nalorphine, and was formerly available in the UK in a preparation containing pethidine (Pethilorfan). The dysphoric and respiratory depressant effects of levallorphan can be antagonized by large doses of naloxone.

Cyclazocine

Many other substituted derivatives of various opioid analgesics have been synthesized, and shown to have mixed agonist/antagonist profiles. The benzomorphan derivative cyclazocine is approximately 100 times more potent than nalorphine as a μ-receptor antagonist, and 40 times more potent than morphine as an analgesic (acting as a $\varkappa$-receptor agonist). Cyclazocine can also produce intense psychotomimetic effects, and abrupt discontinuation after chronic administration causes a withdrawal syndrome similar to nalorphine. Cyclazocine has been used as an antagonist in the treatment of opioid overdosage and drug dependence; when the withdrawal syndrome is controlled, cyclazocine can be used as maintenance therapy. Since it does not produce euphoria, the likelihood of relapse is reduced.

Pure opioid antagonists

Naloxone

Naloxone is the *N*-allyl derivative of oxymorphone. Unlike the *N*-allyl derivatives of other opioids, it has no agonist activity (i.e. it is a 'pure' opioid antagonist). It has a higher affinity for μ-receptors than for other opioid receptors; nevertheless, it can still displace most agonists from $\varkappa$, σ and δ-receptors. Naloxone was originally designed and developed for the treatment of opioid overdosage, and for the prevention of opioid dependence; at first, it was considered to be devoid of any other inherent actions or effects. Nevertheless, 'anti-analgesic' effects may be observed in naive subjects who are given naloxone. Hypertension, pulmonary oedema, and cardiac arrhythmias can also occur. Some of these effects may be related to antagonism of endogenous opioid receptors, or they may reflect generalized central excitation. Both these concepts are possible; thus, naloxone will reverse analgesia produced by classical Chinese acupuncture or placebo analgesia, and can be effective in the treatment of overdosage with CNS depressants (e.g. ethyl alcohol). Naloxone may produce beneficial effects in patients with thalamic pain; its mechanism of action is obscure.

Naloxone is the current drug of choice for the treatment of opioid overdosage. In mild or moderate cases, a single dose (0.4 mg) may be sufficient to antagonize the effects of opioid analgesics. The terminal half-life of naloxone is 2.5 h; the duration of effective antagonism is limited to about 30–45 min. Long-acting agonists will outlast this effect and further bolus doses (or naloxone infusion) will then be required to maintain reversal. Smaller doses ($0.5–1.0\,\mu g\ kg^{-1}$) may be titrated to reverse respiratory depression without significantly affecting the level of analgesia. By contrast, very large bolus doses (up to 2 mg) may be required to antagonize severe opioid overdosage. Naloxone has a low oral bioavailability, due to a large first pass effect. The drug has also been used in the treatment of septic shock (p. 310).

Naltrexone

Naltrexone has an identical mode of action, but has two important pharmacokinetic advantages compared to naloxone. It has a longer duration of action, due to its longer half-life; and it has a low first pass effect (i.e. it is effective after oral administration). It is available in tablet form, and a single dose (50 mg) will remain effective for 24 h.

Nalmefene

Nalmefene is a new pure opioid antagonist derived from naltrexone. It has a terminal half-life of 8–10 h; a dose of 400 μg has a duration of action of approximately 4 h.

Doxapram

Doxapram is a non-specific analeptic which may also be of some value in the prevention or treatment of opioid-induced respiratory depression, particularly in the immediate postoperative period. It is also useful in the management of respiratory depression due to buprenorphine, since its effects are only partially antagonized by naloxone. Doxapram mainly acts by affecting reflex mechanisms mediated via chemoreceptors in the carotid body; it also produces some direct medullary stimulation of the respiratory centre. Doxapram has a higher therapeutic ratio than many other analeptics (e.g. nikethamide), since very high doses are required to produce cortical stimulation. However, it should be used cautiously in patients with hypertension, ischaemic heart disease, thyrotoxicosis, and epilepsy.

Doxapram may antagonize opioid-induced respiratory depression without abolishing analgesia, and its use in combination with opioid analgesics reduces the incidence of postoperative chest complications. It has a short duration of action (5–12 min) and may need to be given by intravenous infusion. The usual intravenous dose ($1.0–1.5 \, mg \, kg^{-1}$) is administered over 30 seconds. It is also available as a ready-made solution ($2 \, mg \, ml^{-1}$) which should be infused at a rate of $2–3 \, mg \, min^{-1}$. The drug may be of some value in the management of respiratory failure in patients with chronic obstructive pulmonary disease.

CHOICE OF ANALGESIC

The use of opioid analgesics is indicated in a wide variety of conditions.

Acute pain states

Acute pain states include abdominal catastrophes, major trauma, the pain of myocardial infarction, and pain associated with labour. In most cases, morphine is the drug of choice, although pethidine is preferred in obstetrics. Morphine should be administered by slow intravenous injection in the shocked patient to produce an optimal effect. In the undiagnosed acute abdomen, half the usual dose of morphine or pethidine may be given; some analgesic effect will be attained without masking vital signs.

Although diamorphine has been widely used to relieve the pain of myocardial infarction, its advantages are doubtful; some clinicians consider that it produces more sedation and euphoria and less vomiting than other analgesics. Codeine and its derivatives are commonly used for the management of traumatic pain associated with head injury, since they are less likely to disturb levels of consciousness and have minimal effects on pupillary signs.

In the management of many types of pain, mixed agonist/antagonist drugs are not as popular as pure agonists, for several reasons. The quality of analgesia is often inferior due to the 'ceiling' effect (which may be reached when the dose is increased). In addition, dysphoria is more common, and mixed agonist/antagonists are less predictable than pure agonists. Finally, their antagonist actions at the μ-receptor may complicate any subsequent change of therapy.

The perioperative period

When pain is present, morphine or pethidine is indicated for premedication. Pethidine, morphine and fentanyl are most frequently used as analgesic supplements. Alternatively, phenoperidine or fentanyl, usually in combination with droperidol, may be used at induction to supplement (or even replace) intravenous anaesthetic agents. Alfentanil is particularly useful during induction, in order to suppress the cardiovascular responses to intubation; it may be also given as an infusion during surgery.

Morphine or pethidine are still the most frequently used opioids for the relief of postoperative pain. Intramuscular injection is not the most effective way of ensuring good postoperative analgesia; during the past decade, numerous techniques have been developed in an attempt to provide more effective pain relief. Current methods now include spinally administered opioids, patient-controlled analgesia, computer-assisted infusions, and transdermal and transmucosal drug delivery by sublingual, buccal, gingival, and nasal administration. The partial agonist buprenorphine has a longer duration of action than most other opioids, and has possible advantages (as well as several disadvantages) as a postoperative analgesic.

Prolonged IPPV

During prolonged IPPV, analgesics may be necessary, both to provide adequate pain relief and to facilitate compliance with mechanical ventilation. In the past, phenoperidine has been extensively used, as it produces marked respiratory depression, analgesia and sedation. In recent years, alfentanil has also been widely used for this purpose. When administered by infusion, it provides good analgesia which may be quickly increased to cover periods of enhanced stimulation (e.g. physiotherapy). When the infusion is stopped, there is much quicker recovery from its effects than from any other opioid in current use.

Chronic pain

Opioid analgesics are widely used for the management of intractable pain associated with malignant disease. In most situations, effective analgesia can be provided by oral or sublingual administration of drugs.

Morphine is the most useful opioid analgesic for the management of terminal pain. It may be given orally as an elixir (e.g. morphine hydrochloride in chloroform water, 4-hourly), or as slow-release tablets. The initial dose should be the minimum that is compatible with adequate pain relief; frequent readjustment may be necessary. It is important to ensure that the drug is given at regular intervals in sufficient dosage to prevent the return of severe pain. Respiratory depression is not usually a problem, although nausea and constipation may require concurrent treatment with other agents (e.g. phenothiazines and laxatives). The oral bioavailability of morphine is poor due to the large first pass effect; nevertheless, small doses of regular oral morphine may be remarkably effective in the management of terminal pain. It has been suggested that the first pass effect of morphine gradually decreases with its chronic oral administration, or that accumulation of an active metabolite (morphine-6-glucuronide) occurs. Although compound elixirs containing diamorphine (e.g. cocaine and diamorphine elixir) have been widely used in the past, they have no significant advantages compared with oral morphine.

Other opioid analgesics are sometimes given by oral administration in terminal pain due to malignant disease. Methadone and its analogues (e.g. dipipanone) may be useful, since they have a relatively long half-life and a high oral bioavailability. Similarly, some derivatives of morphine (e.g. levorphanol) may be of value, since they are effective orally (although they may produce sedation). Drugs that are given sublingually (e.g. phenazocine and buprenorphine) may be particularly useful due to their rapid onset of action.

In advanced malignant disease, problems with swallowing may occur; in these conditions, morphine suppositories can be used, or opioids can be given parenterally. Thus, morphine can be given by continuous subcutaneous infusion, using a battery driven syringe driver. When large doses of opioid analgesics are required, diamorphine hydrochloride (rather than morphine) should be injected or infused; due to its relatively high aqueous solubility, diamorphine hydrochloride can be injected in a smaller volume of solution than the equivalent dose of morphine sulphate. This is a significant factor in underweight and cachectic patients; it is the main advantage of diamorphine in terminal malignant disease.

Simple analgesics

Simple analgesics (also known as antipyretic or non-opioid analgesics) are frequently used in the treatment of mild or moderate musculoskeletal pain. Since most of them also possess a variable degree of anti-inflammatory activity, they are frequently referred to as non-steroidal anti-inflammatory drugs (NSAIDs). Nevertheless, it should be recognized that not all of these drugs have anti-inflammatory effects; for example, paracetamol has little or no effect on inflammatory processes, and may not be an effective analgesic when pain is associated with inflammation. Similarly, relatively high doses of aspirin (>3 g per day) are usually necessary to produce significant anti-inflammatory effects (Table 10.9). NSAIDs mainly act at peripheral sites, and are usually administered orally. They are principally used in the treatment of mild or moderate pain associated with somatic structures; they are of limited value in the treatment of severe visceral pain. Nevertheless, some NSAIDs (e.g. diclofenac) may be used in the management of renal colic, and are increasingly used in the control of pain during the perioperative period. In minor surgery, they may eliminate the need for additional analgesia, and they significantly reduce opioid requirements after major procedures.

Table 10.9 The analgesic, antipyretic and anti-inflammatory activity of simple analgesic drugs.

Drug	Analgesic activity	Antipyretic activity	Anti-inflammatory activity
Aspirin (<3 g/day)	++	++	−
Aspirin (>3 g/day)	+++	+++	++
Paracetamol	++	++	−
Phenylbutazone	+	+	+++
Indomethacin	+	+	+++
Naproxen	+	+	++
Ibuprofen	+	+	+
Diclofenac	+	+	+++

−, absent; +, slight; ++, moderate; +++, marked.

Mode of action

Many NSAIDs modify nociceptive responses induced by certain polypeptides (e.g. bradykinin). Bradykinin is rapidly synthesized during tissue injury from an α_2-globulin in plasma (bradykininogen; plasma kininogen I), which is converted to a decapeptide (lysyl-bradykinin) by a plasma or tissue enzyme (kallikrein). Subsequently, lysyl-bradykinin is converted to the active nonapeptide bradykinin. In the circulation and most tissues, bradykinin has a half-life of 10–20 s; it is rapidly broken down by the enzyme kininase II, also known as angiotensin-converting enzyme (ACE). Consequently, ACE inhibitors (Chapter 13) may prolong the half-life of bradykinin.

The hyperaemia, pain and oedema of the inflammatory response are partly mediated by bradykinin and related polypeptides; high concentrations of bradykinin can be identified in inflammatory exudates and synovial fluid from arthritic joints. Bradykinin stimulates sensory nerve endings, and subcutaneous administration in man causes intense, evanescent, pain. Approximately 20 years ago, it was shown that these effects could be antagonized by aspirin (although the drug has no direct effects on the synthesis, degradation, or action of bradykinin). It was subsequently shown that aspirin inhibited the synthesis of prostaglandins, which normally sensitize nerve endings to the action of bradykinin; the synthesis of both mediators is usually increased by tissue injury. In particular, prostaglandin E_2 sensitizes nerve endings to bradykinin and similar peptides that stimulate peripheral sensory pathways (as well as histamine and 5-hydroxytryptamine). Consequently, subcutaneous infusion of prostaglandin E_2 in man produces oedema and lowers the pain threshold to artificial stimuli, although spontaneous pain does not occur. When bradykinin or histamine is subsequently infused into the site, intense pain is produced.

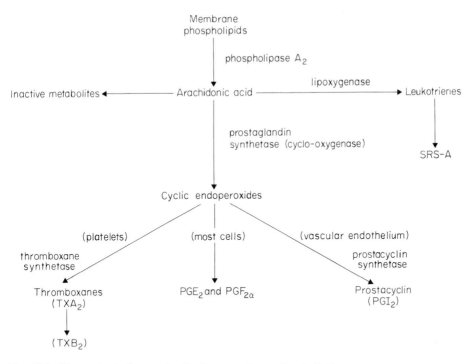

Fig. 10.5 The synthesis of prostaglandins from membrane phospholipids.

In the 1930s, human seminal fluid was shown to cause contraction of isolated smooth muscle. Approximately 30 years later, the active agents were isolated as a series of unsaturated fatty acid derivatives, and given the name prostaglandins; they are sometimes known as eicosanoids, since they are related to the 20C acid, eicosanoic acid. Prostaglandins were subsequently identified in almost all tissues in the body. They are synthesized in increased amounts after tissue injury (from the inactive precursor arachidonic acid) by the enzyme prostaglandin synthetase or cyclo-oxygenase (Fig. 10.5); the conversion of arachidonic acid to precursor prostaglandins (prostaglandin G_2 and prostaglandin H_2, also known as cyclic endoperoxides) is inhibited by aspirin and all NSAIDs. The inactive precursor arachidonic acid is present in the phospholipid membrane of almost all cells, from which it is released by the lysosomal enzyme phospholipase A_2; this step is inhibited by lipocortin (a protein whose synthesis is controlled by glucocorticoids; Chapters 3 and 16). Thus, glucocorticoids inhibit the formation of arachidonic acid, while NSAIDs inhibit its conversion to prostaglandins (Fig. 10.5).

The subsequent formation of prostaglandins depends on the tissue concerned. In most tissues, cyclic endoperoxides are converted to prostaglandins of the D_2, E_2 and $F_{2\alpha}$ series; these prostaglandins have complex effects on inflammation, smooth muscle activity, glandular secretions, peripheral blood vessels, and bone reabsorption. Some of them are formed in bone, and are synthesized in bone metastases.

In platelets, a series of prostaglandin derivatives, the thromboxanes, are formed by the enzyme thromboxane synthetase; thromboxane A_2 (TXA_2) induces platelet aggregation and adhesion, and causes vasoconstriction. By contrast, in vascular endothelial cells, prostacyclin (PGI_2) is formed by the enzyme prostacyclin synthetase; in general, it has opposite effects to the thromboxanes (i.e. it inhibits platelet aggregation and causes vasodilatation). It is believed that the balance between the formation of thromboxanes (by the platelets) and prostacyclin (by the vascular endothelium) plays an important role in maintaining the integrity of platelets in circulating blood. When this balance is disturbed, thrombosis may occur. In gastric mucosal cells, prostacyclin and other prostaglandins are synthesized; they may have a protective role in preventing mucosal damage. A series of related compounds, the leukotrienes, are synthesized in white cells (and other tissues) from arachidonic acid by the enzyme lipoxygenase (Fig. 10.5); SRS-A (slow reacting substance of anaphylaxis) is probably identical with leukotrienes C and D_4. This substance plays an important role in mediating bronchoconstriction in allergic and anaphylactic conditions.

Many prostaglandins are highly unstable, and have extremely short half-lives; for example, thromboxane A_2 and prostacyclin have a half-life of approximately 30 seconds. Prostaglandins of the series E_2 and $F_{2\alpha}$ are almost entirely metabolized in a single passage through the pulmonary circulation. Other prostaglandins are removed to a lesser extent.

Some of the actions of aspirin and other NSAIDs can be explained in terms of their effects on prostaglandin synthesis. Thus, the effects of these drugs on platelet aggregation and adhesiveness may reflect the inhibition of thromboxane synthesis; their anti-inflammatory effects may be due to decreased synthesis of PGE_2 and $PGF_{2\alpha}$; and their effects in promoting gastric irritation and ulceration may reflect decreased prostaglandin synthesis by gastric mucosal cells. It has been suggested that the antipyretic effects of aspirin may be related to inhibition of PGE_2 synthesis, since this substance can raise body temperature in some experimental conditions. Prostaglandins are undoubtedly present in the CNS, where they may play a role in neurotransmission. However, it is doubtful whether increased PGE_2 synthesis is the main factor responsible for hyperpyrexia in common bacterial or viral infections.

Nevertheless, not all of the effects of aspirin are related to inhibition of prostaglandin synthesis, and analgesia may be partly due to the direct action of the drug on central pathways. Thus, in decerebrate animals, the suppression of pain responses may require greater amounts of aspirin than in other conditions. It has been generally believed for many years that aspirin may prevent the transmission and integration of painful stimuli at the thalamic level; however, there is no definitive evidence that aspirin has direct effects on central pathways.

Aspirin (acetylsalicylic acid)

Aspirin (acetylsalicylic acid; Fig. 10.6) is a derivative of salicylic acid, which is produced from the glycoside salicin obtained from willow bark. It was introduced into medicine in 1899; since then, it has become one of the cheapest and most widely used drugs in the world.

Aspirin is most commonly used for its analgesic, antipyretic, and anti-inflammatory effects. It is most effective in low intensity somatic pain, rather than severe visceral pain. Most of its analgesic effects are probably related to inhibition of prostaglandin synthesis in peripheral tissues; nevertheless, it may have some central effects (p. 340). Aspirin has little or no effect on normal body temperature, although it characteristically reduces body temperature rapidly in febrile patients. Toxic doses frequently cause hyperthermia accompanied by an increased metabolic rate and raised oxygen consumption, associated with abnormal cellular respiration. The anti-inflammatory actions of aspirin are due to the decreased production of prostaglandins (particularly prostaglandin E_2) by inflammatory cells (p. 339); however, relatively high doses of aspirin are required to produce these effects. In general, daily dosage of 3 g per day or less does not produce sustained anti-inflammatory effects; dosage of 3–6 g per day usually decreases inflammatory responses, but may produce unacceptable side-effects.

Aspirin produces complex effects on acid–base balance. Therapeutic doses of aspirin commonly increase O_2 consumption and CO_2 production; this is mainly due to the uncoupling of oxidative phosphorylation (i.e. the conversion of ADP to ATP and the conservation of energy during cellular respiration). There is usually a compensatory increase in alveolar ventilation so that Pa_{CO_2} tension remains constant. When the plasma concentration of salicylate is higher (e.g. with high dosage or overdosage), a CSF acidosis occurs; this may affect the activity of

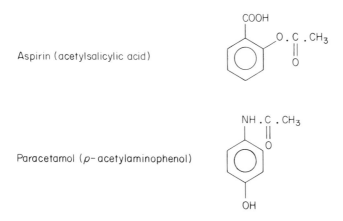

Aspirin (acetylsalicylic acid)

Paracetamol (*p*-acetylaminophenol)

Fig. 10.6 The chemical structure of aspirin and paracetamol.

the medullary centres, producing hyperventilation and respiratory alkalosis. In addition, high concentrations of salicylates directly stimulate the respiratory centre, producing increased ventilation and respiratory alkalosis, with a rise in pH and a fall in $Paco_2$ tension. This may be partially compensated by the increased renal excretion of bicarbonate. Hyperventilation and respiratory alkalosis are common presenting features of aspirin overdosage in adults; terminally, an acidotic state (due to respiratory and metabolic changes) may supervene.

In children, a different clinical picture frequently occurs during aspirin overdosage. Hyperventilation is rare, and the rise in plasma salicylate levels usually depresses the respiratory centre (causing respiratory acidosis). In addition, a true metabolic acidosis develops (due to salicylate dissociation, and the accumulation of lactic and pyruvic acid). These changes are partly due to the uncoupling of oxidative phosphorylation, and partly to vasomotor depression and reduced renal perfusion. Consequently, in childhood aspirin overdosage usually presents as a combination of respiratory and metabolic acidosis.

Aspirin also reduces platelet adhesion and aggregation, due to its effects on prostaglandin production (which indirectly affects the formation of thromboxane by platelets). These effects occur with small single doses (e.g. 150 mg or 300 mg), and may last for as long as 4–7 days. It is believed that aspirin irreversibly acetylates platelet cyclo-oxygenase (Fig. 10.5); consequently, new platelets must be formed from megakaryocytes before normal function is restored. For this reason, aspirin has been widely studied for its possible role in preventing vascular thrombosis. In theory, it should only be of value when the production of thromboxanes and prostacyclin is imbalanced, since these two mediators produce opposing effects on platelets and blood vessels. However, this situation may be present when the vascular endothelium is damaged (e.g. by atheroma). Aspirin is sometimes used after cardiopulmonary bypass surgery to prevent graft occlusion, and may help prevent thrombotic episodes associated with mitral stenosis. In recent years, it has also been used in patients with transient ischaemic attacks, in order to prevent the occurrence of major cerebrovascular embolism or thrombosis. In addition to its effects on platelets, aspirin may also decrease prothrombin synthesis (and possibly that of other clotting factors); however, relatively high doses (more than 3 g per day) may be required to produce hypoprothrombinaemia.

Aspirin may also affect renal function. In low doses (1–2 g per day), it may cause urate retention (due to inhibition of the tubular secretion of urate anions). In high dosage (more than 5 g per day), it is an effective uricosuric agent, since it also inhibits the tubular reabsorption of urates. Unfortunately, these doses usually produce unacceptable side-effects. Aspirin can also produce complex effects on carbohydrate metabolism. In therapeutic doses, it may lower blood glucose (due to increased tissue utilization), and can potentiate the effects of insulin or oral hypoglycaemic agents. Conversely, high doses may cause hyperglycaemia by increasing adrenal cortical and medullary activity.

Unfortunately, the side-effects of aspirin frequently limit its dosage and its therapeutic use. High doses (more than 5–6 g per day) frequently cause the condition of 'salicylism', with confusion, dizziness, nausea and vomiting, tinnitus, deafness, sweating, tachycardia, and hyperventilation. These effects are usually associated with plasma concentrations of $300 \mu g \ ml^{-1}$ or above. In particular, tinnitus may be produced by high therapeutic doses, and may be used as a guide to the plasma concentration of the drug in patients on high-dose aspirin. In addition, aspirin frequently produces gastrointestinal side-effects which limit its dosage (e.g. dyspepsia, gastric erosions, reactivation of peptic ulceration, and gastric bleeding). Approximately 70% of patients on aspirin lose 5–15 ml of blood daily. Occasionally, aspirin causes haematemesis or severe gastrointestinal hae-morrhage, which is probably due to a hypersensitivity reaction. Some of the gastrointestinal effects of aspirin may be related to the inhibition of prostaglandin production (particularly prostacyclin) by gastric mucosal cells. However, physico-chemical factors suggest that high concentrations of acetylsalicylate or salicylate ions may be present in gastric mucosal cells due to non-ionic diffusion and salicylate trapping (see Chapter 1).

Hypersensitivity reactions to aspirin occasionally occur (particularly in atopic individuals with a history of infantile eczema or asthma). These may present as bronchospasm, angio-oedema, skin rashes, or rhinitis; rarely, blood dyscrasias and thrombocytopenia may occur. Drug interactions may occur with oral anti-coagulants or with uricosuric drugs (e.g. probenecid and sulphinpyrazone).

In recent years, it has been suggested that the incidence of Reye's syndrome is commoner in children with febrile illnesses who are given aspirin. Reye's syndrome is a rare condition that produces hepatic damage and encephalopathy, and has a high mortality rate. Consequently, aspirin should not be given to chil-dren under the age of 12 years.

Aspirin poisoning is not uncommon; after aspirin overdosage, patients are usually conscious and the effects on acid–base balance are often an important clinical feature. Gastric lavage may be worthwhile for up to 12 h after over-dosage; in addition, forced alkaline diuresis, using intravenous bicarbonate, may accelerate the renal elimination of salicylates. Haemodialysis and charcoal haemoperfusion may also be of value.

Absorption, distribution and elimination. Aspirin is usually administered orally, and is well absorbed from the gastrointestinal tract. Absorption from the stomach is favoured by the presence of salicylate in a non-ionized form ($pK_a = 3.5$); how-ever, significant amounts may be trapped as salicylate anions in the relatively alkaline mucosal cells (Chapter 1). Absorption from the small intestine is prob-ably more important, due to its larger surface area (Chapter 1).

After absorption, aspirin is rapidly hydrolysed by esterase enzymes in the intestinal mucosa and the liver to salicylate ions; consequently, in the systemic circulation most of the drug is present as salicylate. Both aspirin and salicylate ions are rapidly distributed throughout most tissues, and readily cross most cellular barriers. Binding to plasma proteins occurs; 80–90% is bound to plasma albumin, although the free fraction is increased in patients with hypoalbuminaemia. Salicylates are mainly metabolized in the liver to salicyluric acid, a phenolic glucuronide, and an ester glucuronide. Some steps in the metabolism of salicylates are saturable; in particular, the conversion of salicylate to salicylurate (a glycine conjugate).

The unchanged drug and its metabolites are eliminated by the kidney and their excretion is enhanced by an alkaline urine. The terminal half-life depends on the dosage, since saturation of glycine conjugation occurs; with normal therapeutic doses, the half-life of salicylate is approximately 4–12 h. In drug overdosage, the half-life may increase due to zero-order metabolism, and it can be up to 30 h.

Clinical uses. Aspirin is commonly used for its analgesic and anti-inflammatory effects. It is particularly useful for the non-specific relief of many types of pain of moderate intensity, and for the symptomatic relief of painful conditions associated with inflammatory processes (e.g. rheumatic diseases and musculoskeletal disorders). Its antipyretic effects may provide increased comfort in febrile conditions, but are unlikely to alter the course of the underlying disease.

Aspirin may also be used for its antiplatelet and antithrombotic effects (e.g. in the secondary prevention of myocardial infarction and the prevention of cerebrovascular accidents).

Aspirin is sometimes used in other conditions. Salicylates and related drugs may be used in the management of diarrhoea associated with irradiation of pelvic tumours, or certain bacterial toxins. In these conditions, there may be increased release of prostaglandins from the damaged gut wall. Similarly, certain malignant tumours may synthesize substantial amounts of prostaglandins and their derivatives. These compounds may influence the uptake of metastatic deposits in bone, and the subsequent bone resorption, destruction, and pain. In these conditions, aspirin and related inhibitors of prostaglandin synthesis may be extremely valuable.

Related drugs. In the high dosage required to produce anti-inflammatory effects, aspirin may produce unacceptable and intolerable effects on the gastrointestinal tract. Whenever possible, aspirin should be given in the form of dispersible tablets and dissolved before administration. In addition, various formulations and buffered preparations of aspirin are available. Some of these may increase the pH of gastric juice, and increase the ionization of the parent drug, thus decreasing its absorption from the stomach. The ionized drug dissolves readily in gastric secretions, rapidly passes into the small intestine, and is distributed over the large absorptive surface. Aloxiprin is a polymer of aspirin and aluminium oxide; aspirin is slowly released in the stomach, but more rapidly in the small intestine. Enteric-coated preparations that dissolve in the higher pH of the small intestine are also available (e.g. Nu-Seals). Salsalate is a similar preparation. Benorylate is an ester of aspirin and paracetamol, which is hydrolysed after absorption. These drugs may have an improved gastric tolerance, and a reduced tendency to produce gastrointestinal side-effects.

Sodium salicylate is sometimes used as an anti-inflammatory drug; its properties, mechanism of action, and side-effects are similar to aspirin.

Phenylbutazone and indomethacin

Phenylbutazone and indomethacin have pronounced anti-inflammatory effects (due to inhibition of cyclo-oxygenase). Unfortunately, they are both toxic drugs, and are less effective analgesics than aspirin for pain of non-specific origin. In particular, phenylbutazone produces serious adverse effects (i.e. agranulocytosis and aplastic anaemia); it may also cause sodium retention and precipitate cardiac failure. In the UK, its use is now restricted to hospital practice, and it is only used in the treatment of ankylosing spondylitis. Indomethacin causes headaches and gastrointestinal side-effects; it is less likely to cause blood dyscrasias, and is sometimes used in the treatment of acute gout. Both drugs are extensively bound by plasma proteins, and may be involved in significant drug interactions. Phenylbutazone may also induce or inhibit hepatic enzyme systems. In recent years, the use of both drugs has significantly declined.

Other NSAIDs

In recent years many other NSAIDs have been synthesized and used in the treatment of rheumatic conditions and injuries. All of these drugs inhibit cyclo-oxygenase, and have anti-inflammatory effects; however, most of them are relatively poor analgesics and antipyretics. Many of them were developed as possible alternatives to aspirin, but without its tendency to produce gastrointestinal side-effects (e.g. erosions, bleeding, ulceration, and perforation). However, since their anti-inflammatory effects and gastrointestinal side-effects may both be related to decreased prostaglandin synthesis, they all, to some extent, have these disadvantages. All drugs that decrease the synthesis of prostacyclin by the gastric mucosa may affect the normal balance between gastric acid secretion and mucous production, and may thus be poorly tolerated.

In general, NSAIDs should not be prescribed for patients with a history of peptic ulceration; however, many patients who develop ulcers when given NSAIDs have no previous history of dyspepsia. Complications are much commoner in the over 60s (particularly in women). The incidence of gastrointestinal side-effects may be considerably reduced by the use of histamine (H_2) antagonists. Alternatively, the prostaglandin analogue misoprostol may provide some protection against the development of gastric ulceration in susceptible patients. In addition, NSAIDs should always be taken with food or milk.

Inhibition of prostaglandin synthesis may also cause impairment of renal function. NSAIDs reduce renal blood flow and glomerular filtration rate in some groups of patients, particularly elderly subjects. Other predisposing factors are chronic heart failure, hepatic cirrhosis, hypovolaemia and concurrent treatment with diuretics. NSAIDs may also cause hyperkalaemia and fluid retention. Some of the individual agents are highly protein-bound and can potentiate the action of anticoagulants, hydantoins, lithium, and certain sulphonamides; in addition, various adverse effects such as blood dyscrasias and skin rashes have been reported with their use.

The main differences between individual NSAIDs are concerned with the incidence and the occurrence of side-effects (which in general resemble those produced by aspirin). In addition, there is a marked variability in patient response. In the UK, approximately 15 of these drugs are available; naproxen, ibuprofen, sulindac, azapropazone and diclofenac are among the most commonly used NSAIDs.

Naproxen is an effective anti-inflammatory drug, but has a relatively low incidence of gastrointestinal side-effects. Since it has a relatively long half-life, it can be given twice daily. It is commonly used in the treatment of acute gout.

Ibuprofen is a relatively mild anti-inflammatory drug that produces fewer side-effects than naproxen. Although it is widely used in certain conditions (e.g. in dental pain), it has a low affinity for cyclo-oxygenase, and is not suitable for the management of conditions in which inflammation is a prominent feature (e.g. ankylosing spondylitis).

Sulindac has similar properties to naproxen (although it is closely related chemically to indomethacin). The parent drug is inactive (i.e. it is a prodrug), and only produces slight effects on prostaglandins in the gastrointestinal tract. However, sulindac is metabolized to a sulphide metabolite that is a potent inhibitor of cyclo-oxygenase. It undergoes extensive enterohepatic recirculation, and thus provides a reservoir of the active drug. It is usually given twice daily.

Azapropazone is chemically related to phenylbutazone; however, it does not appear to cause blood dyscrasias (although it may cause skin rashes). It is commonly used in the treatment of acute gout. It is not extensively metabolized, but is eliminated unchanged by the kidney, and may accumulate in renal failure.

Diclofenac is a potent anti-inflammatory drug, and has a greater affinity for cyclo-oxygenase than most other NSAIDs. Consequently, it is most commonly used in treating rheumatic disorders when inflammation is a prominent feature. Unfortunately, it is frequently associated with gastrointestinal side-effects. It has a relatively long duration of action, and may be given by intramuscular injection. Diclofenac has been used in the treatment of renal colic. It is also an effective analgesic when used in the management of postoperative pain; after certain procedures (e.g. tonsillectomy and minor gynaecological surgery) it may eliminate the need for any additional analgesia, and it reduces opiate requirements after major surgery. The use of diclofenac during the perioperative period may well increase in the future.

Paracetamol

Although paracetamol was synthesized more than 100 years ago, it has only been widely used as an analgesic since 1949. Paracetamol has analgesic and antipyretic effects that are similar to aspirin; however, it has little if any anti-inflammatory activity. It has been suggested that it only inhibits prostaglandin synthesis in the CNS; however, it has little effect on cyclo-oxygenase in *in vitro* conditions. Nevertheless, it is usually classified with the NSAIDs, since it has similar effects to aspirin on non-specific pain. Paracetamol is widely used in the treatment of pain of moderate intensity such as headache, toothache, dysmenorrhoea, and pains of musculoskeletal origin. Similarly, it is incorporated into many compound preparations containing aspirin, pentazocine, dextropropoxyphene, or codeine and its derivatives.

Paracetamol is well absorbed from the gastrointestinal tract, and does not cause gastric irritation or bleeding. This is probably related to its low affinity for cyclo-oxygenase, since it also has little effect on platelet activity. Although it is an active metabolite of phenacetin and acetanilide, in normal doses it is relatively free from toxic effects. Occasionally, skin rashes, methaemoglobinaemia, and haemolytic anaemia may occur; in some cases, haematological side-effects may be related to a deficiency of erythrocyte glucose-6-phosphate dehydrogenase.

After absorption, paracetamol is not significantly bound to plasma proteins. It is almost completely metabolized by the liver; approximately 60% is eliminated as a glucuronide conjugate, and the remainder as sulphate and cysteine conjugates. Only trace amounts are eliminated unchanged in urine.

Paracetamol overdosage produces delayed, subacute, liver damage; in the UK, it is involved in approximately 15% of all hospital admissions for drug overdosage (and 7% of all deaths, mainly due to its delayed presentation). Liver damage due to acute overdosage has been reported after the ingestion of as little as 5 g. More commonly, it is produced by more than 10–15 g (i.e. 20–30 tablets) of the drug. Small amounts of paracetamol are metabolized to an aryl metabolite with a high affinity for sulphydryl groups (N-acetyl-p-amino-benzoquinone-imine). After normal doses, this toxic metabolite is innocuous, since it is inactivated by conjugation with hepatic glutathione. In paracetamol overdosage, the hepatic reserves of glutathione (and other –SH donors, e.g. methionine) are conjugated and depleted; in these conditions, the toxic metabolite combines covalently with –SH groups in liver macromolecules, producing subacute hepatic necrosis (Fig. 10.7). If patients are on enzyme-inducing drugs, the risk of sig-

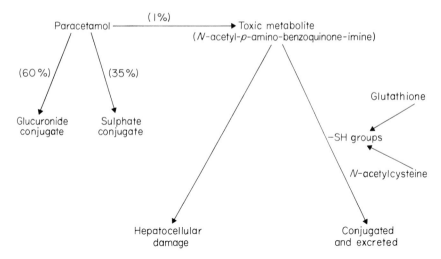

Fig. 10.7 The metabolism of paracetamol. In overdosage, a toxic metabolite produces hepatocellular damage, unless it is conjugated by sulphydryl (–SH) groups.

nificant hepatic damage is considerably greater. Unless specific therapy is given, some degree of centrilobular hepatic necrosis will occur in 10–20% of poisoned patients, and 2–3% will die in hepatic failure. Signs of liver damage are usually delayed for 2–5 days after overdosage; the initial symptoms (e.g. nausea, vomiting, and abdominal pain) may regress, thus engendering a false sense of security.

Immediate treatment is essential in paracetamol overdosage, since sulphydryl donors (e.g. methionine, cysteamine and *N*-acetylcysteine) can conjugate the toxic metabolite and prevent liver damage if given soon after an acute overdose. Treatment includes gastric lavage (if the patient is seen within 4 h of paracetamol ingestion), intravenous fluids, and the cautious use of antiemetics (if there is persistent nausea and vomiting). The sulphydryl donor *N*-acetylcysteine is the treatment of choice; however, it must be given by intravenous infusion within 12–15 hours of ingestion of the drug, since it is ineffective and may be dangerous if given at a later stage. Plasma paracetamol levels are invaluable in the assessment of the severity of overdosage, and provide a guide to the possible effectiveness of treatment with *N*-acetylcysteine. Vitamin K and other clotting factors may be necessary for the management of coagulation defects.

Analgesic nephropathy

Renal papillary necrosis and chronic interstitial nephritis may occur following the prolonged intake of some NSAIDs, particularly compound proprietary analgesic preparations. In the past, phenacetin was frequently implicated as the causative agent; however, nephropathy will probably occur when any analgesic drug

Table 10.10 A chemical classification of simple analgesics and non-steroidal anti-inflammatory drugs.

Enolic acids		Carboxylic acids			
Oxicams	Pyrazolones	Acetic acid derivatives	Fenamates	Salicylates	Propionates
Piroxicam	Phenylbutazone	Diclofenac	Mefenamic acid	Aloxiprin	Fenbufen
	Azapropazone	Etodolac	Flufenamic acid	Aspirin	Fenoprofen
		Indomethacin		Diflunisal	Flurbiprofen
		Sulindac		Salsalate	Ibuprofen
		Tolmetin		Benorylate	Ketoprofen
		Zomepirac			Naproxen
					Tiaprofenic acid

is continually used over a long period of time (hence the term 'analgesic nephropathy'). Renal complications produced by analgesic drugs may be related to impaired synthesis of prostaglandins, since many prostaglandins are produced by the kidney (e.g. PGE_2, which is an important renal vasodilator). After administration of NSAIDs, the response to renal vasoconstrictors (e.g. noradrenaline and angiotensin II) may be enhanced. In practice, analgesic nephropathy is commoner in compulsive drug users who show mild personality disorders, rather than in patients with rheumatic disorders who are on continuous drug therapy. The prognosis is good, and renal function may completely recover if all analgesics are withdrawn.

Nefopam

Nefopam is chemically related to diphenhydramine. Its mode of action is unknown, and it is not usually classified as an opioid or a simple analgesic. It is usually free from opioid side-effects, such as respiratory depression and drug dependence. Nefopam blocks the uptake of noradrenaline by sympathetic nerve endings, and can also produce numerous atropine-like side-effects (such as a dry mouth). However, it may also induce excessive sweating, and its antimuscarinic effects may be mediated within the CNS, rather than peripherally. Nefopam has been successfully used in musculoskeletal and cancer pain.

Specific analgesics

In specific circumstances, many drugs that are not primarily analgesics may be beneficial in the management of pain. Thus, anticholinergic drugs are of value in the treatment of smooth muscle spasms. Similarly, pain which arises due to spasm of striated muscle (e.g. upper motor neurone lesions, spasmodic torticollis, or muscle tension headaches), may be relieved by centrally acting muscle relaxants. These agents, which increase the effectiveness of the inhibitory transmitter γ-aminobutyric acid (GABA), include the benzodiazepines and the GABA agonist baclofen (Chapter 12). Drugs that affect the calibre of blood vessels are also important. Vasodilators will provide symptomatic relief of pain due to ischaemia of somatic or visceral structures; conversely, the ergot alkaloids, which have partial agonist effects on α-receptors in extracranial blood vessels, play an important role in the treatment of migraine.

Some of the chemical excitants of a painful impulse may be inactivated or antagonized by specific drugs. Examples include antacid therapy for peptic ulcer, and the use of 5-hydroxytryptamine antagonists in the prophylaxis of migraine. The hormone calcitonin produces symptomatic relief in patients with Paget's disease, and occasionally in other forms of bone pain; it has been suggested that these effects are related to a translocation of phosphate ions.

Psychotropic drugs are often used as adjuncts in pain therapy. In addition to their action on the reactive components of pain (e.g. anxiety and misery), they may have a more specific effect. Phenothiazines potentiate the effects of opioid analgesics, and may produce analgesia as part of a generalized deafferentation. Tricyclic antidepressants may facilitate transmission in descending fibres that release 5-hydroxytryptamine, which are thought to modify C-fibre input at the substantia gelatinosa.

Treatment of trigeminal neuralgia

In trigeminal neuralgia, the sudden attacks of severe lancinating pain are inadequately managed by conventional analgesic therapy. The aetiology of the condition is unknown, but the paroxysmal nature of the pain suggests that it is a type of focal sensory epilepsy. It is therefore not surprising that several drugs that were originally introduced into clinical practice for the treatment of epilepsy are effective in the condition; their membrane stabilizing activity may be of prime importance (particularly on the spinal trigeminal nucleus).

Carbamazepine is the drug of choice. When taken regularly, it is highly effective in controlling the attacks of pain, and 70% of patients gain relief. The development of drug tolerance may be due to an alteration in its pharmacokinetics, since it is known that carbamazepine induces its own metabolism. Side-effects such as drowsiness and ataxia are common, although these may disappear with continued dosage, and gastrointestinal intolerance may occur; blood dyscrasias are an occasional but more serious problem. Other anticonvulsant agents, such as phenytoin and valproate, are logical alternatives to carbamazepine when unacceptable side-effects are present; however, they are not quite as effective. If the symptoms of trigeminal neuralgia are abolished by a destructive lesion to the

Gasserian ganglion or its appropriate branches, anticonvulsant therapy should be gradually withdrawn, since sudden cessation may induce epileptiform attacks.

Treatment of migraine

Current views suggest that attacks of migraine are caused by the initial release of 5-hydroxytryptamine, which triggers off the cerebral vasoconstriction and the associated prodromal symptoms. Further release of 5-hydroxytryptamine may occur, due to platelet aggregation. The headache corresponds to the phase of dilatation of extracranial vessels; it is probably mediated by the increased production of histamine and plasma kinins, while plasma 5-hydroxytryptamine levels are decreasing.

Acute attacks are managed with NSAIDs; the inhibitory effects on platelet aggregation may be an added advantage. These drugs are often combined with ergot alkaloids, which maintain vessel tone by stimulating α-adrenoceptors. For continuous prophylaxis, drugs which antagonize the peripheral effects of 5-hydroxytryptamine, histamine, and the kinins may be used; these include methysergide, cyproheptadine, and pizotifen. In low dosage, the antihypertensive agent clonidine is also effective, particularly when the attacks are triggered by food containing tyramine. Propranolol is occasionally used in the prophylaxis of migrainous neuralgias and 'atypical' facial pain.

FURTHER READING

Akil H, Watson SJ, Young E, Lewis ME, Khatchturian H, Walker JM. Endogenous opioids: biology and function. *Annual Review of Neuroscience* 1984; **7**: 223–255.

Atweh SF, Kuhar MJ. Autoradiographic localization of opiate receptors in rat brain. I: spinal cord and lower medulla. *Brain Research* 1977; **124**: 53–67.

Atweh SF, Kuhar MJ. Autoradiographic localization of opiate receptors in rat brain. II: the brain stem. *Brain Research* 1977; **129**: 1–12.

Atweh SF, Kuhar MJ. Autoradiographic localization of opiate receptors in rat brain. III: the telencephalon. *Brain Research* 1977; **134**: 393–405.

Behar M, Magora F, Olshwang D, Davidson JT. Epidural morphine in the treatment of pain. *Lancet* 1979; **i**: 527–528.

Bovill JG. The opioids in intravenous anaesthesia. In: Dundee JW, Wyant GM (eds) *Intravenous Anaesthesia*. Edinburgh: Churchill Livingstone, 1988; 206–247.

Brunk SF, Delle M. Morphine metabolism in man. *Clinical Pharmacology and Therapeutics* 1974; **16**: 51–57.

Bullingham RES. Synthetic analgesics. In: Atkinson RS, Adams AP (eds) *Recent Advances in Anaesthesia and Analgesia*, No 15. Edinburgh: Churchill Livingstone, 1985; 43–62.

Carr DB. Opioids. *International Anesthesiology Clinics* 1988; **26**: 273–287.

Carr DB, Murphy MT. Operation, anesthesia, and the endorphin system. *International Anesthesiology Clinics* 1988; **26**: 199–205.

Chadwick HS, Ross BK. Analgesia for post-cesarian delivery pain. In: Oden RV (ed.) *Management of Postoperative Pain Anesthesiology Clinics of North America*. Philadelphia: WB Saunders, 1989; **7**: 133–153.

Duggan AW. Nociception and antinociception: physiological studies in the spinal cord. In: Brena SF, Chapman SL (eds) *Chronic Pain: Management Principles. Clinics in Anaesthesiology.* Philadelphia: WB Saunders, 1985; **3**: 17–40.

Durant PAC, Yaksh TL. Epidural injections of bupivacaine, morphine, fentanyl, lofentanil, and DADL in chronically implanted rats: a pharmacologic and pathologic study. *Anesthesiology* 1986; **64**: 43–53.

Etches RC, Sandler AN, Daley MD. Respiratory depression and spinal opioids. *Canadian Journal of Anaesthesia* 1989; **36**: 165–185.

Finck AD. Opiate receptors and endogenous opioid peptides. In: Current Opinion in Anaesthesiology. *Current Science* 1989; **2**: 428–433.

Fleetwood-Walker S, Mitchell R. Role of Substance P in Nociception. In: Current Opinion in Anaesthesiology. Prys-Roberts C (ed.) *Current Science* 1989; **2**: 645–648.

Gillman MA. Analgesic (sub-anesthetic) nitrous oxide interacts with the endogenous opioid system: a review of the evidence. *Life Science* 1986; **39**: 1209–1221.

Glynn CJ. Intrathecal and epidural administration of opiates. In: Budd K (ed.) *Update in Opioids. Clinical Anaesthesiology.* Edinburgh: Baillière Tindall, 1987; **1**: 915–923.

Goodchild CS, Serrao JM,. Analgesics and the spinal cord dorsal horn. In: Kaufman L (ed.) *Anaesthesia Review*, No 6. Edinburgh: Churchill Livingstone, 1989; 215–229.

Gregg R. Spinal analgesia. In: Oden RV (ed.) *Management of Postoperative Pain. Anesthesiology Clinics of North America.* Philadelphia: WB Saunders, 1989; **7**: 79–100.

Gustafsson LL, Post C, Edvardsen B, Ramsay CH. Distribution of morphine and meperidine after intrathecal administration in rat and mouse. *Anesthesiology* 1985; **63**: 483–489.

Gustafsson LL, Wiesenfeld-Hallin Z. Spinal opioid analgesia. A critical update. *Drugs* 1988; **35**: 597–603.

Hinds CJ, Donaldson MDJ. Endogenous opioids in shock. In: Ledingham IMcA (ed.) *Recent Advances in Critical Care Medicine.* Edinburgh: Churchill Livingstone, 1988; 175–194.

Hug CC Jr, Pharmacokinetics and dynamics of narcotic analgesics. In: Prys-Roberts C. Hug CC Jr (eds) *Pharmacokinetics of Anaesthesia.* Oxford: Blackwell Scientific Publications, 1984; 187–234.

Itzhak Y, Alernand S. Differential regulation of σ and PCP receptors after chronic administration of haloperidol and phencyclidine in mice. *Faseb Journal* 1989; **3**: 1868–1872.

Jordan CC. Opioid receptors. In: Kaufman L (ed.) *Anaesthesia Review*, No. 3. Edinburgh: Churchill Livingstone, 1985; 36–48.

Kaufman L. Pain. In: Kaufman L (ed.) *Anaesthesia Review*, No. 4. Edinburgh: Churchill Livingstone, 1987; 194–206.

Kaufman L. Pain. In: Kaufman L (ed.) *Anaesthesia Review*, No. 6. Edinburgh: Churchill Livingstone, 1989; 203–213.

Konieczko KM, Jones JG, Barrowcliffe MP, Jordan C, Altman DG. Antagonism of morphine-induced respiratory depression with nalmefene. *British Journal of Anaesthesia* 1988; **61**: 318–323.

Mansour A, Khatchaturian H, Lewis ME, Akil H, Watson SJ. Autoradiographic differentiation of mu, delta, and kappa opioid receptors in the rat forebrain and midbrain. *Journal of Neuroscience* 1987; **7**: 2445–2464.

Martin WR, Eades CG, Thompson JA, Huppler RE, Gilbert PE. The effects of morphine- and nalorphine-like drugs in the non-dependent chronic spinal dog. *Journal of Pharmacology and Experimental Therapeutics* 1976; **97**: 517–532.

Melzack R. Hyperstimulation analgesia. In: Brena SF, Chapman SL (eds) *Chronic Pain: Management Principles. Clinics in Anaesthesiology.* Philadelphia; WB Saunders, 1985; **3**: 81–92.

Melzack R, Wall PD. Pain mechanisms: a new theory. *Science* 1965; **150**: 971–979.

Merrell WJ, Gordon L, Wood AJJ, Shay S, Jackson EK, Wood M. The effects of halothane on morphine disposition: relative contributions of the liver and kidney to morphine glucuronidation in the dog. *Anesthesiology* 1990; **72**: 308–314.

Mitchell RWD, Smith G. The control of acute postoperative pain. *British Journal of Anaesthesia* 1989; **63**: 147–158.

Morgan M. Use of intrathecal and extradural opioids. *British Journal of Anaesthesia* 1989; **63**: 165–188.

Nishio Y, Sinatra RS, Kitahata LM, Collins JG. Spinal cord distribution of ^{3}H-morphine after intrathecal administration: relationship to analgesia. *Anesthesia and Analgesia* 1989; **69**: 323–327.

Olson GA, Olson RD, Kastin AJ. Review of endogenous opiates: 1985. *Peptides* 1986; **7**: 907–933.

Olson GA, Olson RD, Kastin AJ. Review of endogenous opiates: 1986. *Peptides* 1987; **8**: 1135–1164.

Pasternak GW. Multiple morphine and enkephalin receptors and the relief of pain. *Journal of the American Medical Association* 1988; **259**: 1362–1367.

Pert CB, Snyder SH. Opiate receptor: demonstration in nervous tissue. *Science* 1973; **179**: 1011–1014.

Pinnock CA. Endorphins. In: Kaufman L (ed.) *Anaesthesia Review*, No. 3. Edinburgh: Churchill Livingstone, 1985; 49–62.

Raja SN, Meyer RA, Campbell JN. Peripheral mechanisms of somatic pain. *Anesthesiology* 1988; **68**: 571–590.

Rance MJ. Multiple opiate receptors — their occurrence and significance. In: Brena SF, Chapman SL (eds) *Chronic Pain: Management Principles. Clinics in Anaesthesiology*. Philadelphia; WB Saunders. 1985; **3**: 183–199.

Rosow C. Newer opioid analgesics and antagonists. In: Fragen RJ (ed.) *New Anesthetic Drugs. Anesthesiology Clinics of North America.* 1988; **6**: 319–333.

Simon EJ, Hiller JM, Edelman I. Stereospecific binding of the potent narcotic analgesic [^{3}H]etorphine to rat-brain homogenate. *Proceedings of the National Academy of Science USA* 1973; **70**: 1947–1949.

Smith AP, Lee NM. Pharmacology of dynorphin. *Annual Review of Pharmacology and Toxicology* 1988; **28**: 123–140.

Smythe DG. Opioid peptides and pain. In: Bullingham RES (ed.) *Opiate Analgesia. Clinics in Anaesthesiology*. Philadelphia; WB Saunders. 1983; **1**: 201–218.

Sorkin LS. Pain pathways and spinal modulation. In: Oden RV (ed.) *Management of Postoperative Pain. Anesthesiology Clinics of North America.* Philadelphia: WB Saunders. 1989; **7**: 17–32.

Staren ED. Cullen ML. Epidural catheter analgesia for the management of postoperative pain. *Surgery, Gynecology and Obstetrics* 1986; **162**: 389–404.

Tempel A, Zukin RS. Neuroanatomical patterns of the μ, σ, and х opioid receptors of rat brain as determined by quantitative *in-vitro* autoradiography. *Proceedings of the National Academy of Science USA* 1987; **84**: 4308–4312.

Terenius L. Stereoscopic interaction between narcotic analgesics and a synaptic plasma membrane fraction of rat cerebral cortex. *Acta Pharmacologica et Toxicologica* 1973; **32**: 317–320.

Thorpe DH. Opiate structure and activity — a guide to understanding the receptor. *Anesthesia and Analgesics* 1984; **63**: 143–151.

Wang JK, Nauss LA, Thomas JE. Pain relief by intrathecally applied morphine in man. *Anesthesiology* 1979; **50**: 149–151.

Woolf CJ. Recent advances in the pathophysiology of acute pain. *British Journal of Anaesthesia* 1989; **63**: 139–146.

Yaksh TL, Al-Rodhan NRF, Mjanger E. Sites of action of opiates in production of analgesia. In: Kaufman L (ed.) *Anaesthesia Review*, No. 5. Edinburgh: Churchill Livingstone, 1988; 254–268.

Yaksh TL, Rudy TA. Analgesia mediated by a direct spinal action of narcotics. *Science* 1976; **192**: 1357–1358.

ELEVEN

Drugs and the Autonomic Nervous System

ANATOMY AND PHYSIOLOGY OF THE AUTONOMIC NERVOUS SYSTEM

Autonomic nerves constitute all the efferent fibres which leave the CNS, apart from those which innervate skeletal muscle, and the system is thus widely distributed throughout the body. In all cases, the autonomic outflow makes synaptic connections with the cell bodies of peripheral neurones; such synapses normally occur in clusters or ganglia. Postganglionic fibres, usually unmyelinated, then innervate the effector organs.

The autonomic nervous system is also known as the visceral or automatic system and in general its activity cannot be influenced by individual will or volition. Cellular functions which are influenced by autonomic transmission include smooth muscle activity in blood vessels and all viscera, the mechanisms of the specialized muscle fibres of the heart and uterus, the secretory role of the salivary, mucus and eccrine sweat glands, and the activity of the adrenal medulla.

Afferent fibres from visceral structures are carried to the CNS usually by major autonomic nerves such as the vagus, splanchnic or pelvic nerves. They are concerned with the mediation of visceral sensation and the regulation of vasomotor and respiratory reflexes. Specialized examples of afferent autonomic fibres arise from the baroreceptors and chemoreceptors in the carotid sinus and the aortic arch; these are important in the control of heart rate, blood pressure and respiratory activity. Autonomic afferent fibres from blood vessels, which transmit pain impulses, may be carried in somatic nerves.

Autonomic reflex activity occurs at a spinal level (as can be demonstrated in animal experiments and observed in man following spinal cord transection), while vital functions such as respiration and the control of blood pressure are mediated via nuclei in the medulla oblongata. However, central integration of autonomic function occurs principally in the hypothalamus. The hypothalamus is itself under regulatory control by the neocortex, has important connections with the limbic system, and exerts a modulatory effect by virtue of efferent pathways to the pituitary gland.

The autonomic nervous system is conveniently divided on anatomical and physiological grounds into two divisions.

Parasympathetic division

The preganglionic outflow of the parasympathetic division is from certain cranial nerves and the sacral region of the spinal cord. The cells of origin of the cranial fibres are in the midbrain and medulla and the axons are contained in the 3rd, 7th, 9th and 10th cranial nerves. The 3rd, 7th and 9th cranial nerves affect ocular accommodation and salivary gland secretion, while the vagus nerve carries fibres to the heart, lungs and bronchi, stomach and upper intestine.

Sacral outflow occurs from the 2nd, 3rd and 4th sacral segments of the spinal cord. These form pelvic plexuses which innervate the distal colon and the rectum, bladder and reproductive organs. Minute ganglia are situated at points of union and in the walls of individual viscera, and postganglionic parasympathetic fibres are thus very short.

In physiological terms, the parasympathetic nervous system is concerned with the conservation and restoration of energy. Thus the heart rate is slowed, the blood pressure falls, and the digestion and absorption of nutrients (plus the excretion of waste material) is facilitated.

Sympathetic division

The cells of origin of this system are located in the lateral horns of the thoracic and upper lumbar segments of the spinal cord. Their axons travel a short distance in the mixed spinal nerves and then branch off as white rami to enter the sympathetic ganglia. These consist of bilateral chains which lie anterolateral to the vertebral bodies and extend from the cervical to the sacral region. The preganglionic fibres which enter the chain may:

1 Make a synaptic connection with a cell body at the same dermatomal level;

2 Traverse to a ganglion at a higher or lower level before forming a synapse (in both (1) and (2) the postganglionic fibres usually return to the adjacent spinal nerve via grey rami); or

3 Emerge through medial branches of the sympathetic chain to synapse with prevertebral ganglia and plexuses in the abdominal cavity.

Some preganglionic fibres which emerge from the lower thoracic segments travel in the greater splanchnic nerve and directly synapse with chromaffin cells in the adrenal medulla.

Experimental studies suggest that an intact sympathetic nervous system, while not essential to life, enables the body to be prepared for 'fear, fight or flight'. Sympathetic responses include increased heart rate and blood pressure, diversion of blood flow from skin and splanchnic vessels to those supplying skeletal muscle,

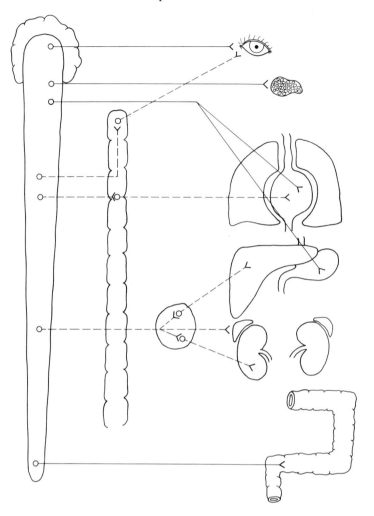

Fig. 11.1   Schematic representation of principal autonomic nerve pathways: ⎯⎯ parasympathetic, ... sympathetic.

an increase in the availability of glucose due to liver glycogenolysis, pupillary and bronchiolar dilatation, and contraction of sphincters.

The principal efferent pathways in the autonomic nervous system are illustrated in Fig. 11.1.

Neurotransmitters

Acetylcholine

This neurotransmitter was synthesized by Baeyer in 1868. In 1914, Dale found that the pharmacological responses to acetylcholine mimicked all the effects of parasympathetic nerve stimulation. The first evidence that neurohumoral transmission occurred was provided by the classical experiments of Otto Loewi in the early 1920s. He stimulated the vagus nerve of a perfused frog's heart and allowed the perfusion fluid to come into contact with a second frog's heart, the rate of which subsequently slowed. He originally called the substance which was released 'Vagustoff', but a few years later it was identified as acetylcholine.

Subsequent investigations showed that acetylcholine was the neurotransmitter released at the following sites:

1 All postganglionic parasympathetic nerve endings.

2 All autonomic ganglia. All preganglionic fibres (sympathetic or parasympathetic) release acetylcholine at their nerve endings; these include the sympathetic fibres which supply the chromaffin cells of the adrenal medulla.

3 Certain postganglionic sympathetic nerves, such as those supplying the sweat glands.

4 Some vasodilator fibres that supply arterioles in skeletal muscle. However, parasympathetic innervation of vascular smooth muscle appears to be limited, and the mechanism of a 'vasovagal' attack may involve both the direct effects of acetylcholine at non-innervated sites and prejunctional inhibitory effects on sympathetic fibres (vide infra). It has also been suggested that acetylcholine may act as an intraneuronal precursor in the release of transmitter at all post-ganglionic sympathetic nerve endings.

In addition, acetylcholine is released at the motor endplate and is an important synaptic transmitter in the CNS.

Nerve fibres that release acetylcholine from their endings are described as cholinergic fibres. The synthesis, storage, release and subsequent fate of acetylcholine is similar at all sites and is more fully described in Chapter 9.

Noradrenaline and adrenaline

In the early years of this century, Langley showed that the actions of an extract of the adrenal gland closely resembled the responses from sympathetic nerve stimulation. He originally suggested that adrenaline was the neurotransmitter involved, although other evidence indicated that the results of stimulation were more accurately mimicked by noradrenaline. Various theories were propounded to explain why injected adrenaline or released 'sympathin' could stimulate some smooth muscle whilst it relaxed others. These included suggestions that the transmitter was modified by receptor substances at the effector site to produce either sympathin I or sympathin E; alternatively it was considered that there were basically two different types of receptors. In the mid-1940s, Von Euler established that noradrenaline was the chemical transmitter released at postganglionic sympathetic nerve endings and that only small quantities of adrenaline (or dopamine) were liberated; such fibres are thus more correctly described as noradrenergic (rather than adrenergic).

Autonomic receptors

Cholinergic receptors

The effects of acetylcholine released from all postganglionic nerve endings (including cholinergic sympathetic fibres) on effector organs can be mimicked by the mushroom alkaloid, muscarine. Such effects have been classically described as 'muscarinic' actions. In clinical practice, the pharmacological effects of para-sympathomimetic agents are mediated via muscarinic receptors; similarly, anti-cholinergic or parasympatholytic agents such as atropine specifically block muscarinic receptors by competitive antagonism.

The cardiovascular responses to muscarinic activity are usually depressant, due to bradycardia and vasodilatation. However, if muscarinic receptors are blocked by adequate doses of atropine, acetylcholine will cause a rise in blood pressure due to stimulation of sympathetic ganglia and the vasoconstrictor and the cardioaccelerator nerves. Release of catecholamines from the adrenal medulla and fasciculation of skeletal muscle will also occur. Similar effects may be produced by administration of the alkaloid nicotine, and postsynaptic receptors in the autonomic ganglia and in the motor endplate have been designated as 'nicotinic'.

Muscarinic receptors

Recent evidence has accumulated from autoradiographic and radioligand binding studies on cholinergic receptors within the CNS, and from observations of the effects of novel muscarinic antagonists (particularly pirenzepine) on lower oesophageal contraction and on gastric acid secretion. This has led to the proposal that at least three subtypes of muscarinic receptors may be present in experimental animals and in man.

M_1-receptors show a high affinity for the antagonists pirenzepine and telenzepine. It was originally considered that M_1-receptors were mainly located at lower oesophageal and gastric sites. Present opinion suggests that M_1-receptors are present in the CNS and in all autonomic ganglia (in addition to the nicotinic receptors). Receptor activation may involve the closure of K^+ channels, or the hydrolysis of phosphatidylinositol bisphosphate (PIP_2) to inositol trisphosphate (IP_3) and diacylglycerol (DAG).

In general, M_1-receptors have facilitatory effects. Although their physiological role is uncertain, they appear to be responsible for the slow depolarization of autonomic ganglion cells during synaptic transmission.

M_2-receptors are present in the myocardium, the cerebellum, and on nerve terminals supplying bronchiolar smooth muscle. They are selectively antagonized by gallamine (and some experimental drugs, e.g. methoctramine and himbucine).

M_2-receptors mainly inhibit the release of noradrenaline from adrenergic nerve terminals (although they may also have a role in the autoregulation of acetylcholine release). Increased acetylcholine release mediated by antagonism at M_2-receptors may be involved in some clinical phenomena (e.g. the initial bradycardia sometimes seen after atropine, bronchoconstriction induced by low dose ipratropium). Experimental evidence suggests that M_2-receptors are coupled to potassium channels, and that the resultant efflux of K^+ leads to membrane hyperpolarization.

M_3-receptors are found at classical postsynaptic sites (e.g. in the smooth muscle of airways and in mucus glands). They are non-selectively antagonized by classical antimuscarinic drugs and selectively antagonized by some experimental drugs (e.g. hexahydrosiladifenidol). When therapeutic doses of atropine or ipratropium are administered, they produce antagonistic effects at M_3-receptors which will overshadow any activity at M_2-receptors. The desired pharmacological result (e.g. antisialogogue activity, bronchodilatation) will thus be achieved. The activation of M_3-receptors is usually coupled to the synthesis of IP_3 and the subsequent mobilization of intracellular calcium ions.

Acetylcholine also produces direct inhibitory effects on vascular smooth muscle. These tissues are not innervated by parasympathetic fibres and the receptor has not been clearly identified. The intracellular mechanism is closely related to production of endothelium derived relaxing factor (EDRF) which has recently been identified as nitric oxide. The enzyme guanylate cyclase is also activated resulting in the intracellular accumulation of cyclic guanosine monophosphate (cGMP).

Table 11.1 Distribution of peripheral acetylcholine receptors, effects produced by their stimulation and intracellular mechanisms postulated (for abbreviations see text).

Type/site of receptor	Pharmacological effects	Intracellular mechanisms
Nicotinic		
Neuromuscular junction	Voluntary muscle contraction	Mobilization of Ca^{2+} from sarcoplasmic reticulum and binding to Troponin C
Autonomic ganglia	Ganglionic transmission (fast channels)	? ↑ cAMP and Ca^{2+} mobilization
Muscarinic		
M_1 (autonomic ganglia)	Ganglionic transmission (slow channels)	Closure of K^+ channels → depolarization
M_2 (prejunctional sites)	Modulation of ACh and ?noradrenaline release	Hyperpolarization of cell membrane due to K^+ efflux
M_3 (postsynaptic)	Smooth muscle contraction (bronchi); SA slowing glandular secretion	Production of IP_3 and mobilization of intracellular Ca^{2+}
Unclassified		
Vascular smooth muscle	Vasodilatation	Production of EDRF and subsequent accumulation of GMP

The distribution of peripheral acetylcholine receptors is summarized in Table 11.1. There is some evidence that intermediary neurones containing purines (ATP-releasing fibres) may also be involved in some aspects of cholinergic transmission.

Noradrenergic receptors

In 1948 Ahlquist compared the relative potencies of six different sympathomimetic agents on a variety of peripheral organ systems and on isolated cardiac and smooth muscle. Contraction of smooth muscle was most marked with adrenaline and least with isoprenaline, while cardiac stimulation and relaxation of smooth muscle was greatest with isoprenaline and least with noradrenaline. On the basis of these studies Ahlquist suggested that there were two types of receptors (thus supporting Langley's original concept), namely the α and β-adrenoceptors. In general terms stimulation of α-receptors produces vasoconstriction, whilst stimulation of β-receptors results in an increase in the force, rate and conduction velocity of the heart, relaxes bronchial and intestinal smooth muscle, and produces vasodilatation.

There are at least two major subgroups of each type of adrenoceptor. In 1967, Lands and his co-workers subdivided the β-receptors on the basis of their differing responses to adrenaline and noradrenaline.

1 β_1-receptors are located in the heart and in the smooth muscle of the intestine, and at these sites adrenaline and noradrenaline have equipotent effects.

2 β_2-receptors are found in bronchial, vascular and uterine smooth muscle and are far more sensitive to the effects of circulating adrenaline than noradrenaline (i.e. β_2-receptors behave as 'hormonal' rather than 'transmitter' receptors).

It has subsequently been shown, using radioligand binding studies, that the myocardium contains both β_1 and β_2-adrenoceptors. They are present in a ratio of $3:1$ in the normal heart. It is thought that β_2-receptors in the myocardium are situated extrajunctionally and act as 'hormonal' receptors. The excess sympathetic drive (principally mediated by noradrenaline) which frequently occurs in heart failure may lead to a downregulation of receptors. In these circumstances β_1-receptors appear to be principally affected, whilst there is a relative sparing of β_2-receptors. It has been shown that in severe heart failure the ratio of β_1 and β_2-receptors may change to $3:2$. The identification of β_2-receptors on lymphocytes has also enabled further study of adrenergic receptors. There is considerable evidence that at many sites β_2-receptors are located presynaptically on the adrenergic neurone; their stimulation appears to promote the release of noradrenaline from the nerve terminal.

Two subgroups of the α-adrenoceptor have also been described. α_1-receptors are those which subserve the classical vasoconstrictor activity from smooth muscle stimulation. Physiological evidence suggests that autoregulation of noradrenaline

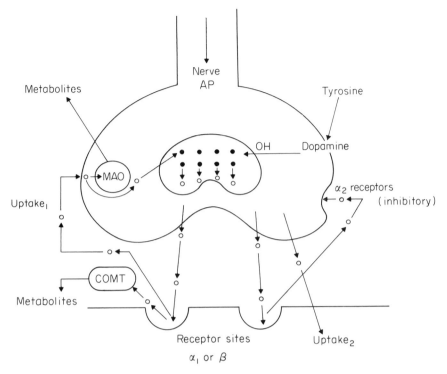

Fig. 11.2 The adrenergic nerve terminal showing the synthesis, release and reuptake of noradrenaline. AP (action potential), ● bound noradrenaline, ○ unbound noradrenaline, MAO (monoamine oxidase), and COMT (catechol-O-methyl transferase).

release occurs at sympathetic nerve endings; noradrenaline is considered to inhibit its own neuronal discharge by an effect mediated on α_2-receptors located at presynaptic sites (Fig. 11.2). A similar ('hormonal') effect at α_2-receptors may be induced by circulating adrenaline.

Studies with radioligands suggest that certain compounds exhibit a selective activity at α_2-receptors, for example clonidine as an agonist and yohimbine as an antagonist. α_2-receptors are also found in platelets (their stimulation results in platelet aggregation) and may exist at other 'hormonally' mediated postsynaptic sites.

It is now generally accepted that the effects of sympathomimetic amines on adrenergic receptors are activated by means of the 'second messenger' system. Stimulation of either β_1 or β_2-receptors on the surface of the cell membrane results in the activation of adenylate cyclase, an enzyme present on the cytoplasmic face of the cell. This acts as a catalyst in the conversion of adenosine triphosphate (ATP) into cyclic adenosine-3,5-monophosphate (cAMP). This mediator subsequently activates a specific protein kinase which leads to phosphorylation of a variety of intracellular proteins. The resultant electrophysiological changes (e.g.

depolarization or hyperpolarization of the cell membrane) and pharmacological effects (e.g. inotropic activity, smooth muscle relaxation) can obviously differ. This may be related to:

1 The nature of the regulatory protein which binds to the enzyme.
2 The type of intracellular protein which undergoes phosphorylation (e.g. troponin C, troponin I, calmodulin, or phospholamban).
3 Subsequent effects on calcium transport and release of intracellular calcium.
4 Possible effects on the cell membrane enzyme Na^+/K^+ ATPase.

Current evidence suggests that the effects mediated via α_1-receptors depend on a different intracellular mechanism. In this case a membrane bound enzyme (phospholipase C) is activated, and hydrolyses PIP_2. IP_3 is subsequently produced and this leads to increased calcium mobilization (and possibly enhanced calcium uptake) in the effector cell.

The effects of stimulation of α_2-adrenoceptors are mediated via a reduction in the activity of cAMP through an inhibitory regulatory protein (Chapter 3).

Dopaminergic receptors

Dopamine is the immediate precursor of noradrenaline and may also stimulate its release from noradrenergic nerve terminals. Dopamine is also an important transmitter within the CNS, and receptors have been located in the basal ganglia, the nigrostriatal pathway and in areas of the anterior and intermediate lobes of the pituitary gland. Two types of dopaminergic receptors, designated D_1 and D_2, have been identified in the CNS; both groups are thought to be located at presynaptic and postsynaptic sites. Activation of D_1-receptors stimulates various hormonal and neurosecretory functions, leading to a modulation of extrapyramidal activity. These effects are induced by an increase in intracellular cAMP probably due to stimulation of adenylate cyclase. Stimulation of D_2-receptors results in inhibition of pituitary hormone output, and modulation of the release of acetylcholine and endorphins within the CNS. The mechanism may involve inhibition of cAMP.

Functional interaction between the two groups of receptors occurs. Alteration of the receptor population may account for the tardive dyskinesia which can occur following the administration of non-selective dopamine agonists in the treatment of parkinsonism.

Two receptors described as DA_1 and DA_2 are found at peripheral sites and may be identical to their CNS counterparts. DA_1-receptors are found in renal and mesenteric vascular smooth muscle; agonist effects lead to an increase in intracellular cAMP content and subsequent vasodilatation. DA_2-receptors appear to be inhibitory autoreceptors and also inhibit the release of noradrenaline from certain postganglionic sympathetic sites.

Table 11.2 Subtypes of peripheral adrenoceptors, principal pharmacological effects and probable intracellular mechanisms involved (for abbreviations see text).

Type of receptor	Principal effects	Intracellular mechanisms
β_1	Positive inotropic and chronotropic	$\uparrow$ cAMP availability $\rightarrow$ phosphorylation of phospholamban and $\uparrow$ Ca^{2+} mobilization
β_2	Relaxation of smooth muscle	$\uparrow$ cAMP availability $\rightarrow$ increase in cell membrane Na^+/K^+ ATPase activity (?phosphorylation of Troponin I in myocardium)
α_1	Contraction of smooth muscle	Activation of phospholipase C $\rightarrow$ production of IP_3 and subsequent $\uparrow$ Ca^{2+} turnover and binding to calmodulin
α_2	Presynaptic inhibition of adrenergic neurone	$\downarrow$ cAMP availability
DA_1	Relaxation of renal vascular and mesenteric smooth muscle	$\downarrow$ cAMP availability and membrane stabilization from effects on Na^+/K^+ ATPase
DA_2	Presynaptic inhibition of dopamine and noradrenaline release	? $\downarrow$ cAMP availability

The subtypes of peripheral adrenergic receptors are summarized in Table 11.2, whilst their involvement in different sympathetic responses is shown in Table 11.3.

AUTONOMIC DRUGS

Drugs may affect autonomic function in a number of ways:

1 By mimicking or modifying the action of the neurotransmitter on the effector organ.

2 By effects on ganglionic transmission or on release of the appropriate transmitter.

3 By modifying central integration of autonomic activity.

4 Occasionally, by an effect on afferent autonomic input. For example the veratrum alkaloids, which were used in the early years of the 20th Century in the treatment of eclampsia and were among the original group of drugs used in the treatment of essential hypertension, appeared to induce their cardio-vascular depressive responses through stimulation of chemoreceptor sensory mechanisms.

Table 11.3 Types of receptors involved in differing sympathetic responses

Tissue/organ	Response	Receptor type
Vascular smooth muscle		
Skin	Constriction	α_1
Muscle	Dilatation or	β_2
	constriction	α_1
Splanchnic	Dilatation or	β_2, DA_1
	constriction	α_1
Renal	Dilatation or	β_2, DA_1
	constriction	α_1
Other smooth muscle		
Bronchial	Relaxation	β_2
Intestinal	Relaxation	α_1, β_2
Sphincters	Contraction	α
Uterine	Relaxation	β_2
Other effects		
Heart	Increase in rate contractility and conduction velocity	Mainly β_1 (also β_2 + ?α and DA_1)
Renin secretion by kidney	Increased	β_1
Liver glycogenolysis	Stimulation	β_2, α
Lipolysis	Stimulation	β_1, α

DA_1 = dopamine receptors; where α only is cited, the subtype has not been definitely identified.

Parasympathomimetic agents

Acetylcholine

The widespread effects and evanescent action of acetylcholine preclude its systemic administration, although it has been used historically to induce convulsions in the treatment of schizophrenia. It may be employed as a topical agent in ophthalmology when a rapid miosis is required.

Synthetic choline esters

These are more stable compounds than the parent drug, and may exhibit a more selective action at certain muscarinic sites. Methacholine is only hydrolysed slowly by cholinesterases; it has been used to decrease the heart rate in cases of supraventricular tachycardia and occasionally as a vasodilator in peripheral vascular disorders. Carbachol and the related compound bethanechol are resistant to enzymatic destruction and have been used in the treatment of postoperative atony of the bladder and the gut, and as locally acting miotics in the treatment of glaucoma.

Naturally occurring cholinomimetic alkaloids

These include muscarine (which is found in various wild mushrooms), arecoline (a constituent of the betel nut), and pilocarpine (an extract of certain South American shrubs) which is employed as a miotic.

Anticholinesterase drugs

These agents may be subdivided into:
1 Carbamate esters (reversible or acid-transferring inhibitors).
2 Organophosphorus compounds, with potentially irreversible effects.

By inhibiting enzymatic degradation of acetylcholine, anticholinesterases will allow accumulation of the neurotransmitter at all its peripheral sites of liberation. In addition the non-polar compounds (e.g. physostigmine, and most organophosphorus substances) may induce significant CNS activity. The nicotinic effects of this group of compounds are essentially dose-related. Thus, the carbamates are used therapeutically to reverse the effects of competitive muscle relaxants and to improve neuromuscular function in myasthenia gravis and related conditions. Conversely, overdosage of the 'reversible' agents, or inadvertent systemic uptake of organophosphorus compounds, can lead to muscular weakness or even paralysis.

Carbamate esters are also employed for their autonomic effects. They may be used for the treatment of paralytic ileus and atony of the urinary bladder; distigmine, which is a combination of two molecules of pyridostigmine and has a relatively long duration of action, is particularly useful in this context. These agents may also be administered by topical instillation in the management of glaucoma. Ecothiopate, a quaternary ammonium organophosphorus compound, has also been used as a miotic but has now been withdrawn in the UK. The anticholinesterase agents are further discussed in Chapter 9.

ANTAGONISTS OF PARASYMPATHOMIMETIC ACTIVITY

Several naturally occurring and synthetic compounds competitively antagonize the muscarinic effects of acetylcholine and other parasympathomimetic drugs. Their principal site of action is at effector organs innervated by postganglionic parasympathetic fibres, although some members of the group may inhibit ganglionic transmission or have significant CNS activity. Pharmacological effects at the neuromuscular junction are not significant, although in experimental studies high doses of atropine have been shown to inhibit depolarization of the motor endplate.

Naturally occurring antagonists

These compounds are organic esters which are derived from solanaceous plants and are chemically related to cocaine; an aromatic acid (tropic acid) is combined with a complex base (tropine or scopine) to form atropine or hyoscine respectively.

Atropine

This drug has been used in anaesthetic practice for many years both for pre-medication and to antagonize the muscarinic effects from the administration of anticholinesterase drugs; these aspects are considered more fully in the appropriate chapters (9 and 12). Atropine is sometimes employed topically as a mydriatic in the treatment of iritis and choroiditis; the effects may last up to 2 weeks and profound cycloplegia (paralysis of accommodation) occurs. Atropine is frequently administered with narcotic analgesics in the treatment of biliary and renal colic, in the hope that smooth muscle relaxation will contribute to pain relief. Likewise, it has been used in the management of acute pancreatitis to reduce the volume and tryptic activity of pancreatic secretion, and thus produce an analgesic effect. There is little evidence that such measures are of value. The use of atropine is indicated in myocardial infarction where there is bradycardia associated with hypotension or where the prolonged AV conduction results in ventricular 'escape' and multiple extrasystoles ensue.

Atropine is a specific antidote in the treatment of mushroom poisoning caused by the alkaloid muscarine; it is also a valuable agent in the management of organophosphorus poisoning.

Therapeutic doses of atropine can produce slight stimulation of the CNS, and larger doses give rise to excitement, hallucinations, and hyperpyrexia (although in the untreated case respiratory depression and coma will supervene). Children are most frequently affected by atropine poisoning as they may accidentally consume 'deadly nightshade' berries. Treatment may include gastric lavage, methods to reduce body temperature, the administration of physostigmine and the use of controlled ventilation.

Hyoscine

In contrast to atropine, hyoscine produces a depressant effect on the CNS when administered in therapeutic doses. The amnesic property may be advantageous when hyoscine is used in combination with morphine to induce 'twilight sleep', or when it is given by intravenous injection after clamping of the cord to minimize awareness during obstetric anaesthesia. When used in anaesthetic practice, hyoscine appears to induce less tachycardia than an equipotent dose of atropine; it also has greater antisialogogue activity and more pronounced ocular effects. However, the administration of hyoscine may lead to undue excitation or confusion in elderly patients.

Hyoscine is of proven value when used prophylactically in the management of motion sickness and other vestibular disorders. The mechanism of action probably involves inhibition of cholinergic pathways from the labyrinthine apparatus to the medullary centres.

Atropine and hyoscine were the first drugs that were available for the treatment of Parkinson's disease. The imbalance of cholinergic/dopaminergic activity within the CNS was corrected, and tremor and rigidity were particularly benefited. In more recent years drugs which effectively improve dopaminergic transmission, such as levodopa and bromocriptine, have been developed, and found to be more beneficial in alleviating the akinesia (immobility) associated with parkinsonism. However, in patients who are intolerant of the side-effects of dopaminergic agents, and particularly in drug-induced parkinsonism, anticholinergic drugs may still be valuable.

Synthetic antagonists

Benzhexol (Artane) which appears to produce less peripheral antimuscarinic side-effects than atropine, is commonly used as an antiparkinsonian agent. Homatropine has a shorter duration of action than atropine when applied locally, and is preferred as a mydriatic when diagnostic examination of the eye is necessary.

Many synthetic and semi-synthetic drugs have been developed as antispasmodics for the management of various gastrointestinal and genitourinary disorders. They differ from the parent drug in that they are quaternary amines; they are poorly absorbed from the gut and do not effectively cross the blood–brain barrier. They also show some affinity for ganglionic (nicotinic) receptors and may abolish the effects of sympathetic nerve activity on muscle tone, particularly in the sphincters. Drugs in this group include propantheline, dicyclomine and ipratropium; the last compound is a common constituent of inhalant mixtures used in the treatment of bronchospasm. A similar drug, glycopyrrolate, may confer a number of advantages when used in premedication prior to anaesthesia and during the reversal of neuromuscular blockade. It appears to be devoid of any CNS effects and placental transfer is not significant. It is an effective antisialogogue with a long duration of action; changes in heart rate and pupillary size appear to be minimal.

Pirenzepine, which demonstrates a high affinity for M_1-receptors, has been developed for the treatment of peptic ulceration; pirenzepine appears to reduce gastric acid secretion and prevent reflux without other significant antimuscarinic effects. The varying affinities of anticholinergic drugs for the three types of receptors at both central and peripheral sites may help to explain the different clinical responses observed when equipotent doses of atropine and hyoscine are used.

SYMPATHOMIMETIC AGENTS

Endogenous substances

Adrenaline, noradrenaline and dopamine are the sympathomimetic amines which exist in the body as neurotransmitters. The synthesis of adrenaline from the amino acid phenylalanine *in vivo* has been demonstrated using radiolabelled techniques, and the pathway involved in this process also leads to the formation of dopamine and noradrenaline (Fig. 11.3). As 3,4-dihydroxybenzene is also known as catechol, these three substances are commonly referred to as catecholamines.

Adrenaline

Adrenaline is considered to have only a minor role in the conduction of peripheral autonomic impulses. However, adrenaline is the major constituent (80–90%) of the adrenal medulla in adults and may produce 'hormonally' mediated effects on both α_2 and β_2-receptors. Furthermore, adrenaline is an important neurotransmitter within the CNS.

The physiological responses to an infusion of adrenaline are mediated via both α and β-receptors. The heart rate, force of contraction and conduction velocity are invariably increased, and arrhythmias are likely. The systolic blood pressure is elevated, but depending on the dose and rate of administration there may be a fall in diastolic pressure due to effects mediated via β_2-receptors on splanchnic and muscle blood vessels. At higher dose levels, effects at α-receptors at these sites will predominate and peripheral resistance will be increased. In all instances skin blood flow will be reduced. Coronary arterioles will be dilated as a consequence of the metabolic changes brought about by the increased work of the heart. This effect will overshadow the responses mediated through α-receptors in the coronary vascular smooth muscle.

The systemic uses of adrenaline are limited. However, it may be employed as the first-line approach in the treatment of status asthmaticus or anaphylactic shock; 0.5 mg of adrenaline, administered subcutaneously or intramuscularly, is recommended. Following cardiac arrest, 5–10 ml of a 1 in 10 000 solution of adrenaline may be given intravenously or by the intratracheal route when there is ECG evidence of asystole, or when fine fibrillation (high frequency, low amplitude waves) needs to be coarsened prior to DC cardioversion.

Adrenaline is commonly incorporated into local anaesthetic solutions in con-

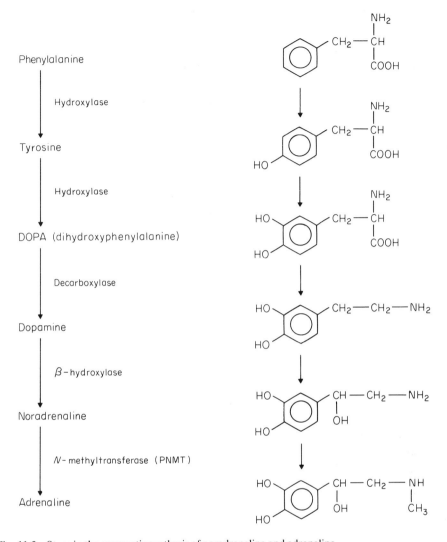

Fig. 11.3 Steps in the enzymatic synthesis of noradrenaline and adrenaline.

centrations varying from 1 in 80 000 (12.5 μg ml^{-1}) to 1 in 200 000 (5 μg ml^{-1}). The vasoconstrictor effect will diminish local blood flow and decrease the rate of absorption of the local anaesthetic agent, thus prolonging its pharmacological action and reducing systemic toxicity.

Adrenaline may also be used as a local decongestant or as a topical haemostat, and is also found in various proprietary mixtures used for bronchodilator therapy. Adrenaline eye-drops may be of value in the treatment of wide-angle glaucoma, where the vasoconstrictor effect will reduce the secretion of aqueous humour.

Noradrenaline

The effects of noradrenaline are exerted almost exclusively via α-receptors. Peripheral resistance and both systolic and diastolic blood pressure are raised due to generalized vasoconstriction. Although noradrenaline has direct effects on the heart, these are usually obscured by baroreceptor responses (mediated via the vagus nerve) to the increase in blood pressure. In consequence the heart is little affected, although slight bradycardia may occur.

Noradrenaline infusions were formerly used in the treatment of hypotensive 'shock' states. Blood pressure levels were maintained at the expense of reduced tissue perfusion, and the state of shock actually worsened; furthermore, extravasation of the infusion into the tissues often produced severe necrosis.

Noradrenaline was also employed as a vasoconstrictor in local anaesthetic solutions; this is no longer recommended as severe and occasionally fatal pressor responses have been associated with its use.

Dopamine

Dopamine has developed a role as an inotropic agent in the treatment of low output states associated with renal insufficiency; clinical indications for its use include endotoxic or cardiogenic shock, refractory congestive cardiac failure, and the support of the circulation following cardiac surgery. Dopamine is administered by continuous infusion; when a low dose regime ($1-2 \mu g \ kg^{-1} \ min^{-1}$) is employed, renal blood flow is enhanced and urinary output increased due to a direct effect on the renal vasculature. With higher dose levels ($2-10 \mu g \ kg^{-1} \ min^{-1}$) cardiac output is improved due to an effect mediated via β-receptors. In these circumstances, dopamine is considered to have a more specific effect on the force of contraction (inotropic) than the heart rate (chronotropic), although tachycardia can sometimes be a problem, particularly in underhydrated patients. If the rate of infusion is further increased, α-receptor effects may supervene and lead to profound vasoconstriction and a decreased renal blood flow; arrhythmias are also likely.

Replenishment of dopamine stores in the CNS is a logical approach to the treatment of parkinsonism. Dopamine does not effectively cross the blood–brain barrier; its precursor, levodopa is usually prescribed, and may be used in combination with a dopa-decarboxylase inhibitor (carbidopa or benserazide) to minimize side-effects such as nausea, vomiting and cardiac arrhythmias which may occur due to the formation of extracerebral dopamine. Other drugs which may be used to increase dopaminergic activity within the CNS include bromocriptine (which has analogous effects), amantidine (which stimulates the release of dopamine presynaptically), and selegiline (which selectively inhibits the principal enzyme (MAO_B) concerned in the destruction of dopamine at central sites).

Exogenous substances acting principally via β-receptors

Isoprenaline

Isoprenaline is a synthetic catecholamine which has a powerful action on β-receptors. Following infusion of isoprenaline both heart rate and cardiac output are increased; there does not appear to be a selective inotropic effect and arrhythmias are likely. There is a fall in peripheral resistance, but renal blood flow is not specifically increased as with dopamine; furthermore, coronary perfusion may be embarrassed because of a tachycardia and a reduced diastolic blood pressure.

Isoprenaline infusions $(0.5-10\,\mu g\,min^{-1})$ are sometimes used in the management of 'shock' although dopamine is usually preferred. Isoprenaline is of more value in the management of bradyarrhythmias, and particularly in Stokes–Adams attacks.

Isoprenaline exhibits a powerful bronchodilator effect and has been administered by sublingual routes and as an inhalant in the treatment of bronchospasm. However, the excessive use of isoprenaline inhalers has been associated with an increased incidence of sudden death in asthmatic patients. This has been assumed to be due to the cardiotoxicity of isoprenaline (although the effects of the propellant have sometimes been implicated); safer drugs are now available.

Selective β₂-agonists

These agents were developed primarily for their use in bronchial asthma. They are relatively specific for β₂-receptors and normally have little effect on the heart. Tachycardia and palpitations may occur occasionally, and were previously thought to be compensatory mechanisms following β₂-vasodilatation. Present evidence would indicate that a direct action on the myocardium may be involved. Such effects may be enhanced in heart failure when there is a relative preponderance of β₂-receptors.

Salbutamol is available as an oral preparation, an injection form, and as a nebulized solution. Salbutamol may be given intravenously as a bolus dose $(250\,\mu g$ repeated 4-hourly if necessary) or by continuous infusion $(3-20\,\mu g$ $min^{-1})$ in the treatment of severe bronchospasm. Alternatively, salbutamol may be administered as a 'respirator' solution either intermittently $(5\,mg\,ml^{-1})$ or continuously $(50-100\,\mu g\,ml^{-1})$ through a suitably driven nebulizer in severe asthmatic states. Closely related drugs include terbutaline, isoetharine, isoxsuprine and ritodrine.

β₂-agonists will relax uterine smooth muscle, and may be administered by continuous infusion to delay delivery in premature labour. Isoxsuprine is occasionally employed as a cerebral or peripheral vasodilator. β₂-agonists will cross the blood–brain barrier and central side-effects, including tremor and nervous tension, are associated with their use.

β_2-agonists may cause hypokalaemia. The mechanism involved is likely to be a stimulation of membrane bound Na^+/K^+ ATPase which is linked to the receptor.

Exogenous substances acting via α-receptors

Phenylephrine

This has a close structural relationship to the endogenous catecholamines and exhibits pharmacological effects which resemble those of noradrenaline. Phenylephrine may be employed as a mydriatic or as a topical decongestant; it may also be incorporated into local anaesthetic solutions as a vasoconstrictor.

Methoxamine

Methoxamine has similar effects mediated via α-receptors. It is of proven value when administered intravenously (2–10 mg) in the management of untoward hypotension occurring during anaesthesia, particularly following subarachnoid or extradural blockade or when ganglion-blocking drugs have been employed. Metaraminol is an alternative drug of choice in this context.

α_2-adrenoceptor agonists

Drugs with significant α_2-agonist activity, such as clonidine and α-methyldopa (via its active metabolite α-methylnoradrenaline) have been used in the treatment of hypertension. Their principal therapeutic effects appear to be mediated via α_2-adrenoceptors which inhibit vasomotor responses in the medulla oblongata. More selective α_2-agonists include azepexole and dexmedetomidine. Such agents may eventually achieve significance in anaesthetic practice. They appear to have significant hypnotic properties and reduce the MAC requirements of certain inhalational agents. Such effects are presumably due to inhibition of central adrenergic pathways. Furthermore, their peripheral actions at presynaptic receptors could prove valuable in the attenuation of reflex sympathetic responses which may occur during anaesthesia.

Exogenous synthetic agents with a mixed effect on receptors

Ephedrine

Ephedrine occurs naturally in various plants but can also be synthesized. The drug exhibits both α and β (β_1 and β_2) effects and its pharmacological actions are partly dependent on the displacement of noradrenaline from sympathetic nerve endings, and partly due to direct stimulation of receptors. Ephedrine may also inhibit the action of monoamine oxidase on the metabolism of noradrenaline. Tachyphylaxis will occur with the continuous use of ephedrine due to depletion of noradrenergic stores.

Ephedrine readily crosses the blood–brain barrier, and is employed for its effects on the CNS in the management of narcolepsy and nocturnal enuresis. It is still occasionally used in the treatment of bronchospasm and in the management of arrhythmias associated with AV conduction defects. Ephedrine is usually preferred to methoxamine for the management of hypotensive complications which may occur during obstetric anaesthesia and analgesia, as the combined α and β_2-effects are less likely to compromise placental perfusion and subsequent fetal oxygenation. However, ephedrine is more likely to cross the placental barrier.

Amphetamine and related compounds, such as methylphenidate and phentermine, which may be used as analeptics or anorectics, have a peripheral action which resembles that of ephedrine. Fenfluramine, which unlike these agents is not subject to abuse and is thus free from controlled drug regulations, is often used as an appetite suppressant. Drug interactions have been reported in patients who are also receiving MAOIs or various antihypertensive agents and dangerous arrhythmias have been described when halothane has been administered to patients who are also taking fenfluramine.

Miscellaneous agents

Aminophylline

Aminophylline, a mixture of theophylline and ethylenediamine, is a methylxanthine derivative. Although it is not strictly speaking a sympathomimetic amine it is a potent inhibitor of the enzyme phosphodiesterase, and many of its pharmacological effects appear to be due to the accumulation of intracellular cAMP. Other modes of action which may have some import include a reduction in the translocation of calcium ions, blockade of adenosine receptors, effects on the release and subsequent availability of catecholamines and potentiation of prostaglandin synthetase activity.

Aminophylline is a highly effective bronchodilator, and was the drug of choice for the treatment of severe bronchospasm before the advent of the β_2-selective agonists. Aminophylline has both inotropic and chronotropic effects on the heart and has often been used in the treatment of asthma when the distinction between a respiratory or cardiac cause was not clear cut.

Aminophylline may be given by slow intravenous injection (250–500 mg over 20 min) or as an infusion 500 µg kg^{-1} h^{-1}). Tachyarrhythmias may occur, and nausea, vomiting and other gastrointestinal disturbances are sometimes encountered. At high dose levels convulsions may be induced and plasma levels should be monitored during such therapy. Aminophylline is also of value when administered prior to anaesthesia as a slow-release oral preparation or in suppository form, or as a prophylactic measure in patients with a history of bronchospasm.

Ergot alkaloids

Ergotamine has more than 300 times the affinity of noradrenaline for α-receptors and initially acts as a partial agonist to induce direct stimulation of smooth muscle. Prolonged administration of ergot alkaloids can produce symptoms of vascular insufficiency and may lead to gangrene of the extremities; marked CNS effects, including headache, loss of consciousness and convulsions, may also occur. Endemic episodes of ergotism ('St Anthony's fire') have resulted following the ingestion of rye bread manufactured from grain infected with the ergot fungus.

The agonist effect is followed by α-adrenoceptor blockade, but this is of little therapeutic value. The principal use of ergotamine is in the treatment of an acute attack of migraine. Some of the beneficial effects may be also due to an interaction with 5-HT receptors. Ergometrine, which has powerful oxytocic activity, and is used in obstetrics to control postpartum bleeding, has considerably less effect on vascular smooth muscle (either as a partial agonist or as an antagonist) than ergotamine; however, the drug should be administered with special care to hypertensive patients or those with pre-existing cardiac disease.

Drugs used as inotropic agents

The use of dopamine and isoprenaline in this context has been discussed previously. Digitalis and related glycosides also produce a positive inotropic effect. This appears to be principally due to direct inhibition of membrane bound Na^+/K^+ ATPase (with subsequent effects on calcium mobilization) combined with enhancement of vagal activity on the myocardium. Digitalis is discussed more fully in Chapter 14.

Dobutamine

This is a synthetic catecholamine which resembles dopamine. It is also used in the treatment of 'shock' states which result in a low cardiac output; dobutamine appears to have a more selective inotropic action than dopamine, and thus leads to less increase in myocardial oxygen requirements. Unlike dopamine, it does not appear to have any effect on the renal vasculature and does not directly increase urinary output.

Dobutamine has a very short plasma half-life due to rapid metabolism in the liver to inactive conjugates. The drug must therefore be administered by continuous intravenous infusion; the normal dose range which is required is $2.5-10\,\mu g\ kg^{-1}\ min^{-1}$.

Dobutamine is frequently infused in combination with 'renal' doses of dopamine in low cardiac output states. More recently, there has been a reappraisal of the use of supplementary noradrenaline infusions in hypotensive patients who are unresponsive to plasma expansion and dopamine alone. It would appear that when relatively low doses $(0.5-1.5\,\mu g\ kg^{-1}\ min^{-1})$ of noradrenaline are used, excessive vasoconstriction is not a problem and that there are no deleterious effects on renal function.

Dopexamine

Dopexamine hydrochloride, an analogue of dopamine, is a potent β_2-agonist and also acts on peripheral dopaminergic (DA_1) receptors. In contrast to dopamine it lacks α and β_1-agonist activity. Dopexamine exerts a positive inotropic effect, presumably due to effects on cardiac β_2-adrenoceptors. Clinical trials of dopexamine in patients with cardiac failure have proved inconclusive.

Enoximone

Enoximone belongs to the imidazole group of cardioactive compounds. The mode of action of this drug has not been precisely defined, but is considered to be principally mediated by inhibition of the enzyme phosphodiesterase, thus increasing the availability of cAMP. The intracellular concentration of calcium ions in the myocardium is enhanced, whilst calcium uptake into the sarcoplasmic reticulum is also promoted. In peripheral vascular smooth muscle, the increase in cAMP induces vasodilatation.

Enoximone would thus appear to be a positive inotropic agent, but with the additional benefits of a decrease in systemic vascular resistance and more efficient ventricular wall relaxation during diastole (due to increased calcium binding). Consequently, the administration of enoximone does not lead to a significant increase in myocardial oxygen requirements.

Enoximone has been used in the treatment of congestive cardiac failure which has proved refractory to other therapies (e.g. ACE inhibitors). It is administered by slow intravenous injection or by infusion; the solution provided in the ampoules must be diluted beforehand and mixing performed in plastic syringes or infusion containers as crystal formation has been observed when glass apparatus is used. The drug is principally eliminated by the kidney as a sulphoxide metabolite; the elimination half-lives of both the parent drug and the metabolite are approximately 20 times greater in patients with congestive cardiac failure than in healthy volunteers.

Sustained haemodynamic and clinical benefits have been observed in patients treated for up to 48 h, but as yet there is no conclusive evidence of a reduction in mortality. Furthermore, the use of enoximone has been associated with a significant number of side-effects which include tachyarrhythmias, hypotension, nausea and vomiting, fever, oliguria, and limb pain.

Milrinone, a dipyridine derivative with similar properties to those of enoximone, has recently been introduced as an inotropic agent.

Xamoterol

This drug, which was recently introduced into clinical practice, is a partial agonist at β_1-adrenoceptors. Clinical responses to this agent are dependent on the resting sympathetic tone. Thus xamoterol appears to exert a moderate inotropic effect at rest, but during exercise can partly attenuate the β-adrenergic response. Xamoterol has been used in patients with mild to moderate chronic heart failure due to ischaemic disease, and where there is no evidence of sympathetic overactivity xamoterol augments myocardial contractility, and reduces left ventricular filling pressure. Myocardial relaxation during diastole is enhanced and there is no increase in resting oxygen consumption. However, the use of this drug is absolutely contraindicated in more severe forms of cardiac failure when sympathetic 'drive' is presumed to be high, and the depressant effects of the drug will supervene. In these circumstances, xamoterol reduces cardiac output and can precipitate cardiac failure.

Xamoterol does not exhibit any significant β_2-agonist activity and tachyphylaxis is not associated with the continued use of the drug.

Glucagon

Glucagon is a polypeptide which is secreted by the α-cells of the pancreatic islets. The positive inotropic effects were first described in 1960. The effects on adenylate cyclase with subsequent cAMP production and intracellular calcium mobilization are similar to those of catecholamines, although a different receptor may be involved. Glucagon is still used occasionally when an inotropic action is required following cardiac surgery, or in heart failure complicating acute myocardial infarction. Glucagon appears to be relatively ineffective in congestive cardiac failure. Hyperglycaemia and hyperkalaemia are likely problems during its use.

ANTAGONISTS OF SYMPATHETIC ACTIVITY

Centrally acting agents

There is little doubt that the activity of central catecholamine containing neurones will determine peripheral sympathetic responses. For example, the tricyclic antidepressant drugs which effectively increase the availability of noradrenaline within the CNS by inhibiting neuronal uptake may produce manifestations of overactivity at peripheral sites, including excessive sweating (which is mediated via cholinergic sympathetic fibres). Conversely, there is evidence that the cardio-accelerator and vasomotor areas in the medulla oblongata are under modulatory control by α_2-receptors. The antihypertensive properties of both α-methyldopa and clonidine are considered to be due to agonistic effects on centrally situated receptors.

Ganglion-blocking agents

Drugs in this group were initially believed to act as competitive antagonists of the effects of acetylcholine on postsynaptic ('nicotinic') receptors in autonomic ganglia. Originally used in the treatment of essential hypertension, initial members of the group included tetraethylammonium chloride and salts of the bisquaternary ammonium compound hexamethonium (C6); at a later stage secondary (mecamylamine) and tertiary (pempidine) amines were introduced. Current evidence suggests that they block ion channels in the postsynaptic membrane.

Marked disadvantages associated with the use of these compounds included irregular absorption following oral administration, postural hypotension and numerous side-effects (e.g. cycloplegia, intestinal ileus and disturbances of sexual function) due to the indiscriminate blockade of both sympathetic and parasympathetic ganglia.

They are no longer used as antihypertensive agents in the UK. However, the related compound, trimetaphan, is used to produce controlled hypotension in surgery, in the treatment of hypertensive crises and in the management of autonomic hyperreflexia associated with spinal cord injuries.

Drugs that affect postganglionic sympathetic nerve endings

In sympathetic nerve terminals, dopamine and recirculating noradrenaline are taken up from the cytoplasm into storage vesicles by active transport mechanisms. In the vesicles, these catecholamines mainly exist in a bound form and are linked to various proteins described as chromogranins. One type of chromogranin contains the enzyme dopamine β-hydroxylase which catalyses the conversion of dopamine to noradrenaline. The arrival of an action potential at the nerve terminal causes the release of noradrenaline into the synaptic gap when it acts on the receptor of the appropriate effector organ (Fig. 11.2). As mentioned previously, the released noradrenaline may inhibit further output from the nerve terminal by an effect on α_2-receptors located at presynaptic sites. The subsequent fate of the noradrenaline which has been discharged into the synaptic gap involves two alternative mechanisms:

1 Re-uptake into the neurone (Uptake$_1$) where some of the noradrenaline is inactivated by the enzyme monoamine oxidase, while the remainder is transported back into the storage vesicles.

2 Uptake into extraneuronal tissues (Uptake$_2$); noradrenaline is then metabolized chiefly by the enzyme catechol-*O*-methyl-transferase. Both enzymes involved are widely distributed throughout the body and the metabolism of noradrenaline will eventually involve two pathways as shown in Fig. 11.4.

Urinary metabolites include *O*-methylnoradrenaline and *O*-methyladrenaline (resulting from the conversion of adrenaline by COMT), small amounts of which are conjugated as sulphates and glucuronides. 3-methoxy-4-hydroxymandelic acid (VMA) and 3-methoxy-4-hydroxyphenylethylene glycol (MHPG) can also be recovered from urine and changes in urinary MHPG levels may reflect differing activity within the CNS, where it is the major metabolite of noradrenaline. Drugs which are classified as adrenergic neurone blocking agents are thought to act by interfering with the storage of intraneuronal catecholamines. Reserpine appears to inhibit the transport of noradrenaline (and its precursor dopamine) from the cytoplasm into the storage granules. The action of guanethidine and its analogues (bethanidine, debrisoquine) is probably more complex. They may act partially as 'false transmitters' and also prevent storage of noradrenaline by competing

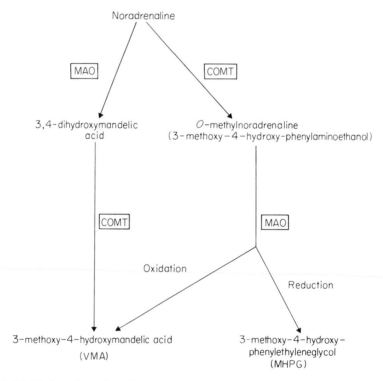

Fig. 11.4 Metabolism of noradrenaline.

for granular binding sites. Guanethidine requires active transport for neuronal uptake; the pathway involved appears to be identical to that required for the reuptake of noradrenaline. This provides further evidence for the pharmacological action of guanethidine, and explains why its own effects are antagonized in the presence of drugs which block $Uptake_1$ mechanisms (e.g. phenothiazines, tricyclic antidepressants). Drugs of this type are still employed as antihypertensive agents and this role is discussed more fully in Chapter 13.

Adrenoceptor blocking agents

α-receptor antagonists

This group of drugs will bind selectively to α-adrenergic receptors and inhibit the sympathetic responses involved at these sites. However they show considerable variation with regard to their affinity for the two subgroups involved. Those agents which indiscriminately block both $α_1$ and $α_2$-receptors (e.g. phentolamine, tolazoline) will facilitate the further release of noradrenaline. As only α-receptors are blocked, there will be an enhanced response to the circulating catecholamines mediated via β-receptors and tachycardias are likely; postural hypotension may also be a problem. Such drugs are thus of little use in lowering the blood pressure of patients with essential hypertension, but are of some value in the control of secondary hypertension due to a high level of circulating catecholamines. In particular, phentolamine is a useful drug for the management of hypertensive episodes associated with surgical removal of a phaeochromocytoma, and is occasionally employed to ablate the sympathetic responses to anaesthesia and surgery which may occur in uncontrolled hypertensive patients.

Phenoxybenzamine exhibits a more selective $α_1$-blockade. A covalent linkage is formed with the receptor and the effects of a single dose of this agent can last for several days. Phenoxybenzamine is used in the preoperative preparation of patients with phaeochromocytoma and in the long-term management when surgery is precluded. At one time it was employed (usually in combination with an inotropic agent such as dopamine) to improve peripheral perfusion in 'shock' states. Neuroleptic agents (e.g. phenothiazines, butyrophenones) have significant α-blocking activity and have sometimes been used in a similar context.

Prazosin appears to be relatively devoid of $α_2$-blocking activity and has been developed as an antihypertensive agent; prazosin has also been used in the management of urinary outflow obstruction. Yohimbine is a selective $α_2$-antagonist and has been shown experimentally to block the hypotensive responses to clonidine.

β-receptor antagonists

In recent years, many agents with β-blocking properties have been introduced into clinical practice for the treatment of cardiovascular disorders. The prototype,

Table 11.4 Properties of β-adrenoceptor antagonists.

Drug	Cardio-selectivity	Partial agonist activity	Membrane stabilizing effect	Lipid solubility
Acebutolol	±	+	+	Moderate
Atenolol	+	−	−	Low
Betaxolol	+	−	+	Moderate
Bisoprolol	+	−	−	Low
Esmolol	+	−	−	High
Labetalol*	−	±	+	High
Metoprolol	+	−	±	High
Nadolol	−	−	−	Low
Oxprenolol	−	+	+	High
Penbutolol	−	+	+	Moderate
Pindolol	−	++	±	Moderate
Propranolol	−	−	++	High
Sotalol	−	−	−	Low
Timolol	−	+	+	High

* A combined α and β-adrenoceptor antagonist. −, absent; ±, minimal; +, present; ++, marked.

dichlorisoprenaline, was not used clinically as it produced considerable partial agonist effects prior to blockade of the receptors. The closely related compound, pronethalol, was developed commercially as an antiarrhythmic and antianginal agent, but was later withdrawn when teratogenic effects had been observed following prolonged administration to mice. Propranolol, which differs chemically from the two aforementioned agents in that it has an oxymethylene ($-O-CH_2-$) bridge between the benzene ring and the ethanolamine side-chain, was then undergoing clinical trials. Propranolol and other analogues have subsequently been developed commercially and are identified in Table 11.4.

Pharmacological properties

The varying members of this group of drugs may differ with respect to three distinct pharmacological actions:

1 *Cardioselectivity.* The majority of these agents, including propranolol, oxprenolol and alprenolol, are non-selective antagonists of both β_1 and β_2-receptors. β_2-receptor blockade will account for the principal undesirable effects associated with the use of these drugs, notably bronchospasm in susceptible individuals and symptoms of peripheral vascular insufficiency; in addition β_2-receptor activity mediates the secretion of insulin following a glucose load and potentiation of the effects of hypoglycaemic agents may occur when these drugs are used concurrently. Relatively specific β_1-antagonists, such as atenolol and acebutolol, are usually preferred when therapy is required in patients with bronchial asthma, insulin-dependent diabetes and peripheral vascular disorders, although cardio-selectivity should be regarded as a relative and a dose-dependent phenomenon.

2 *Intrinsic sympathomimetic activity.* Some of these drugs (e.g. acebutolol and pindolol) display a partial agonist effect as well as antagonistic activity at β-adrenoceptors. In theory, they should be less likely to induce severe bradyarrhythmias or to induce cardiac failure. However, the significance of this property in clinical practice is less clear, although drugs with a much greater partial agonist effect (e.g. xamoterol) have been introduced and used in the treatment of mild to moderate cardiac failure.

3 *Local anaesthetic effect.* Some of the drugs in this group can decrease the rate of depolarization and increase the refractory period of cardiac muscle; this is a membrane stabilizing or local anaesthetic effect. However, this property is observed with β-blockers only at doses 100 times the therapeutic range.

Pharmacokinetic properties

The degree of lipid or water solubility is the most important determinant of the subsequent pharmacokinetic behaviour of the β-adrenoceptor antagonists. In general terms, lipid-soluble β-blockers (e.g. propranolol and metoprolol) are well absorbed following oral administration but are subject to a considerable 'first-pass' effect due to hepatic metabolism. Thus the bioavailability of such drugs is susceptible to a number of factors including pharmacogenetic influences, liver disease and concomitant therapy with other drugs. Subsequently, drugs in this category usually have a short elimination half-life and are subject to wide variations in their plasma levels. Transfer across the blood–brain barrier is also more easily attained and such agents are more likely to induce side-effects such as sedation and bizarre dreams.

In contrast, water-soluble and relatively lipophobic agents (e.g. atenolol, nadolol) are less well absorbed from the gut, but are unlikely to be subject to first pass effects in the liver. They are usually eliminated unchanged by the kidney, and thus have considerably longer plasma half-lives, so that less frequent dosage regimes are required. They are relatively impermeable to the blood–brain barrier and in consequence, CNS effects are unlikely.

Clinical uses

β-receptor antagonists have developed a widespread role in the treatment of hypertension and in the management of angina pectoris and of certain cardiac arrhythmias. In almost all cases the therapeutic benefits achieved are due to blockade of β_1-receptors.

Hypertension. β-adrenoceptor antagonists are now regarded as 'first-line' therapy in the treatment of essential hypertension. However the mechanism of this anti-hypertensive action is not entirely clear and may involve:
1   A reduction in cardiac output.
2   A resetting of baroreceptor activity at a lower blood pressure level.
3   Inhibition of the renin–angiotensin–aldosterone system.
4   An effect on plasma volume.
5   Presynaptic inhibition of noradrenaline release.
6   A CNS effect by those compounds which can effectively traverse the blood–brain barrier.
    Present opinion suggests that the therapeutic benefits achieved in hypertension relate principally to the reduction in cardiac output and to the inhibition of renin release. This topic is also discussed in Chapter 13.

Angina pectoris. The use of β-receptor antagonists in the prophylaxis of attacks of exertional angina is logical. The negative inotropic effect reduces the work of the heart, whilst the concomitant slowing of the cardiac rate effectively improves coronary perfusion; furthermore the effect of lowering the blood pressure will reduce the cardiac 'afterload'. Similar pharmacological mechanisms also underlie the numerous trials of various β-blocking agents for the prevention of reinfarction and the reduction of mortality following myocardial infarction.
    However, not all the effects of β-receptor antagonists in this context can be considered to be beneficial. The lowering of the heart rate and the decrease in contractility will lead to a prolongation of the systolic ejection time with a result-ant increase in the left ventricular end-diastolic volume; oxygen consumption may therefore be greater. In those cases in which the attacks of angina are primarily due to spasm of the coronary vasculature ('Prinzmetal's angina') the administra-tion of β-blockers can actually worsen the symptoms, as the unopposed effects mediated via the α-receptors will further reduce coronary perfusion. Finally, there is a danger that these agents may precipitate heart failure in patients with a poor cardiac reserve.

Arrhythmias. β-receptor antagonists are defined as class II antiarrhythmic agents. These agents prevent the increase in the rate of diastolic (phase 4) depolarization which is induced by catecholamines and decrease the rate of spontaneous firing of the SA node in the presence of excess sympathetic activity; of considerable therapeutic import is the increase in the effective refractory period of the AV node which results from blockade of β-receptor activity.
    β-receptor antagonists are thus particularly useful in the management of

tachyarrhythmias related to abnormal catecholamine activity such as those induced by exercise, emotion or thyrotoxicosis. They may also be used in the treatment of dysrhythmias induced by cardiac glycosides; conversely propranolol is sometimes used in association with digoxin to control the ventricular rate in the presence of atrial fibrillation or flutter.

Other less common uses of β-receptor antagonists include the control of the peripheral responses to stress, the management of pathological anxiety states, the prophylaxis of migraine and the treatment of schizophrenia. β-blocking agents are also used as topical preparations in the treatment of chronic simple glaucoma. Intraocular pressure is reduced by a mechanism which is not entirely clear but probably involves a reduction in the rate of production of aqueous humour.

β-receptor antagonists in anaesthetic practice

β-blocking agents have been employed in the preoperative preparation and intra-operative management of patients undergoing cardiac or vascular procedures, surgery for the removal of a phaeochromocytoma, thyroidectomy, and in the prevention of dysrhythmias which may occur during dental extractions under general anaesthesia. They may also be used to minimize reflex tachycardia during induced hypotension with ganglion-blocking agents (e.g. trimetaphan). Trimetaphan may release histamine, and its use in combination with a non-cardioselective β-blocker can accentuate the risk of bronchospasm. A β-receptor antagonist may also be used to suppress the dysrhythmias observed during induced hypothermia.

Those patients who are on established therapy with β-adrenoceptor antagonists should continue to receive their medication until a few hours prior to surgery and should recommence treatment as soon as is practical in the postoperative period. Acute withdrawal of such therapy may cause ventricular dysrhythmias, severe angina, myocardial infarction and even sudden death. Furthermore, pretreatment with β-blockers prior to surgery and anaesthesia has been advised for patients with uncontrolled or inadequately treated hypertension. Such an approach may considerably modify the pressor responses which can occur, particularly during induction of anaesthesia and endotracheal intubation. Conversely, excessive β-blockade during anaesthesia can produce its own complications of bradyar-rhythmias and hypotension; the administration of atropine and occasionally the use of a β-receptor agonist such as isoprenaline may be necessary.

FURTHER READING

Adgey AA Jennifer, Geddes JS, Mulholland HC *et al.* Incidence, significance and management of early bradyarrhythmia complicating acute myocardial infarction. *Lancet* 1968; **ii**: 1097–1101.

Ahlquist RP. A study of adrenotropic receptors. *American Journal of Physiology* 1948; **153**: 586–600.

Ask JL, Stene-Larsen G, Helle KB, Resch F. Functional β_1 and β_2 receptors in the human myocardium. *Acta Physiologica Scandinavica* 1985; **123**: 81–88.

Barger G, Dale HH. Chemical structure and sympathomimetic action of amines. *Journal of Physiology* (London) 1910; **41**: 19–59.

Barnett DB. Myocardial β-adrenoceptor function and regulation in heart failure: implications for therapy. *British Journal of Clinical Pharmacology* 1989; **27**: 527–538.

Breckenridge A. Which beta-blocker? *British Medical Journal* 1987; **286**: 1085–1088.

Burn JH, Rand MJ. Sympathetic postganglionic mechanisms. *Nature* (London) 1959; **184**: 163–165.

Chamberlain DA, Williams JH. Immediate care of cardiac emergencies. *Anaesthesia* 1976; **31**: 758–763.

Cohen LH, Thale T, Tissenbaum MJ. Acetylcholine treatment of schizophrenia. *Archives of Neurology and Psychiatry* 1944; **51**: 171–175.

Dale HH. The action of certain esters and ethers of choline, and their relation to muscarine. *Journal of Pharmacology and Experimental Therapeutics* 1914; **6**: 147–190.

DeJong W, Zandberg P, Bohus PH. Central inhibitory noradrenergic cardiovascular control. *Progress in Brain Research* 1975; **42**: 285–298.

Desjars P, Pinaud M, Bugnon D, Tasseau F. Norepinephrine has no deleterious renal effects in human septic shock. *Critical Care Medicine* 1989; **17**: 426–429.

Farah AE, Tuttle R. Studies on the pharmacology of glucagon. *Journal of Pharmacology and Experimental Therapeutics* 1960; **129**: 49–55.

Föex P. Beta-blockade in anaesthesia. *Journal of Clinical and Hospital Pharmacy* 1983; **8**: 183–190.

Furchgott RF. The role of endothelium in the responses of vascular smooth muscle to drugs. *Annual Review of Pharmacology and Toxicology* 1984; **24**: 175–197.

Goldberg LI. Dopamine — clinical uses of an endogenous catecholamine. *New England Medical Journal* 1974; **291**: 707–710.

Grant WM. Action of drugs on movements of ocular fluids. *Annual Review of Pharmacology* 1969; **9**: 85–94.

Greenberg MJ, Pines A. Pressurised aerosols in asthma. *British Medical Journal* 1967; **1**: 563.

Gurin S, Delluva A. The biological synthesis of radioactive adrenalin from phenylephrine. *Journal of Biology and Chemistry* 1947; **170**: 545–550.

Hammer R, Giachetti A. Muscarinic receptor subtypes; biochemical and functional characterisation. *Life Sciences* 1982; **31**: 2992–2998.

Jewitt J, Birkhead J, Mitchell A, Dollery C. Clinical cardiovascular pharmacology of dobutamine. *Lancet* 1974; **ii**: 363–367.

Kebabian JW, Agui T, van Oene JC *et al.* The D_1 dopamine receptor: new perspectives. *Trends in Pharmacological Sciences* 1986; **7**: 96–99.

Lands AM, Arnold A, McAuliff JP *et al.* Differentiation of receptor systems activated by sympathomimetic amines. *Nature* 1967; **214**: 597–598.

Lands AM, Luduena FP, Buzzo HJ. Differentiation of receptors responsive to isoproterenol. *Life Sciences* 1967; **6**: 2241–2249.

Langer SZ. Presynaptic receptors and their role in the regulation of transmitter release. *British Journal of Pharmacology* 1977; **60**: 481–497.

Langer SZ, Hicks PE. Physiology of the sympathetic nerve ending. *British Journal of Anaesthesia*. 1984; **56**: 689–700.

Langley JN. On the reaction of cells and of nerve-endings to certain poisons, chiefly as regards the reaction of striated muscles to nicotine and to curare. *Journal of Physiology* (London) 1905; **33**: 374–413.

Leff SE, Creese I. Dopamine receptors re-explained. *Trends in Pharmacological Sciences* 1983; **4**: 483–487.

Lewis RV, McDevitt DG. Adverse reactions and interactions with beta-adrenoceptor blocking drugs. *Medical Toxicology* 1986; **1**: 343–361.

Loewi O, Navratil P. Über humorale Übertragbarkeit der Herznervenwirkung. X. Mitterling. Über das Schicksal des Vagusstoffs. *Pflügers Archiv für die gesamte Physiologie* 1926; **214**: 678–688.

Maclagan J, Barnes PJ. Muscarinic pharmacology of the airways. *Trends in Pharmacological Sciences* (Supplement IV) 1989; **10**: 88S–92S.

Mitchell JR, Oates JA. Guanethidine and related agents I. Mechanisms of the selective blockade of adrenergic neurones and its antagonism by drugs. *Journal of Pharmacology and Experimental Therapeutics* 1970; **172**: 100–107.

Moncada S, Radomski MW. Endothelium derived relaxing factor. Identification as nitric oxide and role in the control of vascular tone and platelet function. *Biochemical Pharmacology* 1988; **37**: 2495–2502.

Okospki JV. Recent advances in pharmaceutical chemistry—review III. A new wave of beta-blockers. *Journal of Clinical Pharmacy and Therapeutics* 1987; **12**: 369–388.

Parker JO, West RO, Digiori S. Haemodynamic effects of propranolol in coronary heart disease. *American Journal of Cardiology* 1968; **21**: 11–19.

Powell CE, Slater IH. Blocking of inhibitory adrenergic receptors by a dichloro analogue of isoproterenol. *Journal of Pharmacology and Experimental Therapeutics* 1958; **122**: 480–488.

Prys-Roberts C. Developments in adrenergic receptor pharmacology and their relevance to anaesthesia. *Current Opinion in Anaesthesiology* 1990; **3**: 89–97.

Putney JW Jr. Calcium mobilising receptors. *Trends in Pharmacological Sciences* 1987; **8**: 481–485.

Rhoden KJ, Meldrum LA, Barnes PJ. Inhibition of cholinergic neurotransmission in human airways by beta$_2$-adrenoceptors. *Journal of Applied Physiology* 1988; **65**: 700–705.

Rosenblum R. Physiological basis for the therapeutic use of catecholamines. *American Heart Journal* 1974; **87**: 527–530.

Sen G, Bose KC. Rauwolfia Serpentina, a new Indian drug for insanity and high blood pressure. *Indian Medical World* 1931; **2**: 194–201.

Smith LDR, Oldershaw PJ. Inotropic and vasopressor agents. *British Journal of Anaesthesia* 1984; **56**: 767–780.

Snow HM. The pharmacology of xamoterol: a basis for modulation of the autonomic control of the heart. *British Journal of Clinical Pharmacology* 1989; **28**: 3S–13S

Speizer FE, Doll R, Strang LG. Investigation into use of drugs preceding death from asthma. *British Medical Journal* 1968; **1**: 339–343.

Starke K. Regulation of noradrenaline release by presynaptic receptor systems. *Review of Physiology, Biochemistry and Pharmacology* 1977; **77**: 1–124.

Stoof JF, Kebabian JW. Dopaminergic receptors. *Life Sciences* 1984; **35**: 2281–2296.

Sutherland EW, Rall TW. The relation of adenosine-3′5′ phosphate and phosphorylase to the actions of catecholamines and other hormones. *Pharmacological Reviews* 1959; **12**: 265–269.

Symposium (various authors). Subtypes of muscarinic receptors. Hirschowitz BI, Hammer R, Giachetti A, Keirns JJ, Levine RR (eds) *Trends in Pharmacological Sciences* 1984; (Suppl 1): 1–103.

Von Euler US. A specific sympathomimetic ergone in adrenergic nerve fibres (sympathin) and its relations to adrenaline and nor-adrenaline. *Acta Physiologica Scandinavica*. 1946; **12**: 73–97.

Weiner N. Multiple factors regulating the release of norepinephrine consequent to nerve stimulation. *Federation Proceedings* 1979a; **38**: 2193–2202.

Whyte KF, Addis GJ, Whitesmith R, Reid JF. The mechanism of salbutamol-induced hypokalaemia. *British Journal of Clinical Pharmacology* 1987; **23**: 65–71.

Wilmshurst P. Phosphodiesterase inhibitors. *Current Opinions in Anaesthesiology* 1989; **2**: 83–87.

Yaksh TL. Pharmacology of spinal adrenergic systems which modulate spinal nociceptive processing. *Pharmacology, Biochemistry and Behaviour* 1985; **22**: 845–848.

Yeo J, Southwell P, Hindmarsh E. Preliminary report on the effect of distigmine on the neurogenic bladder. *Medical Journal of Australia* 1973; **1**: 116–120

TWELVE

Drugs used in Premedication and Antiemetic Agents

The principal aims of premedication are usually considered to be:

1　The reduction of fear and anxiety.

2　The suppression of unwanted autonomic activity (particularly certain parasympathetic responses).

3　The prevention or diminution of undesirable effects produced by the administration of anaesthetic agents.

DEVELOPMENT OF PREMEDICATION

For many years opioid analgesics were routinely used as premedicant drugs. Their sedative and analgesic effects had considerable advantages in facilitating the induction and maintenance of anaesthesia in the era prior to the introduction of intravenous barbiturates, neuromuscular blocking agents, and potent inhalational anaesthetics.

Nevertheless, there are several disadvantages associated with opioid premedication:

1　Dysphoria may occur in the absence of preoperative pain.

2　Gastric emptying time is prolonged, and nausea and vomiting may occur.

3　Interaction with other CNS depressants may be undesirable.

4　There may be difficulty in timing drug administration to produce an optimal effect during routine operating lists.

5　Parenteral administration is usually essential.

Opioid analgesics are less widely used for premedication in present-day anaesthetic practice, but are still a valuable choice in small children; in these conditions, parenteral administration is usually necessary, and some 'hangover' analgesia into the postoperative period is particularly desirable. Morphine ($0.25\,\text{mg kg}^{-1}$) or pethidine ($1\,\text{mg kg}^{-1}$) are commonly used and may be administered with atropine ($0.02\,\text{mg kg}^{-1}$ up to a maximum dose of $0.6\,\text{mg}$) by intramuscular injection 30–45 min prior to surgery. Some anaesthetists consider that the 'twilight sleep' induced by a combination of papaveretum (Omnopon; $20\,\text{mg}$)

and hyoscine (scopolamine; 0.4 mg) (adult doses) confers marked advantages when used as premedication prior to cardiac surgery.

At one time, preanaesthetic sedation or basal narcosis was induced by the rectal administration of powerful CNS depressants during the preoperative period. The agents used included tribromethyl alcohol (bromethol; 'Avertin'), paraldehyde, or thiopentone sodium suspension, in large doses (approximately 45 mg kg^{-1}). This method was considered to be particularly useful in uncooperative children, or in patients with uncontrolled thyrotoxicosis ('stealing the thyroid'). However, there is the likelihood of profound depression of vital reflexes and delayed recovery from anaesthesia, and the technique is now considered obsolete. Similarly, the use of orally administered barbiturates as hypnotics or preoperative sedatives has declined. Barbiturates potentiate the CNS effects of anaesthetic agents, and increased restlessness in the presence of pain may be anticipated.

In recent years, benzodiazepine tranquillizers have been widely used for premedication (particularly in adult patients). They may be used as night hypnotics (i.e. to promote drowsiness and sleep), or administered during the day to produce sedation (a state conducive to sleep) or anxiolysis (the reduction of fear, anxiety, and apprehension). Benzodiazepines have a low toxicity and do not affect the pain threshold; drug interactions, or potentiation of other agents administered during anaesthesia, are of little practical significance.

GENERAL HAZARDS OF HYPNOTIC AND PREMEDICANT DRUGS

Some potential hazards and side-effects are common to all hypnotic and sedative drugs, including those that are commonly used as agents for premedication. All hypnotic drugs characteristically impair judgement and increase reaction time; ambulant patients should always be warned of their hazards in relation to car driving, working at heights, and operating dangerous machinery. Even short-acting hypnotics may impair psychomotor performance or produce hangover effects on the day after their administration. In normal dosage, currently used hypnotic drugs do not usually affect respiration (except, perhaps, in elderly patients with impaired respiratory function). Nevertheless, hypnotic overdosage (particularly with barbiturates and their derivatives) is classically associated with severe respiratory depression. All hypnotic drugs may interact with other central depressants, including ethyl alcohol. Some hypnotic drugs (e.g. the barbiturates and dichloralphenazone) are enzyme-inducing agents, and may potentially interact with other drugs (e.g. oral anticoagulants, antidepressants, anticonvulsants, and contraceptives). The elimination of all hypnotics may be compromised in hepatic and/or renal impairment, and in patients over 60 years old. In general, hypnotics are poorly tolerated by elderly patients, and drowsiness, disorientation and unsteadiness may result in slurred speech, falls and fractures, poor memory, and acute confusional states. The increased susceptibility of elderly patients is partly due to pharmacokinetic factors (i.e. decreased hepatic oxidative drug metabolism), and partly to enhanced sensitivity at neuronal sites in the CNS. All hypnotic drugs may also induce tolerance and drug dependence, and they may alter the pattern of physiological sleep. During their administration, the intensity and duration of stage 3, stage 4, and REM sleep (rapid eye movement sleep or 'dreaming sleep') is reduced. When the hypnotic is stopped, a rebound phenomenon occurs, and there is subsequent compensation for the earlier loss of REM sleep. This is sometimes associated with unpleasant dreams and nightmares due to more intense REM mentation. Since the function of non-REM sleep is unknown, the significance of these changes is a matter of conjecture.

BENZODIAZEPINES

Benzodiazepines are the most commonly prescribed drugs in the Western world; in the UK alone, there may be three million chronic users of these agents. They have significant advantages compared with the barbiturates, which they have largely replaced as hypnotics, sedatives, tranquillizers, and premedicant agents. They are less dangerous in overdosage; they are less likely to interact with other drugs (apart from other hypnotic drugs); and their side effects are less frequent. Nevertheless, performance of psychomotor skills, such as driving a car, may be impaired; and the potentiation of the effects of other CNS depressants, such as ethyl alcohol, may be a problem. At present 19 benzodiazepines are currently available in the UK as hypnotics, sedatives, or tranquillizers (Table 12.1), and some of them are widely used as premedicants. Although their pharmacological actions are similar, there are significant differences in their pharmacokinetics.

Mode of action

Benzodiazepines are generally considered to produce sedation and hypnosis by depressing the excitability of the limbic system. This loosely defined area of the brain consists of the hippocampus, the septal region, the amygdaloid nuclei, and part of the cerebral cortex and the hypothalamus, and is believed to be concerned with the integration of emotional responses. Consequently, benzodiazepines generally produce:

1 Modification of emotional responsiveness and behaviour, due to suppression of neuronal activity between the limbic system and the hypothalamus.

2 A decrease in alertness and arousal reactions, since interaction between the limbic system and the reticular activating system is depressed.

3 Anticonvulsant properties, probably due to effects on the amygdaloid nuclei.

4 Suppression of polysynaptic reflexes in the spinal cord.

Table 12.1 Relative potencies, terminal half-lives, and active metabolites of benzodiazepines currently available as hypnotics or sedatives in the UK.

	Approximate normal hypnotic or sedative dose (mg)	Approximate potency	Terminal half-life of parent drug (h)	Active metabolites	Half-lives of significant active metabolites (h)
Hypnotics					
Flunitrazepam	1	30	12–20	Yes	25–30
Flurazepam	30	1	2–3	Yes	50–100
Lormetazepam	2	15	8–12	No	
Loprazolam	2	15	6–8	Yes	6–8
Nitrazepam	10	3	18–34	Doubtful	
Temazepam	20	1.5	4–10	No‡	
Triazolam	0.25	120	1–3	Yes	3–5
Midazolam	10	3	1–3	No	
Sedatives					
Alprazolam	0.5	60	10–12	Yes	†
Bromazepam	6	5	8–19	Yes	†
Chlordiazepoxide	20	1.5	5–30	Yes	6–25 50–120
Clobazam	20	1.5	10–30	Yes	35–45
Clorazepate	15	2	*	Yes	50–120
Diazepam	10	3	24–48	Yes	4–10 6–25 50–120
Ketazolam	15	2	*	Yes	50–120
Lorazepam	1	30	10–20	No	
Medazepam	10	3	1–2	Yes	50–120
Oxazepam	30	1	6–25	No	
Prazepam	20	1.5	*	Yes	50–120

* Clorazepate, ketazolam, and prazepam are rapidly metabolized in the gut or the liver to desmethyldiazepam.

† Alprazolam and bromazepam have active metabolites, but they are probably not clinically significant.

‡ Minor amounts of temazepam (about 2–5%) may be metabolized to oxazepam.

Benzodiazepines may be regarded as centrally acting muscle relaxants.

Although initial electrophysiological studies demonstrated that benzodiazepines depressed the reticular activating system, recent neurochemical evidence suggests that they produce more widespread effects by facilitating inhibitory transmission mediated by GABA (γ-aminobutyric acid). Benzodiazepines also decrease dopamine and 5-hydroxytryptamine turnover in specific brain regions, and the increase in noradrenaline turnover induced by stress is prevented. It is now believed that these changes represent indirect and secondary effects on brain metabolism. Benzodiazepines appear to act at specific receptor sites in the CNS (although these are not particularly numerous in the limbic system). Benzodiazepine receptors are heterogeneous; at least two subgroups (BZ_1 and BZ_2) have been identified, which may be separate proteins or different conformational states of the same receptor. They are closely related to GABA receptors in a benzodiazepine receptor–GABA receptor–chloride channel complex in the neuronal membrane (Fig. 12.1). GABA is probably the main inhibitory neurotransmitter in the CNS, and is believed to mediate both presynaptic and postsynaptic inhibition at 20–40% of all synapses. In the presence of GABA, chloride channels in normally impermeable neuronal membranes open. Chloride ions subsequently diffuse from the external environment into the neurone, resulting in hyperpolarization and decreased neuronal excitability (i.e. inhibition). In the presence of benzodiazepines, the effects of GABA are facilitated, probably by increasing the frequency of chloride channel opening in response to a given GABA stimulus; in contrast, channel opening times are unchanged or only slightly increased. There is no evidence that benzodiazepines affect the synthesis or the breakdown of GABA, or influence the action of the inhibitory transmitter in any other way.

Benzodiazepines differ greatly in potency (Table 12.1); for instance, triazolam (normal hypnotic dose = 0.25 mg) is approximately 80 times as potent as temazepam (normal hypnotic dose = 20 mg). These differences in potency appear to be related to the variable affinity of benzodiazepines for receptors in the CNS.

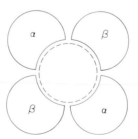

Fig. 12.1 Diagrammatic representation of the benzodiazepine (BZD) receptor–GABA receptor–chloride channel complex in the postsynaptic neuronal membrane. The α-subunits contain benzodiazepine receptors: the β-subunits contain GABA receptors.

Thus, in experimental conditions there is a close relation between receptor occupancy in *in vivo* conditions and anticonvulsant activity. Nevertheless, not all drugs that have a high affinity for benzodiazepine receptors have hypnotic and tranquillizing effects. Some extensively bound drugs (e.g. carboxylic acid esters of β-carboline) may even have proconvulsant or overt convulsant effects in experimental animals, although their actions are opposed by benzodiazepine antagonists. These compounds are sometimes known as contra-agonists or inverse agonists.

Pharmacokinetics

In general, benzodiazepines that are used to produce hypnosis and premedication have variable and different half-lives (Table 12.1). In addition, some drugs have metabolites with considerable pharmacological activity, which may cumulate during chronic administration. Differences between the terminal half-lives of the benzodiazepines and their metabolites have been used to divide them into hypnotics (with a relatively short terminal half-life) and sedatives/tranquillizers (with a relatively long terminal half-life). Although this distinction is rather artificial and arbitrary, it may be valuable in practice. Benzodiazepines with short terminal half-lives (and whose active metabolites have short half-lives) have considerable advantages as hypnotic or premedicant drugs. They are less likely to produce impaired psychomotor performance and hangover effects (e.g. ataxia, motor incoordination, muscle weakness, poor memory and concentration, and mental confusion) on the day after their administration.

Most benzodiazepines have a large apparent volume of distribution due to their high lipid solubility. Most of them are extensively bound to plasma proteins; diazepam, for example, is 96–97% bound, mainly by albumin. Only the unbound (free) fraction can cross the blood–brain barrier and affect the CNS. Although protein-displacement reactions can be demonstrated in *in vitro* conditions, little is known of their significance in anaesthetic practice. In general, benzodiazepines are non-polar, lipid-soluble drugs, and are not extensively excreted unchanged in urine. Consequently, they do not usually cumulate in renal failure. Benzodiazepines are almost entirely eliminated from the body by hepatic metabolism. This usually involves oxidative reactions that are primarily carried out by microsomal enzymes associated with the hepatic endoplasmic reticulum. Nevertheless, some benzodiazepines (e.g. oxazepam) are almost entirely eliminated by glucuronide conjugation. Most benzodiazepines have a low intrinsic hepatic clearance which is not restricted by hepatic blood flow (with the possible exception of midazolam). Many of the metabolic pathways of the benzodiazepines are closely interrelated; to some extent, this may account for the similarity in their actions. Thus medazepam, diazepam, ketazolam, prazepam, and clorazepate are all converted to the active compound desmethyldiazepam (nordiazepam), which has a half-life of several days (Table 12.1; Fig. 12.2). Elderly patients are more sensitive and vulnerable

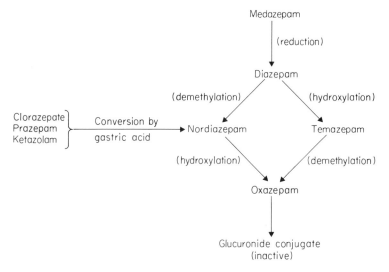

Fig. 12.2 Metabolic relationships between some commonly used benzodiazepines.

to benzodiazepines; this is partly due to decreased oxidative metabolism by the liver.

Although most benzodiazepines are extensively bound to plasma proteins, the unbound ('free') drug can diffuse across the placental barrier and may affect the fetus. There is little or no definite evidence that the benzodiazepines cause fetal abnormalities; nevertheless, some of these drugs can cause complications when used during pregnancy or labour. For instance, when diazepam is used in late pregnancy (e.g. in the treatment of pre-eclampsia and eclampsia), it readily crosses the placenta, and may be metabolized by the fetus. Some of its active metabolites (including desmethyldiazepam, temazepam, and oxazepam) may accumulate in fetal tissues, and can cause neonatal depression, hypotonia, and hypothermia. In addition, chronic exposure of the fetus to benzodiazepines can result in withdrawal symptoms after birth.

Use in anaesthetic practice

In anaesthetic practice, benzodiazepines are often used as premedicant agents in adult patients prior to elective surgery. Regimes have been designed to provide sedation and hypnosis during the preoperative period; they are usually started on admission to hospital and continue until the morning of the operation. Combinations of nitrazepam (10 mg at night) and diazepam (5 mg three times daily) have been commonly used for this purpose. This combination is satisfactory, as assessed by subjective and objective measurements of the level of anxiety (although either drug, used alone, would probably be equally effective). Nightmares, disorientation, and a pronounced hangover effect may occur in elderly patients. In these cases, the dose of nitrazepam should not exceed 5 mg, or an alternative hypnotic drug should be prescribed.

For day-case surgery, including endoscopic procedures and out-patient dental treatment, benzodiazepines with a shorter duration of action (e.g. temazepam 20 mg) may be equally effective and have some advantages. Alternatively, diazepam (5–10 mg) or lorazepam (1–2.5 mg), which usually has a more pronounced amnesic effect, may be given 1.5–2 h before the procedure. There is little advantage in using the intramuscular route, which is painful and is associated with a reduced bioavailability.

Although benzodiazepines have been used as intravenous induction agents, they have a relatively slow onset of action, and produce variable and unpredictable effects on the level of consciousness. They are generally less satisfactory than intravenous barbiturates, but are occasionally of value in patients known to be hypersensitive to other agents. Some benzodiazepines are widely used to produce sedation and anterograde amnesia during unpleasant or painful procedures (e.g. during endoscopy, dentistry, or minor surgery under local anaesthesia). Intravenous preparations of lorazepam, diazepam, and midazolam have been mainly used for this purpose.

Intravenous lorazepam has a relatively slow onset of action (usually within 10–20 min) and a prolonged duration of action (up to 6 h) due to its slow distribution to, and redistribution from, the CNS. It usually produces intense and prolonged anterograde amnesia within 30 min which lasts for up to 4 h. It is less likely to cause pain, thrombophlebitis, and venous thrombosis than aqueous diazepam. Despite the disadvantage of its slow onset of action, it may be of value in prolonged procedures under local anaesthesia, in intensive care, or to diminish the psychotomimetic effects of other drugs.

Diazepam has been widely used as an intravenous sedative. It usually acts within 2–3 min, producing sedation (for up to 60 min) and amnesia (for 10–30 min). Nevertheless, active metabolites of the drug can usually be detected for at least 24–48 h, and ambulant patients must be warned of the possible hazards during this period. The drug was widely used prior to regional anaesthesia, therapeutic nerve blocks, uncomfortable diagnostic procedures, conservative dentistry, and sometimes as a prelude to general anaesthetic techniques. There is wide individual variation in the response to this agent, and the injection should be given very slowly (2.5 mg every 30 s) until drooping of the eyelids is observed. Diazepam was sometimes used in this way in combination with opioid agents (e.g. pentazocine) to produce sedation and analgesia during dental treatment. In these conditions, respiratory depression is a real possibility and facilities for artificial ventilation should always be available when this technique is used.

Like most benzodiazepines, diazepam is poorly soluble in water; in the UK, aqueous preparations are acidic and viscous, and contain various organic solubilizers (e.g. propylene glycol, ethanol and benzoic acid). Local complications can be produced by these preparations; pain on injection, thrombophlebitis, and venous thrombosis are not uncommon, particularly when the drug is injected into small diameter veins on the hand. Occasionally, hypersensitivity reactions may occur. The incidence of local complications can be reduced by appropriate techniques (e.g. the injection of the drug into a fast-running infusion, the use of veins in the antecubital fossa, or by 'barbotage') or by the use of other preparations of diazepam. Diazemuls is a white opaque soybean oil-in-water emulsion of diazepam similar to Intralipid. It only rarely causes pain and thrombophlebitis after injection, but in other respects is similar to aqueous diazepam.

Midazolam has several advantages compared with diazepam; in recent years, it has largely replaced diazepam as an intravenous sedative and amnesic agent. At an acid pH (i.e. pH 4 or less) midazolam is ionized in aqueous solution and is relatively water-soluble. After intravenous injection, the chemical structure of the drug is modified, increasing its lipid solubility and facilitating its diffusion into the CNS. Consequently, pain on injection and thrombophlebitis are infrequent complications. Midazolam has a rapid onset of action, and usually causes more profound amnesia than diazepam. The relatively short terminal half-life of the drug (approximately 2 h) is associated with rapid recovery and the absence of hangover effects. Midazolam is almost entirely metabolized by the liver. Its metabolism (unlike that of other benzodiazepines) may be partly dependent on liver blood flow; one of its metabolites may have slight hypnotic activity. Midazolam is also available as an oral preparation, which may be suitable for premedication.

Other uses

Benzodiazepines are the hypnotics and sedatives of choice for short-term oral administration. They are particularly useful in the treatment of insomnia associated with anxiety. In most subjects, they are relatively safe in overdosage, and patients have recovered from as much as 80 times the normal hypnotic dose. Nevertheless, they can produce dangerous respiratory depression in the elderly, or in patients with impaired pulmonary function (for example, in chronic bronchitis). They do not induce hepatic microsomal enzymes, and do not usually interact with other drugs (apart from other hypnotics and sedatives, including ethyl alcohol). Similarly, side-effects (apart from drowsiness and related central phenomena) are rare; occasionally they cause nightmares, nausea, skin rashes, or an increase in body weight. Although most benzodiazepines are suitable hypnotics, a drug with a short half-life (e.g. temazepam) may be preferred when hangover effects impair performance. Unfortunately, there is increasing evidence that drug tolerance and dependence are not uncommon, and their use as hypnotics and sedatives should be restricted to less than 1 month, if possible. It is usually stated that tolerance to their hypnotic effects may occur after 3–14 days continual administration; during their chronic use, physical dependence is said to occur in 15% of patients.

Benzodiazepines are widely used for other purposes. It is generally accepted that intravenous diazepam is the drug of choice in status epilepticus, whether idiopathic or drug-induced (except, perhaps, when thiopentone and facilities for artificial ventilation are immediately available). An initial dose of 10–30 mg can be given intravenously, but repeated administration or continuous infusion may be necessary; a total dose of 200 mg in 24 h should not be exceeded, unless controlled ventilation has been instituted. Although benzodiazepines are effective in the prophylaxis of many forms of epilepsy (particularly those associated with a generalized EEG discharge), the doses required often cause an unacceptable degree of sedation and drowsiness. Clonazepam and clobazam have been most widely used for the prophylaxis of seizures. They may be useful for short-term prophylaxis, or as an addition to other anticonvulsant regimes. Clonazepam may be particularly effective in the long-term control of myoclonic disorders, although problems with oversedation can occur. Like certain other anticonvulsant drugs, it may be of value in the management of trigeminal neuralgia and other painful conditions. Clobazam (a 1,5-benzodiazepine) may cause less psychomotor disturbance than clonazepam and other 1,4-benzodiazepines. It should be remembered that most benzodiazepines can provoke seizures, and may cause irritability and hyperactivity in children. Benzodiazepines are also useful in the management of muscle hypertonicity or spasticity, due to their central muscle relaxant effects. Thus, they may be of value in painful spasms associated with spinal cord injury or demyelinating disorders, 'muscle contraction' headaches, and in the management of tetanus. In addition, they are used in the treatment of alcohol withdrawal, and the control of night terrors and sleep walking.

Benzodiazepine antagonists

Flumazenil is a competitive, reversible antagonist of most other benzodiazepines; it may also stimulate benzodiazepine receptors, and some of its actions appear to be unrelated to benzodiazepine antagonism. It is mainly metabolized in the liver, and has a rapid onset but relatively brief duration of action, due to its short half-life (approximately 1 h). Consequently, it may require to be given by repeated injection or continuous intravenous infusion in order to antagonize sedation and respiratory depression produced by longer acting benzodiazepines. It may be used to reverse the effects of benzodiazepines after anaesthesia, or after short diagnostic procedures, although careful supervision will be required until recovery is complete.

It sometimes causes anxiety, and can precipitate convulsions in epileptic patients. The duration of anterograde amnesia produced by benzodiazepines is usually reduced by flumazenil. The initial dose is 0.2 mg, with further 0.1 mg increments at 1 min intervals until recovery is complete.

OTHER HYPNOTIC DRUGS

Chlormethiazole

Chlormethiazole is a hypnotic drug that is chemically related to vitamin B_1 (thiamine). Its proprietary name (Heminevrin) reflects this structural similarity. Although its mode of action has not been precisely defined, it is believed to have direct or indirect effects on GABA-dependent pathways in the CNS. Approximately 50% of the drug is normally bound by plasma proteins, and its terminal half-life is usually 3–5 h. After oral administration, it induces sleep within 30–40 min, and is particularly useful for the management of agitation, confusion, restlessness, and insomnia in elderly patients. Chlormethiazole has also been used for the control of delirium tremens and acute withdrawal symptoms in alcoholic patients, and as an anticonvulsant for the management of status epilepticus and pre-eclamptic toxaemia. It is available as an oral preparation and as an intravenous infusion (0.8%). The hypnotic dose is 250–500 mg.

Although chlormethiazole is a relatively safe hypnotic drug with a low systemic toxicity, it may potentiate the effects of other CNS depressants, and may cause respiratory embarrassment, especially in acute or chronic pulmonary disease. Nevertheless, hangover effects are infrequent, and acute overdosage is uncommon. Chlormethiazole can cause nasal congestion, increased secretions, and conjunctivitis. These effects usually occur within 20–30 min of oral administration, and are commoner in younger patients with an allergic diathesis. They appear to be mainly due to local histamine release from mast cells in the nasal mucosa.

Chloral hydrate and its derivatives

Chloral hydrate is one of the oldest and safest hypnotic drugs. It is a halogenated hydrocarbon, and is closely related to chloroform and trichlorethylene. Indeed, its introduction as a hypnotic drug by Liebreich in 1869 was based on the assumption that chloral would slowly release chloroform in the body. Although this is incorrect, it is believed that chloral hydrate and its derivatives act like general anaesthetics, i.e. they produce hypnosis by acting at non-polar sites on lipid or protein components of neuronal membranes. In this manner, they may interfere with ion transport and prevent depolarization. In electrophysiological studies, both chloral hydrate and its main metabolite reduce synaptic activity in the reticular activating system, causing a de-activating response in the EEG.

When taken orally, chloral hydrate acts within 30–40 min and produces hypnosis for 6–8 h. It has little effect on respiration or on reflex activity in the spinal cord. Although tolerance and dependence may develop, they are uncommon; side-effects are also infrequent. Chloral hydrate is metabolized by the liver to trichlorethanol, which is subsequently eliminated as a glucuronide conjugate ('urochloralic acid'). Trichlorethanol itself has considerable hypnotic activity, and is probably mainly responsible for the effects of chloral hydrate.

When used as an oral hypnotic drug, chloral has several important disadvantages. After oral administration it has an unpleasant taste and an irritant effect on the gastric mucosa, and may cause nausea and vomiting. In addition, it is hygroscopic and deliquescent, and cannot be prepared or preserved as tablets. Nevertheless, mixtures, elixirs, and capsules of chloral hydrate are sometimes used in children and in elderly patients. Alternatively, 'stabilized' preparations of chloral may be used. These preparations do not have the disadvantages of chloral hydrate, since the drug is present as a complex which is not dissociated until absorption is complete. Dichloralphenazone is a stabilized preparation of chloral and the analgesic phenazone, and generally causes fewer gastrointestinal side-effects than chloral hydrate. Unfortunately, phenazone ('antipyrine') may induce drug metabolizing enzymes in the liver, and can cause interactions with other drugs (e.g. oral anticoagulants). The occasional development of hypersensitivity reactions and blood dyscrasias is probably due to phenazone. An alternative preparation is trichlorethanol phosphate, which is a stabilized form of the main metabolite of chloral hydrate.

Phenothiazines

Some hypnotic and sedative drugs that are chemically classified as phenothiazines (e.g. promethazine and trimeprazine) are used as premedicant drugs, particularly in children. Both these drugs have considerable antimuscarinic ('anticholinergic') effects and indirect evidence suggests that their hypnotic activity is related to the antagonism of acetylcholine at central synapses. There are numerous cholinergic neurones in the brain and the spinal cord, and acetylcholine is an important excitatory transmitter at many sites in the CNS (including the reticular activating system and the cerebral cortex). Many drugs that produce sedation have antimuscarinic activity (e.g. antidepressants, antipsychotics, H_1-histamine antagonists and scopolamine). In general phenothiazines produce varying degrees of sedation that are closely related to their antimuscarinic effects.

Most phenothiazines may antagonize or affect a wide range of central neurotransmitters (as well as acetylcholine). Consequently, they have multiple actions on the CNS, and are generally unsuitable as sedative or hypnotic drugs. Nevertheless, promethazine and trimeprazine have reasonably selective effects and are widely used as hypnotic and premedicant agents in children.

Promethazine (a structural analogue of promazine) is a H_1-histamine antagonist with a prolonged duration of action (up to 24 h). After oral administration it is well absorbed and widely distributed, and usually acts within 30–60 min. It is relatively safe in overdosage, and therapeutic doses have little effect on the cardiovascular or respiratory system. Promethazine may produce dizziness and disorientation (particularly in the elderly). In addition to its sedative and hypnotic effects, it has antiemetic and antisecretory properties, which contribute to its usefulness as a premedicant drug in children. Promethazine is sometimes indicated as a hypnotic-premedicant drug in asthmatic patients; the drug has bronchodilator effects, and may also prevent responses due to histamine release by certain anaesthetic agents. It may be useful in the symptomatic relief of various hypersensitivity reactions, although hypnotic and antimuscarinic side-effects are common. Promethazine may be valuable in the prophylaxis of motion sickness, and can be used as an antiemetic drug in early pregnancy. Like other antihistamines and certain phenothiazines with marked antimuscarinic activity, promethazine may be useful in Parkinsonism.

Trimeprazine is a H_1-histamine antagonist with more powerful sedative and hypnotic effects than promethazine. It is widely used as a premedicant agent in children. The palatable apricot-flavoured elixir may be administered in a dosage of 1.5–2.0 mg kg^{-1} (depending on the degree of sedation required) 1.5–2 h prior to surgery. Some delay in the recovery from anaesthesia may be anticipated. Trimeprazine can antagonize the effects of 5-hydroxytryptamine, dopamine, and noradrenaline, and high doses may produce extrapyramidal effects, hypothermia and hypotension. Other central side-effects (e.g. disturbing dreams and possibly hallucinations) have also been reported.

Barbiturates

Barbiturates were widely used as hypnotics and premedicant agents for many years, although their use for this purpose is currently considered to be undesirable. Nevertheless, proprietary preparations of amylobarbitone, butobarbitone, cyclobarbitone, pentobarbitone and quinalbarbitone are still available, and appear to be widely used to induce sleep. In some patients with long-standing and intractable insomnia, they may produce more predictable and reliable effects than benzodiazepines. Unfortunately, there are many hazards and disadvantages associated with their use. Barbiturates readily depress respiration, and may be dangerous in patients with pulmonary disease (e.g. chronic bronchitis or asthma). Overdosage is hazardous and may be fatal, particularly when ethyl alcohol is a complicating factor. The action of many barbiturates is prolonged in hepatic and renal disease; in addition, they induce hepatic enzymes concerned with drug metabolism, and may affect the breakdown of other drugs (e.g. anticoagulants, oestrogens and corticosteroids). Central and peripheral adverse effects are relatively common, and barbiturates may antagonize the effects of analgesics, and induce physical and psychological dependence. Acute withdrawal of barbiturate therapy prior to surgery is unwise, as a withdrawal syndrome or epilepsy may be induced; in addition, there may be problems if concurrent therapy with oral anticoagulants is necessary. In general, benzodiazepines are much safer hypnotic and premedicant drugs.

Pentobarbitone is an example of a barbiturate with a medium duration of action; its hypnotic effect lasts for up to 6 h. Pentobarbitone is the oxygen analogue of thiopentone, but has a much lower lipid solubility. It is well absorbed after oral administration, is 50% bound to plasma proteins, and undergoes extensive distribution and metabolism. Pentobarbitone is very occasionally used as a premedicant drug prior to general or regional anaesthesia. The usual dose is 100–200 mg by mouth, 2 h prior to surgery.

Recent studies have clarified the neurochemical effects of the barbiturates. It has been known for many years that they modify cellular metabolism in the CNS; it is now believed that these changes may be secondary effects. Thus barbiturates decrease cerebral oxygen consumption and mitochondrial respiration, increase glycogen and phosphate levels, and depress dopamine, noradrenaline, and 5-hydroxytryptamine turnover in certain areas of the brain. More recent electro-physiological studies suggest that the primary action of barbiturates is to increase the duration of GABA-dependent chloride channel opening, and thus produce hyperpolarization and diminished neuronal excitability. Barbiturates inhibit the binding of radiolabelled picrotoxin analogues at sites related to chloride channels, and the chronic administration of phenobarbitone in the rat increases GABA levels in all regions of the CNS. These neurochemical effects may well account for the hypnotic, anaesthetic, and anticonvulsant effects of the barbiturates.

ANTIMUSCARINIC DRUGS

Premedication with antimuscarinic drugs (in particular, atropine and hyoscine) has been an established clinical practice for many years. The main advantages are a reduction in the amount of bronchial and salivary secretions, a diminution in the cardiac responses to inhalational anaesthetics with significant vagomimetic activity, and a decrease in reflex stimulation during endotracheal intubation and visceral traction.

In present day circumstances, the routine use of these agents may no longer be considered necessary. Anaesthetic agents which induced pronounced salivation and respiratory secretions (diethyl ether) or vagomimetic activity (cyclopropane) are rarely administered, and neuromuscular blocking agents are used to provide optimal conditions for laryngoscopy and intubation. In addition, the subjective discomforts of a dry mouth, palpitations, and blurring of vision are obviously undesirable.

Current indications for the use of antimuscarinic drugs as premedicants are not well defined. In many instances they are omitted, or are given intravenously at the time of induction of anaesthesia. However, they may have some advantages in the following situations:

1 In small children, when the presence of copious secretions in the airway may be a particular embarrassment.

2 When effects mediated through the cardiac vagus may be enhanced (e.g. in patients receiving treatment with β-adrenoceptor antagonists or cardiac glycosides; during ophthalmic surgery, in order to prevent oculocardiac reflexes; during D and Cs and cholecystectomies; and when techniques involving intermittent suxamethonium are used).

3 In patients with obstructive airways disease, in order to prevent reflex or drug-induced bronchospasm.

4 In order to minimize the risk of the acid ·aspiration syndrome in obstetric anaesthesia. Although antimuscarinic drugs do not significantly alter gastric pH in the doses normally used in man, the total volume of secretion is considerably reduced; consequently, the buffering capacity of concurrent antacid therapy is enhanced, and treatment with antacids is more effective.

The action of antimuscarinic drugs in preventing the regurgitation of stomach contents is less clearly understood. In theory, the tone of the cardiac sphincter is increased by antimuscarinic drugs; this should impede the entry of gastric contents into the oesophagus. However, current concepts suggest that the cardiac valve is produced by the apposition of folds of gastric mucosa at the acutely angled cardiooesophageal junction. Thus, antimuscarinic drugs may produce relaxation of smooth muscle and facilitate regurgitation (i.e. they may lower the barrier pressure).

The antimuscarinic drugs most commonly used as premedicant agents are the naturally occurring alkaloids atropine and hyoscine (Chapter 11). These tertiary amines readily cross the blood–brain barrier; however, they produce different central effects, and also have differential effects on acetylcholine receptors in some effector organs (which results in variable sensitivity to atropine and hyoscine).

Atropine

When administered intramuscularly in man in the dose conventionally used for premedication (0.6 mg), atropine may produce initial slowing of the heart prior to the development of tachycardia. This may be due to central effects on the vagal nucleus, or to a partial agonist effect at peripheral muscarinic receptors. However, bradycardia is not usually observed after intravenous injection; indeed, tachyarrhythmias may be produced. In these circumstances, moderate antisialogogue effects occur, and some mydriasis may be observed. In normal conditions, significant elevation of intra-ocular pressure does not occur. Bronchodilatation results in an increase in the physiological dead space. This effect, which is associated with slight stimulation of the cerebral cortex and the medullary centres, leads to an increase in the rate and the depth of respiration.

Atropine has a relatively short duration of action (1–1.5 h); it is extensively metabolized by liver esterases, and only small amounts of the unchanged drug are normally identified in urine. After oral administration, atropine is extensively (60–70%) absorbed from the small intestine; it is frequently administered orally, with a sedative such as trimeprazine, as premedication for elective surgical procedures in children. The recommended dose is 0.05 mg kg^{-1}, up to a maximum dose of 1.2 mg.

Hyoscine

Hyoscine (scopolamine) may also be used as a premedicant drug. In the doses normally used in adults (0.4 mg), it has a shorter duration of action than atropine, and produces less tachycardia; cardiac arrhythmias are unlikely to occur after its use. It is a more powerful antisialogogue than atropine, and has more pronounced effects on the eye.

In contrast, it has less bronchodilator activity. In therapeutic doses, it causes depression of the CNS; drowsiness, amnesia, and confusion (particularly in elderly patients) may occur. The central actions of hyoscine may be useful in the management of motion sickness and other vestibular disorders, and it has been used with opioid analgesics to produce 'twilight sleep'. It also has a short duration of action (1–1.5 h), and is extensively metabolized by liver esterases; only trace amounts of hyoscine (approximately 1% of the dose) are eliminated unchanged in urine. Although hyoscine may be given orally, it is less extensively absorbed from the small intestine than atropine.

Glycopyrrolate

Glycopyrrolate is an antimuscarinic drug which has been widely used in premedication in recent years. Unlike atropine and hyoscine, glycopyrrolate is an ionized quaternary amine, and does not readily cross cell membranes. Thus, it does not readily cross the blood–brain barrier, and does not produce central effects; similarly, placental transfer of the drug is insignificant.

Glycopyrrolate is an effective antisialogogue with a prolonged duration of action (approximately 6 h); sweat gland activity is also affected for a similar period of time. However, moderate doses do not tend to cause other antimuscarinic effects. Heart rate may not increase; indeed, a slight but insignificant bradycardia may occur, and arrhythmias are rare. Similarly, changes in pupillary size are minimal. Nevertheless, larger doses will cause typical antimuscarinic effects.

Glycopyrrolate may be given by intramuscular or intravenous injection, in doses ranging from 0.1–0.4 mg in the adult. It is usually considered that 0.2 mg i.m. produces optimal premedicant effects. Larger doses (2–8 mg) may be given orally, but there is a predictable delay in the onset of action.

Other uses of antimuscarinic drugs

These drugs are used to prevent muscarinic effects produced by the administration of anticholinesterase drugs (Chapters 9 and 11). Atropine is often given with opioid analgesics in the management of biliary and renal colic, in the belief that it will relax smooth muscle; it probably does not contribute greatly to the relief of pain. It is commonly used as a mydriatic in the treatment of iridocyclitis or choroiditis; when locally applied to the eye, it may produce pupillary dilatation for 1–2 weeks. A shorter acting analogue (homatropine or tropicamide) is commonly preferred for diagnostic examination of the eye. It is also used in myocardial infarction, when bradycardia is associated with hypotension or premature ventricular beats. It may be used to increase heart rate in sinus bradycardia due to other causes.

Semi-synthetic and synthetic derivatives of naturally occurring alkaloids, such as atropine methonitrate, hyoscine *N*-butylbromide, and propantheline have been used as antispasmodics in various gastrointestinal and genitourinary disorders; atropine methonitrate is a common constituent of various inhalant mixtures used in the treatment of bronchospasm.

Antimuscarinic drugs which are selectively localized in the CNS are widely used in the treatment of Parkinson's disease; they are particularly valuable in patients who are intolerant of levodopa and its analogues, and in the management of drug-induced extrapyramidal disorders. Atropine was originally used in the treatment of Parkinson's disease more than 100 years ago; some other antimuscarinic drugs produce fewer peripheral side-effects (e.g. orphenadrine, benztropine, and benzhexol). Many other drugs have antimuscarinic ('anticholinergic') properties, including tricyclic antidepressants, phenothiazines, antihistamines, and some analgesics and antiarrhythmic drugs.

NEUROLEPTIC DRUGS

Promethazine (a phenothiazine derivative with antihistamine, sedative, and hypnotic properties) was introduced into anaesthetic practice in France in 1952; it was primarily used as a premedicant drug, and to supplement the action of other anaesthetic agents. At that time, the related phenothiazine, chlorpromazine, had recently been synthesized, and its ability to potentiate other anaesthetic agents had been investigated. It was also recognized that chlorpromazine produced profound sedation without loss of consciousness, and the absence of any interest in the immediate environment. Consequently, promethazine and chlorpromazine (in combination with pethidine) were used as a 'lytic cocktail' to induce a state of artificial hibernation or neurovegetative block. This method, with little or no supplementation, was used as an alternative to conventional anaesthetic techniques. The main advantages were said to be the reduction in bleeding, the absence of shock, and a decreased requirement of postoperative analgesic drugs. However, a profound degree of hypotension and a prolonged depression of autonomic reflexes tended to restrict the use of this technique.

Chlorpromazine was subsequently shown to have marked antipsychotic properties, and was the first effective drug to be used in the treatment of schizophrenia. The term 'neuroleptic' (supporting the nervous system) was introduced to describe chlorpromazine and its analogues in 1957. At this time, various phenylpiperidine derivatives related to pethidine were shown to have properties similar to chlorpromazine; subsequent chemical modification led to the development of the butyrophenones (i.e. haloperidol and droperidol). Other phenyl-piperidine derivatives were shown to be extremely potent analgesics, and had an extremely short duration of action. Some of these drugs (e.g. fentanyl and phenoperidine) were subsequently introduced into clinical practice.

The concept of neuroleptanalgesia was introduced in 1959, and the use of a butyrophenone (e.g. droperidol) and a potent opioid analgesic (e.g. phenoperidine) became popular as an alternative to general anaesthesia. There were frequent problems of respiratory depression associated with the use of these drugs, and the applications and use of neuroleptanalgesia have diminished in recent years. However, a remarkable degree of cardiovascular stability is commonly produced by this technique. Thus, these drugs may be used to supplement light anaesthesia in the elderly or poor risk patient, during induction and maintenance of anaesthesia for cardiac and vascular surgery, and in neurosurgery (although droperidol may cause some reduction in cerebral blood flow). Neuroleptanalgesia is also valuable as an adjunct to regional anaesthesia, and for procedures in which patient cooperation is an advantage (e.g. percutaneous cordotomy).

In recent years, chlorpromazine and related phenothiazines have assumed a more specific role in anaesthetic practice; in particular, they are widely used for their antiemetic properties.

ANTIEMETIC DRUGS

Nausea and vomiting can be induced by many physiological and pathological factors. These include pregnancy; acute pain; raised intracranial pressure; ionizing radiation; psychogenic factors; labyrinthine or vestibular disturbances; metabolic disorders; and inflammation or irritation of the gastrointestinal tract. In addition, many drugs or ingested toxins can induce nausea and vomiting. Some of these agents (e.g. ipecacuanha, squill, non-steroidal anti-inflammatory analgesics, chloral hydrate, ammonium chloride, and other simple salts) act immediately after oral administration. Indeed, ipecacuanha emetic mixtures are sometimes used in the management of acute drug overdosage in children. These drugs have a local irritant effect on the stomach, or they activate abdominal visceral afferent nerves in the intestinal mucosa or the portal vein. Afferent stimuli are mainly conducted to the brain via the vagus nerves. Other emetic drugs (e.g. opioid analgesics, digitalis glycosides, levodopa, bromocriptine and some inhalational anaesthetics) predominantly affect central pathways concerned with the control of nausea and vomiting. Cytotoxic drugs with pronounced emetic properties (i.e. mustine, cisplatin, dacarbazine and streptozotocin) act by both peripheral and central mechanisms.

For many years, it has been generally accepted that nausea and vomiting are primarily controlled and coordinated by the vomiting centre, which is situated in the dorsolateral reticular formation of the medulla. More recent evidence suggests that the existence of a discrete vomiting centre is doubtful; physiologically, it can be considered as the area in the brainstem that integrates emetic responses. Its functions are probably dependent on complex interactions between the reticular formation, the nucleus tractus solitarius, and certain autonomic nuclei (particularly the dorsal vagal nucleus). Similarly, its neurochemistry is extremely complex, since almost 40 different neurotransmitters have been identified in this area of the brain. Efferent impulses from these medullary centres influence related brainstem nuclei (e.g. the vasomotor, respiratory, and salivary nuclei) and pass to the gastrointestinal tract to initiate the vomiting reflex.

The activity of the vomiting centre is affected by afferent stimuli from chemoreceptors and pressure receptors in the gut and the CNS, as well as peripheral pain receptors (Fig. 12.3). In addition, it has an afferent input from other sites

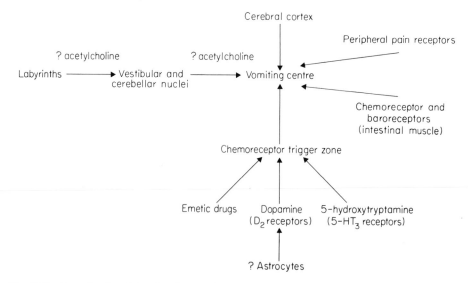

Fig. 12.3 Central and peripheral pathways affecting the activity of the vomiting centre.

in the CNS (i.e. the cerebral cortex, vestibular and cerebellar nuclei and the chemoreceptor trigger zone). Stimuli from the labyrinths, mediated by vestibular and cerebellar nuclei, increase the excitability of the vomiting centre and may cause nausea and vomiting. At least one of the synaptic connections in this afferent pathway is cholinergic, and is susceptible to antagonism by centrally acting antimuscarinic drugs. There is also some evidence that noradrenaline may be an inhibitory neurotransmitter in the brain stem reticular system and the vestibular nuclei. However, the activity of the vomiting centre is primarily dependent on other neurotransmitters; in particular, it is affected by the activity of the chemoreceptor trigger zone (Fig. 12.3).

The chemoreceptor trigger zone (CTZ) is a group of cells close to the area postrema on the floor of the fourth ventricle; it normally has a tonic effect on the activity of the vomiting centre. The area postrema is a highly vascular area of the brain stem; physiologically, it is outside the blood–brain and CSF–brain barriers, and is extremely sensitive to systemic emetic stimuli. It may also be concerned with the control of blood pressure, sleep, and the regulation of food intake. Many emetic drugs increase the excitability of the CTZ and only indirectly affect the vomiting centre. At least two neurotransmitters (i.e. dopamine and 5-HT) play an important functional role in the activity of the CTZ.

Dopamine is probably released physiologically from the peripheral processes of astrocytes that synapse with the CTZ, and can directly influence neurones in the area postrema by the activation of specific receptors. Current concepts suggest that the dopamine receptors in the area postrema and the CTZ are mainly dopamine D_2-receptors, i.e. they are not associated with adenylate cyclase, are sensitive to apomorphine and dopaminergic ergots, and are antagonized by metoclopramide and sulpiride. Most centrally acting emetic drugs are D_2-receptor agonists in the CTZ. There is also considerable evidence that dopamine may act as an inhibitory transmitter in the gastrointestinal tract, and may affect peripheral mechanisms concerned with nausea and vomiting.

More recent evidence suggests that 5-HT may also play a crucial role in drug-induced emesis. One subtype of 5-HT receptors ($5-HT_3$ receptors) appears to play an important part in the mediation of nausea and vomiting induced by high doses of cytotoxic agents. These receptors are present in the small intestine, the CTZ, and the area postrema, and can be stimulated by emetic drugs. Preliminary experimental and clinical evidence suggests that $5-HT_3$ receptor antagonists are highly effective antiemetic drugs; indeed, the effectiveness of high-dose metoclopramide in cisplatin-induced emesis appears to be due to antagonism of 5-HT at $5-HT_3$ receptors.

Thus, experimental evidence suggests that the neurotransmitters acetylcholine (via central cholinergic pathways and vestibular nuclei), dopamine (via D_2-receptors in the CTZ), and 5-HT (via $5-HT_3$ receptors in the area postrema and the CTZ) may play an important part in the central control of nausea and vomiting. Consequently, most antiemetic drugs act as antagonists of one or more than one of these neurotransmitters. In addition, they may affect peripheral pathways concerned with nausea and vomiting. Unfortunately, most antiemetic drugs do not selectively or specifically antagonize these neurotransmitters (either at vestibular pathways or at the CTZ). Drugs with central antimuscarinic activity invariably produce peripheral parasympathetic blockade, causing pupillary dilatation and cycloplegia, decreased salivary and respiratory secretions, tachycardia, and relaxation or decreased motility of smooth muscle in the respiratory tract, the gut, and the bladder. Central side-effects, such as drowsiness and sedation, may be due to competitive blockade of cholinergic pathways in the reticular activating system and the cerebral cortex. In contrast, dopamine antagonists may act on the pituitary gland, the hypothalamus, the mesolimbic system, and the corpus striatum, causing hyperprolactinaemia, decreased body temperature, and extrapyramidal effects (e.g. tremors, dystonias, and oculogyric crises). Dopamine antagonists may affect 5-HT$_3$ receptors in high dosage (e.g. metoclopramide); however, some 5-HT$_3$ receptor antagonists appear to have relatively specific effects.

Individual antiemetic drugs can be classified pharmacologically as:
1 Antimuscarinic ('anticholinergic') drugs.
2 Dopamine antagonists.
3 Other agents.

Antimuscarinic drugs

In general, all drugs that antagonize the muscarinic effects of acetylcholine and that can cross the blood–brain barrier may have antiemetic properties (particularly in motion sickness, labyrinthine disease, or vestibular disorders). In practice, atropine, hyoscine, and some antihistamine drugs (i.e. H$_1$-histamine antagonists) have been mainly used for this purpose.

The antiemetic effects of atropine and hyoscine are mainly due to their central antimuscarinic effects; however, both drugs decrease muscle tone and secretions in the gut, which may contribute to their effects. In general, atropine is a less potent and less effective antiemetic agent than hyoscine (although its activity on intestinal motility and secretions is greater). Both drugs decrease the opening pressure of the lower oesophageal sphincter ('barrier pressure') and thus predispose to gastrooesophageal regurgitation. They also produce characteristic autonomic side-effects, and hyoscine may cause profound sedation. Both atropine and hyoscine may suppress the emetic effects of therapeutic doses of opioid analgesics, and are used for premedication (p. 399).

Some antihistamine drugs (i.e. competitive antagonists of histamine at H$_1$-receptors) have antiemetic properties; in the UK, cinnarizine, cyclizine, diphenhydramine, dimenhydrinate, and promethazine have been most widely used in the management of nausea and vomiting. Cyclizine and cinnarizine usually produce less sedation than diphenhydramine and promethazine. Nevertheless, promethazine (a phenothiazine) has a longer duration of action than other anti-histamines, and is commonly used for its antiemetic effects. These drugs are frequently of value in the prophylaxis and treatment of motion sickness, and in the management of labyrinthine disorders (e.g. Ménière's disease). When nausea and vomiting are due to other causes, their effectiveness is limited. Nevertheless, antihistamines may suppress the emetic effects of opioid analgesics, and some of them (e.g. cyclizine and promethazine) have been used in anaesthetic practice. In particular, promethazine has been used for premedication in children (p. 397), and cyclizine is commonly used as an antiemetic drug in the perioperative period. The drug is available as a compound preparation with morphine ('Cyclimorph'), and is also present with the methadone analogue dipipanone in 'Diconal' for use in chronic pain therapy.

Although these drugs are primarily competitive antagonists at H_1-receptors, there is little or no evidence that histamine plays any part in peripheral and central mechanisms concerned with nausea and vomiting. Many antihistamines also have significant antimuscarinic activity, which accounts for many of their side-effects (e.g. dryness of the mouth, urinary retention and drowsiness). Their antiemetic effects (particularly in nausea and vomiting of labyrinthine origin) are probably entirely due to the central antagonism of acetylcholine. Antihistamines that do not cross the blood–brain barrier (e.g. terfenadine and astemizole) are of no value as antiemetic drugs.

Dopamine antagonists

Since dopamine plays an important physiological role in the CTZ and the area postrema, almost all drugs that antagonize its effects at D_2-receptors have anti-emetic properties. The dopamine antagonists that are used clinically for their antiemetic effects are usually phenothiazines, butyrophenones, metoclopramide, or domperidone.

Phenothiazines

In general, phenothiazines have many pharmacological effects and can modify responses to a wide range of central and peripheral neurotransmitters. Most phenothiazines antagonize the effects of dopamine at central synapses, and have a variable degree of antimuscarinic activity. Consequently, they are often use-ful in the control of nausea and vomiting, whether induced by drugs or other causes (e.g. uraemia, neoplastic disease, or radiotherapy). Phenothiazines are usually divided into three groups, depending on their chemical structure. Type 1 phenothiazines (e.g. chlorpromazine) cause sedation and have some tendency to produce extrapyramidal side-effects, particularly at high dose levels. Type 2 phenothiazines (e.g. thioridazine) are usually less potent; they have only moderate sedative effects and little tendency to produce extrapyramidal side-effects. Type 3 phenothiazines (e.g. fluphenazine) are more potent drugs with little sedative effect, but have a marked tendency to produce extrapyramidal effects.

The classical Type 1 phenothiazine, chlorpromazine, has a wide range of actions (as suggested by its proprietary name Largactil). These are mainly related to its widespread effects on different central and peripheral receptors. Thus, chlorpromazine can cause antagonism of dopamine (at D_1 and D_2-receptors), acetylcholine (at muscarinic receptors), noradrenaline (at α_1 and α_2-receptors), histamine (at H_1-receptors), and 5-hydroxytryptamine (at some 5-HT receptors). In addition, chlorpromazine has membrane stabilizing (local anaesthetic) activity and prevents the uptake of noradrenaline at sympathetic neurones (Uptake$_1$). Some of the central effects of chlorpromazine are due to its relatively selective action on the brainstem alerting system. This consists of ascending neurones in the pontine and medullary reticular formation, which project to thalamic and hypothalamic nuclei, and transmit arousal impulses to the sensory cortex. Chlorpromazine does not directly inhibit the reticular activating system, but isolates it from numerous collateral afferents (including auditory and visual impulses) which are constantly impinging on it. The resultant effects are classically described as neurolepsy, i.e. sedation, indifference to external stimuli, and a reduction in motor activity. The electroencephalograph shows a characteristic sleep pattern (although patients can be roused by moderate stimulation). Paradoxically, chlorpromazine may induce epileptic attacks in susceptible individuals, and convulsions may be a prominent feature of phenothiazine overdosage. Reduction in muscle tone may also occur, due to suppression of reticular afferents from proprioceptive fibres in muscle spindles.

Other central effects of chlorpromazine are probably mainly due to dopamine antagonism. Extrapyramidal effects (e.g. acute dystonia, akathisia, and tardive dyskinesia) are usually seen with high and continuous dosage; classical Parkinsonism (i.e. rigidity, tremor, and akinesia) is less common. The hypothalamic regulation of pituitary function is modified; the secretion of growth hormone and pituitary gonadotrophins is decreased, and hyperprolactinaemia occurs. (Dopamine inhibits the release of prolactin from the anterior pituitary, i.e. it is prolactin release-inhibitory factor; consequently central dopamine antagonism invariably increases plasma prolactin.) Hypothalamic activity is also affected in other ways. Temperature regulation is impaired, and a fall in body temperature may occur. Similarly, interference with autonomic regulation by the hypothalamus (as well as α-adrenoceptor blockade) may cause profound hypotension. In addition, chlorpromazine produces antiemetic effects by competitive antagonism of dopamine D_2-receptors in the area postrema and the CTZ.

Chlorpromazine may potentiate the actions of other central depressants, including analgesics. Indeed, one phenothiazine (methotrimeprazine; levomepromazine) has analgesic effects that are similar to morphine, and schizophrenic patients who are receiving long-term treatment with phenothiazines may have a stoical indifference to pain.

Hypersensitivity reactions to chlorpromazine are not uncommon. Cholestatic jaundice may develop during chronic treatment; it is less common with other phenothiazines. Agranulocytosis can also occur, and skin reactions in patients and nursing staff may be due to handling tablets containing the drug. Photosensitivity and pigmentation of the skin and the cornea occasionally develop. Like other phenothiazines, chlorpromazine may cause the malignant neuroleptic syndrome.

Chlorpromazine is well absorbed after oral administration. It is extensively metabolized by the liver to a large number of breakdown products; it has been suggested that some of these can be detected in urine for as long as 18 months. Only small amounts of the active drug are eliminated unchanged in bile or urine. After oral administration, the drug has a large and variable first pass effect, and its metabolism is affected by enzyme-inducing agents. Consequently, it is commonly given by intramuscular injection. Chlorpromazine has a relatively long terminal half-life, and a large total apparent volume of distribution.

Chlorpromazine is the classical phenothiazine used in the treatment of psychotic disorders. In schizophrenic patients, it controls violence and hyperactivity, and also has a beneficial effect on other symptoms, such as thought disorders, delusions, and hallucinations. It is useful in the treatment of mania and drug-induced psychoses; small doses may be used in the treatment of psychoneurotic disorders associated with agitation. Chlorpromazine can also be used in the treatment of intractable hiccup, and in the management of tetanus.

In anaesthetic practice, chlorpromazine may be used with opioid analgesics during the perioperative period, or in the management of pain due to malignant disease. It may also be used as an adjunct to induce hypotension or hypothermia. It is sometimes indicated in the treatment of shock; the α-adrenoceptor antagonism results in increased tissue perfusion, and the anti-shivering and deafferentation properties may also be useful.

More commonly, chlorpromazine is used in the symptomatic treatment of nausea and vomiting; it has a protective effect against emesis induced by opioid analgesic drugs. It is less effective in motion sickness or the vomiting which occurs after radiotherapy. In the doses required to control nausea and vomiting, antimuscarinic and extrapyramidal side-effects are usually moderate; unfortunately, sedation and drowsiness may be severe and disabling. Consequently, phenothiazines without marked sedative properties are more commonly used as antiemetic drugs (e.g. perphenazine, prochlorperazine and trifluoperazine). These drugs are all Group 3 phenothiazines, and do not usually have significant antimuscarinic effects. Unfortunately, extrapyramidal effects due to dopamine antagonism (e.g. tremors, dystonia, and dyskinesias) are relatively common, particularly when high doses are used over a prolonged period. Prochlorperazine is less potent than perphenazine and trifluoperazine, and is widely used for its antiemetic effects during the postoperative period. The usual dose is 12.5 mg, by intramuscular injection; after oral administration, the drug has a large and variable first pass effect (like most other phenothiazines).

Butyrophenones

Some butyrophenones are relatively selective dopamine receptor antagonists, and have similar effects to Group 3 phenothiazines. This may be related to their uptake and localization in the CNS. The chemical structure of the butyrophenones is related to the inhibitory transmitter GABA, and it has been suggested that they may compete with GABA at postsynaptic receptor sites (although it is not clear how this is related to dopamine antagonism).

Butyrophenones have powerful tranquillizing and antiemetic effects. Although they are commonly administered with opioid analgesics, they do not appear to potentiate their analgesic and respiratory depressant effects. In low doses, they do not produce significant sedation or pronounced peripheral antimuscarinic effects; unfortunately, extrapyramidal signs (e.g. dystonias and oculogyric crises) and hypothalamic dysfunction are relatively common. They have less peripheral activity than most phenothiazines, and adverse haemodynamic effects are infrequent.

Two butyrophenones (haloperidol and droperidol) have been extensively used in medical practice. Haloperidol is potent, effective and long-acting, and is sometimes used as an antiemetic agent; the effects of a single dose may last for 24–48 h. It is also used in the treatment of various psychoses, behavioural disorders, and motor tics. Droperidol has a shorter duration of action (6–12 h) and is often used with opioid drugs to produce neuroleptanalgesia (p. 403). It should not be used alone, as the occurrence of apparent tranquillization may conceal a state of inner anxiety with psychotic features (e.g. hallucinations, and bizarre symptoms of body transference). Droperidol may cause a slight fall in blood pressure, due to α-adrenoceptor blockade. Premedication with droperidol may be of value in preventing the emergence of delirium after the administration of ketamine.

Metoclopramide

The antiemetic properties of metoclopramide are mainly due to dopamine antagonism; however, in high doses it also antagonizes the effects of 5-HT at 5-HT_3 receptors in the area postrema and the CTZ. Unfortunately, metoclopramide does not have a selective action at these sites; consequently, it may cause extrapyramidal effects (e.g. dyskinesias, dystonias, restlessness and oculogyric crises). These can be prevented or treated by drugs with antimuscarinic properties (e.g. diphenhydramine, promethazine or benztropine). Other toxic reactions, apart from drowsiness, are relatively rare. Metoclopramide has also significant peripheral effects on the gastrointestinal tract. It increases the rate of gastric emptying by enhancing fundal and antral contractility, relaxes the pyloric sphincter, stimulates peristalsis, and increases lower oesophageal sphincter pressure ('barrier pressure'). These effects may be due to the peripheral antagonism of dopamine in the gastrointestinal tract. Metoclopramide has been used in the prophylaxis of Mendelson's syndrome, and to prevent nausea and vomiting during cancer chemotherapy.

Domperidone

Domperidone is also an antiemetic drug with central and peripheral effects, which are mainly due to dopamine antagonism. Like metoclopramide, it increases the rate of gastric emptying and increases the lower oesophageal sphincter pressure. Domperidone also prevents the effects of dopamine and dopamine agonists on the CTZ, and may cause increased prolactin secretion. It is less likely to produce acute dystonic reactions than metoclopramide, since it does not cross the blood–brain barrier readily and affect the corpus striatum. In large doses, domperidone may cause cardiac arrhythmias which are sometimes fatal. It is mainly used as an antiemetic drug during chemotherapy with cytotoxic drugs; in these conditions, it may have some advantages over metoclopramide. It is not available as an intravenous preparation.

Other antiemetic drugs

Nabilone is a synthetic cannabinoid with antiemetic properties, and is chemically related to tetrahydrocannabinol. Experimental evidence suggests that it acts on opioid receptors in the area postrema, since its antiemetic effects can be competitively antagonized by naloxone. It has been suggested that the activation of opioid receptors may lead to persistent inhibition of the vomiting centre. It has been used to prevent nausea and vomiting during cancer chemotherapy, although it is probably less effective than other drugs during cisplatin therapy. Unwanted effects (particularly drowsiness, dizziness, and dry mouth) and psychotic reactions (e.g. dysphoria, depression, nightmares, and hallucinations) are relatively common. Nabilone should only be used as an antiemetic drug during cancer chemotherapy, due to the possibility of drug dependence and misuse.

Lorazepam is a potent benzodiazepine with profound sedative and amnesic properties. It has also been used as an antiemetic drug during cancer chemotherapy. Its mode of action is obscure; presumably it modifies central pathways concerned with the control of nausea and vomiting. In addition, the powerful amnesic action of lorazepam prevents anticipatory vomiting, which occurs in approximately 20% of patients during repeated courses of therapy with cytotoxic drugs.

Some corticosteroids (e.g. i.v. dexamethasone) have been used as antiemetic drugs during cancer chemotherapy. In these conditions, dexamethasone is well tolerated and is as effective as prochlorperazine or metoclopramide. The mode of action of corticosteroids is uncertain. It has been suggested that their action depends on the decreased release of arachidonic acid, reduced turnover of 5-hydroxytryptamine, or decreased permeability of the blood–brain barrier.

In recent years, a number of specific 5-HT$_3$ antagonists have been synthesized, and are currently under investigation (e.g. BRL 43694, GR 38032F and ICS 205–930). These compounds may have selective and specific effects on nausea and vomiting, and should have considerable advantages over currently available antiemetic drugs. One of these 5-HT$_3$ antagonists (Ondansetron) is now available in the UK.

FURTHER READING

Andrews PLR, Rapeport WG, Sanger GJ. Neuropharmacology of emesis induced by anti-cancer therapy. *Trends in Pharmacological Sciences* 1988; **9**: 334–341.

Ashton H. Benzodiazepine withdrawal: an unfinished story. *British Medical Journal* 1984; **288**: 1135–1140.

Betts TA, Birtle J. Effect of two hypnotic drugs on actual driving performance next morning. *British Medical Journal* 1982; **285**: 852.

Bowcock SJ, Stockdale AD, Bolton JAR, Kang AA, Retsas S. Antiemetic prophylaxis with high dose metoclopramide or lorazepam in vomiting induced by chemotherapy. *British Medical Journal* 1984; **288**: 1879.

Braestrup C, Schmiechen R, Nielsen M, Petersen EN. Benzodiazepine receptor ligands, receptor occupancy, pharmacological effect and GABA receptor coupling. In: Usdin E, Skolnick P, Tallman JF, Greenblatt D, Paul SM (eds) *Pharmacology of Benzodiazepines*. London: Macmillan Press, 1982; 71–85.

Brand ED, Harris TD, Borison HL, Goodman LS. The anti-emetic effect of 10-(α-dimethyl-aminopropyl)-2-chlorophenothiazine (chlorpromazine) in dog and cat. *Journal of Pharmacology and Experimental Therapeutics* 1954; **110**: 86–92.

Brandt AL, Oakes FD. Preanaesthesia medication: double-blind study of a new drug, diazepam. *Anesthesia and Analgesia* 1965; **44**: 125–129.

Breimer DD. Clinical pharmacokinetics of hypnotics. *Clinical Pharmacokinetics* 1977; **2**: 93–109.

Brogden RN, Carmine AA, Heel RC, Speight TM, Avery GS. Domperidone: a review of its pharmacological activity, pharmacokinetics and therapeutic efficacy in the symptomatic treatment of chronic dyspepsia and as an anti-emetic. *Drugs* 1982; **24**: 360–400.

Butler TC. Theories of general anaesthesia. *Pharmacological Reviews* 1950; **2**: 121–160.

Calvey TN. Hypnotics, sedatives and antiemetics. In: Nimmo WS, Smith G (eds) *Anaesthesia*. Oxford: Blackwell Scientific Publications, 1989; 22–33.

Castleden CM, George CF, Marcer D, Hallett C. Increased sensitivity to nitrazepam in old age. *British Medical Journal* 1977; **1**: 10–12.

Clift AD. Factors leading to dependence on hypnotic drugs. *British Medical Journal* 1972; **3**: 614–617.

Conney AH. Pharmacological implications of microsomal enzyme induction. *Pharmacological Reviews* 1967; **19**: 317–366.

Cook P. How drug activity is altered in the elderly. *Geriatric Medicine*; 1979; **9**: 45–46.

Cree JE, Meyer J, Hailey DM. Diazepam in labour: its metabolism and effect on the clinical condition and thermogenesis of the newborn. *British Medical Journal*; 1973; **4**: 251–255.

Davis CJ, Lake-Bakaar GV, Grahame-Smith DG. *Nausea and Vomiting: Mechanisms and Treatment*. Berlin: Springer-Verlag; 1986.

Dent SJ, Ramachandra V, Stephen CR. Postoperative vomiting: incidence, analysis and therapeutic measures in 3000 patients. *Anesthesiology* 1955; **16**: 564–572.

Doughty A. The evaluation of premedication in children. *Proceedings of the Royal Society of Medicine* 1959; **52**: 823–833.

Fenton GW. Clinical disorders of sleep. *British Journal of Hospital Medicine* 1975; **14**: 120–145.

Gee KW, Yamamura HI. Benzodiazepine receptor heterogeneity: a consequence of multiple conformational states of a single receptor or multiple population of structurally distinct macromolecules? In: Usdin E, Skolnick P, Tallman JF, Greenblatt D, Paul SM (eds) *Pharmacology of Benzodiazepines*. London: Macmillan Press, 1982; 93–108.

Haefely WE. Central actions of benzodiazepines: general introduction. *British Journal of Psychiatry* 1978; **133**: 231–238.

Iversen LL, Bloom FE. Studies on the uptake of ^{3}H-GABA and ^{3}H-glycine in slices and homogenates of rat brain and spinal cord by electron microscopic autoradiography. *Brain Research* 1972; **41**: 131–143.

Joss RA, Goldhirsch A, Brunner KW, Galeazzi RL. Sudden death in cancer patient on high-dose domperidone. *Lancet* 1982; **1**: 1019.

Kanto JH. Use of benzodiazepines during pregnancy, labour and lactation, with particular reference to pharmacokinetic considerations. *Drugs* 1982; **23**: 354–380.

Kawar P, Dundee JW. Frequency of pain on injection and venous sequelae following the i.v. administration of certain anaesthetics and sedatives. *British Journal of Anaesthesia* 1982; **54**: 935–939.

Kebabian JW, Calne DB. Multiple receptors for dopamine. *Nature* 1979; **277**: 93–96.

Kesson CM, Gray JMB, Lawson DH. Benzodiazepine drugs in general medical patients. *British Medical Journal* 1976; **1**: 680–682.

Klotz U, Antonin K-H, Bieck PR. Pharmacokinetics and plasma binding of diazepam in man, dog, rabbit, guinea pig and rat. *Journal of Pharmacology and Experimental Therapeutics* 1976; **199**: 67–73.

Kris MG, Tyson LB, Gralla RJ, Clark RA, Allen JC, Reilly LK. Extrapyramidal reactions with high dose metoclopramide. *New England Journal of Medicine* 1983; **309**: 433–434.

Lader MH. How tranquillisers work. *British Journal of Hospital Medicine* 1976; **16**: 622–628.

Lader MH, Petursson H. Benzodiazepine derivatives — side effects and dangers. *Biological Psychiatry* 1981; **16**: 1195–1201.

Laduron PM. Leysen JE. Domperidone, a specific *in vitro* dopamine antagonist, devoid of *in vivo* central dopaminergic activity. *Biochemical Pharmacology* 1979; **28**: 2161–2165.

Lidbrink P, Corrodi H, Fuxe K, Olson L. The effects of benzodiazepines, meprobamate, and barbiturates on central monoamine neurons. In: Garrattini S, Mussini E, Randall LO (eds) *The Benzodiazepines*. New York: Raven Press, 1973; 203–223.

Lind JF, Crispin JS, McIver DK. The effect of atropine on the gastro-oesophageal sphincter. *Canadian Journal of Physiology and Pharmacology* 1968; **46**: 233–238.

McKay AC, Dundee JW. Effect of oral benzodiazepines on memory. *British Journal of Anaesthesia* 1980; **52**: 1247–1257.

Malagelada J-R. Gastric emptying disorders: clinical significance and treatment. *Drugs* 1982; **24**: 353–359.

Martin IL. The benzodiazepine receptor: functional complexity. In: Lamble JW, Abbott AC (eds) *Receptors Again*. Amsterdam: Elsevier Science Publications, 1984; 214–220.

Mazzi E. Possible neonatal diazepam withdrawal: a case report. *American Journal of Obstetrics and Gynecology* 1977; **129**: 586–587.

Mirakhur RK. Anticholinergic drugs. *British Journal of Anaesthesia* 1979; **51**: 671–679.

Mohler H, Okada T. Benzodiazepine receptor: demonstration in the nervous system. *Science* 1977; **198**: 849–851.

Murphy SM. Owen RT, Tyrer PJ. Withdrawal symptoms after six weeks treatment with diazepam. *Lancet* 1984; **2**: 1389.

Olesen AS, Huttel MS. Local reactions to i.v. diazepam in three different formulations. *British Journal of Anaesthesia* 1980; **52**: 609–611.

Olsen RW. Drug interactions at the GABA receptor–ionophore complex. *Annual Review of Pharmacology* 1982; **22**: 245–277.

Owen RT, Tyrer P. Benzodiazepine dependence: a review of the evidence. *Drugs* 1983; **25**: 385–398.

Padfield NL, Twohig M McD, Fraser ACL. Temazepam and trimeprazine compared with placebo as premedication in children. *British Journal of Anaesthesia* 1986; **58**: 487–493.

Patsalos PN, Lascelles PT. Changes in regional brain levels of amino acid putative transmitters after prolonged treatment with the anticonvulsant drugs diphenylhydantoin, phenobarbitone, sodium valproate, ethosuximide and sulthiame in the rat. *Journal of Neurochemistry* 1981; **36**: 688–695.

Patton CM, Moon MR, Dannemiller FJ. The prophylactic antiemetic effect of droperidol. *Anesthesia and Analgesia* 1974; **53**: 361–364.

Przybyla AC, Wang SC. Locus of central depressant action of diazepam. *Journal of Pharmacology and Experimental Therapeutics* 1968; **163**: 439–447.

Ricou B, Forster A, Bruckner A, Chastonay P, Gemperle M. Clinical evaluation of a specific benzodiazepine antagonist (Ro 15–1788). *British Journal of Anaesthesia* 1986; **58**: 1005–1011.

Sage DJ, Close A, Boas RA. Reversal of midazolam sedation with anexate. *British Journal of Anaesthesia* 1987; **59**: 459–464.

Schacht U, Backer G. In vitro studies on GABA release. *British Journal of Clinical Pharmacology* 1979; **7**: 25–31S.

Skegg DCG, Richards SM, Doll R. Minor tranquillisers and road accidents. *British Medical Journal* 1979; **1**: 917–919.

Smith DE, Wesson DR. Benzodiazepine dependency syndromes. *Journal of Psychoactive Drugs* 1983; **15**: 85–96.

Smith MT, Eadie MJ, Brophy TO'R. The pharmacokinetics of midazolam in man. *European Journal of Clinical Pharmacology* 1981; **19**: 271–278.

Squires RF, Braestrup C. Benzodiazepine receptors in rat brain. *Nature* 1977; **266**: 732–734.

Study RE, Barker JL. Diazepam and (−)pentobarbital: Fluctuation analysis reveals different mechanisms for potentiation of γ-aminobutyric acid responses in cultured central neurons. *Proceedings of the National Academy of Sciences USA* 1981; **78**: 7180–7184.

Study RE, Barker JL. Cellular mechanisms of benzodiazepine action. *Journal of the American Medical Association* 1982; **247**: 2147–2151.

Thomas DL, Vaughan RS, Vickers MD, Mapleson WW. Comparison of temazepam elixir and trimeprazine syrup as oral premedication in children undergoing tonsillectomy and associated procedures. *British Journal of Anaesthesia* 1987; **59**: 424–430.

Wilkinson GR. Factors influencing the disposition of benzodiazepines. In: Usdin E, Skolnick P, Tallman JF, Greenblatt D, Paul SM (eds) *Pharmacology of Benzodiazepines*. London: Macmillan Press, 1982; 285–297.

Wilson J, Ellis FR. Oral premedication with lorazepam (Ativan); a comparison with heptabarbitone (Medomin) and diazepam (Valium). *British Journal of Anaesthesia* 1973; **45**: 738–744.

Wood CD. Antimotion sickness and antiemetic drugs. *Drugs* 1979; **17**: 471–479.

Wood CD, Graybiel A. A theory of motion sickness based on pharmacological reactions. *Clinical Pharmacology and Therapeutics* 1970; **11**: 621–629.

Young WS, Kuhar MJ. Autoradiographic localisation of benzodiazepine receptors in the brains of humans and animals. *Nature* 1979; **280**: 393–395.

THIRTEEN

Antihypertensive Agents and Drugs Used to Induce Hypotension

Hypertension has been recognized as a disease for over a century, but it is only in the last 3 or 4 decades that effective pharmacological therapy has become generally available. Prior to this time, treatment was directed principally to those patients with only the most severe forms of the disease; remedies included prolonged bed rest, the use of sedative drugs and surgical attempts to extirpate the sympathetic nervous system.

The World Health Organization has defined hypertension as a condition which exists when the blood pressure persistently exceeds 160/95. There appears to be little doubt that specific therapy aimed at reducing diastolic levels will decrease morbidity and mortality resulting from the disease. In particular, large-scale studies have demonstrated that the incidence of renal complications, haemorrhagic stroke, and cardiac failure is diminished; recent surveys have also indicated that myocardial infarction is less likely to ensue. There is current agreement on the value of treating diastolic levels greater than 105 mmHg. However, there still remains some controversy with regard to specific therapy when diastolic measurements range between 95–104 mmHg, and the management of high systolic levels alone has not been clearly defined. In these circumstances the following factors may be taken into consideration:

1 The age of the patient, as the undesirable effects of antihypertensive agents may outweigh the possible benefits in the elderly.

2 The existence of related diseases (e.g. diabetes, hypercholesterolaemia) which if more effectively treated may provide improved control of the hypertensive disorder.

3 The use of non-specific measures (e.g. cessation of smoking and excessive alcohol consumption, reduction of weight and salt intake) where appropriate.

In more than 80% of patients with hypertension no aetiology is apparent although there is some evidence to suggest that morphological changes in the arteriolar wall may be an important precipitating factor. Alterations in either sodium or calcium 'balance' have also been implicated in having a causal relationship with essential hypertension. However, in 10–20% of cases an identifiable and

Table 13.1   Sites of action of the various antihypertensive agents.

Inhibitors of sympathetic nervous system activity:
Centrally acting drugs (e.g. methyldopa, clonidine)
Ganglion-blocking compounds (trimetaphan)
Adrenergic neurone-blocking agents (e.g. guanethidine, bretylium)
α-adrenoceptor antagonists (e.g. prazosin, phenoxybenzamine)
β-adrenoceptor antagonists (e.g. propranolol, atenolol)
Combined α and β-antagonists (labetalol)

Inhibitors of the renin–angiotensin–aldosterone system:
Reduction of renin secretion (by β-adrenergic blockade)
Angiotensin-converting enzyme inhibitors (e.g. captopril, enalapril)
Angiotensin antagonists (saralasin)
Aldosterone antagonists (e.g. spironolactone, potassium canrenoate)

Drugs with non-autonomic effects on peripheral resistance:
Vasodilators (e.g. calcium-channel blockers, hydralazine)
Diuretics (thiazides and loop diuretics)

---

sometimes curable cause of their hypertension may be found. Disease processes resulting in secondary hypertension include coarctation of the aorta, renal artery stenosis, phaeochromocytoma and hyperaldosteronism.

The level of arterial blood pressure is determined by the cardiac output and the impedance of the resistance vessels (arterioles) and is principally maintained by the efficiency of both the sympathetic nervous system and the renin–angiotensin–aldosterone system. Pharmacological methods of reducing blood pressure frequently involve the modification of these pathways at various sites. In addition, drugs which act directly to relax vascular smooth muscle or alter vessel wall compliance by effects on extracellular fluid volumes (thus decreasing peripheral resistance) are effective antihypertensive agents. In some instances drugs of this class may also reduce cardiac output secondary to their effects on capacitance vessels (thus diminishing venous return) or by negative inotropic or chronotropic effects on the heart. The sites of action of the various drugs which may be employed in the treatment of hypertension is shown in Table 13.1. It must be stressed that this physiological classification is not in any way correlated with their importance in practice. The clinical implications are discussed at a later stage of the chapter.

CENTRALLY ACTING DRUGS

Methyldopa

Methyldopa was originally shown to be a dopa decarboxylase inhibitor, and it was considered that the antihypertensive effect was due to failure of conversion of dopa to dopamine and then to noradrenaline. It was subsequently demonstrated that methyldopa itself acted as a substrate for the enzyme and was converted into α-methylnoradrenaline which was thought to act as a 'false transmitter' at noradrenergic nerve terminals. Further evidence indicated that this substance displayed significant intrinsic sympathomimetic activity. Methyldopa readily traverses the blood–brain barrier and is converted into α-methylnoradrenaline which subsequently inhibits cardioregulatory centres in the tractus solitarius in the medulla oblongata, through effects mediated via α_2-receptors situated at these sites.

In recent years the use of methyldopa in the treatment of hypertension has declined. Side-effects include drowsiness and depression, oedema, drug rashes and hepatotoxicity. With prolonged therapy 10–20% of patients show a positive direct Coombs test and in a small proportion of these haemolytic anaemia will occur. In contrast, postural hypotension rarely occurs with methyldopa therapy.

Clonidine

Clonidine was originally designed as a topical vasoconstrictor and its potent antihypertensive activity was discovered accidentally. The intravenous administration of clonidine produces a transient increase in blood pressure and peripheral vasoconstriction, an effect which appears to be mediated via α_1-adrenoceptors. The secondary responses of bradycardia and hypotension are principally due to a CNS effect; clonidine has an agonistic effect on α_2-receptors in the medulla oblongata and inhibits central vasomotor activity. Clonidine may also act as an agonist on peripheral presynaptic (α_2) receptors to inhibit the release of noradrenaline.

Clonidine produces some degree of sedation, and a dry mouth (which appears to be due to central inhibition of salivation) is a common side-effect. Postural hypotension is not usually a problem. However the use of this drug in the therapy of hypertension has been considerably restricted by the severe 'rebound' phenomena which have occurred following the sudden withdrawal of the drug. A life-threatening hypertensive crisis associated with hyperexcitability can ensue and may require treatment with a combination of α and β-adrenoceptor antagonists.

Clonidine has been used in low dosage in the prophylaxis of migraine; presumably the peripheral vasoconstrictor effect is considered to predominate in these circumstances. The administration of clonidine has also been shown to reduce the MAC value of anaesthetic agents. Furthermore, clonidine appears to exhibit an antinociceptive effect and has been administered by intrathecal routes for the relief of intractable pain. The drug has also been used in the management of the Gilles de la Tourette syndrome.

GANGLION-BLOCKING COMPOUNDS

These were the first drugs used specifically for the treatment of essential hypertension. Marked disadvantages to the use of these drugs include:

1   Irregular absorption after oral administration.

2   Non-selective blockade of nicotinic receptors in all autonomic ganglia leading to a variety of side-effects, including dry mouth, blurred vision, paralytic ileus and disturbances of sexual function.

3   The problem of postural hypotension; the receptors on the chromaffin cells of the adrenal medulla are also blocked, and adequate compensation for postural changes is not possible.

Mecamylamine is still available in the USA and pentolinium and hexamethonium are used to a limited extent for the treatment of hypertension in some countries. These drugs are no longer used in the UK, where the role of ganglion-blocking agents is now limited to the more rapid reduction of blood pressure in hypertensive emergencies, or to provide a relatively bloodless field during surgical procedures. Trimetaphan is commonly used in this context and is discussed later in the chapter (p. 431).

ADRENERGIC-NEURONE BLOCKING AGENTS

In sympathetic nerve terminals, noradrenaline which has been taken up by $Uptake_1$ mechanisms, together with dopamine which is available for its further synthesis, undergo active transport from cytoplasm into storage vesicles. Drugs which lower the blood pressure by acting at postganglionic sympathetic nerve endings appear to have complex mechanisms affecting the transport, storage and subsequent release of noradrenaline.

Guanethidine

Guanethidine is an antihypertensive agent which acts principally on the storage vesicles in sympathetic nerve terminals by displacing noradrenaline from binding sites and preventing its further uptake from the axoplasm. Intravenous administration of guanethidine appears to produce a triphasic effect. Initially there is a fall in blood pressure which is due to a direct effect on resistance vessels (in this respect guanethidine may be regarded as a 'false transmitter'). A slight rise of blood pressure then occurs because noradrenaline is displaced into the synaptic gap. A progressive fall of both systolic and diastolic blood pressure subsequently ensues because of failure of release of further neurotransmitter. Following oral administration of guanethidine a rise in blood pressure is unlikely to occur; the fall is slow in onset and usually develops over several days. The drug has a long duration of action; the effects of a single dose persist for up to 4 days and cumulation is likely. Side-effects include postural hypotension, diarrhoea and failure of ejaculation; CNS effects are uncommon as guanethidine does not readily penetrate the blood–brain barrier. Transport of the drug into the neurone and the subsequent antihypertensive effect is prevented by drugs which block Uptake$_1$ mechanisms (e.g. tricyclic antidepressants, cocaine, amphetamines). Conversely, those patients receiving long-term therapy with guanethidine exhibit a marked 'supersensitivity' to pressor amines.

Guanethidine is also used to produce intravenous regional sympathetic blockade in the treatment of intractable pain involving a limb in which there is evidence of autonomic dysfunction; the drug also has significant local anaesthetic activity.

Bethanidine and debrisoquine are closely related drugs with a shorter duration of action. Bretylium, another analogue, has now found a role in the management of ventricular dysrhythmias resistant to other treatment and is described as a Class 3 antiarrhythmic agent.

Reserpine

Reserpine is an alkaloid which has been extensively used in the treatment of hypertension. It acts by preventing the uptake of noradrenaline from the axoplasm into the storage granules. The uptake of dopamine into the vesicles is similarly inhibited and storage of 5-hydroxytryptamine also appears to be impaired. The amines are thus more vulnerable to the mitochondrial monoamine oxidase, and eventually depletion of the neurotransmitter occurs. Reserpine readily crosses the blood–brain barrier, and undoubtedly produces similar effects on adrenergic neurones within the CNS. Deficiency of dopamine and noradrenaline at central sites would account for the main side-effects of reserpine which include depression, extrapyramidal disturbances and the manifestations of hyperprolactinaemia. These effects appear to be dose dependent and reserpine is still sometimes used in the treatment of hypertension.

Metyrosine (α-methyl-*p*-tyrosine) is a competitive inhibitor of the enzyme tyrosine hydroxylase. Metyrosine thus prevents the conversion of tyrosine to dopa with a consequent reduction in the formation of dopamine and noradrenaline at central and peripheral sites, including the adrenal medulla.

Metyrosine may be used in the preoperative preparation of patients scheduled for the removal of a phaeochromocytoma, or in the long-term management of those unsuitable for surgery. Side-effects associated with the use of the drug include moderate or severe sedation and the appearance of extrapyramidal disorders; diarrhoea is also a common complaint. Metyrosine is not recommended for the treatment of esssential hypertension.

Other drugs which can produce a hypotensive effect which is probably due to the production of a 'false transmitter' at the noradrenergic nerve terminal include the monoamine oxidase inhibitor pargyline and the experimental agent 6-hydroxydopamine.

α-ADRENOCEPTOR BLOCKING AGENTS

In general, drugs of this group have been of more value in treating secondary hypertension due to a high level of circulating catecholamines than for the management of essential hypertension. They have also been used to improve organ blood flow in the treatment of 'shock', and occasionally as peripheral vasodilators.

Many of these agents indiscriminately block both α_1 and α_2-receptors so that further release of noradrenaline is facilitated. As only α-receptors are blocked, there will be an enhanced response to the circulating catecholamines mediated via β-receptors and tachycardias are likely; postural hypotension can also be a problem.

Phenoxybenzamine forms a covalent linkage with the α-receptor and a potentially irreversible blockade results. The effects of a single dose of this agent may last for several days. Phenoxybenzamine is used in the preoperative management of patients with phaeochromocytoma or in the long-term treatment when surgery is precluded. The drug has also been employed in the control of hypertensive episodes associated with MAOI–food interactions, or those following the sudden withdrawal of antihypertensive therapy with, for example, clonidine. Phenoxy-benzamine has also been used to improve splanchnic and renal perfusion in 'shock' states; in such circumstances monitoring of the central venous pressure is essential.

Indoramin is an α-adrenoceptor antagonist which has local anaesthetic properties (including a quinidine-like effect on the myocardium) and antihistamine activity. It is used in the treatment of hypertension, usually in combination with a thiazide diuretic or a β-blocker ànd has also been shown to reduce the frequency of migraine attacks in some patients.

Phentolamine was formerly employed as a diagnostic agent for phaeochro-mocytomata. However, false-positive responses may occur, and a dangerous degree of hypotension may ensue; this effect may be due to a direct action of the drug on vascular smooth muscle, or is possibly mediated via receptors at these sites. Estimations of the levels of urinary metabolites of catecholamines and radiological techniques, in particular the use of computerized axial tomography (CT scans) to localize the tumour, are more rational approaches to diagnosis. Nevertheless, phentolamine infusions $(0.1-2\,\mathrm{mg\ min^{-1}})$ are still useful in the management of hypertensive crises which may occur with surgical removal of a phaeochromocytoma, especially during manipulation of the tumour.

Prazosin has a highly selective action on α_1-receptors. It is therefore about ten times more potent than phentolamine in controlling the vasoconstrictor responses to noradrenaline, and rarely produces tachycardia. Prazosin is available as an oral preparation for the treatment of essential hypertension. A number of incidents of fainting with loss of consciousness have occurred when a course of treatment with this agent is initiated ('first-dose phenomenon'). It is unclear whether this effect is due to severe postural hypotension from peripheral receptor blockade or whether central mechanisms are involved. This untoward response can be minimized by commencing treatment with a low dose which is taken on retiring to bed.

Terazosin has similar properties to those of prazosin. Other agents which exhibit α-adrenoceptor blocking activity include the neuroleptic phenothiazines and the ergot alkaloids (see Chapter 11).

β-ADRENOCEPTOR ANTAGONISTS

The value of β-blocking agents in the treatment of hypertension is well established and most of the drugs in this group have been used for this purpose. The mechanism of the antihypertensive effect is not entirely clear and it may be that more than one pharmacological action is involved. These may include the following:

1 A reduction in cardiac output which occurs fairly rapidly following the administration of a β-blocker. However, the peripheral resistance will rise initially due to compensatory mechanisms and the hypotensive response will occur more slowly.

2 A resetting of baroreceptor activity at a lower blood pressure level.

3 Inhibition of the renin–angiotensin system particularly in those patients showing high plasma renin activity (PRA).

4 Presynaptic inhibition (via β_2-adrenoceptors) of noradrenaline release from sympathetic nerve terminals.

5 A CNS effect. A hypotensive response can be shown experimentally following the intraventricular injection of a β-blocker. However, some drugs in this group (e.g. atenolol and nadolol) have a low lipid solubility and do not cross the blood–brain barrier significantly. Nevertheless they are effective antihypertensive agents.

Present opinion suggests that the most important effects are those influencing cardiac output and the renin–angiotensin system. The release of renin from the juxtaglomerular apparatus is stimulated via β_1-receptors and is thus inhibited by propranolol and related compounds. There is evidence to show that hypertensive patients who exhibit elevated levels of PRA can be more effectively controlled with low doses of β-blockers.

Propranolol was the first β-blocker to be widely used for the treatment of hypertension. It is non-selective with regard to β_1 and β_2 effects and is devoid of intrinsic sympathomimetic activity (ISA). Propranolol is a highly lipid-soluble compound which undergoes significant first pass metabolism. It readily crosses the blood–brain barrier and has a large volume of distribution, a high clearance rate and a relatively short elimination half-life (approximately 4 h). Related compounds which are poorly lipid-soluble (e.g. atenolol and nadolol) can be advantageous when central side-effects (sedation, depression, unpleasant dreams) are a problem; their pharmacokinetic properties also allow blood pressure to be controlled on a once-daily dose regime. One exception is the hydrophilic agent esmolol, which has a plasma half-life of less than 10 min. The relatively evanescent effects of esmolol are due to its rapid destruction by plasma enzymes.

Cardioselective agents (e.g. acebutolol and metoprolol) should be chosen for those patients in whom β_2-effects such as bronchospasm, intermittent claudication and hypoglycaemia are likely to occur. However, even selective β_1-antagonists demonstrate significant degrees of β_2-adrenoceptor blockade at high doses. Drugs with ISA (e.g. oxprenolol and alprenolol) are theoretically superior when there is a risk of heart failure developing.

β-adrenoceptor antagonists are also discussed in Chapters 11 and 14.

Labetalol produces competitive blockade at α_1 (postsynaptic), β_1 and β_2-receptors. When given intravenously it is approximately seven times more active at β-receptors than at α-receptors; following oral administration the relative activities are 3 to 1. Labetalol is used in the management of hypertensive disorders; it may be administered by mouth in a twice daily regime. Like propranolol it is subject to first pass metabolism and sometimes produces CNS side-effects and occasional skin rashes. Intravenous administration of labetalol may also be of value in hypertensive emergencies, and is occasionally used to produce controlled hypotension during anaesthesia and surgery. It may be given by injection or infusion up to a maximum dose of 200 mg. A fall in peripheral resistance, principally due to a reduction in arteriolar tone, occurs. Reflex tachycardia does not ensue as cardiac β-receptors are blocked. The hypotensive effects can be readily reversed by atropine and tachyphylaxis has not been observed.

THE RENIN–ANGIOTENSIN–ALDOSTERONE SYSTEM

Angiotensin II is the most potent pressor substance known. In addition to having a direct vasoconstrictor effect, particularly on arterioles, it promotes the release of catecholamines from the adrenal medulla and facilitates sympathetic nervous system activity by central and peripheral mechanisms. Furthermore, it blocks the reuptake of noradrenaline into the adrenergic nerve terminal and has a stimulatory effect on autonomic ganglia cells. Angiotensin II also stimulates the production of aldosterone by the adrenal cortex. This mineralocorticoid enhances sodium reabsorption and potassium excretion in the distal tubule.

The production of angiotensin II itself depends upon the release of renin, a proteolytic enzyme which is produced in the cells of the juxtaglomerular apparatus of the renal cortex. The substrate for renin is a plasma protein, angiotensinogen, which is present in the α_2-globulin fraction.

Angiotensin I, a decapeptide which has limited intrinsic pharmacological activity is then formed but is almost immediately converted to angiotensin II; this reaction is catalysed by an angiotensin-converting enzyme (ACE) which is present in the vascular endothelium and lung tissue. Angiotensin II is metabolized under the influence of various peptidases to produce a number of breakdown products, one of which (angiotensin III) retains some pressor activity.

There are three principal mechanisms which appear to control the release of renin from the juxtaglomerular apparatus:

1 *Mechanical.* A fall in renal perfusion pressure will reduce the tension within the wall of the afferent arteriole and signal the release of renin.

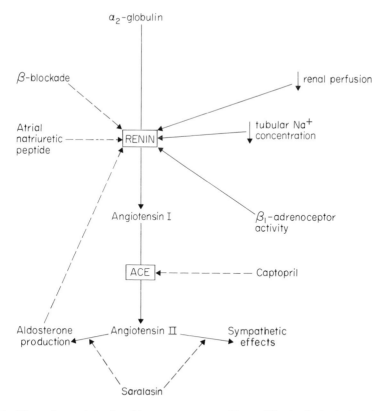

Fig. 13.1 The renin–angiotensin–aldosterone system and its modification by intrinsic and extrinsic factors. ☐ enzymes; —— stimulatory effects; - - - - antagonistic activity.

2 *Ionic.* A lowering of the sodium concentration in the distal tubule situated in the adjacent macula densa is considered to stimulate the secretion of renin. This implies that the increased production of aldosterone, which promotes the retention of sodium ions at this site, will result in a negative 'feedback' effect.

3 *Neurogenic.* Stimulation of the nerves of the renal plexus will result in the release of renin; this secretomotor effect is mediated via β_1-adrenoceptors.

The renin–angiotensin–aldosterone system can be inhibited at a number of sites and by a variety of mechanisms; these are summarized in Fig. 13.1. The production of both renin and aldosterone appears to be antagonized by *atrial natriuretic peptide* (ANP) a hormone which is stored (in an inactivated form) by atrial myocyte granulocytes and whose rate of secretion into the plasma appears to be dependent on atrial wall tension. Thus, elevated levels have been observed following expansion of the blood volume ·and in congestive cardiac and renal failure. Specific high-affinity receptors for ANP have been identified in vascular, renal and adrenal tissue. ANP appears to produce an increase in both glomerular filtration rate and fractional excretion of sodium, and experimental evidence suggests that it is an arterioselective vasodilator. Furthermore, there appears to be now little doubt that the antihypertensive effects of the β-blockers are at least partially due to inhibition of renin secretion.

Captopril

Captopril is an ACE inhibitor which prevents the conversion of Angiotensin I to Angiotensin II. Captopril produces a fall in blood pressure initially by reducing peripheral resistance; arteriolar tone is more predominantly affected than venous tone. Heart rate is usually unchanged or slightly increased and postural hypotension is infrequent. Renal blood flow is usually increased — aldosterone secretion is thus further inhibited and sodium excretion is promoted. Initial dosage may produce a profound fall in blood pressure particularly when there is a pre-existing deficit of sodium. Side-effects which may be induced by captopril include a persistent dry cough, loss of taste sensation, gastrointestinal disturbances, proteinuria and occasionally bone marrow depression. Captopril is used in the treatment of mild to moderate hypertension, usually as an adjunct to diuretic therapy, and in severe hypertension resistant to other treatment.

ACE inhibitors will undoubtedly produce vasodilatation in patients with normal or low levels of plasma renin. The mechanism of this action is not completely clear but may involve a potentiation of the inhibitory effects of bradykinin (by inhibiting its breakdown) and possibly other 'relaxing' factors on smooth muscle. Captopril has thus developed a useful role in the management of chronic congestive cardiac failure by reducing both preload and afterload. Originally used when fluid retention proved refractory to other forms of treatment (e.g. digitalis, diuretics) it is now sometimes introduced as first-line therapy.

Enalapril (a prodrug ester which is hydrolysed to the pharmacologically active parent dicarboxylic acid, enalaprilat) and lisinopril are related compounds with a more prolonged duration of action.

Saralasin is a competitive antagonist of Angiotensin II which has been used in the USA as an aid in the differential diagnosis of hypertension, although partial agonist effects would appear to preclude its more general use as a therapeutic agent. Antagonists of renin activity are also being investigated.

Spironolactone is a diuretic which selectively binds to aldosterone receptors in the distal tubule and thus inhibits the mineralocorticoid effect. At one time, it was extensively used in the management of essential hypertension. There is now some evidence that spironolactone is carcinogenic to animals when it is administered over a prolonged period; side-effects such as gastrointestinal disturbances, gynaecomastia and those related to potassium retention can also be a problem. The role of this drug is now normally restricted to the management of primary hyperaldosteronism (Conn's syndrome) and in the treatment of refractory oedema associated with cirrhosis of the liver, congestive cardiac failure or the nephrotic syndrome. Potassium canrenoate has similar properties (it is hydrolysed to canrenone, which is the major metabolite of spironolactone) and is available as a preparation for parenteral use.

VASODILATORS

Calcium-channel blockers

This class of drugs will antagonize the cardiovascular effects mediated via voltage-dependent calcium channels. They have become widely used in the management of angina pectoris and have developed an established role as antiarrhythmic agents (see Chapter 14). Class 2 calcium-channel blockers (dihydropyridine derivatives), which include nifedipine and nicardipine, do not appear to affect the rate of recovery of the 'slow' calcium channel in the myocardium, in contrast to papaverine derivatives (e.g. verapamil). Thus they will produce arteriolar vasodilatation at concentrations which appear to have little effect on cardiac conduction. Coronary blood flow and subendocardial perfusion are also improved and there is a reduction in the work of the left ventricle. Nifedipine has been used in the treatment of essential hypertension usually in combination with a β-blocker. Side-effects related to peripheral vasodilatation, such as headache, flushing and postural hypotension are sometimes a problem and ankle oedema may occur.

Hydralazine

Initial studies of this agent suggested that its antihypertensive activity was mediated within the CNS. However, present evidence indicates that its major effect is to produce a direct relaxation of smooth muscle. The mechanism is thought to be similar to that of the organic nitrates, as it produces intracellular accumulation of cGMP. However, arteriolar tone is more selectively inhibited and postural hypotension does not usually occur during treatment with this agent. Reflex tachycardia and fluid retention are common accompaniments; thus, in the treatment of hypertension it is normally administered in combination with a β-blocker and a diuretic. Hydralazine is a valuable drug, when administered intravenously, in the treatment of hypertensive emergencies and is a popular agent for the management of severe hypertension associated with pregnancy. Chronic therapy with a high daily dosage may produce a lupus-like syndrome. Hydralazine is subject to pharmacogenetic influences and 'slow acetylators' of the drug are more prone to develop this condition.

Minoxidil has a similar spectrum of activity to that of hydralazine and its mechanism of action is probably identical. One interesting side-effect of this agent is hypertrichosis and it has been used by topical application for the treatment of baldness.

DIURETICS

Many drugs which are used as diuretics can induce a moderate fall in blood pressure when the plasma volume decreases consequent to enhanced renal elimination of water and electrolytes. Thiazide diuretics are most commonly employed in the long-term management of oedema associated with congestive cardiac failure, hepatic cirrhosis and the nephrotic syndrome. They are acidic compounds which are structurally related to the sulphonamides and are actively secreted in the proximal tubule. Their principal site of action is in the distal tubule, where they inhibit the active transport (reabsorption) of sodium ions. Thiazide diuretics may also stimulate the secretion of potassium at a more distal site, and potassium supplementation is sometimes necessary during continuous therapy. Drugs in this group include hydrochlorothiazide, bendrofluazide and hydroflumethazide.

However, thiazide diuretics and closely related analogues (e.g. chlorthalidone, metolazone) are commonly used in the long-term therapy of mild to moderate hypertension. They exert this therapeutic effect at doses far lower than those required to induce significant loss of free water, sodium or potassium ions. In this context, thiazide diuretics appear to act as peripheral vasodilators although the mechanism probably involves a reduction in interstitial fluid volume resulting in an increase in vascular compliance. The use of low-dose regimes appears to be safe and effective; in particular the many side-effects associated with this group of agents when 'diuretic' doses are required (e.g. hypokalaemia, urate retention, hyperglycaemia and elevated plasma lipid levels) are considerably reduced.

Furthermore, thiazide diuretics appear to potentiate the antihypertensive effects of other drugs with different mechanisms of action.

In contrast, both the diuretic and antihypertensive effects of the thiazides may be antagonized in patients who are concomitantly treated with NSAIDs. Inhibition of the synthesis of prostaglandins, which have significant effects on renal blood flow, glomerular filtration and tubular ion transport, is undoubtedly a causal factor.

The carboxylic acid derivatives (frusemide, ethacrynic acid, and bumetanide) are highly potent diuretics with a relatively short duration of action. In contrast to the thiazides which produce a diuretic effect by inhibiting reabsorption in the distal tubule, the site of action of frusemide and related compounds is in the ascending loop of Henle and they are commonly referred to as 'loop' diuretics. In addition an increase in renal blood flow frequently occurs following intravenous administration of these agents. They are most effective for producing a rapid diuresis in severe cardiac failure, pulmonary or cerebral oedema. They are also valuable when administered with blood transfusions for severe anaemia where cardiac failure due to fluid overloading may be anticipated. Loop diuretics are not used for their antihypertensive effects.

Other diuretics of clinical importance include the carbohydrate derivative mannitol. Mannitol is a polyhydric alcohol which is produced by reduction of the monosaccharide mannose and has a molecular weight of approximately 200. Mannitol is widely distributed throughout the vascular bed and interstitial tissues. Its volume of distribution (0.2 litre kg^{-1}) thus reflects the volume of the extracellular fluid. Mannitol is pharmacologically inert; it is freely filtrable at the glomerulus and is not significantly reabsorbed. When administered intravenously as a hypertonic infusion (usually 250 ml of a 10 or 20% solution given over 20 min) it produces a rapid diuresis due to an osmotic effect which reduces water and electrolyte absorption in the renal tubule. Mannitol is of value in the prophylaxis of renal failure (e.g. during surgery for aortic aneurysm or for operations in the presence of severe jaundice), in the treatment of cerebral oedema and glaucoma, and to promote forced diuresis in cases of drug overdose.

Carbonic anhydrase inhibitors, such as acetazolamide, are now rarely used as diuretics. However, they reduce bicarbonate production and consequently the secretion of aqueous humour, and may be useful in the management of glaucoma.

Potassium-sparing diuretics (e.g. triamterene, amiloride) may be used as an alternative to potassium supplements to prevent the hypokalaemia associated with thiazide or loop diuretic therapy.

TREATMENT OF HYPERTENSION

In many patients with moderate or severe essential hypertension, blood pressure can be slowly and gradually controlled by oral therapy. Thiazide diuretics or β-adrenoceptor antagonists are recommended as 'first-line' therapy. The choice of such drugs may be determined by the presence of coexisting disorders (e.g. angina pectoris, obstructive airways disease, peripheral vascular insufficiency, diabetes, gout) but they may be used in combination when they are ineffective alone. A peripheral vasodilator such as hydralazine may be added to this regime in resistant cases and supplementation by centrally acting drugs (e.g. methyldopa) or adrenergic-neurone blocking agents (e.g. bethanidine) may also be valuable.

More recently introduced drugs which are proving effective in the treatment of hypertension include ACE inhibitors (e.g. captopril, enalapril), calcium-channel blockers (e.g. nifedipine, nicarpidine) and α-adrenoceptor antagonists (e.g. prazosin, indoramin). Minor side-effects are perhaps more common with these latter agents and their use in long-term management is less well established. Drugs in this category are perhaps more specifically of value in the presence of associated disease; examples include the use of ACE inhibitors where there is evidence of incipient heart failure, calcium-channel blockers in patients with peripheral vascular insufficiency, and the use of α_1-adrenoceptor antagonists where there is a history of prostatism.

Thiazide diuretics and β-blockers both produce adverse effects on the plasma lipid profile. In contrast, selective α_1-blockers slightly reduce the levels of risk factors associated with coronary heart disease, namely total cholesterol, its low-density sub-fraction (LDL-C) and triglycerides, whilst elevating the high-density cholesterol levels.

In certain hypertensive emergencies, the blood pressure must be lowered immediately. Such situations include hypertensive encephalopathy, intracranial haemorrhage, dissecting aortic aneurysm, acute congestive cardiac failure and severe hypertension associated with toxaemia of pregnancy. Parenteral therapy is usually indicated in such cases although precipitous falls in blood pressure should be avoided to minimize further complications from the reduction in cerebral, myocardial or renal blood flow. Drugs which may be used for this purpose include hydralazine, labetalol, diazoxide, sodium nitroprusside, and trimetaphan (the two last mentioned drugs are discussed more fully in a subsequent section of this chapter).

Diazoxide has a close structural resemblance to the thiazide diuretics, although paradoxically the drug itself has sodium retaining effects. Diazoxide produces its hypotensive effects by relaxation of arteriolar smooth muscle; there appears to be little effect on capacitance vessels. The baroreceptor response evoked by the fall in blood pressure may lead to an increase in heart rate and stroke volume; the release of renin is also enhanced. When used in the treatment of a hypertensive crisis, diazoxide is administered by rapid intravenous injection in a dose of $1-3\,mg\,kg^{-1}$ to a maximal single dose of 150 mg. The optimal depressor response occurs after a few minutes and if further treatment is not instituted the blood pressure will return to its original level within 4–24 h. The concomitant use of a rapidly acting diuretic, such as frusemide may be necessary if the hypertensive emergency is associated with pulmonary oedema or renal failure. As with the thiazide diuretics, diazoxide has diabetogenic properties and may antagonize the effects of insulin and other hypoglycaemic agents. Conversely, it is sometimes used as an oral preparation in the management of chronic hypoglycaemia associated with hyperplasia or tumours of the islet cells of the pancreas.

Hypertension in pregnancy

The presence of hypertension during pregnancy is one of the leading causes of maternal death and of fetal mortality and morbidity. There is a considerable amount of evidence to show that an increase in the incidence of stillbirths and intra-uterine growth retardation may be associated with only a moderate increase in the diastolic or mean arterial blood pressure during the middle trimester. Maternal risks appear to correlate with rises in blood pressure which occur during the third trimester.

It is thus important to control an elevated blood pressure which occurs during pregnancy, whether this is due to pre-existing essential or secondary hypertension or to pre-eclampsia. Non-pharmacological methods (e.g. strict bed rest) are sometimes of value, but drug treatment will often be required. However, the choice of an appropriate antihypertensive agent will need careful consideration. Thiazide diuretics are probably not indicated in pregnancy. They do not prevent the development of toxaemia and may lead to hypovolaemia and to a decrease in placental perfusion. In the neonate thrombocytopenia, jaundice, hyponatraemia and an increased risk of hypertension developing at maturity have been reported.

Propranolol readily crosses the placental barrier; a number of fetal complications have been reported in association with its use; these include intra-uterine growth retardation, severe neonatal hypoglycaemia, bradycardia and respiratory depression. Reserpine has also been associated with a number of fetal abnormalities including lethargy, disturbances of temperature control, and engorgement of the mucous membranes, whilst clonidine has been shown to be teratogenic in animal studies. ACE inhibitors such as captopril may adversely affect fetal and neonatal blood pressure control and renal function, whilst the use of calcium-channel blockers such as nifedipine may inhibit the progress of labour.

Methyldopa and β-adrenoceptor antagonists with low lipophilic properties (e.g. atenolol) are safe to administer during pregnancy and oral hydralazine is useful as second-line therapy; the intravenous administration of this drug may be necessary to control hypertensive crises associated with eclampsia.

Antihypertensive drugs and anaesthesia

It is evident that many of the agents used in anaesthetic practice can exert significant activity on the autonomic nervous system and can theoretically potentiate the effects of established antihypertensive therapy. At one time it was considered desirable that whenever possible antihypertensive drugs should be withdrawn for up to 14 days prior to anaesthesia and surgery. Various tests were used to assess the magnitude of residual sympathetic activity; these included the measurement of blood pressure responses to the Valsalva manoeuvre or to postural changes, or to the administration of indirectly acting sympathomimetic amines such as ephedrine or tyrosine.

This view is no longer tenable. The attendant dangers of a rising blood pressure are an obvious disadvantage, and the enhanced pressor responses which are observed during laryngoscopy and intubation in uncontrolled hypertensive patients is particularly hazardous. Furthermore, the sudden withdrawal of clonidine, β-blockers and possibly other agents may lead to dangerous rebound phenomena.

It is now standard practice to continue antihypertensive therapy until a few hours prior to surgery. However, special vigilance is still necessary to prevent excessive hypertension and tachycardia which may result from airway manipulation or surgical stimulation. In this context, the depth of anaesthesia is of considerable import; however, the concentrations of volatile agents required to suppress such haemodynamic responses are considerably greater than their MAC values, and may lead to depression of an already compromised myocardium.

In such a situation, the use of rapidly acting narcotic analgesics (e.g. fentanyl, alfentanil) during induction may be especially valuable. Topical lignocaine applied to the larynx before intubation and, on occasions, the prior administration of glyceryl trinitrate would also appear to be beneficial.

In this context, the ultrashort acting β-adrenoceptor antagonist, esmolol, may also prove to be of value. Esmolol is a cardioselective blocker with no intrinsic sympathomimetic or membrane stabilizing activity. Esmolol has a rapid onset of action following intravenous administration; no significant blockade can be detected 20 min after termination of treatment. The short $t_{\frac{1}{2}\beta}$ (approximately 9 min) is due to rapid biotransformation of the drug, by esterases present in the red blood cells, to an inactive acid metabolite and methyl alcohol (less than 2% is excreted unchanged in the urine). Such properties would suggest that the drug would be particularly suitable for the management of hypertensive responses which may occur during the induction or recovery phases of anaesthesia. Esmolol has also been used in the treatment of supraventricular tachycardias, and may be effective in the management of acute myocardial ischaemia and unstable angina. A non-cardioselective analogue flestolol, which may have an even briefer action, is also being developed. α_2-adrenoceptor agonists (e.g. clonidine and azepexole) which can reduce anaesthetic requirements, and also decrease adrenergic activity by both central and peripheral mechanisms, may also develop a role in the modification of cardiovascular reflex responses which may occur during anaesthesia (see Chapter 11).

In both treated and untreated hypertensive patients, untoward changes in cardiovascular parameters are more prone to occur during anaesthesia than in normotensive subjects. Special attention must thus be paid to the maintenance of blood volume, ventilatory parameters and positioning the patient on the operating table.

Induced hypotension

Deliberate hypotension has been employed for many years to reduce bleeding during surgical procedures. Techniques which were originally used included controlled arteriotomy, the application of negative pressures to the lower limbs and the production of 'high' spinal or extradural blockade with local anaesthetic agents. The inhalational agents now in common use (halothane, enflurane, isoflurane) all produce dose-related effects on blood pressure and may be employed to produce moderate and predictable hypotension during anaesthesia. Controlled ventilation is necessary for this technique and the combined use of tubocurarine as the muscle relaxant may be particularly beneficial. Other drugs which have been specifically employed to produce controlled hypotension during surgery include trimetaphan, sodium nitroprusside, and glyceryl trinitrate.

Trimetaphan

Trimetaphan is a sulphonium compound containing two tertiary amine groups. When used to produce a 'bloodless field' during surgery, it is usually administered in physiological saline at a rate of $1-4\,mg\,min^{-1}$. Trimetaphan is incompatible in solution with some other drugs commonly used in anaesthesia (e.g. intravenous barbiturates and gallamine). Its hypotensive effects are due to several different actions of the drug. Trimetaphan causes blockade of both sympathetic and parasympathetic ganglia and releases histamine from mast cells. Furthermore, it decreases peripheral resistance by a direct action on blood vessels; experimental evidence suggests that this may be an important factor in the hypotensive response. Arteriolar and venular tone are both decreased, so that both afterload and preload are reduced and venous pooling may occur. These changes are frequently associated with a compensatory tachycardia; the pulse rate may increase by 20% and the cardiac output is variably affected. Although the tachycardia may be controlled by β-adrenoceptor blockade (e.g. with propranolol) this may result in a fall in cardiac output and the occurrence of bronchospasm in susceptible patients. The administration of trimetaphan is unlikely to lead to a fall in cerebral blood flow unless the mean arterial blood pressure falls below 60 mmHg; however, renal and splanchnic perfusion are usually decreased. Trimetaphan does not cross the blood–brain barrier.

The use of trimetaphan may be associated with several problems:

1 The effects of the drug are often unpredictable. It may cause a dramatic fall in blood pressure in susceptible patients. Conversely, continued infusion of trimetaphan may lead to the occurrence of tachyphylaxis or acute tolerance with a diminution in response to the drug. This may be partially related to the compensatory tachycardia or to increased neurotransmitter release.

2 Trimetaphan can cause the release of histamine from mast cells and produce local oedema, bronchospasm, and an accentuated fall in blood pressure. Histamine release may also account for a delay in the return of the blood pressure to normal values which sometimes occurs after the infusion is stopped.

3 Trimetaphan causes pupillary dilatation which may persist and thus complicate observations during recovery from anaesthesia.

4 Postoperative complications such as paralytic ileus and urinary retention may result from the autonomic blockade.

5 Trimetaphan may potentiate and thus prolong the effects of competitive neuromuscular blocking agents and produce variable responses to reversal by anticholinesterases. Although trimetaphan is not an ester, it may be broken down by plasma cholinesterase and can enhance the effects of suxamethonium. The use of trimetaphan is contraindicated in patients with genetic variants in plasma cholinesterase or in the presence of liver disease and other drugs which may inhibit the enzyme.

Sodium nitroprusside

Sodium nitroprusside (SNP) was first shown to reduce blood pressure in 1929. Over 30 years elapsed before it was used in anaesthetic practice to provide controlled hypotension. SNP causes arteriolar and venular dilatation by a direct action on the blood vessels. This results in a fall in peripheral resistance and an increase in venous capacitance with a reduction in blood pressure which is not posture dependent. SNP has little or no direct effect on cardiac function although reflex tachycardia may occur following its administration. Renal blood flow is usually unaltered, but the effects of SNP on the cerebral circulation are complex and controversial. There has been some concern that the drug may increase cerebral blood flow and intracranial pressure and that autoregulation of the cerebral circulation may be impaired. A fall in arterial oxygen tension may also occur.

The mechanism of the hypotensive action is probably similar to that of the organic nitrates and is mediated by the nitroso group ($-N{=}O$) contained in the drug. Sulphydryl receptors may be implicated and the influx, binding or translocation of calcium ions with effects on excitation–contraction coupling appear to be involved.

SNP must be given parenterally. It has a rapid onset and a short duration of action and is an extremely potent and toxic drug. SNP is normally administered as a 0.01% solution in 5% dextrose. It is available as crystals (50 mg per ampoule); the solution, which should be freshly prepared, has a faint orange-brownish tint. When exposed to light, SNP is broken down to cyanide ions and other derivatives; solutions become dark brown or blue and must then be discarded. The infusion solution should be protected by wrapping the container in aluminium foil or other opaque material. SNP is normally infused until a mean arterial pressure of 50–60 mmHg (6.7–8.0 kPa) is reached. It is suggested that the dose used to provide controlled hypotension during anaesthesia should not normally exceed $1.5\,\mu g\,kg^{-1}\,min^{-1}$.

The brief duration of action of SNP is due to its rapid breakdown. Initially cyanide ions are produced, but under the influence of the enzyme rhodanase and in the presence of thiosulphate (which provides sulphydryl groups) cyanide is converted into thiocyanate which is excreted by the kidney. An 'alternative pathway' for removal of cyanide ions is by combination with hydroxocobalamin to form cyanocobalamin.

Cyanide may accumulate when high rates of infusion are employed or when elimination is impaired. Cyanide toxicity inhibits cellular oxidative processes; the resultant metabolic acidosis may present as sweating, hyperventilation, cardiac arrhythmias and an accentuated fall in blood pressure. The appearance of toxic effects is sometimes delayed until 1–3 h after the administration of SNP.

If the diagnosis of cyanide intoxication is clearly established, the infusion should be stopped immediately and an antidote (either sodium thiosulphate or dicobalt edetate) administered. Hydroxocobalamin is sometimes given prophylactically to provide another route for the removal of cyanide. Conversely, the use of SNP should be avoided in patients with disorders of vitamin B_{12} metabolism. Thiocyanate inhibits the uptake of iodide by the thyroid gland; thus SNP is contraindicated in hypothyroid states or in renal failure (when this potentially toxic metabolite can accumulate).

Glyceryl trinitrate

Glyceryl trinitrate (nitroglycerine) can be used to enhance or induce controlled hypotension. This agent causes peripheral vasodilatation by a direct action on vascular smooth muscle. In contrast to SNP, there appears to be a more selective effect on capacitance vessels. Thus venular tone and preload are decreased to a greater extent than arterial tone and afterload; in consequence the hypotensive action of glyceryl trinitrate is highly susceptible to alterations in posture. Furthermore, glyceryl trinitrate is less likely to induce direct effects on cerebral blood flow than SNP.

Glyceryl trinitrate is normally diluted prior to use, with either normal saline or isotonic dextrose, to give a final concentration not greater than $400\,\mu g\,ml^{-1}$. Loss of activity may occur if glyceryl trinitrate is prepared in packs or bags composed of polyvinyl chloride. The resulting solution is normally infused using a dose range between $10-200 \, \mu g \, min^{-1}$ until the desired level of blood pressure is achieved. The onset of action is usually within 2–3 min, because of rapid formation of the active free radical nitric oxide (NO), and tolerance to the effects of the drug (see Chapter 14) is not usually a problem with short-term use.

By virtue of the effects of glyceryl trinitrate (principally on preload) left ventricular end-diastolic pressure and myocardial wall tension are reduced and there is a resultant decrease in myocardial oxygen demand. Glyceryl trinitrate can be administered by a number of routes (sublingual, buccal or percutaneous) in the management of anginal attacks and may also be given by intravenous infusion in the treatment of unstable angina, the management of congestive cardiac failure following myocardial infarction, or to control myocardial ischaemia during and after cardiovascular surgery.

Labetalol has occasionally been used to facilitate controlled hypotension during surgery. This drug is discussed more fully with the β-receptor antagonists.

Induced hypotension is not infrequently required to facilitate neurosurgical procedures but its use in other fields has probably declined in recent years. The consequences of cerebral ischaemia which may occur in the absence of any evidence of cardiac ischaemic changes are particularly hazardous. Loss of autoregulation of cerebral blood flow, rebound hypertension and significant haemorrhage occurring during the procedure may add to the difficulties. Induced hypotension is probably best avoided in hypovolaemic states, cardiovascular, hepatic and renal diseases and during pregnancy. When such techniques are used meticulous attention to detail with accurate drug administration (when possible by means of an infusion pump) and the continuous monitoring of blood pressure are essential.

FURTHER READING

Aitken D. Cyanide toxicity following nitroprusside induced hypotension. *Canadian Anaesthetists Society Journal* 1977; **24**: 651–660.

Alper MH, Flacke W, Krayer O. Pharmacology of reserpine and its implications for anaesthesia. *Anesthesiology* 1963; **24**: 524–542.

Ames RP. The effects of antihypertensive drugs on serum lipids and lipoproteins. II: Non-diuretic drugs. *Drugs* 1986; **32**: 335–357.

Andrews G, MacMahon SW, Austin A, Byrne DG. Hypertension: comparison of drug and non-drug treatments. *British Medical Journal* 1982; **284**: 1523–1526.

Antonaccio MJ. Angiotensin-converting-enzyme (ACE) inhibitors. *Annual Review of Pharmacology and Toxicology* 1982; **27**: 57–87.

Bagnall WE, Salway JG, Jackson EW. Phaeochromocytoma with myocarditis managed with α-methyl-*p*-tyrosine. *Postgraduate Medical Journal* 1976; **52**: 653–656.

Barlow RB, Ing HR. Curare-like action of polymethylene bis-quaternary ammonium salts. *British Journal of Pharmacology and Chemotherapy* 1948; **3**: 298–304.

Bloor BC, Flacke WE. Reduction in halothane anaesthetic requirement by clonidine, an alpha-adrenergic agonist. *Anesthesia and Analgesia* 1982; **61**: 741–745.

Braunwald E. Mechanism of action of calcium-channel blocking agents. *New England Journal of Medicine* 1982; **307**: 1618–1627.

Chestnut JS, Albin NS, Gonzalez-Aboda E, Newfield P, Maroon JC. Clinical evaluation of intravenous nitroglycerine for neurosurgery. *Journal of Neurosurgery* 1978; **48**: 704–711.

Clive DM, Stoff JS. Renal symptoms associated with non-steroidal anti-inflammatory drugs. *New England Journal of Medicine* 1984; **310**: 563–572.

Conolly ME, Briant RH, George CF, Dollery CT. A crossover comparison of clonidine and methyldopa in hypertension. *European Journal of Clinical Pharmacology* 1972; **4**: 222–227.

Crandell D Le R. The anesthetic hazards in patients on antihypertensive therapy. *Journal of the American Medical Association* 1962; **179**: 495–500.

Dale HH. On some physiological actions of ergot. *Journal of Physiology* (London) 1906; **34**: 163–206.

Deacock AR de C, Hargrove RL. The influence of certain ganglionic blocking agents on neuromuscular transmission. *British Journal of Anaesthesia* 1962; **34**: 357–362.

Enderby GEH. A report on the mortality and morbidity following 9107 hypotensive anaesthetics. *British Journal of Anaesthesia* 1961; **33**: 109–113.

Feneck R. Cardiovascular function and the safety of anaesthesia. In: Taylor TH, Major E (eds) *Hazards and Complications of Anaesthesia.* Edinburgh: Churchill Livingstone, 1987; 11–32.

Folkow B. The haemodynamic consequence of adaptive structural changes of the resistance vessels in hypertension. *Clinical Science* 1971; **41**: 1–7.

Fries ED, Rose JC, Riggins TF *et al.* The haemodynamic effects of hypotensive drugs in man IV. I-Hydrazinophthalazine. *Circulation* 1953; **8**: 188–204.

Garcia JY Jr, Vidt DG. Current management of hypertensive emergencies. *Drugs* 1987; **34**: 263–278.

Goldberg LI. Current therapy of hypertension — a pharmacological approach. *American Journal of Medicine* 1974; **58**: 489–494.

Goldman L, Caldera DL. Risks of general anaesthesia and elective operation in the hypertensive patient. *Anesthesiology* 1979; **50**: 285–292.

Gorczynski RJ. Basic pharmacology of esmolol. *American Journal of Cardiology* 1985; **56**: 3F–13F.

Graham RM, Thornell IR, Gain JM *et al.* Prazosin: the first-dose phenomenon. *British Medical Journal* 1976; **2**: 1293–1294.

Hannington-Kiff JG. Intravenous regional sympathetic block with guanethidine. *Lancet* 1974; **i**: 1019–1020.

Heise A, Kroneberg G. Central nervous alpha-adrenergic receptors and the mode of action of α-methyldopa. *Archives of Pharmacology* 1973; **279**: 285–300.

Hellewell J, Potts MW. Propranolol during controlled hypotension. *British Journal of Anaesthesia* 1966; **38**: 794–801.

Janssen PAJ. 5-HT$_2$ receptor blockade to study serotonin-induced pathology. *Trends in Pharmacological Sciences* 1983; **5**: 198–206.

Johnson CI, Arnolde L, Hiwatari M. Angiotensin-converting inhibitors in the treatment of hypertension. *Drugs* 1984; **27**: 271–277.

Lang RE, Unger T, Ganten D. Atrial natriuretic factor: a new factor in blood pressure control. *Journal of Hypertension* 1987; **5**: 255–271.

Larson AG. Deliberate hypotension. *Anesthesiology* 1964; **25**: 682–706.

Leigh JM. The history of controlled hypotension. *British Journal of Anaesthesia* 1975; **47**: 745–749.

Low J, Harvey J, Prys-Roberts C, Dagnino J. Studies of anaesthesia in relation to hypertension. *British Journal of Anaesthesia* 1986; **58**: 471–477.

McDowall DG. Induced hypotension and brain ischaemia. *British Journal of Anaesthesia* 1985; **57**: 110–119.

Mehta J, Cohn JN. Haemodynamic effects of labetalol, an alpha and beta adrenergic blocking agent, in hypertensive subjects. *Circulation* 1977; **55**: 370–375.

Murphy MB, Scriven AJI, Dollery CT. Role of nifedipine in the treatment of hypertension. *British Medical Journal* 1983; **287**: 257–259.

Murthy VS, Patel KD, Elangovar RG *et al*. Cardiovascular and neuromuscular effects of esmolol during general anaesthesia. *Journal of Clinical Pharmacology* 1986; **26**: 351–357.

Paton WDM, Zaimis E. The methonium compounds. *Pharmacological Reviews* 1952; **4**: 219–253.

Peach MJ. Renin–angiotensin system; biochemistry and mechanisms of action. *Physiological Reviews* 1977; **57**: 313–370.

Prichard BNC. Beta-adrenergic receptor blockade in hypertension; past present and future. *British Journal of Clinical Pharmacology* 1978; **5**: 379–399.

Prys-Roberts C, Green LT, Meloche R, Foex P. Studies of anaesthesia in relation to hypertension; II Haemodynamic consequences of induction and endotracheal intubation. *British Journal of Anaesthesia* 1971; **43**: 531–547.

Regoli D, Park WK, Rioux F. Pharmacology of angiotensin. *Pharmacological Reviews* 1974; **26**: 69–123.

Robertson D, Nies AS. Antihypertensive drugs. In: Turner P, Shand DG (eds) *Recent Advances in Clinical Pharmacology*, No 1. Edinburgh: Churchill Livingstone, 1978; 55–92.

Rogers MC, Troystman RJ. Cerebral haemodynamic effects of nitroglycerine and nitroprusside. *Anesthesiology* 1979; **51**: 199S.

Salem MR. Therapeutic uses of ganglion blocking drugs. *International Anaesthesiology Clinics* 1978; **16**: 171–200.

Stamler J, Stamler R. Intervention for the prevention and control of hypertension and arteriosclerotic disease: United States and International experience. *American Journal of Medicine* 1984; **77** (Supplement 12): 13–36.

Stanaszek WF, Kellerman D, Brogden RN, Romankiewitz JA. Prazosin update; a review of its pharmacological properties and therapeutic use in hypertension. *Drugs* 1983; **25**: 339–384.

Tamsen A, Gordh TE. Epidural clonidine produces analgesia. *Lancet* 1984; **ii**: 231–232.

Tinker JH, Michenfelder JD. SNP: pharmacology, toxicology and therapeutics. *Anesthesiology* 1976; **45**: 340–354.

Tobian L. Why do thiazide diuretics lower blood pressure in essential hypertension? *Annual Review of Pharmacology* 1967; **7**: 399–408.

Turlapaty P, Laddu A, Murthy VS *et al*. Esmolol: a titratable short-acting intravenous beta blocker for acute critical care settings. *American Heart Journal* 1987; **114**: 866–885.

Vanhoutte PM, Auch-Schwelk W, Biondi ML *et al*. Why are converting enzyme inhibitors vasodilators? *British Journal of Clinical Pharmacology* 1989; **28**: 95S–104S.

Vesey CJ, Cole PV, Linnell JC, Wilson J. Some metabolic effects of sodium nitroprusside in man. *British Medical Journal* 1974; **2**: 140–142.

Webb DJ, Benjamin N, Allen MJ *et al*. Vascular responses to local atrial natriuretic peptide infusion in man. *British Journal of Clinical Pharmacology* 1988; **26**: 245–252.

Wilson AL, Matzke GR. The treatment of hypertension in pregnancy. *Drug Intelligence and Clinical Pharmacy* 1981; **15**: 21–26.

Wolf RL, Mendslowitz M, Fruchter A. Diagnosis and treatment of phaeochromocytoma. *Mount Sinai Journal of Medicine (N.Y.)* 1970; **37**: 549–567.

FOURTEEN

Antiarrhythmic and Antianginal Drugs

ANTIARRHYTHMIC DRUGS

Cardiac arrhythmias may be defined as irregular or abnormal heart rhythms. By convention, they also include bradycardias or tachycardias outside the physiological range (i.e. 55–90 beats per minute in adults). Arrhythmias may be present prior to surgery, and are commonly seen in patients admitted to intensive care units. During anaesthesia, they may be precipitated by surgical stimuli, or by physiological and pharmacological factors. In all these circumstances, the use of antiarrhythmic drugs may be necessary to control cardiac irregularities or maintain cardiac output.

Electrophysiology of normal cardiac muscle

The understanding of the mode of action of antiarrhythmic drugs is dependent on an appreciation of cardiac electrophysiology, and the manner in which this is modified by disease. During recent years, microelectrode studies on single muscle fibres in the heart have clarified these concepts. The heart consists of conducting pathways (i.e. the SA node, the internodal tracts, the AV node, the bundle of His, and the Purkinje network) which initiate or preferentially conduct cardiac impulses; and contractile cells (atrial and ventricular muscle fibres) which subsequently respond to these impulses by depolarization, resulting in muscle contraction. There are important structural differences between conducting tissues and contractile muscle fibres; these are paralleled by electrophysiological differences that are responsible for the sequential conduction of the cardiac impulse. Conducting pathways consist of elongated, delicate, fusiform cells which are usually embedded in dense connective tissue; they contain relatively few myofibrils and are only faintly striated. In contrast, typical cardiac muscle cells contain numerous myofibrils, which are responsible for the prominent striations seen on light microscopy. The myofibrils consist of filaments of myosin and actin, which interact when the intracellular calcium concentration increases above the resting level ('excitation–contraction coupling'). Each muscle cell is partly divided at numerous sites by the transverse (T) tubular system. The sarcolemmal membrane contains numerous ion channels which regulate the concentration of potassium, sodium, and calcium ions in the cytoplasm, and thus control the gradient across the cell membrane. Cardiac muscle fibres form a syncytium; the cells branch frequently and are separated from each other by intercalated discs.

During inactivity, the inside of all conducting tissues and cardiac muscle fibres is electrically negative compared to the outside, i.e. there is a potential difference across the cell membrane (the resting membrane potential). As in all other excitable tissues, the potential difference reflects the balance between two opposing forces; these are (1) the tendency of potassium ions to diffuse from cells along selectively permeable potassium channels, and (2) the attraction of potassium ions for negatively charged phosphate groups on intracellular proteins. The resting membrane potential represents the balance between these forces, i.e. it is a potassium diffusion potential. In conducting tissues and cardiac muscle fibres, the resting membrane potential is approximately -60 to -80 mV.

In the SA node (and to a lesser extent in the AV node and Purkinje tissue) the changes in electrical potential during the cardiac cycle are different from those in atrial and ventricular muscle. The resting membrane potential is unstable, and decreases from approximately -60 mV to -40 mV during atrial diastole (Fig. 14.1). This change in potential (sometimes known as the prepotential or the pacemaker potential) is probably due to changes in sodium and/or calcium permeability of the cells in the SA node. When the resting potential reaches -40 mV, depolarization occurs; the action potential in the SA node is usually bell-shaped and lasts for 150–200 ms. The action potential in the SA node during each cardiac cycle is mainly due to the slow entry of calcium ions along specific slow calcium channels (L channels) in the cytoplasmic membrane. The slow calcium channels are voltage-dependent and tend to open at a membrane potential of approximately 40 mV. Repolarization is due to closure of slow calcium channels and the unopposed diffusion of potassium ions, which re-establishes the normal resting potential.

In contrast, in atrial and ventricular muscle the resting potential is stable at approximately -80 mV. The changes in electrical potential during the cardiac cycle are usually divided into five phases (Fig. 14.1). During phase 0, the myocardial cell depolarizes from -80 mV to appoximately $+30$ mV, due to the rapid influx of sodium ions (and to a lesser extent, of calcium ions). This phase usually lasts for less than 1 ms. In phase 1, the amplitude of the action potential transiently decreases as the fast sodium channels are inactivated, and chloride ions are passively extruded. During phase 2 (the plateau phase), the action potential is maintained between 0 and -20 mV, mainly due to the slow influx of calcium ions along voltage-dependent and receptor-regulated channels. This phase usually lasts for 100–150 ms. In phase 3 (repolarization), the action

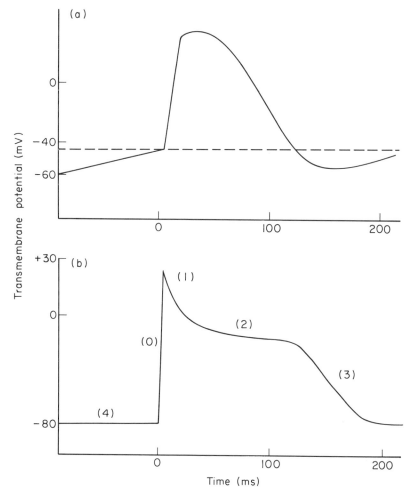

Fig. 14.1 Characteristic transmembrane potentials in (a) the SA node, and (b) ventricular muscle. Figures in parentheses correspond to the five phases of the action potential in cardiac muscle fibres. The events shown in (a), and (b) are not intended to be simultaneous or synchronous.

potential rapidly returns to its resting value of −80 mV (Fig. 14.1), due to calcium channel inactivation and the increased loss of intracellular potassium ions through specific ion channels. In phase 4, the potential is maintained at a value of approximately −80 mV, since atrial and ventricular muscle fibres are effectively impermeable to sodium and calcium ions during diastole. During phase 4, the ionic movements across the myocardial membrane are reversed due to the activity of the ion pump (Na^+/K^+ ATPase), which exchanges three sodium ions for two potassium ions, resulting in a negative intracellular potential.

These electrophysiological differences between the SA node and ventricular muscle are reflected in other conducting tissues. Thus, the action potential of the AV node and the His–Purkinje system have characteristics that are intermediate between those of the SA node and normal ventricular muscle. The duration of the cardiac action potential (i.e. the beginning of phase 1 to the end of phase 3) is shorter in the bundle of His and ventricular muscle (150–200 ms) than in the terminal Purkinje fibres (250–300 ms). It is approximately equal in duration to the refractory period; this is the time after excitation during which cardiac muscle cells will not respond to a second stimulus. In myocardial cells, the refractory period is almost as long as the contractile response. In consequence, cardiac muscle (unlike skeletal muscle) cannot be tetanized (i.e. it will not rapidly respond to repeated electrical stimulation so that summation of the mechanical response occurs).

The origin and propagation of the cardiac impulse can be interpreted in terms of the electrophysiological differences between conducting tissues and contractile myocardial cells. The diastolic membrane potential reaches its threshold value in the SA node earlier than in other cardiac tissues (Fig. 14.1). Consequently, the SA node is depolarized sooner than other cells, and therefore initiates the cardiac impulse. Excitation is propagated over the right atrium by means of the internodal tracts, which are preferentially depolarized before atrial muscle cells. Similarly, the AV node and the His–Purkinje system are normally depolarized before ventricular muscle, since their threshold potential is closer to the resting value.

Physiology of cardiac arrhythmias

The occurrence of tachycardia and some tachyarrhythmias may be related to enhanced pacemaker activity or automaticity (i.e. to an increase in the rate of diastolic depolarization in the SA node). However, arrhythmias are usually due to the presence of an ectopic focus. When there is marked bradycardia or SA block, the cardiac impulse may be initiated by other junctional tissues (e.g. the AV node, the bundle of His, or the His–Purkinje system). These cardiac impulses are known as escape beats; they may be induced by excessive vagal tone, and are responsible for the phenomenon of 'vagal escape'. They are also commonly seen during halothane anaesthesia, which is frequently associated with sinus bradycardia and AV junctional escape rhythms (Chapter 7).

Cardiac arrhythmias that originate in ectopic foci may also be due to abnormal physiological mechanisms that are related to pathological changes in cardiac muscle. This type of arrhythmia may originate in the AV node, the His–Purkinje system, or in atrial or ventricular muscle. In general, they are related to three different phenomena. These are:

1 Enhanced automaticity in conducting tissues or myocardial cells.
2 Re-entry or reciprocating mechanisms in abnormal cardiac cells.
3 The occurrence of pathological after-potentials.

These phenomena are believed to be concerned in the production of many tachyarrhythmias, e.g. atrial flutter, atrial fibrillation, ventricular extrasystoles, ventricular tachycardia and supraventricular tachycardias (including the Wolff–Parkinson–White syndrome).

Enhanced automaticity

Pathological damage to conducting tissues or myocardial cells may cause the development of an unstable membrane potential, resulting in spontaneous de-polarization during diastole. Damaged myocardial cells may be slightly permeable to sodium ions during diastole (i.e. during phase 4 of the action potential). In consequence, their membrane potential may decrease (i.e. become less electro-negative) during phase 4, and reach the threshold for depolarization before the cells of the SA node. Thus, ischaemia may produce pathological changes in myocardial muscle cells, and cause them to assume the electrical characteristics of pacemaker cells. Similar changes may be produced by hypokalaemia, which tends to cause an unstable resting membrane potential during phase 4. These conditions will favour the development of an ectopic focus in atrial or ventricular muscle (or in conducting tissues).

Re-entry and reciprocating mechanisms

Re-entry and reciprocating mechanisms usually arise in anatomical sites that possess the opportunity for differential rates of conduction along alternative pathways. These are particularly likely to occur when impulses can pass down alternative pathways with different conduction times and refractory periods, and when impulses can be blocked. These may be present in the AV node and in terminal Purkinje fibres, as well as in damaged atrial and ventricular muscle. Terminal Purkinje fibres frequently branch as they approach the myocardium, so that a single cardiac muscle fibre can be innervated by more than one terminal (Fig. 14.2). If there is no delay in conduction, impulses can pass down both ter-minal arborizations and are extinguished in the muscle fibre. By contrast, if one of these terminals has a longer refractory period than the other (due to physiological or pathological causes), conduction may only occur down one branch, since the other may still be refractory. The impulse is not extinguished in the muscle fibre, and can approach the previously refractory arborization in a retrograde manner. If this branch has recovered, retrograde conduction of the impulse occurs, followed by anterograde conduction in the contralateral limb (Fig. 14.2). A reciprocal rhythm is set up due to re-entry of the impulse; this phenomenon is probably responsible for many common atrial and ventricular arrhythmias.

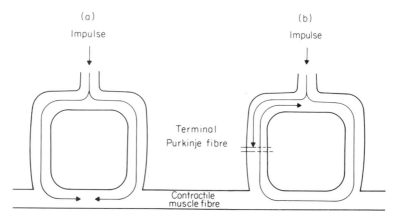

Fig. 14.2 The probable mechanism for the establishment of re-entrant arrhythmias. In (a) the impulse is conducted along two alternative pathways with normal conduction times in the terminal arborization of the Purkinje system. Normal conduction occurs down both pathways and the impulse is extinguished in the contractile muscle fibre. In (b) one of the terminal branches has a prolonged conduction time and refractory period. If this branch is refractory on the arrival of the impulse, conduction only occurs down the opposite terminal. The impulse is not extinguished in the muscle fibre, and can approach the previously refractory arborization in a retrograde manner. If this branch has recovered, retrograde conduction of the impulse continues, followed by anterograde conduction in the opposite branch. In this manner, an ectopic focus is set up.

Pathological after-potentials

Pathological changes in ischaemic myocardium may cause the generation of spontaneous after-potentials after the action potential. These changes may be related to entry of calcium or sodium ions along ion-specific channels.

Classification of antiarrhythmic drugs

In atrial flutter and atrial fibrillation, treatment is usually directed towards a reduction in the rate of ventricular response by the suppression of AV conduction. In most other arrhythmias, the aim of antiarrhythmic treatment is the restoration of sinus rhythm, either by decreasing the enhanced automaticity of ectopic foci, or by interruption (dissociation) of the process of re-entry. Drugs that produce these effects are usually divided into four groups, depending on their action on the ionic and electrophysiological properties of cardiac muscle.

Class 1 antiarrhythmic activity

Drugs with class 1 antiarrhythmic activity reduce the entry of sodium ions into cardiac muscle fibres during depolarization, and thus decrease the maximum rate of rise of phase 0 of the action potential. Drugs with class 1 antiarrhythmic activity often affect other excitable tissues, and have local anaesthetic and membrane stabilizing activity.

They can be divided into three groups, depending on their effect on the refractory period of cardiac muscle. Class 1a drugs (e.g. quinidine and procainamide) increase the refractory period; class 1b drugs (e.g. lignocaine and mexilitine) reduce the refractory period; class 1c drugs (e.g. flecainide) do not affect the duration of the refractory period. The effects of class 1a and class 1b drugs on the duration of the refractory period are probably due to their action on the phase of repolarization (phase 3 of the cardiac action potential). Class 1a and 1b drugs presumably modify calcium entry and/or potassium loss, affecting the duration of the action potential and the refractory period in opposite ways.

These drugs modify arrhythmias that are due to enhanced automaticity or to re-entry mechanisms. When cardiac arrhythmias are due to enhanced automaticity, class 1 drugs reduce the entry of sodium ions into cardiac cells, and reduce the rate of diastolic depolarization in abnormal, ectopic foci. In these conditions, the diastolic potential in the ectopic focus reaches the threshold for depolarization less rapidly, and this may allow the SA node to reassume its normal role as a pacemaker. Some drugs with class 1 activity may also raise the threshold for depolarization. When cardiac arrhythmias are due to re-entry, drugs with class 1a activity may increase the refractory period of the pathway that is responsible for re-entry; this may prevent retrograde conduction of the impulse (Fig. 14.2) and produce bidirectional (rather than unidirectional) block in the pathway concerned. Conversely, drugs with class 1b activity may prevent the occurrence of unidirectional block and restore normal conduction, since they reduce the refractory period of cardiac muscle fibres.

Class 2 antiarrhythmic activity

Drugs with class 2 antiarrhythmic activity prevent the release, or antagonize the effects of endogenous catecholamines on the heart. They may affect the terminal postganglionic sympathetic neurone and prevent the release of noradrenaline (e.g. bretylium); alternatively, they may produce β-adrenoceptor blockade and protect the heart from circulating adrenaline, as well as the β-effects of locally released noradrenaline. β-adrenoceptor agonists (e.g. adrenaline) increase the rate of diastolic depolarization (i.e. the slope of phase 4 of the action potential) in the SA node and conducting tissue, and increase the slow inward calcium current. Thus, β-adrenoceptor antagonists produce antiarrhythmic effects by slowing the rate of diastolic depolarization and decreasing the slow inward movement of calcium ions which is responsible for the prolonged duration of the action potential. Drugs with class 2 antiarrhythmic effects (in particular, the β-adrenoceptor antagonists) are most useful in the management of arrhythmias produced by

Table 14.1 The antiarrhythmic activity of some common drugs.

	Antiarrhythmic activity			
Drug	Class 1	Class 2	Class 3	Class 4
Lignocaine	+			
Disopyramide	+		+	
Mexiletine	+			
Atenolol		+		
Metoprolol	+	+		
Oxprenolol	+	+		
Propranolol	+	+		
Sotalol	+	+	+	
Verapamil				+
Amiodarone			+	

endogenous or administered catecholamines. Many adrenoceptor antagonists possess both class 1 and class 2 antiarrhythmic activity; sotalol has class 1, class 2, and class 3 antiarrhythmic activity (Table 14.1).

Class 3 antiarrhythmic activity

Drugs with class 3 antiarrhythmic activity prolong the duration of the action potential in both conducting tissue and in cardiac muscle. Most drugs with class 3 activity probably prolong the phase of repolarization (phase 3 of the cardiac action potential) by modifying the rate of calcium entry or decreasing the rate of potassium loss through ion-specific channels. This effect is most marked in the bundle of His, anomalous AV conduction pathways, and in atrial and ventricular muscle. Some drugs with class 3 activity also antagonize the effects of catecholamines and may modify the ionic changes responsible for the generation of the action potential. Nevertheless, these drugs primarily increase the duration of the action potential and consequently prolong the refractory period of the His–Purkinje system and cardiac muscle. Ectopic foci due to enhanced automaticity in atrial and ventricular muscle are suppressed; in addition, drugs with class 3 activity tend to interrupt reciprocal rhythms that are due to re-entry by preventing retrograde conduction in pathways with a prolonged refractory period. Antiarrhythmic agents with class 3 activity are usually of value in the management of patients with supra-ventricular tachyarrhythmias, or of arrhythmias associated with anomalous conduction pathways (e.g. the Wolff–Parkinson–White syndrome or the Lown–Ganong–Levine syndrome).

Class 4 antiarrhythmic activity

Drugs with class 4 antiarrhythmic activity are calcium antagonists (also known as calcium-channel blockers), i.e. they prevent the voltage-dependent and receptor-

Table 14.2 The site of action of some antiarrhythmic drugs.

SA node	Atrium and anomalous pathways	AV node	Ventricle
β-adrenoceptor antagonists	Disopyramide	β-adrenoceptor antagonists	Lignocaine
Verapamil	Amiodarone	Verapamil	Disopyramide
Digoxin		Digoxin	Mexiletine
			Phenytoin
			Amiodarone

operated entry of calcium ions into cardiac muscle cells during depolarization. Certain cardiac cells (in particular, cells in the SA and the AV node) are almost entirely dependent on the slow inward calcium current for depolarization; calcium antagonists prevent this process and are particularly effective in preventing re-entrant arrhythmias in the AV node (including nodal tachycardia). Calcium ions also play an important part in the excitation of vascular smooth muscle; consequently, calcium antagonists may decrease vascular tone and induce vasodilatation.

Although the classification of antiarrhythmic drugs by electrophysiological criteria emphasizes the differences between their modes of action, it does have certain disadvantages. For instance, it does not correspond to the clinical use of drugs in cardiac arrhythmias, and it does not include certain drugs with antiarrhythmic properties (e.g. digoxin, or drugs that modify vagal tone). In addition, many drugs possess more than one type of antiarrhythmic activity (Table 14.1). More than 40 drugs with antiarrhythmic properties are currently available in Britain; the site of action of the more commonly used antiarrhythmic drugs is shown in Table 14.2. In the UK, most cardiac arrhythmias are currently treated with lignocaine, disopyramide, mexiletine, β-adrenoceptor antagonists, calcium antagonists, or digoxin; other drugs may be of value, particularly in arrhythmias that are resistant to treatment.

Lignocaine

The amide local anaesthetic lignocaine is widely used as an antiarrhythmic drug (particularly in the treatment of ventricular arrhythmias). It produces at least two effects on the action potential in cardiac muscle; these probably account for its antiarrhythmic effects.

In the first place, lignocaine prolongs the rise time of phase 0 of the action potential by reducing the entry of sodium ions into cardiac muscle fibres during depolarization (i.e. it has class 1 antiarrhythmic effects). It may also increase the threshold for the depolarization of cardiac muscle cells. These effects reduce physiologically or pathologically enhanced automaticity in ventricular muscle fibres.

In addition, lignocaine decreases the duration of the action potential and the refractory period of cardiac muscle, particularly in the preterminal Purkinje fibres. Consequently, lignocaine tends to suppress arrhythmias that are due to re-entry or established reciprocal rhythms. These effects are due to shortened repolarization (phase 3) of the cardiac action potential, and may reflect effects on calcium or potassium channels in the myocardial cell.

In general, therapeutic concentrations of lignocaine do not significantly affect AV conduction. Rarely, the drug may precipitate or exacerbate intraventricular conduction blockade. Moderate doses have little effect on heart rate, blood pressure, or myocardial contractility.

Lignocaine is primarily used in the management of ventricular arrhythmias (particularly when induced by myocardial infarction or cardiac surgery). It is of little use in the treatment of atrial arrhythmias. It may produce toxic effects on the CNS, which are usually associated with high plasma concentrations of the drug (Chapter 8). Its safe and effective use in the control of cardiac arrhythmias depend on its accurate and controlled administration. The optimal antiarrhythmic effects are usually present at plasma concentrations of 2–4 μg ml^{-1}. These plasma concentrations can usually be produced by a bolus injection of 75–100 mg, followed by a constant infusion of 2–4 mg min^{-1}. After 2 h, a slower rate of infusion (e.g. 1 mg min^{-1}) is preferable. The terminal half-life of lignocaine in patients with normal hepatic function usually ranges from 100–120 min. Thus, when the drug is infused at a constant rate, cumulation may occur for at least 7 h before a steady-state is reached. In the presence of liver disease or drugs that impair hepatic blood flow, this period may be prolonged.

Disopyramide

Disopyramide is an antiarrhythmic drug with quinidine-like properties. It has mainly class 1 antiarrhythmic activity, and prolongs the rise time of phase 0 of the cardiac action potential; the threshold potential required to initiate phase 0 may also be increased. Disopyramide prolongs the effective refractory period of conducting tissue as well as atrial and ventricular muscle. It also has class 3 antiarrhythmic activity, and increases the duration of the action potential in cardiac muscle fibres, by prolonging repolarization (phase 3) of the cardiac action potential. Disopyramide has considerable antimuscarinic (anticholinergic) activity, and may produce atropine-like effects in tissues innervated by the parasympathetic nervous system. Overdosage may cause depression of myocardial contractility, AV block, increased ventricular excitability and cardiac arrest.

Disopyramide has been mainly used in the prevention and treatment of ventricular arrhythmias (particularly when they are induced by myocardial infarction, surgical procedures or digoxin overdosage). It is sometimes useful in arrhythmias that do not respond to lignocaine or mexiletine. Disopyramide is sometimes used in supraventricular tachycardia, atrial arrhythmias, or in arrhythmias associated with anomalous conducting pathways. A maximum dose of 800 mg per day should be used.

Disopyramide is well absorbed from the gastrointestinal tract, and can be given by oral or intravenous administration. After intravenous administration, the elimination half-life of disopyramide is 4–6 h; this is increased to 10–12 h in patients with cardiac failure. The drug is mainly eliminated unchanged by the kidney; in renal failure, the half-life of disopyramide is prolonged and the dosage of the drug should be modified.

Mexiletine

Mexiletine is chemically related to lignocaine, and has considerable class 1 antiarrhythmic activity. It slows the rise time of phase 0 of the cardiac action potential (i.e. it reduces the maximum rate of depolarization) without significantly affecting the resting membrane potential. The duration of the cardiac muscle action potential is slightly reduced, due to shortening of repolarization (phase 3).

Mexiletine (like lignocaine) is mainly used in the prevention and treatment of arrhythmias induced by coronary artery disease and myocardial infarction. It is effective when given orally or intravenously.

Mexiletine is used cautiously in patients with cardiac conduction defects. Its therapeutic ratio is low and the drug commonly causes side-effects. These may affect the CNS or the cardiovascular system.

Mexiletine is mainly eliminated by hepatic metabolism. Small amounts of the drug (approximately 10% of the dose) are excreted unchanged in urine. The terminal half-life of the drug is usually 10–15 h.

β-adrenoceptor antagonists

β-adrenoceptor antagonists have been widely used in the prevention and treatment of cardiac arrhythmias (particularly those associated with myocardial infarction or precipitated by endogenous or exogenous catecholamines). By definition, these drugs have class 2 antiarrhythmic effects (i.e. they prevent the diastolic depolarization that is induced in cardiac cells by catecholamines). Most β-adrenoceptor antagonists (with the exception of atenolol and nadolol) also have a variable degree of class 1 antiarrhythmic activity; this is usually referred

Table 14.3 The selectivity, local anaesthetic activity, and partial agonist activity of some common β-adrenoceptor antagonists.

	Selectivity	Local anaesthetic activity (membrane stabilizing activity)	Partial agonist activity (intrinsic sympathomimetic activity)
Acebutolol	CS	+	+
Atenolol	CS	−	−
Metoprolol	CS	+	−
Alprenolol	NS	+	+
Labetalol	NS	+	−
Nadolol	NS	−	−
Oxprenolol	NS	+	+
Pindolol	NS	+	++
Propranolol	NS	++	−
Sotalol	NS	−˚	−
Timolol	NS	+	−

CS, cardioselective (i.e. only produces blockade at β_1 receptors); NS, non-selective (i.e. produces blockade at β_1 and β_2 receptors). Nevertheless, the difference is only relative. −, absent; +, present; ++, marked.

to as local anaesthetic or membrane-stabilizing activity (Table 14.3). One β-adrenoceptor antagonist (sotalol) also has class 3 antiarrhythmic effects. Sotalol prolongs repolarization (phase 3) and thus increases the duration of the action potential in cardiac muscle fibres (probably by producing blockade of potassium channels in cardiac muscle fibres). In general, other β-adrenoceptor antagonists do not affect repolarization or the duration of the action potential.

Most β-adrenoceptor antagonists are structurally related to adrenaline and isoprenaline, and interfere with the effects of sympathomimetic amines by competitive antagonism at β-receptors. Consequently, the characteristic effects of β-agonists on adenylate cyclase and the generation of cAMP (Chapter 3) are attenuated or prevented. Some of them have partial agonist activity ('intrinsic sympathomimetic activity') at β-receptor sites (Table 14.3), and may therefore produce agonist or antagonist effects (depending on the degree of sympathetic tone and the presence or absence of other drugs). In experimental conditions, β-adrenoceptor antagonists with partial agonist activity (e.g. pindolol, oxprenolol, alprenolol and acebutolol) increase heart rate and myocardial contractility. In man, they may produce less bradycardia than pure competitive antagonists, and may have advantages in patients with congestive cardiac failure. Other drugs with partial agonist effects at cardiac β-receptors are predominantly agonists (e.g. xamoterol), and are sometimes used in patients with congestive cardiac failure for their positive inotropic effects.

β-adrenoceptor antagonists are commonly subdivided into two main groups, depending on their relative affinity for β-receptors in different tissues (Table 14.3).

Non-selective antagonists (β_1 and β_2-antagonists) produce adrenoceptor blockade at most β-receptors. Due to competitive antagonism at cardiac β_1-receptors, they reduce heart rate, cardiac excitability, and myocardial contractility. In addition, they may produce blockade at β_2-receptor sites, resulting in bronchospasm, decreased peripheral blood flow, hypoglycaemia, and an increase in uterine tone. Non-selective β-adrenoceptor antagonists (e.g. alprenolol, nadolol, oxprenolol, pindolol, propranolol, sotalol and timolol) are often used in the treatment of hypertension, angina and cardiac arrhythmias. They may also be used in hypertrophic cardiomyopathy, thyrotoxicosis, migraine and essential tremor. One non-selective β-adrenoceptor antagonist (labetalol) blocks both α and β-receptors; it is used in the treatment of hypertension, and is sometimes used to produce controlled hypotension during surgery.

In contrast, cardioselective β-adrenoceptor antagonists possess some degree of selectivity for β_1-receptors, and blockade of β_2-receptors is less likely. Consequently, such drugs (i.e. acebutolol, atenolol, and metoprolol) should be used in preference to other agents in patients with obstructive airways disease, peripheral vascular disease, and diabetes. Nevertheless, cardioselectivity is only relative, and blockade of β_2-receptors may occur with high doses of all β_1-selective antagonists. In addition, the subdivision of β-adrenoceptors is based on the binding affinity of agonists and antagonists in *in vitro* conditions, and not on the biological effects produced by receptor occupation. Almost all tissues (including the heart) contain varying proportions of β_1 and β_2-receptors, which may be situated at different distances from capillary blood vessels and sympathetic nerve endings; consequently, the response to cardioselective and non-selective drugs may be extremely complex.

The pharmacokinetics of β-adrenoceptor antagonists is partly dependent on their polarity (i.e. their lipid solubility).

Relatively lipid-soluble β-adrenoceptor antagonists (e.g. acebutolol, alprenolol, labetalol, metoprolol, oxprenolol, pindolol, propranolol and timolol) are well absorbed from the small intestine and extensively bound to plasma proteins (Table 14.4). They are extensively metabolized by the liver, and have a significant first pass effect, and some of them have active metabolites (e.g. acebutolol and propranolol). Consequently, their bioavailability is usually low, their clearance is similar to liver blood flow, and their terminal half-life is short (approximately 4 h). In addition, lipid-soluble β-adrenoceptor antagonists readily cross the placenta and the blood–brain barrier; consequently, they may affect the fetus (causing bradycardia and hypoglycaemia) and the central nervous system (resulting in hallucinations, depression, and drowsiness). The accumulation of lipid-soluble β-adrenoceptor antagonists in cardiac muscle during prolonged treatment may play an important part in their antiarrhythmic effects.

Table 14.4 The pharmacokinetics and elimination of some common β-adrenoceptor antagonists.

	Absorption (%)	Bioavailability (%)	Protein binding (%)	Terminal half-life (hours)	Significant active metabolites	Eliminated by metabolism (M) or renal excretion (RE)
Alprenolol	90	20	80	3	No	M
Labetalol	70	30	50	4	No	M
Metoprolol	90	50	20	4	No	M
Oxprenolol	80	50	80	2	No	M
Pindolol	90	90	50	4	No	M
Propranolol	90	30	80	5	Yes	M
Timolol	90	50	10	4	No	M and RE
Acebutolol	90	50	20	8	Yes	M and RE
Atenolol	50	50	0	8	No	RE
Nadolol	20	20	30	20	No	M and RE
Sotalol	80	60	0	15	No	RE

The data for absorption, bioavailability, protein binding and terminal half-lives represent median values.

In contrast, more polar β-adrenoceptor antagonists (e.g. atenolol, nadolol, and sotalol) are less completely absorbed from the small intestine, and are not extensively bound to plasma proteins (Table 14.4). They are not significantly metabolized by the liver or affected by changes in hepatic blood flow, and their bioavailability is dependent on their oral absorption. Their terminal half-life is relatively long, so that once daily oral administration may produce adequate β-blockade for 24 h. In addition, their clearance is dependent on renal function; in renal failure, atenolol, nadolol, sotalol, and *N*-acetyl-acebutolol (the active metabolite of acebutolol) may accumulate in the body. Polar β-adrenoceptor antagonists do not readily cross the placenta or the blood–brain barrier, and are unlikely to affect the fetus or cause central side-effects.

All β-adrenoceptor antagonists characteristically produce bradycardia, decrease cardiac excitability, prolong AV conduction, and reduce myocardial contractility. Consequently, they may be used in the treatment of certain atrial tachyarrhythmias (e.g. paroxysmal supraventricular tachycardia) as well as some ventricular arrhythmias. They are particularly useful when arrhythmias are due to increased sympathetic activity, or the presence of endogenous or exogenous catecholamines. They are also used in patients after myocardial infarction, in order to suppress arrhythmias and to decrease the possibility of a recurrent attack. They should be avoided in patients with incipient or definitive heart block, since they increase the refractory period of the AV node and the bundle of His. They may also precipitate or exacerbate congestive cardiac failure. Their antiarrhythmic activity is probably mainly due to their class 2 antiarrhythmic effects; the suppression of ventricular arrhythmias is usually associated with plasma concentrations of β-adrenoceptor antagonists that are insufficient to produce significant class 1 effects. Nevertheless, during prolonged therapy with lipid-soluble drugs, class 1 antiarrhythmic effects may be of some significance.

Calcium antagonists

Calcium ions are intermediate mediators in many cellular processes, including glandular secretion, neurotransmitter release, EC coupling, and blood coagulation. In addition, they play an important role in the excitation and depolarization of cardiac muscle and vascular smooth muscle. During excitation, calcium ions pass from extracellular fluid into junctional and myocardial cells, resulting in depolarization. Drugs that prevent calcium entry during depolarization are usually known as calcium antagonists or calcium-channel blockers; they may interfere with cardiac excitation or conduction, decrease the force of myocardial contraction, or cause relaxation of vascular smooth muscle. The effects of individual calcium antagonists are different (possibly due to the relative affinity of different drugs for junctional tissues, cardiac muscle, and vascular smooth muscle). Calcium antagonists selectively prevent ion entry through voltage-sensitive slow channels (L channels); they do not affect T (transient) channels or N (neuronal) channels. They are usually classified as:

1 Class 1 antagonists (phenylalkylamines), e.g. verapamil.
2 Class 2 antagonists (dihydropyridines), e.g. nifedipine, nicardipine and isradipine.
3 Class 3 antagonists (benzothiazepines), e.g. diltiazem.

Class 1 and class 3 antagonists have significant direct effects on myocardial contractility and AV conduction, and are used in the treatment of cardiac arrhythmias. Class 2 drugs predominantly affect peripheral blood vessels (including the coronary circulation), and are mainly used in hypertension and angina; they are considered here for the sake of completeness. Other drugs may have non-selective effects on calcium channels (e.g. lidoflazine, prenylamine, perhexilene, and possibly halothane, enflurane, and isoflurane).

Verapamil

Verapamil primarily prevents calcium entry in AV nodal cells; it has less marked effects on myocardial contractile tissue and vascular smooth muscle. In most of the AV node, calcium influx mainly determines the speed of impulse conduction; consequently, verapamil decreases conduction velocity and increases the refractory period of nodal cells. Verapamil can precipitate AV block in patients on other drugs that depress AV conduction (e.g. β-adrenoceptor antagonists, quinidine and procainamide). In addition, verapamil may cause bradycardia and can precipitate or intensify cardiac failure. Although the drug has only limited effects on vascular smooth muscle, it may reduce the afterload on the heart and cause hypotension (Table 14.5).

Verapamil can be given orally or intravenously; the usual oral dose ranges from 120–360 mg per day, given in divided doses. There may be considerable individual variability in the response to the drug. Although verapamil is well

Table 14.5 The effect of calcium channel antagonists on the heart and the circulation.

	Heart rate	AV conduction	Myocardial contractility	Peripheral and coronary blood vessels
Class 1 antagonist (e.g. verapamil)	Decreased	Prolonged	Decreased	Slight vasodilatation
Class 2 antagonists (e.g. nifedipine)	Increased	Enhanced*	Increased*	Marked vasodilatation
Class 3 antagonist (e.g. diltiazem)	Decreased	Prolonged	Decreased	Slight vasodilatation

* Mainly due to reflex effects induced by hypotension.

absorbed after oral administration, it is subject to extensive presystemic metabolism, and its systemic bioavailability is only 20–30%. The half-life of verapamil is usually 3–7 h, and the drug is extensively (80–90%) bound to plasma protein. Verapamil is mainly metabolized by the liver to inactive metabolites, which are eliminated in urine.

Verapamil has been mainly used in the treatment of acute and chronic supraventricular tachycardias; it is particularly effective in the re-entrant tachycardia associated with the Wolff–Parkinson–White syndrome. In atrial fibrillation and atrial flutter, it slows the ventricular rate and may restore sinus rhythm. Verapamil is not usually effective in ventricular arrhythmias. In addition to its use as an antiarrhythmic drug, verapamil has been used in the treatment of angina, hypertension, and cardiomyopathy. Unfortunately, it may cause bradycardia, hypotension, and congestive cardiac failure (particularly in patients on β-adrenoceptor antagonists and other drugs which depress AV conduction).

Nifedipine

Nifedipine is a class 2 calcium antagonist, and is chemically related to dihydropyridine. It inhibits the entry of calcium ions into vascular smooth muscle during depolarization, and mainly affects systemic blood vessels and the coronary circulation. It has little or no direct effect on myocardial contractility or AV conduction. It is unclear whether this is related to the preferential localization of nifedipine in vascular smooth muscle, or to differential effects on calcium channels in the heart and the peripheral circulation. Current evidence suggests that nifedipine (and other class 2 antagonists) reduce the duration of channel opening, while class 1 and class 3 antagonists control the change from the open to the closed state. These differences may account for the selective effects of class 2 antagonists on vascular smooth muscle (Table 14.5).

Nifedipine is a powerful vasodilator; it is approximately 30–50 times more potent than verapamil on vascular smooth muscle. It mainly affects calcium channels in arterioles, and has little or no effect on capacitance vessels. Nifedipine decreases systemic resistance and blood pressure, and increases peripheral and coronary blood flow. In the isolated heart, nifedipine has direct depressant effects; thus, it decreases myocardial contractility and AV conduction. In *in vivo* conditions, these effects are overshadowed by reflex tachycardia and increased stroke volume, resulting in a rise in cardiac output (Table 14.5). Most of the side-effects of nifedipine are due to the reduction in blood pressure (e.g. headache, flushing, dizziness, postural hypotension and palpitations).

Nifedipine may be given by oral, sublingual, or intravenous administration. After oral administration, the drug is well absorbed although approximately 50% is eliminated by presystemic metabolism. The terminal half-life of nifedipine is approximately 5–6 h, and its clearance is 20–30% of liver blood flow. The drug is widely used in the treatment of angina and hypertension, but is of little or no value in the management of cardiac arrhythmias.

Nicardipine

Nicardipine is a dihydropyridine derivative closely related to nifedipine. It was originally used in Japan as a cerebral vasodilator, and was subsequently used in the treatment of essential hypertension.

Nicardipine is a potent dilator of vascular smooth muscle; thus, it decreases systemic vascular resistance and diastolic blood pressure, and increases peripheral and coronary blood flow. It has less direct depressant effects on the heart than nifedipine; in *in vivo* conditions, it causes reflex tachycardia and an increase in cardiac output.

After oral administration, nicardipine is rapidly absorbed and extensively metabolized by the liver. The systemic bioavailability is approximately 50%, due to extensive presystemic metabolism; little or none of the unchanged drug is eliminated in urine. The terminal half-life of nicardipine is 4–5 h, and its clearance is approximately 30–50% of liver blood flow.

Although nicardipine is used in the treatment of hypertension and angina, it is of no value in the management of cardiac arrhythmias.

Isradipine

Isradipine is also a derivative of dihydropyridine; it is a class 2 calcium antagonist with similar effects to nicardipine. It produces selective effects on calcium channels in vascular smooth muscle, and is of no value in the treatment of cardiac arrhythmias.

Diltiazem

Diltiazem is a benzothiazepine derivative that affects calcium channels in the heart and the peripheral circulation (i.e. it is a class 3 calcium antagonist). Thus, it impairs cardiac conduction and contractility, and also causes vasodilatation in coronary and peripheral blood vessels (Table 14.5). Diltiazem reduces the automaticity of the SA node, and impairs conduction of the cardiac impulse in the AV node; the PR interval is usually prolonged, and heart rate is usually reduced.

Diltiazem also affects calcium channels in vascular smooth muscle and the coronary circulation, and peripheral resistance is decreased. Systolic and diastolic blood pressure falls, due to the decrease in cardiac output and the reduction in peripheral resistance.

After oral administration, diltiazem is almost completely absorbed from the small intestine, but is subject to considerable presystemic metabolism. Consequently, the oral bioavailability of the drug is only 50–70%. Approximately 60% is metabolized by the liver (mainly to the active metabolite desacetyldiltiazem), while 40% is eliminated unchanged by the kidney. The terminal half-life of diltiazem is 4–6 h.

Although diltiazem has antiarrhythmic effects, it is mainly used in the treatment of angina, hypertension, and peripheral vascular disease (including Raynaud's disease).

Digoxin

Digoxin is one of the most commonly used antiarrhythmic drugs. It is a glycoside derived from the dried leaves of the foxglove (*Digitalis lanata*); its parent glycoside (lanatoside C) is occasionally used as an alternative antiarrhythmic drug. Digoxin consists of a sugar (digitoxose) combined with an aglycone (digoxigenin). The pharmacological and therapeutic effects of the drug are mainly dependent on the properties of digoxigenin. Digoxin has little effect on the normal heart; its actions are most evident in patients with atrial flutter or atrial fibrillation.

The effects of digoxin can be divided into: (1) indirect effects, which are mediated by the vagus and antagonized by atropine; and (2) direct effects, which are due to the inherent action of the drug on cardiac muscle and conducting tissue.

The indirect effects of digoxin cause bradycardia (by slowing the rate of phase 4 depolarization in the SA node), reduce the atrial refractory period, but increase the refractory period of the AV node and the bundle of His. These actions are all antagonized by atropine, and are not observed in the denervated heart.

Digoxin also acts directly on the heart, increasing the refractory period of the AV node and the bundle of His, but decreasing the ventricular refractory period. Ventricular excitability and the force of cardiac contraction are also increased (although digoxin does not affect the rate of contraction or the rate of relaxation). Some of the direct effects of digoxin are probably due to inhibition of sodium/potassium activated adenosine triphosphatase (Na^+/K^+ ATPase), which plays a crucial role in governing the ionic balance in cardiac cells. Enzyme inhibition causes a rise in intracellular sodium; this is followed by sodium/calcium ion exchange (i.e. sodium efflux coupled to calcium entry), which increases the availability of calcium ions in myocardial cells, and increases the excitability and force of contraction.

Digoxin is widely used in the treatment of atrial flutter and fibrillation. In these conditions, numerous impulses impinge on the AV node; a proportion of them are conducted to the His–Purkinje system, resulting in a rapid and irregular ventricular rate. Digoxin (both indirectly and directly) increases the refractory period of the AV node and the bundle of His, and reduces their conductivity. The ventricular rate is decreased, allowing more time for ventricular filling to occur.

Digoxin may increase the rate of the atrial arrhythmia, since it reduces the duration of the atrial refractory period.

Digoxin may also be used in the treatment of paroxysmal atrial tachycardia; it slows the heart by increasing vagal tone and may convert the arrhythmia to sinus rhythm. Digoxin should not be given to patients with ventricular extrasystoles or ventricular tachycardia, since it increases cardiac excitability and may precipitate fibrillation.

The use of digoxin in the treatment of chronic heart failure in patients in sinus rhythm has recently been challenged. Although it increases myocardial contractility and cardiac output in the short-term, its positive inotropic effects may not be maintained during chronic treatment. In mild and moderate heart failure, diuretics and vasodilators may be more effective than digoxin.

Digoxin has a low therapeutic ratio (i.e. the relation between the therapeutic dose and the toxic dose is reasonably close). The initial effects of digoxin toxicity are often gastrointestinal (i.e. anorexia, nausea, vomiting, and abdominal discomfort). Neurological side-effects (headache, fatigue, and visual disturbances) occur frequently, and skin rashes and gynaecomastia are occasionally seen.

In addition, digoxin has serious toxic effects on the heart; almost any arrhythmia may be induced and can simulate cardiac disease. The commonest arrhythmias induced by digoxin are ventricular extrasystoles (including coupled beats), ventricular tachycardia, and various types of AV block. Atrial arrhythmias are less frequent. Digoxin toxicity may be precipitated by electrolyte abnormalities (i.e. hypokalaemia or hypercalcaemia) or acid–base changes; it is particularly common in elderly subjects, and in patients with poor renal function. Digoxin therapy should be controlled (when possible) by the measurement of the serum concentration of the drug by radioimmunoassay. Serum concentrations of less than 1 ng ml^{-1} are usually ineffective; concentrations greater than 2.5 ng ml^{-1} are commonly associated with toxic effects.

Digoxin or digitoxin overdosage can be treated with digoxin-specific antibody fragments (Digibind). This preparation consists of the F (ab) fragments of IgG antibodies to digoxin, raised in sheep. The affinity of digoxin for the antibody fragments is more than ten times greater than its affinity for Na^+/K^+ ATPase; consequently, digoxin is removed from the enzyme and other digoxin receptors and eliminated in urine as a protein-bound complex. Treatment with digoxin-specific antibody fragments is potentially hazardous, and should be restricted to severe and life-threatening cases of digoxin and digitoxin overdosage.

Digoxin is usually administered orally. Patients are commonly digitalized by the administration of 0.75–1.0 mg digoxin daily, until an optimum effect is obtained. Maintenance doses are usually 0.25–0.5 mg in 24 h. Digoxin is usually completely absorbed from the small intestine (as long as drug dissolution is complete). Maximum plasma concentrations are present within 30–60 min (although therapeutic effects are not observed for several hours). The plasma half-life of digoxin is approximately 36 h, and the drug is almost entirely eliminated by glomerular filtration. Consequently, cumulation may occur in elderly subjects or in patients with renal failure. Digoxin has a large volume of distribution (approximately 10 litres kg^{-1}); the concentration of the drug in skeletal or cardiac muscle may be 20–30 times greater than the plasma level.

Anticholinergic agents

Anticholinergic drugs (e.g. atropine and glycopyrrolate) are widely used to prevent or antagonize bradycardia during general anaesthesia. These drugs are considered in detail in Chapters 11 and 12.

Other antiarrhythmic drugs

Quinidine

Quinidine is an isomer of quinine with more powerful antiarrhythmic effects. It has four main actions in cardiac arrhythmias. In the first place, it prevents sodium entry into myocardial cells, and slows the rise time of phase 0 of the action potential (i.e. it has local anaesthetic effects); secondly, it increases the threshold potential required for the electrical excitation of myocardial cells. Thirdly, it directly prolongs the refractory period of conducting tissue and myocardial cells (without significantly affecting the duration of the action potential). Finally, it has antimuscarinic effects on the heart and antagonizes the effects of increased vagal tone.

At one time, quinidine was widely used in the management of certain arrhythmias (particularly supraventricular arrhythmias). In recent years, it has largely been replaced by other agents (or by cardioversion using direct current electric shock), since there are several disadvantages associated with its use.

In the first place, quinidine may cause tachycardia in patients with atrial flutter or fibrillation, and can precipitate ventricular arrhythmias. It is dangerous to use quinidine in patients with heart block or with digoxin-induced arrhythmias. Secondly, the therapeutic ratio of quinidine is relatively low, and the antiarrhythmic dose of the drug (1–3 g per day) is close to the toxic dose. Quinidine may affect the central nervous system or produce various hypersensitivity responses; it may also potentiate the effects of non-depolarizing muscle relaxants. Quinidine has a large apparent volume of distribution, and its concentration in cardiac and skeletal muscle is greater than the plasma level. It has a relatively short terminal half-life (4–5 h) which is decreased to 2–3 h by enzyme-inducing agents. Approximately 40% of the dose is eliminated unchanged in urine, and drug dosage does not require modification in renal and hepatic failure.

Procainamide

The actions of procainamide are similar to quinidine. Procainamide:
1 Decreases the rise time of phase 0 of the action potential.
2 Increases the threshold for electrical activation of cardiac muscle.
3 Increases the refractory period of cardiac cells (with minimal effects on the duration of the action potential).
4 Has antimuscarinic (atropine-like) effects on the heart (although these are usually less marked than the effects of quinidine).

Procainamide is also said to have less myocardial depressant effects than quinidine.

Procainamide has been most commonly used in the management of ventricular arrhythmias. When the drug is injected intravenously, it may cause a dramatic fall in blood pressure. Oral administration is sometimes associated with minor gastrointestinal side-effects; occasionally drug rashes and central effects occur. A long-term hazard of chronic oral treatment is the development of antinuclear antibodies and a syndrome similar to SLE. The condition usually improves slowly when drug therapy is stopped.

Procainamide is partly metabolized and partly eliminated unchanged in urine (60%). The drug is slowly hydrolysed by amidases in the liver and in the plasma; it is also acetylated to an active metabolite with antiarrhythmic properties (*N*-acetylprocainamide). The acetylation of procainamide (like other drug acetylations) is controlled by genes that show polymorphism, so that patients can be divided into slow and fast acetylators. Slow acetylators may be more liable to develop signs of drug toxicity, including SLE. The plasma half-life of procainamide is relatively short (3–4 h), and the drug must be administered frequently in order to maintain a constant plasma concentration.

Due to the problems associated with its use, procainamide is not commonly used as an antiarrhythmic agent.

Flecainide

Flecainide decreases sodium entry into myocardial cells, and prolongs the rise time of phase 0 of the action potential; however, it does not affect the duration of the cardiac action potential or the refractory period. It also affects conduction in all junctional tissues, and thus prolongs intra-atrial, nodal and intraventricular conduction times. It also has negative inotropic effects, and may precipitate cardiac failure in susceptible patients.

Flecainide has been used in the treatment of atrial, junctional and ventricular arrhythmias. There is some evidence that its use is associated with an increased incidence of arrhythmias in patients with symptomless ventricular ectopic beats after myocardial infarction. In these circumstances, its use should probably be avoided.

Flecainide may cause minor unwanted effects (e.g. nausea, dizziness and tremor) in approximately 25% of patients. Its half-life is approximately 14 h, but may be prolonged in the elderly and renal failure. Approximately 50% of the drug is metabolized by the liver; the remainder is eliminated unchanged in urine.

Phenytoin sodium

Phenytoin sodium depresses abnormal pacemaker activity and enhances conduction in the His–Purkinje system (particularly when conductivity is depressed by digitalis glycosides). Consequently, it depresses ectopic rhythms that are due to the escape of conducting tissue from the influence of the SA node. It is particularly useful in the management of cardiac arrhythmias that are associated with digoxin toxicity. Approximately 200–300 mg of phenytoin should be injected intravenously over 10 min. Although some of the antiarrhythmic effects of phenytoin are due to class 1 (and possibly class 4) actions, the drug has complex effects on excitable tissues that are dissimilar to other agents.

Amiodarone

Amiodarone is an iodinated drug with class 3 antiarrhythmic activity. It increases the duration of the action potential in the conducting system and the myocardium by approximately 20–30%. Repolarization is delayed and the maximum rate of repolarization is decreased. The refractory period of the myocardium and the entire conducting system is increased.

Amiodarone has been mainly used in arrhythmias associated with anomalous conducting pathways, and in ventricular and supraventricular arrhythmias. It commonly causes mild sinus bradycardia; when used with other drugs that slow the heart (e.g. digoxin, β-adrenoceptor antagonists and halothane), marked bradycardia and a reduction in cardiac output occurs. Amiodarone commonly causes the formation of microdeposits of lipofuscin in the cornea; photosensitivity and pigmentation of the skin may also occur. It also affects thyroid function, and occasionally causes hypothyroidism.

Amiodarone is extensively bound to plasma protein, but has a large apparent volume of distribution, and a relatively long elimination half-life (approximately 28 days). The drug is usually given orally, and may accumulate for some time after administration is commenced. An antiarrhythmic response usually occurs within 1 week, and may persist for 4–6 weeks after administration is stopped. Metabolites of amiodarone have not been definitely identified, although the drug is deiodinated in the body.

Antiarrhythmic drugs and general anaesthesia

General anaesthesia presents special hazards in patients on antiarrhythmic drug therapy. They may be related to the existence of cardiovascular disease (e.g. coronary artery disease, myocardial ischaemia, congenital or acquired valvular disease, or hypertension) or to its treatment with antiarrhythmic drugs. Calcium antagonists and β-adrenoceptor antagonists reduce cardiac output, and the use of drugs that produce similar effects (e.g. intravenous barbiturates and many inhalational anaesthetics) may be hazardous. Similarly, many antiarrhythmic drugs (e.g. quinidine, procainamide, disopyramide, amiodarone, β-adrenoceptor antagonists, calcium antagonists and digoxin) delay AV conduction by increasing the refractory period of the AV node and the bundle of His. These effects may be potentiated by drugs used in anaesthesia that depress AV conduction (e.g. suxamethonium, neostigmine, halothane, enflurane, and β-adrenoceptor antagonists), and partial or complete heart block may be precipitated.

Cardiac arrhythmias are not uncommon during general anaesthesia; they are often relatively benign and may require little or no intervention or treatment. Occasionally, they are dangerous or life-threatening and require the immediate administration of antiarrhythmic drugs. Although they may have no identifiable cause, they are often precipitated by physiological or pharmacological factors associated with general anaesthesia. Thus, arrhythmias may be due to electrolyte abnormalities (particularly in calcium or potassium levels), increased secretion of catecholamines (due to hypoxia or hypercarbia), surgical stimulation under light anaesthesia, or operative manipulations that reflexly alter vagal or sympathetic tone. Stimulation of the upper airways is associated with a reflex increase in sympathetic activity and increased catecholamine secretion; consequently, arrhythmias may occur during laryngoscopy, bronchoscopy, endotracheal intubation and extubation, and dental surgery. Traction or stimulation of the heart, the lungs, and many intra-abdominal viscera may also cause reflex effects, including arrhythmias. Neurosurgical procedures in the posterior fossa, ocular surgery, and stimulation of the carotid sinus may also cause bradycardia or arrhythmias. Alternatively, drugs used during anaesthesia (e.g. adrenaline, β-adrenoceptor blocking agents, suxamethonium and atropine) may precipitate arrhythmias. Cyclopropane and halogenated hydrocarbons (e.g. trichlorethylene and halothane) sensitize the heart to the effects of administered or endogenous adrenaline, and may cause abnormalities in cardiac rhythm. Arrhythmias associated with catecholamines or increased catecholamine sensitivity are usually treated with propranolol (1.0 mg) injected over 1 min. The dose should be repeated at 2 min intervals until a response is observed, or a maximum dose of 5 mg has been given. In patients with obstructive airways disease, diabetes, or peripheral vascular disease, a cardioselective β-adrenoceptor antagonist (e.g. atenolol or metoprolol) should be used instead of propranolol. Arrhythmias produced by suxamethonium invariably respond to atropine (0.3–0.6 mg). Although atropine itself may produce arrhythmias, these are usually benign and of little importance.

Patients with pre-existing cardiovascular disease or with certain endocrine disorders (e.g. hyperaldosteronism, thyrotoxicosis or phaeochromocytoma) may develop arrhythmias during surgery. Arrhythmias associated with thyrotoxicosis, thyroid surgery, or phaeochromocytomata usually respond to intravenous propranolol.

DRUGS USED IN THE TREATMENT OF ANGINA

Anginal pain occurs when coronary blood flow cannot meet the metabolic demands of the myocardium (i.e. there is an imbalance between the oxygen supply and the oxygen requirement of the myocardium). Myocardial hypoxia leads to the accumulation of local metabolites, such as potassium ions, adenosine, prostaglandins, bradykinin, or related mediators, resulting in precordial pain. Drugs are mainly useful in the prophylaxis rather than the treatment of anginal attacks (since the precordial pain usually rapidly responds to termination of the precipitating stimulus). Occasionally, anginal attacks are prolonged, and drug treatment is necessary.

Three groups of drugs are commonly used to prevent attacks of anginal pain. These are:
1 Nitrates.
2 Calcium antagonists.
3 β-adrenoceptor antagonists.

These drugs have different modes and sites of action, and their use in combination may therefore be beneficial. Nitrates primarily dilate the venous system, and thus reduce the preload; calcium antagonists mainly affect the heart and the peripheral arterioles, decreasing the afterload; while β-adrenoceptor antagonists reduce the work and the oxygen demand of the myocardium.

Nitrates

Nitrates selectively dilate venules and small veins, and thus cause the pooling of blood in capacitance vessels. Ventricular filling pressure (ventricular end-diastolic pressure) is reduced; this in turn decreases ventricular size and myocardial wall tension. Consequently, myocardial work and oxygen requirement are reduced, while coronary perfusion is increased. Larger doses or concentrations of nitrates also act on arterial trunks, arteries, and arterioles, and peripheral resistance is reduced. These effects may decrease cardiac work (although compensatory tachycardia frequently occurs). Finally, nitrates can directly dilate coronary arteries; collateral flow in atherosclerotic areas may be increased, and the oxygenation of ischaemic myocardium is enhanced.

Since nitrates primarily affect capacitance vessels, they may produce postural hypotension. In supine patients, they have only minor effects on the blood pressure, although profound hypotension occurs on standing (particularly in younger subjects). The effects of nitrates on pulse rate is variable. Small doses may cause bradycardia; higher concentrations commonly produce tachycardia, due to a compensatory increase in sympathetic tone.

It has been recently recognized that the vasodilator effects of all nitrates (including sodium nitroprusside) are due to their intracellular metabolism to nitric oxide ('endothelium-derived relaxing factor'). All organic nitroesters have the general formula $R-C-O-NO_2$, and are lipid-soluble compounds that readily penetrate smooth muscle cells. They are metabolized intracellularly to nitric oxide (NO), which reacts with sulphydryl groups to form reactive intermediates (S-nitrosothiols). These reactive intermediates activate soluble guanylate cyclase, and thus increase the conversion of GTP to cGMP (cyclic guanosine monophosphate). This intermediate messenger subsequently activates protein kinases, resulting in the phosphorylation of membrane proteins and the relaxation of vascular smooth muscle (Fig. 14.3).

All nitrates may rapidly induce the development of tolerance to their vasodilator effects. This phenomenon was first observed in munition workers, who were continually exposed to organic nitrates during the manufacture of nitroglycerine. It was also noticed that tolerance to nitrates was rapidly lost during the course of a drug-free weekend, resulting in 'Monday morning headache'. Tolerance to the vascular effects of nitrates may develop within 24–48 h; it commonly occurs during continuous treatment with nitrates, unless a daily drug-free period of 6–8 h occurs. It has been suggested that tolerance to the vascular effects of nitrates is due to the depletion of sulphydryl ($-SH$) groups from vascular smooth muscle cells (which thus prevents the formation of S-nitrosothiols from nitric oxide) (Fig. 14.3). In some studies, nitrate tolerance has been delayed or prevented by the infusion of $-SH$ donors (e.g. acetylcysteine).

Preparations of glyceryl trinitrate have been most widely used in the management of anginal pain. They are mainly used to provide brief and rapid prophylaxis against anginal attacks, and to provide short-term extension of exercise tolerance, and should be taken sublingually approximately 1–2 min before any activity that is liable to provoke angina. After sublingual administration, the action of glyceryl trinitrate is almost immediate, and usually lasts for 20–30 min. (Oral administration of glyceryl trinitrate tablets has little effect, due to the extensive presystemic metabolism of the drug by the gut wall and the liver.) Glyceryl trinitrate tablets may begin to deteriorate within 2–6 months of preparation.

In recent years, other preparations of glyceryl trinitrate have been widely used in the prophylaxis of anginal pain. Sustained-release tablets have an equally rapid onset but a longer duration of action than conventional preparations of glyceryl trinitrate. A metered aerosol spray is also available for buccal administration;

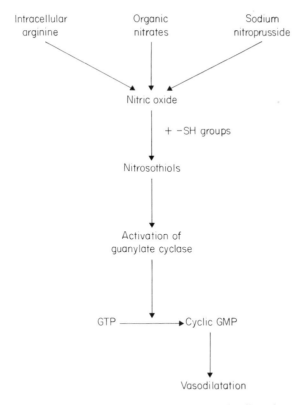

Fig. 14.3 The mechanism of vasodilatation induced by nitrates and sodium nitroprusside.

this preparation is relatively stable, and may be useful in patients who require infrequent prophylaxis. Since glyceryl trinitrate is an extremely potent and lipid-soluble drug, it can also be significantly absorbed across the skin (although skin permeability may affect the degree of absorption). A patch containing a slow release formulation of glyceryl trinitrate produces acceptable bioavailability after application to any area of hairless skin in the body; the rate of drug delivery is controlled by a semi-permeable membrane between the drug and the skin, and usually releases 5–10 mg of glyceryl trinitrate over a 24-h period. This preparation may be particularly useful in patients who suffer from nocturnal anginal attacks. An ointment containing glyceryl trinitrate is also available; after application, it should be covered by a dressing. This preparation provides short-term prophylaxis for 2–3 h, but it is inconvenient to apply and is unsuitable for long-term use. All of these preparations are associated with the rapid and sustained systemic absorption of glyceryl trinitrate, and avoid extensive presystemic metabolism by the liver. Although oral sustained-release tablets of glyceryl trinitrate are also available, they are generally of lesser value in the prophylaxis of anginal attacks.

Oral preparations of organic nitrates have also been widely used in the prophylaxis of anginal pain. In general, these preparations decrease the frequency of anginal attacks and may extend exercise tolerance, but they are of no value in the treatment of anginal pain. For many years, pentaerythritol tetranitrate was widely used; this preparation slowly releases nitrate ions and may provide sustained prophylaxis. More recently, oral preparations of isosorbide dinitrate and isosorbide mononitrate have been used. After oral administration, isosorbide dinitrate is variably absorbed from the small intestine; it is converted by the gut and the liver into two active metabolites (isosorbide-2-mononitrate and isosorbide-5-mononitrate). Most of the drug is present in the systemic circulation as isosorbide-5-mononitrate, which has a terminal half-life of approximately 5 h (i.e. about ten times longer than the parent drug). Consequently, the prolonged prophylaxis produced by isosorbide dinitrate is mainly due to its active metabolite, isosorbide-5-mononitrate. This compound has also been used in its own right in the management of angina. Isosorbide mononitrate has a systemic bioavailability of 100%; it avoids the variable absorption and unpredictable presystemic metabolism of isosorbide dinitrate, and has a longer duration of action. It is probably preferable to isosorbide dinitrate in the management of angina. Isosorbide dinitrate may also be absorbed after sublingual administration (thus potentially avoiding any first pass effects); however, its duration of action is usually no greater than sublingual glyceryl trinitrate.

Intravenous infusions of glyceryl trinitrate are also used to produce controlled hypotension during surgical procedures (Chapter 13).

Calcium antagonists

Calcium antagonists (p. 451) reduce the tone of vascular smooth muscle, and may decrease myocardial contractility. Drugs with predominantly peripheral effects on vascular smooth muscle (e.g. nifedipine, nicardipine and nisoldipine) are of most value in the treatment of angina. These drugs mainly dilate resistance vessels, including those in the coronary circulation; they relax blood vessels in spasm, and may be particularly useful in variant (Prinzmetal's) angina. Occasionally, calcium antagonists with peripheral effects may increase the frequency of anginal attacks and prolong ischaemic pain, due to the fall in peripheral resistance and the associated reflex tachycardia. Verapamil is primarily an antiarrhythmic drug, but may be useful in the treatment of classical and variant angina.

β-adrenoceptor antagonists

β-adrenoceptor antagonists (p. 447) reduce the work of the heart, decrease oxygen consumption, and reduce the afterload. In addition, the associated bradycardia improves coronary and myocardial perfusion. Consequently, both cardioselective and non-selective β-adrenoceptor antagonists are widely used to decrease the frequency and severity of attacks of exertional angina. They may restore the relationship between oxygen supply and oxygen demand, and decrease cardiac activity to a level that does not induce attacks of angina. Unlike calcium antagonists, they are not usually of value in variant (Prinzmetal's) angina; occasionally they may exacerbate or provoke the condition by promoting vasoconstriction of the coronary vasculature.

Nitrates, calcium antagonists, and β-adrenoceptor antagonists have different modes and sites of action on the heart and the circulation, and their use in combination may therefore be beneficial. Nitrates primarily dilate the venous system, and thus reduce the preload; calcium antagonists mainly affect the heart and the peripheral arterioles, decreasing the afterload; while β-adrenoceptor antagonists reduce the work and the oxygen demand of the myocardium. Combinations of nitrates and β-adrenoceptor antagonists are usually additive, and the drugs are often used together in the treatment of angina. Indeed, their disadvantages may be diminished by combined therapy, since β-receptor antagonists decrease tachycardia due to nitrates, while nitrates limit the alterations in ventricular size produced by β-adrenoceptor antagonists. Similarly, combinations of peripherally acting calcium antagonists (e.g. nicardipine, nifedipine, and nisoldipine), β-antagonists, and nitrates are sometimes used in the control of anginal pain. However, combinations of verapamil with other antianginal drugs are potentially dangerous, due to its effects on cardiac conduction and myocardial contractility. This may precipitate heart failure in susceptible patients.

Classical angina is a sensitive and specific indication of the presence of coronary artery disease. Consequently, patients with angina usually have pre-existing cardiovascular pathology, and general anaesthesia may present special hazards. In general, the aim of anaesthetic management is to preserve a balance between myocardial supply and demand, and to maintain the circulation in a slightly hypodynamic state without prejudicing myocardial function. In particular, tachycardia and significant changes in blood pressure should be avoided. Preoperative drug therapy with nitrates, β-adrenoceptor antagonists, or calcium antagonists should be maintained until surgery, and resumed as soon as possible after surgery. Patients on low doses of β-adrenoceptor antagonists may require the dose to be slightly increased. Premedication should be sufficient to allay the undesirable haemodynamic effects of preoperative anxiety, and intravenous opioids may be useful in decreasing the requirements for intravenous agents and in suppressing the undesirable haemodynamic responses to laryngoscopy and intubation. Muscle relaxants that produce tachycardia should be avoided, while the choice of inhalational anaesthetics is controversial. Isoflurane may cause the redistribution of coronary blood flow away from ischaemic areas (Chapter 7), while nitrous oxide may reduce coronary perfusion. Both intravenous anaesthetics, inhalational agents, and other drugs may affect the cardiovascular response to antianginal drug therapy, and haemodynamic changes that are of little significance in healthy patients may result in serious morbidity or death.

FURTHER READING

Abrams J. Glyceryl trinitrate (nitroglycerin) and the organic nitrates: choosing the method of administration. *Drugs* 1987; **34**: 391–403.

Abshagen U (ed.) Clinical pharmacology of antianginal drugs. In: *Handbook of Experimental Pharmacology*. Berlin: Springer-Verlag, 1985; **76**: 1–552.

Abshagen U, Betzien G, Endele R, Kaufmann B. Pharmacokinetics of intravenous and oral isosorbide-5-mononitrate. *European Journal of Clinical Pharmacology* 1981; **20**: 269–275.

.Aellig WH, Hedges A, Turner P, Waite R. Pindolol: the relevance of intrinsic sympathomimetic activity after 12 years of experience. *British Journal of Clinical Pharmacology* 1982; **13** (Suppl. 2): 143S–450S.

Amezcua JL, Dusting GJ, Palmer RMJ, Moncada S. Acetylcholine induces vasodilatation in the rabbit isolated heart through the release of nitric oxide the endogenous nitrovasodilator. *British Journal of Pharmacology* 1988; **95**: 830–834.

Antman EM, Stone PH, Muller JE, Braunwald E. Calcium channel blocking agents in the treatment of cardiovascular disorders. I. Basic and clinical electrophysiologic effects. *Annals of Internal Medicine* 1980; **93**: 875–885.

Aronow WS. Use of nitrates as antianginal agents. In: Neddleman PH (ed.) Organic nitrates. *Handbook of Experimental Pharmacology*. Berlin: Springer-Verlag, 1975; **40**: 163–174.

Barnett DB. Myocardial ischaemia: progress in drug therapy. *British Journal of Anaesthesia* 1988; **61**: 11–23.

Barnett DB. Myocardial β-adrenoceptor function and regulation in heart failure: implications for therapy. *British Journal of Clinical Pharmacology* 1989; **27**: 527–537.

Benfield P, Clissold SP, Brogden RX. Metoprolol: an updated review of its pharmacodynamic and pharmacokinetic properties, and therapeutic efficacy, in hypertension, ischaemic heart disease and related cardiovascular disorders. *Drugs* 1986; **31**: 376–429.

Bennett DH. Acute prolongation of myocardial refractoriness by sotalol. *British Heart Journal* 1982; **47**: 521–526

Bennett PN, John VA, Kendall MJ (eds) Oros drug delivery systems for the β-adrenoceptor antagonists: oxprenolol and metoprolol. *British Journal of Clinical Pharmacology* 1985; **19** (Suppl. 2): 63S–250S.

Black JW, Prichard BNC. Activation and blockade of β-adrenoceptors in common cardiac disorders. *British Medical Bulletin* 1973; **29**: 163–167.

Braunwald E. Mechanism of action of calcium-channel blocking agents. *New England Journal of Medicine* 1982; **307**: 1618–1627.

Breckenridge AM, Davies HC (eds) β-adrenoceptor blocker/drug interactions. *British Journal of Clinical Pharmacology* 1984; **17** (Suppl. 1): 1S–114S.

Brichard G, Zimmerman PE. Verapamil in cardiac dysrhythmias during anaesthesia. *British Journal of Anaesthesia* 1970; **42**: 1005–1072.

Britt BA. Diltiazem. *Canadian Anaesthetists' Society Journal* 1985; **32**: 30–40.

Brogden RN, Todd PA. Disopyramide: a reappraisal of its pharmacodynamic and pharmacokinetic properties, and therapeutic use in cardiac arrhythmias. *Drugs* 1987; **34**: 151–187.

Carson IW, Lyons SM, Shanks RG. Antiarrhythmic drugs. *British Journal of Anaesthesia* 1979; **51**: 659–670.

Castleden CM, George CF. The effect of ageing on the hepatic clearance of propranolol. *British Journal of Clinical Pharmacology* 1979; **7**: 49–54.

Cranefield PF. Action potentials, after potentials and arrhythmias. *Circulation Research* 1977; **41**: 415–423.

Dhalla NS, Pierce GN, Panagia V, Singal PK, Beamish RE. Calcium movements in relation to heart function. *Basic Research in Cardiology* 1982; **77**: 117–139.

DiCarlo FJ. Nitroglycerin revisited: chemistry, biochemistry, interactions. *Drug Metabolism Reviews* 1975; **4**: 1–38

Dominic JA, Bourne DWA, Tan TG, Kirsten EB, McAllister RG. The pharmacology of verapamil. III. Pharmacokinetics in normal subjects after intravenous drug administration. *Journal of Cardiovascular Pharmacology* 1981; **3**: 25–38.

Fabiato A, Fabiato F. Calcium and cardiac excitation–contraction coupling. *Annual Review of Physiology* 1979; **41**: 473–484.

Feely J, de Vane PJ, Maclean D. Beta-blockers and sympathomimetics. *British Medical Journal* 1983; **286**: 1043–1047.

Fleckenstein A. History of calcium antagonists. *Circulation Research* 1983; **52** (Supplement 1): 3–16.

Foex P. Channel blockers. In: Feldman SA, Scurr CF, Paton W (eds) *Drugs in Anaesthesia: Mechanisms of Action.* London: Edward Arnold, 1987; pp. 353–379.

Foex P. The heart and autonomic nervous system. In: Nimmo WS, Smith G (eds) *Anaesthesia.* Oxford: Blackwell Scientific Publications 1989, 115–161.

Freedman SB, Richmond DR, Ashley JJ, Kelley DT. Verapamil kinetics in normal subjects and patients with coronary artery spasm. *Clinical Pharmacology and Therapeutics* 1981; **30**: 644–652.

Georgopoulos AJ, Markis A, Georgiadis H. Therapeutische Studien mit Nitroderm-TTS. In: Bussman W-D, Taylor SH (eds) *Nitroderm — Neue Horizonte in der Nitrat-therapie.* Munchen: Medizin-Verlag, 1984; 23–32.

Gibson DG. Pharmacodynamic properties of β-adrenoceptor blocking drugs in man. In: Avery GS (ed.) *Cardiovascular Drugs.* Vol. 2. Sydney: ADIS-Press, 1–39.

Gibson DG, Sowton GE. The use of beta-adrenergic blocking drugs in dysrhythmias. *Progress in Cardiovascular Diseases* 1969; **12**: 16–38.

Gintant GA, Hoffman BF. The role of local anesthetic effects in the actions of antiarrhythmic drugs. In: Strichartz, GR (ed.) *Handbook of Experimental Pharmacology, Vol. 81. Local Anaesthetics.* Berlin: Springer-Verlag, 1987; 213–251.

Gugler R, Bodem G. Single and multiple dose pharmacokinetics of pindolol. *European Journal of Clinical Pharmacology* 1978; **13**: 13–16.

Harrison DC. Current classification of antiarrhythmic drugs as a guide to their rational clinical use. *Drugs* 1986; **31**: 93–95.

Hashimoto T, Shiina A, Toyoka T, Hosoda S, Kondo K. The cardiovascular effects of xamoterol, a β_1-adrenoceptor partial agonist, in healthy volunteers at rest. *British Journal of Clinical Pharmacology* 1986; **21**: 259–265.

Henry PD. Comparative pharmacology of calcium antagonists: nifedipine, verapamil, and diltiazem. *American Journal of Cardiology* 1980; **46**: 1047–1058.

Hess P, Lansman JB, Tsien RW. Different modes of Ca channel gating behaviour favoured by dihydropyridine Ca agonists and antagonists. *Nature* 1984; **311**: 538–544.

Hoffman BF, Cranefield PF. The physiological basis of cardiac arrhythmias. *American Journal of Medicine* 1964; **37**: 670–684.

Hoffman BF, Rosen MR. Cellular mechanisms for cardiac arrhythmias. *Circulation Research* 1981; **49**: 1–15.

Ijzerman AP, Soudijn W. The antiarrhythmic properties of β-adrenoceptor antagonists. *Trends in Pharmacological Sciences* 1989; **10**: 31–36.

Johnsson G, Regardh C-G. Clinical pharmacokinetics of β-adrenoceptor blocking drugs. *Clinical Pharmacokinetics* 1976; **1**: 233–263.

Jones RM. Calcium antagonists. *Anaesthesia* 1984; **39**: 747–749.

Jones RM. Calcium antagonists. In: Atkinson RS, Adams AP (eds) *Recent Advances in Anaesthesia and Analgesia.* London: Churchill Livingstone, 1985; 89–106.

Klein HO, Kaplinsky E. Digitalis and verapamil in atrial fibrillation and flutter. Is verapamil now the preferred agent? *Drugs* 1986; **31**: 185–197.

Krikler DM. A fresh look at cardiac arrhythmias. *Lancet* 1974; **i**: 851–854, 913–918, 974–976, 1034–1037.

McDevitt DG, Brown HC, Carruthers SG, Shanks RG. Influence of intrinsic sympathomimetic activity and cardioselectivity on beta adrenoceptor blockade. *Clinical Pharmacology and Therapeutics* 1977; **21**: 556–566.

Nestico PF, Morganroth J, Horowitz LN. New antiarrhythmic drugs. *Drugs* 1988; **35**: 286–319.

Opie L. The heart. *Physiology, Metabolism, Pharmacology and Therapy.* London: Grune & Stratton; 1986.

Palmer RMJ, Ashton DS. Moncada S. Vascular endothelial cells synthesize nitric oxide from L-arginine. *Nature* 1988; **333**: 664–666.

Palmer RMJ, Rees DD. Ashton DS. Moncada S. L-arginine is the physiological precursor for the formation of nitric oxide in endothelium-dependent relaxation. *Biochemical and Biophysical Research Communications* 1988; **153**: 1251–1256.

Peach MJ, Singer HA, Loeb AL. Mechanisms of endothelium-dependent vascular smooth muscle relaxation. *Biochemical Pharmacology* 1985; **34**: 1867–1874.

Platzer R, Reutemann G, Galleazzi RL. Pharmacokinetics of intravenous isosorbide dinitrate. *Journal of Pharmacokinetics and Biopharmaceutics* 1982; **10**: 575–585.

Prys-Roberts C. Anaesthetic considerations for the patient with coronary artery disease. *British Journal of Anaesthesia* 1988; **61**: 85–96.

Rasmussen H, Barrett PQ. Calcium messenger system: an integrated view. *Physiological Reviews* 1984; **64**: 938–984.

Rees DD, Palmer RMJ, Hodson HF, Moncada S. A specific inhibitor of nitric oxide formation from L-arginine attenuates endothelium-dependent relaxation. *British Journal of Pharmacology* 1989; **96**: 418–424.

Regardh CG. Pharmacokinetics of β-adrenoceptor antagonists. In: Poppers PJ, van Dijk B, van Elzakker AMH (eds) *B-blockade in Anaesthesia.* Rijswijk, The Netherlands: Astra Pharmaceutica, 1980; 29–45.

Reid JL, Prichard BNC, Bridgman KM (eds) Calcium antagonists and their future clinical potential. *British Journal of Clinical Pharmacology* 1986: **21** (Suppl. 2): 93S–204S.

Reiz S, Myocardial ischaemia associated with general anaesthesia. *British Journal of Anaesthesia* 1988; **61**: 68–84.

Richards DA. Prichard BNC (eds) Proceedings of the second symposium on labetalol — March 1979. *British Journal of Clinical Pharmacology* 1979; **8** (Suppl. 2): 85S–244S.

Rotmensch HH, Rotmensch S, Elkayam U. Management of cardiac arrhythmias during pregnancy: current concepts. *Drugs* 1987; **33**: 623–633.

Shand DG. The pharmacokinetics of propranolol: a review. *Postgraduate Medical Journal* 1976; **52**: 22–25.

Singh BN, Jewitt DE. β-adrenoceptor blocking drugs in cardiac arrhythmias. In: Avery GS (ed.) *Cardiovascular Drugs*, Vol. 2. Sydney: ADIS-Press, 119–159.

Sorkin EM, Clissold SP. Nicardipine: a review of its pharmacodynamic and pharmacokinetic properties, and therapeutic efficacy, in the treatment of angina pectoris, hypertension, and related cardiovascular disorders. *Drugs* 1987; **33**: 296–345.

Sowton E, Dajgupta DS, Baker I. Comparative effects of β-adrenergic blocking drugs. *Thorax* 1975; **30**: 9–18.

Taylor SH. α- and β-blockade in angina pectoris. *Drugs* 1984; **28** (Suppl. 2): 69–87.

Thomas GR, Thiemermann C, Walder C, Vane JR. The effects of endothelium-dependent vasodilators on cardiac output and their distribution in the anaesthetized rat: a comparison with sodium nitroprusside. *British Journal of Pharmacology* 1988; **95**: 986–992.

Thompson RH. The clinical use of transdermal delivery-devices with nitroglycerin. *Angiology* 1983; **34**: 23–31.

Turner P, Feely J, Barrett P (eds) Nicardipine: a new calcium antagonist. *British Journal of Clinical Pharmacology* 1986; **22** (Suppl. 3): 191S–352S.

Vaughan Williams EM. Electrophysiological basis for a rational approach to antidysrhythmic drug therapy. *Advances in Drug Research* 1974; **9**: 69–102.

Vaughan Williams EM. Some factors that influence the activity of anti-arrhythmic drugs. *British Heart Journal* 1978; **40** (Suppl.): 52–61.

Weidmann S. Heart: electrophysiology. *Annual Review of Physiology* 1974; **36**: 155–169.

Wit AL, Rosen MR. Pathophysiological mechanisms of cardiac arrhythmias. *American Heart Journal* 1983; **106**: 798–811.

Woosley RL, Rumboldt TZ. Anti-arrhythmic drugs. In: Turner P, Shand DG (eds) *Recent Advances in Clinical Pharmacology*, Vol. 1. Edinburgh: Churchill Livingstone, 1978; 93–122.

Zipes DP, Heger JJ, Prystowski EN. Pathophysiology of arrhythmias: clinical electrophysiology. *American Heart Journal* 1983; **106**: 812–827.

FIFTEEN

Anticoagulants, Antiplatelet Drugs and Fibrinolytic Agents

MECHANISMS OF HAEMOSTASIS AND COAGULATION

Blood coagulation is a complex biological process which is intended to conserve blood volume in the event of vascular injury. Following tissue damage, arterioles contract immediately, and within a short time platelets become bound to collagen in the vessel wall and to each other. This process is stimulated by the release of adenosine diphosphate (ADP) and subsequently thromboxane from the platelets themselves. Local stimulation of the coagulation process is initiated by a lipo-protein released from the vessel wall (tissue thromboplastin — Factor III) and by phospholipids released from platelets. These interact with several components in the plasma (Factors V, VII, X, and calcium ions) to convert a glycoprotein, prothrombin, into the active proteolytic enzyme thrombin. The subsequent action of thrombin on the plasma protein fibrinogen results in the formation of fibrin (two peptide fragments are liberated during this process). Fibrin subsequently forms cross-links with adjacent monomers to produce an insoluble fibrin clot.

A different sequence of events occurs initially when blood is allowed to contact a foreign surface. More than a dozen proteins are involved in a cascading series of proteolytic reactions. Individual factors are considered as proenzymes; they are converted to active enzymes by each preceding action and then catalyse a subsequent reaction.

The two coagulation mechanisms described above are usually distinguished as the *intrinsic system*, in which all the activating factors are present in the circulating plasma, and the *extrinsic system* which is initiated by tissue injury. However, this distinction is largely artificial as there is no clear demarcation between the systems in physiological events. Both systems lead to the formation of the thrombin activating complex (Factor Xa) and then proceed identically. Both pathways, which must be intact for adequate haemostasis, are further illustrated in Fig. 15.1.

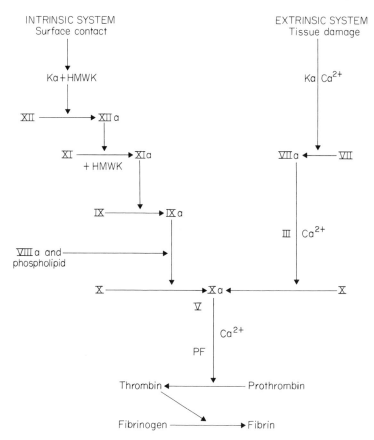

Fig. 15.1 Intrinsic and extrinsic systems of coagulation: the suffix a indicates the activated factor. PF = Platelet factor (phospholipid), Ka = kallikrein, HMWK = high molecular weight kininogen.

DISORDERS OF COAGULATION

Dietary factors

Vitamin K is a dietary constituent which is essential for the synthesis of certain coagulation factors in the liver. This was originally discovered during feeding experiments on chicks in which it was noted that deficiency of an ether-soluble substance caused a bleeding disease. It was subsequently elicited that there are at least two distinct natural forms of vitamin K: vitamin K_1 (phytomenadione), which is found in plants and is the only natural vitamin K available for therapeutic use, and vitamin K_2 (menaquinones), one or more compounds that are synthesized in the alimentary tract by Gram-negative bacteria. Both these types of vitamin K are fat-soluble, and intestinal absorption is dependent on the presence of bile salts in the duodenum.

Vitamin K deficiency may result from inadequacy of dietary intake or intestinal synthesis, failure of absorption or impaired utilization by the liver. The resultant effects will be a reduced availability of prothrombin and Factors VII, IX and X, thus producing a bleeding tendency. Clinical situations in which this can occur include haemorrhagic disease of the newborn, various malabsorption syndromes, obstructive jaundice, biliary fistulae, and cirrhosis of the liver. Phytomenadione (1 mg i.m.) is the treatment of choice in neonatal deficiency; larger doses (>10 mg daily for 3 days preoperatively) should restore prothrombin levels to normal in the jaundiced patient, although if there is severe hepatocellular damage infusion of fresh frozen plasma may be necessary. Vitamin K_3 (menadione) is a synthetic compound which can be converted into a water-soluble derivative; this may be administered orally in order to prevent vitamin K deficiency in malabsorption syndromes.

Hereditary disorders

Haemophilia is the classical example of a sex-linked coagulation defect. There are two types of haemophilia; haemophilia A (classical haemophilia), in which there is a deficiency of Factor VIII (antihaemophilic globulin or AHG) and haemophilia B (Christmas disease) in which there is a deficiency of Factor IX. Von Willebrand's disease is an autosomal dominant trait in which both males and females may be affected. In this condition, there is a deficiency of von Willebrand factor, which acts as a protective carrier for Factor VIII in the circulation and is also involved in platelet adhesion to subendothelium. The haemostatic defect is therefore due to a lowering of Factor VIII as well as a prolonged bleeding time. When such patients require surgery, concentrates of the appropriate factors will need to be administered in the perioperative period.

Thrombogenesis

Thrombogenesis is an altered state of haemostasis which results in the formation of an intravascular thrombus. The classical triad of Virchow implicates changes in the vessel wall, stasis and hypercoagulability as the main precipitating factors. Thrombi can form:

1   In arteries, leading to ischaemic changes in vital tissues or organs.
2   In veins, where there is a high risk of emboli becoming detached and occluding the pulmonary circulation.
3   As intramural deposits in the chambers of the heart, which can lead to embolic complications in systemic vessels.

Thromboembolic disease is a common cause of mortality and morbidity which may have special implications in the postoperative period. Undoubtedly, there are a number of preventable and treatable causes of vessel wall pathology (e.g.

cigarette smoking, hypercholesterolaemia, and other diseases such as essential hypertension) which produce the 'at-risk' patient. Furthermore, the venous stasis induced by prolonged surgery and postoperative immobilization may be remedied by a number of non-pharmacological measures (e.g. careful positioning during surgery, leg exercises, adequate hydration and the use of elasticated stockings).

A hypercoagulable state may be associated with changes which are conducive to thrombosis formation if additional factors, such as stasis, are present. Hyper-coagulability can occur due to changes in coagulation factors, platelets, the fibrinolytic system or physiological inhibitors of haemostasis. Although increased levels of unactivated clotting factors do not increase the rate of fibrin formation, raised concentrations of Factor VIII and fibrinogen are predictive of an increased risk of ischaemic heart disease. Diminished fibrinolysis constitutes a risk factor for venous thrombosis and results from insufficient availability or dysfunction of plasminogen activators, plasminogen (see Fig. 15.3) and fibrin cofactor activity.

Physiological inhibitors of the clotting mechanism include α_2-macroglobulin, α_1-antitrypsin, C1 esterase inhibitor, antithrombin III, protein C and protein S. Congenital deficiencies of antithrombin III, protein C and protein S are characterized by a predisposition to thrombotic disease.

In most cases of this type, the initial episode of venous thrombosis occurs between the ages of 20 and 30, and a precipitating factor can be determined in approximately 50% of these. If surgery is contemplated in such patients, the use of short-term anticoagulation should be considered (if long-term therapy is not already being used). Concentrates of antithrombin III or plasma administered on the day of surgery may also be useful.

There is also an increased risk of thromboembolism in the postoperative period in young women who are taking the contraceptive pill; oestrogens have been shown to accelerate blood clotting and to raise the concentration of some coagulation factors. However the role of factors influencing platelet aggregation may be of more significance. It has been shown that the abnormal coagulatory 'state' may not revert to normal until about 3 months following cessation of oestrogen therapy. The problem is likely to be lessened when the oestrogen content of the oral contraceptive is low. Present opinion suggests that, when such patients present for elective surgery, low-dose heparin regimes should be administered prophylactically. This is preferable to attempts to discontinue medication in the preoperative period.

In the remainder of this chapter drugs which may be used in the prevention and treatment of thromboembolic disorders will be discussed. In general, they can be divided into three groups:

1 Drugs that interfere with the coagulation process (anticoagulant agents).
2 Drugs that inhibit platelet aggregation (antiplatelet or antithrombotic agents).
3 Drugs which promote the dissolution of thrombi (thrombolytic or fibrinolytic agents).

Anticoagulants

Two main types of anticoagulants are used in clinical practice. These are:(1) heparin, and (2) oral anticoagulants.

Heparin

Heparin, as its name implies, is a naturally occurring substance which was originally found in the liver. It can also be obtained in large amounts from mast cells in the lung and intestinal mucosa. Heparin is a mucopolysaccharide containing many sulphate residues, and has a molecular weight of approximately 16 000. The physiological significance of heparin is not clear. It may be released in a macromolecular form from mast cells in the vascular endothelium in anaphylactic shock, and render the blood less coagulable.

Heparin produces immediate effects, both *in vivo* and *in vitro*, but acts indirectly via a cofactor, an α_2-globulin which is present in plasma and known as antithrombin III.

1 In low concentrations, heparin binds to antithrombin III and accelerates its combination with thrombin to form an inactive complex. The activated Stuart factor (Factor Xa), which promotes the conversion of prothrombin to thrombin, may be inhibited by a similar mechanism. These effects form the basis of action of 'low-dose' heparin regimes.

2 When more elevated plasma levels of heparin are achieved, other activated clotting factors (IXa, XIa, XIIa) may also be neutralized. The synthesis of thrombin is thus further suppressed.

3 In high doses, heparin, in combination with antithrombin III, also inhibits the platelet aggregation which can be induced by thrombin.

Heparin also lowers plasma triglyceride levels, and thus reduces plasma turbidity, by releasing a lipoprotein lipase from tissues. The resultant increase in free fatty acid levels which ensues can interfere with the plasma binding of certain drugs (e.g. propranolol, phenytoin) when blood is sampled from cannulae which are intermittently flushed with heparin.

Heparin crosses membranes poorly because of its polarity and large molecular size. It is ineffective when administered orally or sublingually and does not readily traverse the placental and blood–brain barriers. When given as a single intravenous dose, the effect of heparin usually lasts for 4–6 h, although the half-life of the anticoagulant activity does appear to be dependent upon the amount administered. Heparin is metabolized in the liver by the enzyme heparinase, and the metabolites are excreted in the urine. The effects of the anticoagulant may thus be prolonged in renal failure or hepatic cirrhosis.

Heparin has a large number of anionic groups present at physiological pH which are essential for its anticoagulant action. Neutralizing these negatively charged groups with basic substances such as protamine or toluidine blue will rapidly abolish the pharmacological effects of heparin.

Commercial preparations of heparin are normally obtained from bovine and porcine lung tissue. Biological assay is necessary for standardization and the activity is measured in units. The potency of preparations of heparin is usually expressed in terms of $u\,g^{-1}$ and the concentration of solutions as $u\,ml^{-1}$.

As heparin is derived from animal tissue, hypersensitivity responses may be anticipated and are occasionally observed, particularly in those patients with a history of an allergic disorder. Manifestations include fever, urticaria and anaphylactic shock. Thrombocytopenia may also occur. Hypersensitivity responses which occur immediately following the administration of heparin (and may include a mild form of thrombocytopenia) are thought to be anaphylactoid reactions and may involve the 'alternate' complement pathway (see Chapter 5). A more severe form of thrombocytopenia which presents at a later stage is considered to be a cytolytic (Type II hypersensitivity) response. Patients who receive continuous or intermittent therapy with heparin will have a progressive reduction in antithrombin III activity and there is a possibility that a paradoxical increase in the thrombotic tendency may eventually occur. Alopecia and osteoporosis have also been reported after long-term use.

Clinical uses Heparin is used in the prophylaxis and treatment of deep venous thrombosis, pulmonary embolism and myocardial infarction. Therapeutic doses of heparin are used to prevent thrombosis occurring during cardiac and major vascular surgery and during haemodialysis. 'Low-dose' heparin is frequently advocated in the prophylaxis of thromboembolic complications in patients who undergo a wide variety of surgical procedures, particularly those who may be considered at special risk. Important factors include major surgery with prolonged immobilization, obesity, congestive cardiac failure, venous stasis in the lower limbs, and previous thrombotic episodes. Heparin is contraindicated in haemorrhagic states, following recent ophthalmic or neurosurgery, in hypertensive patients with a diastolic pressure greater than 110 mmHg, peptic ulceration or oesophageal varices, and in cases of known hypersensitivity to heparin.

Dose regimes. **1** Standard i.v. regime for the treatment of established thrombosis. Whenever possible, heparin should be administered intravenously and preferably by continuous infusion. A loading dose of 5000 units of heparin sodium is given, followed by $1000-2000\,u\,h^{-1}$. The dose is adjusted to maintain the activated partial thromboplastin time (APTT) between 1.5 and 2.5 times the normal value. In most instances where prolonged anticoagulation is required, oral anticoagulants (*vide infra*) are started at the same time and heparin can be withdrawn after these have achieved their therapeutic effect (this usually takes a minimum of 3 days). **2** Alternative regimes when i.v. administration is not feasible or oral anticoagulants are contraindicated (e.g. pregnancy).

In these instances heparin can be given by the subcutaneous route using a high concentration preparation ($25\,000$ u· ml^{-1}). It is recommended that such injections are given into the anterolateral wall of the abdomen adjacent to the iliac crest or thigh. An initial dose of $10\,000–20\,000$ u 12-hourly is administered and adjusted daily by laboratory monitoring.

3 Prophylactic regimes in 'high-risk' surgical patients. In these circumstances, heparin is usually administered subcutaneously. A dose of 5000 u is given 2 h before operation and repeated at 8–12-hourly intervals for 7 days, or until the patient is mobile. When subcutaneous routes are employed calcium heparin preparations, which are thought to produce less haematomata at tissue injection sites, are often preferred. Laboratory monitoring of clotting activity is not necessary with low-dose regimes.

4 Anticoagulation during surgical procedures. It is essential that anticoagulants are administered before cardiopulmonary bypass is commenced. The usual recommended dose is 300 u kg^{-1} given 4 min before the insertion of the cannulae. Further increments (50–100 u kg^{-1} for each hour of bypass) may be necessary; an *in vitro* test of coagulation, such as the activated clotting time (ACT), performed in theatre is helpful. A value approximately three times the control is desirable. Heparinization is also required prior to aortic clamping during peripheral vascular surgery. A dose of 150 u kg^{-1} is used initially and again measurement of the ACT in the operating theatre is of value in verifying control and the need for subsequent dosage.

Heparin may also be of value in the treatment of disseminated intravascular coagulation (DIC). This condition is commonly associated with the introduction of thromboplastic material into the circulation and can occur following obstetric accidents, major trauma, severe infections, neoplastic disorders and liver failure. The widespread development of thrombi will consume clotting factors; fibrin degradation products are also liberated, the circulating blood becomes incoagulable and a haemorrhagic diathesis will ensue. Heparin may arrest the coagulation process by allowing the accumulation of clotting factors and lead to cessation of bleeding. However the bleeding tendency may actually worsen; infusions of fresh whole blood or plasma and concentrates of platelets and other coagulation factors will also be necessary, inhibitors of fibrinolysis (*vide infra*) may be indicated and in some cases reversal of the effects of heparin by protamine will be required. In this context, the use of heparin is now usually restricted to the treatment of incompatible blood transfusion and the early stages of amniotic fluid embolism, and as induction therapy for acute promyelocytic leukaemia.

Protamine

Protamine is a highly basic compound which will rapidly neutralize the effects of heparin. Protamine is commercially available as a sulphate salt which is always administered by the intravenous route; slow rates of injection are employed in order to reduce the likelihood of anaphylactoid reactions. The dose required will depend on the time at which the heparin has been given previously but should not exceed 1 mg per 80–100 u of heparin (to a maximum dose of 50 mg). Overdosage may exacerbate any bleeding problems as protamine is itself a weak anticoagulant which can inhibit the formation and activity of thromboplastin.

Oral anticoagulants

Oral anticoagulants were eventually introduced into clinical practice following the accidental discovery that cattle fed on a spoiled sweet clover silage developed a haemorrhagic disorder. The cause was traced to a severe reduction in plasma prothrombin, and it was shown that the defect could be prevented by adding alfalfa, which is a rich source of vitamin K, to the diet. The haemorrhagic agent which was present in the silage was subsequently identified as dicoumarol. Dicoumarol was first used clinically as an anticoagulant in 1941. A racemic analogue, warfarin sodium, which was originally utilized as a rat poison and considered to be too toxic for use in man, is now the drug of choice. A related group of compounds, the indanediones, are more likely to cause hypersensitivity responses than the coumarins.

Oral anticoagulants antagonize the action of vitamin K, which is involved in the synthesis of prothrombin and of Factors VII, IX, and X. The precursors of these clotting factors, which are produced in the liver and appear in the plasma, have antigenic properties but are biologically inactive. Their subsequent activation requires carboxylation of glutamic acid residues on the molecule; the resultant products can then chelate calcium (which allows them to bind to phospholipid membranes and produce their coagulant effects).

Carboxylation of the inactive precursors is coupled to the conversion of vitamin K from the reduced (hydroquinone) to the oxidized (epoxide) form. Subsequent regeneration (and thus further availability) of the hydroquinone requires the presence of a cofactor, NADH (the reduced form of nicotinamide adenine dinucleotide) and an enzyme, diaphorase (epoxide reductase). This latter reaction is considered to be inhibited by the oral anticoagulants (Fig. 15.2).

Oral anticoagulants will be without influence on previously activated clotting factors and thus be ineffective *in vitro*. Furthermore, their activity *in vivo* will be delayed whilst these circulating factors are removed from the plasma. The elimination half-lives of the various factors range from 5 to 60 h. The therapeutic effect of the initial dose will thus be delayed for up to 12 h, whilst the maximal required response may take 48 to 72 h to develop.

Warfarin is rapidly and completely absorbed from the gastrointestinal tract and peak plasma concentrations are achieved within 1 h. Warfarin is almost completely bound (95–98%) to plasma proteins. Diffusion across various mem-

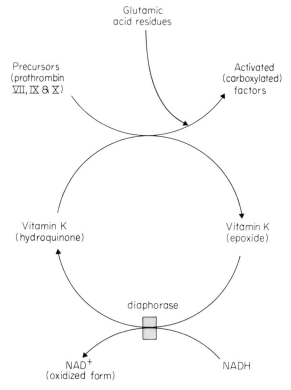

Fig. 15.2   The mode of action of vitamin K and its modification by oral anticoagulants. ▢ indicates the principal site of action of warfarin and related compounds.

brane barriers (e.g. blood–brain barrier, placenta, glomerular membrane) is thus largely, but not completely, restricted and the volume of distribution (0.1 litre kg^{-1}) reflects the volume of the vascular bed. The elimination half-life of warfarin is normally about 35 h; the isomers undergo both oxidative and reductive metabolism and subsequently form glucuronide conjugates which are excreted in the urine.

Considerable variability may be observed in the response to oral anticoagulants, and three factors may be implicated:
1   The availability of vitamin K and the various clotting factors.
2   Pharmacogenetic differences.
3   The influence of other drugs administered concurrently.

Availability. Any condition which reduces the availability of vitamin K (e.g. dietary deficiency, decreased synthesis or absorption in the gastrointestinal tract) will enhance the response to oral anticoagulants. Similarly, patients with liver disease will exhibit augmented effects, presumably due to impaired synthesis of the various clotting factors. Biotransformation of the vitamin K-dependent clotting factors is considerably influenced by the metabolic rate; thus the response to oral anticoagulants is decreased in myxoedema but enhanced in fever and hyperthyroidism.

Pharmacogenetic differences. Resistance to the effects of oral anticoagulants in some instances appears to be due to hereditary factors. The mechanism of action in these circumstances is unclear. Genetic variations in a suppressor substance which inhibits the synthesis of clotting factors, or the development of resistant forms of the enzyme diaphorase (epoxide reductase) which reduces vitamin K epoxide to its active form, have both been suggested.

The influence of other drugs. Oral anticoagulants may be involved in a number of drug interactions which can have serious clinical consequences. Aspirin and most NSAIDs will enhance the pharmacological effects of oral anticoagulants. Even a single dose of aspirin will reduce platelet aggregation, prolong bleeding time and impair haemostasis, whilst larger doses will inhibit prothrombin synthesis and decrease plasma levels. In addition to these mechanisms phenylbutazone and related compounds will potentiate the anticoagulant effects by displacing warfarin from plasma-binding sites and by inhibiting the metabolism of the drug.

A number of other drugs can also prolong and enhance the response to oral anticoagulants and increase the likelihood of bleeding. In most instances competition for protein binding sites and metabolizing enzymes appears to be implicated. Drugs in this category include cimetidine, chloramphenicol, disulfiram, metronidazole and ketoconazole. Alcohol may prolong the clearance of warfarin.

Drugs with significant enzyme inducing activity (e.g. barbiturates, dichloralphenazone, rifampicin and oral contraceptives) will stimulate the metabolism of oral anticoagulants and thus increase the dose requirement if these drugs are being used concomitantly. When the administration of the inducing agent is stopped the activity of the anticoagulant is increased, and dangerous or fatal haemorrhage may occur if the dosage is not adjusted accordingly.

Oral anticoagulants are used in the prophylaxis and treatment of deep venous thrombosis, pulmonary embolism, transient ischaemic attacks and in the management of poorly controlled atrial fibrillation. They are also used to prevent the deposition of thrombi on prosthetic heart valves and vascular grafts. When oral anticoagulant therapy is instituted, a baseline prothrombin time should be determined. The usual induction dose of warfarin is 10 mg daily for 3 days but this should be reduced in small or elderly subjects, in patients with liver disease or cardiac failure, or if the control prothrombin time is prolonged. The aim of treatment is to increase the prothrombin time so that the international normalized ratio (INR) is maintained between 2 and 4.5. In the treatment of deep vein thrombosis, pulmonary embolism and transient ischaemic attacks, the ratio should be maintained between 2 and 3. However, in the management of recurrent deep vein thrombosis or pulmonary embolism, arterial grafts and cardiac prosthetic valves, a higher level (INR 3–4.5) is necessary. The maintenance dose will thus depend on the laboratory results desired and achieved; the INR should be determined on the second and third days of treatment and subsequently on alternate days until a stable level is achieved. As previously mentioned, heparin must be administered simultaneously until the therapeutic effects of the oral anticoagulant have been achieved.

When surgery is contemplated on patients receiving oral anticoagulants the INR should be measured. A level not greater than 2 is acceptable (and may even be desirable) as prophylaxis against further thrombotic episodes. However, the problems of perioperative control of warfarin levels due to surgical interference, and possible interactions with drugs which are administered during anaesthesia, suggest that in most cases a low-dose heparin regime should be substituted. When the INR is greater than 2, management will depend upon the urgency of the surgery and the need for anticoagulant control. An acceptable prothrombin level may be attained by withholding warfarin therapy for a day or two. If this cannot be achieved because of surgical necessity vitamin K_1 (phytomenadione) may be administered by i.v. injection. It is preferable to use a small dose (say 1 mg) to bring about a partial correction of the INR ratio as subsequent anticoagulation may be difficult. Alternatively, the infusion of fresh frozen plasma (FFP) is more rapidly effective in correcting the coagulation defect.

Absolute or relative overdosage of oral anticoagulants can lead to frank haemorrhage. Bleeding may occur at various sites, including the gastrointestinal tract, lung, central nervous system and skin. In these circumstances, the administration of fresh frozen plasma or the various clotting factors is necessary and the cause must be investigated. In addition, phytomenadione is given in a dose of 2.5–10 mg by slow intravenous injection.

Antiplatelet drugs

Drugs in this group will exert their effects by inhibiting platelet function. Platelets have long been known to play an important role in the production of arterial thrombi in patients with pre-existing vascular damage due to atheroma; there is some evidence to suggest that platelets may be involved in the process of atherogenesis itself. However, the role of platelets in the production of venous thrombi is less clear. Thus the principal indication for the use of antiplatelet agents is the prevention or management of thromboembolic episodes which originate on the arterial side of the circulation. These will include prophylaxis following cardiac or arterial surgery, the prevention and treatment of cerebral ischaemia or myocardial infarction and the inhibition of thrombus formation in haemodialysis equipment or in pump oxygenators. Accelerated atherosclerosis in

coronary arteries after heart transplantation and small vessel occlusion in trans-
planted kidneys have been attributed to immune-mediated endothelial injury and
may also be preventable by antiplatelet drugs.

Aspirin

Aspirin exerts an antiplatelet effect by acetylating and irreversibly inhibiting
platelet cyclo-oxygenase. This enzyme promotes the synthesis of thromboxane A_2
(TXA_2), a potent vasoconstrictor (which also induces platelet aggregation by
promoting the release of ADP). The production by vascular endothelium of
prostacyclin (PGI_2), an autacoid whose biological effects are diametrically opposed to those of thromboxane, is similarly inhibited by aspirin. However, both
clinical and experimental evidence suggests that the overall effect is a reduction in
platelet aggregation, as the inhibition of cyclo-oxygenase present in the vascular
endothelium appears to be much less sensitive to aspirin than the platelet enzyme.

A large number of studies have been undertaken to assess the long-term effect
of variable doses of aspirin (from 75 to 325 mg daily) in the prevention of primary
and secondary myocardial infarction or cerebral ischaemia. Encouraging results
have been obtained in reducing the frequency of transient ischaemic attacks and
the incidence of strokes in male patients. Aspirin also appears to reduce the
incidence of myocardial infarction in patients with unstable angina.

There is some evidence that the perioperative use of aspirin can reduce the
incidence of thromboembolic phenomena following certain surgical procedures.
In particular, an impressive and statistically significant reduction of these complications has been demonstrated after hip replacement surgery in male patients
pretreated with aspirin.

Dipyridamole

Dipyridamole is a drug which has many similar effects to those of papaverine, and
was originally introduced into clinical practice for the treatment of angina. It is a
potent coronary vasodilator, but apparently has little effect on vascular resistance
and is therefore no longer used for this purpose. Dipyridamole appears to reduce
platelet aggregation by two mechanisms:
1 Reversible inhibition of phosphodiesterase enzyme activity in platelets occurs. The resultant increase in cAMP levels may impair platelet aggregation by
sequestrating calcium ions in the cytosol and inhibiting phospholipase activity.
2 Uptake of adenosine into erythrocytes is blocked by dipyridamole. The
increased plasma concentration of adenosine may then reach a level at which
ADP-induced platelet aggregation is inhibited.

Dipyridamole is used with oral anticoagulants to prevent thrombus formation
on prosthetic heart valves, or independently as a prophylactic measure against

transient ischaemic attacks. The drug is administered orally in 3–4 divided doses before food; the daily requirement is usually 300–600 mg. Side-effects include throbbing headache and postural hypotension. Dipyridamole can potentiate the effects of oral anticoagulants and special care must be taken in monitoring prothrombin activity when these drugs are used in combination.

Sulphinpyrazone

Sulphinpyrazone is a uricosuric agent which is used in the treatment of gout to prevent tubular reabsorption of urates. It has also been shown to be a reversible inhibitor of prostaglandin synthetase (cyclo-oxygenase) and to impair platelet aggregation. Initial studies suggested that long-term treatment with this drug significantly reduced the incidence of myocardial reinfarction, but these have not been substantiated. Sulphinpyrazone may potentiate the effects of oral anti-coagulants, oral hypoglycaemic agents and phenytoin.

A number of other drugs have been in vogue at various times for their antiplatelet effect, and have been used either alone or in combination for the prophylaxis of deep venous thrombosis, particularly in the perioperative period. These include the antimalarial agent hydroxychloroquine, the lipid-lowering agent clofibrate, biguanide hypoglycaemic agents and certain anabolic steroids. In many cases the underlying mechanism of action is obscure and the likelihood of undesirable effects or drug interactions high. They can no longer be recommended in this context.

Dazoxiben

Dazoxiben is a drug which has been shown to selectively inhibit synthesis of thromboxane (TXA_2) *in vitro*. However, it does not appear to reduce platelet aggregation unless used in combination with low doses of aspirin, and has not as yet been introduced into clinical practice in the UK.

Ticlopinide

Ticlopinide appears to inhibit platelet aggregation independently of any effect on prostaglandin synthesis and has undergone clinical trials in the USA. It may be useful to prevent thrombus formation in heart–lung bypass machines.

Low molecular weight dextrans

Dextrans, which are sometimes used as plasma expanders, are polysaccharides which contain long chains of glucose units and are produced by fermentation of a sucrose medium with the bacterium *Leuconostoc mesenteroides*. These glucose polymers have molecular weights which range from 10 000 to 50 000 daltons and a number of preparations are commercially available.

Dextran 40 is prepared as a 10% solution in either 5% glucose or 0.9% saline. The resulting compound contains glucans with an average molecular weight of 40 000 daltons and has a slightly higher osmotic pressure than that due to plasma proteins.

Dextran 70 is produced as a 6% solution in either isotonic saline or dextrose; the average molecular weight of the contained glucans is of the order of 70 000 daltons and the osmotic pressure of the solution equates with that of plasma.

When added to blood *in vitro*, dextrans appear to have no effect on platelet function. However, following the infusion of these solutions bleeding time may be prolonged, polymerization of fibrin impaired and platelet function reduced. Thus in addition to their use as plasma substitutes to maintain blood volume in hypovolaemic shock, dextrans are sometimes administered in the prophylaxis of thromboembolic complications following surgical procedures. Furthermore, the infusion of Dextran 40 can reduce the viscosity of plasma and the intravascular agglutination of erythrocytes and may be indicated to enhance peripheral flow in small blood vessels.

The administration of dextrans is not without possible hazards. Overloading of the circulation may be especially dangerous in patients with pre-existing cardiac or renal disease. Anaphylactoid reactions which may manifest as urticaria, bronchospasm or hypotension may occur occasionally, and hypersensitivity responses observed in unconscious subjects are considered to be more extensive. Dextrans with higher molecular weights induce erythrocyte aggregation into rouleaux formation and increase the sedimentation rate; they may also interfere with blood grouping and cross-matching and certain biochemical tests.

Other colloidal volume expanders such as hydroxyethyl starch and urea-bridged gelatin (Haemaccel) may also diminish platelet aggregation to some extent.

Epoprostenol

Epoprostenol (prostacyclin) is a naturally occurring prostaglandin which is produced by the intima of blood vessels. It is a potent vasodilator and produces dose-related inhibitory effects on platelet aggregation. Epoprostenol is now commercially available and is used as an alternative to heparin during renal dialysis. The plasma half-life of this agent is only about 3 min, so that it must be given by continuous intravenous infusion, usually at a rate of 5 ng kg^{-1} min^{-1}.

Side-effects include flushing, headache, and hypotension, whilst bradycardia, pallor, and sweating may occur with higher doses.

Fibrinolytic agents

When the clotting mechanism is activated an opposing process, the fibrinolytic system, is also initiated by tissue damage and results in the formation of a proteolytic enzyme (plasmin) which breaks down fibrin with subsequent dissolution of the clot. Plasmin itself is not normally present in the circulation but exists as an inactive precursor, plasminogen, contained in the α_2-globulin fraction of plasma protein. The conversion of plasminogen to plasmin results from the effects of tissue-bound plasminogen activators which are released from the endothelium of damaged blood vessels, e.g. the active form of the Hageman Factor (Factor XII), and from similar substances present in the circulation. The rate of fibrinolysis is normally controlled by antiplasmins which are also present in the

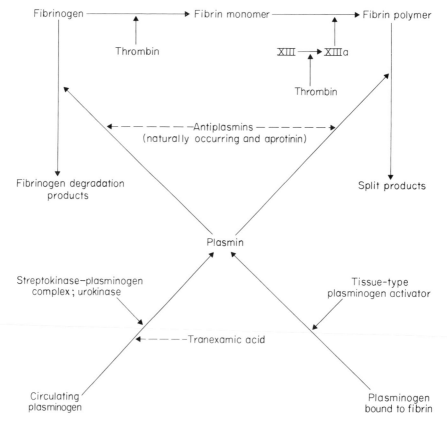

Fig. 15.3 The fibrinolytic system. ⟶ stimulatory processes. – – ⟶ inhibitory effects.

plasma and may be released from the platelets. The principal steps involved in the fibrinolytic process are shown in Fig. 15.3.

Plasminogen activators are also produced at a number of other tissue sites and can be recovered from various secretions such as urine, milk, tears and sweat where they may play a normal physiological role in preventing fibrin deposition in the ducts. One such substance, urokinase, was originally identified in human urine in 1885 and later prepared from cultures of human renal cells; a related compound, streptokinase, was obtained from group C haemolytic streptococci in 1945. Both of these agents have subsequently been introduced into clinical practice for the treatment of widespread venous thrombosis associated with pulmonary embolism, the management of myocardial infarction and for localized thrombolytic effects.

Urokinase

Urokinase is a globulin which directly converts plasminogen to plasmin in a two-stage reaction. It has been used in clinical trials for the treatment of pulmonary embolism, but the resultant systemic bleeding disorders have precluded its more generalized use. Urokinase is currently recommended for its local thrombolytic effects and may be instilled into an AV shunt to lyse a clot, or irrigated into the anterior or vitreous chambers of the eye in the treatment of refractory thrombi. In these circumstances a dose range of 5000–25 000 iu is used and haematological monitoring is not required. More recently, the use of genetic technology has led to the production of recombinant pro-urokinase or single-chain urokinase plasminogen activator (rscu-PA); this has undergone trials in the treatment of acute myocardial infarction.

Streptokinase

Streptokinase forms a complex with plasminogen and this complex is rapidly converted to plasmin. Streptokinase can be administered by intravenous infusion in the treatment of major thromboembolic disorders. Anticoagulant therapy should be withdrawn, a loading dose of 250 000–600 000 iu administered into a peripheral vein over 30–60 min and therapy maintained for up to 72 h, using a dose of 100 000 iu hourly. Haematological monitoring, including estimations of thrombin and prothrombin times, haematocrit and platelet levels is necessary before commencing treatment and during infusion. Following this regime, and when the thrombin time has returned to a value of less than twice the normal, heparin should be administered (preferably by continuous infusion) to prevent recurrent thrombosis.

Streptokinase is antigenic and may produce drug fever, allergic manifestations and overt anaphylaxis. The incidence of such side-effects is reduced by the use of slow infusion rates and the administration of prophylactic steroids. Treatment of major hypersensitivity responses may involve the use of adrenaline and both H_1 and H_2-receptor antagonists.

Streptokinase has also been administered locally in the treatment of myocardial infarction. Therapy is ideally given within 6 h following the onset of symptoms. Standard techniques for selective coronary angiography by either the brachial or femoral approach are used to identify the presence and location of the thrombus. In these circumstances a bolus dose of up to 250 000 iu is administered, followed by a continuous infusion of 4000 iu min^{-1} for up to 75 min until vessel patency is restored. Subsequent heparin therapy will again be necessary.

Intracoronary administration of streptokinase is a highly skilled and potentially hazardous procedure, which of necessity must be restricted to regional cardiology centres and other highly specialized units. Intravenous therapy with streptokinase involves a simpler and easily performed regime, although there is some evidence that recanalization of the occluded vessel is less likely with this method. Furthermore, there is theoretically an increased risk of bleeding complications due to a greater availability of plasmin in the systemic circulation. One attempt to circumvent this problem has been the use of improved drug-delivery systems for streptokinase.

APSAC (anisoylated plasminogen–streptokinase activator complex) is a compound in which streptokinase forms a complex with an acylated (and thus a temporarily inactivated) form of plasminogen. Following i.v. injection of APSAC, deacylation to the activated form of plasminogen occurs by hydrolysis. The half-life of this deacylation process is approximately 40 min and it is considered that APSAC is relatively well protected during its passage in the circulation to sites of recent thrombosis, where it acts preferentially on clot fibrin, whilst less systemic fibrinolysis occurs.

An alternative approach to more selective 'targeting' of fibrinolytic therapy is in the development of tissue type plasminogen activator (t-PA) for clinical use. t-PA has a much lower affinity for circulating plasminogen than for that which is bound to fibrin. Thus very little plasmin is produced in the general circulation, even at high plasma concentrations of t-PA. This activator has been purified from cultured human melanoma cells and an identical material (rt-PA) reproduced using recombinant DNA techniques. However it is as yet unclear whether APSAC or rt-PA produces a greater long-term benefit or a reduction in bleeding complications as compared with systemic streptokinase.

Stanozolol is an anabolic steroid with relatively low androgenic activity which can enhance endogenous fibrinolysis by increasing the synthesis and release of plasminogen activator in the vessel wall. Stanozolol is administered daily in a dose of 10 mg orally. Stanozolol is used in the treatment of Behçet's disease, (Raynaud's syndrome associated with systemic sclerosis, and lipodermatosclerosis) and in the management of adhesive arachnoiditis associated with 'failed' disc surgery.

Inhibitors of fibrinolysis

Drugs in this category can inhibit the conversion of plasminogen to plasmin, and in higher doses antagonize the effects of plasmin. They have been used as antidotes for the treatment of overdosage of a fibrinolytic agent. On occasions they have also been administered in the treatment of pathological states associated with hyperfibrinolytic activity, as may occur following obstetric accidents or prostatic surgery, and in the management of haemorrhage in haemophilic disorders.

Aminocaproic acid is a synthetic compound which is structurally related to lysine. It has been used as an oral preparation and also administered intravenously; in the latter case a slow rate of injection is important to avoid hypotension and arrhythmias. It is no longer commercially available in the UK.

Tranexamic acid, a cyclohexyl analogue of aminocaproic acid, is a more potent inhibitor of plasmin and has been used in similar circumstances. The occurrence of renal, hepatic and occasionally cardiac necrotic lesions have been reported following the use of these agents, and these have been attributed to failure of the fibrinolytic system to remove clots which have formed spontaneously. This undoubtedly accounts for the decline in their popularity and availability and they should only be administered, if at all, following expert haematological advice.

Miscellaneous agents

Ancrod is a proteolytic enzyme which has been isolated from the venom of the Malayan pit-viper. Ancrod reduces plasma fibrinogen by promoting the cleavage of fibrin. Microemboli are produced which are rapidly removed from the circulation; fibrinogen is depleted and the blood becomes less coagulable. The effect observed can be considered as a benign and controlled form of disseminated intravascular coagulation. Ancrod has been used on occasions in the prevention and treatment of deep venous thrombosis. The drug can be given by i.m. or i.v. routes; in the latter case a slow rate of infusion is necessary to avoid the rapid release of fibrin degradation products. Response can be monitored by observing clot size or by measuring plasma fibrinogen levels. The effects of overdosage can be reversed by a specific antivenom (which is itself antigenic) or by replacement of fibrinogen.

Ethamsylate is sometimes used as a haemostatic agent in the treatment of menorrhagia and to control capillary bleeding during a variety of surgical procedures. Following systemic administration the bleeding time is reduced although platelet levels and clotting factors are unaffected. Ethamsylate is considered to act by improving capillary stability and by promoting the aggregation of platelets. The mechanism of action is unclear but may be related to an inhibitory effect on prostacyclins. The drug is marketed in the UK as Dicynene and is available both in tablet form and as a parenteral preparation. Side-effects are rare but may include headache, nausea and skin rashes; transient falls of blood pressure have been reported following intravenous administration.

Aprotinin is a proteolytic enzyme inhibitor which exerts antiplasmin activity. It has been recommended for the treatment of hyperfibrinolytic states, in particular those associated with malignant disease. Aprotinin is also a kallikrein (trypsin) inhibitor which has been used in the treatment of acute pancreatitis. Aprotinin is always administered by slow i.v. infusion; localized thrombophlebitis has occasionally been associated with its use and severe hypersensitivity responses have occurred.

Desmopressin acetate (also known as DDAVP) is a synthetic analogue of vasopressin which lacks vasoconstrictor activity. It has been used to improve haemostasis in patients with mild haemophilia or von Willebrand's disease; in these conditions it apparently induces the release of the required coagulation factors. Desmopressin has also been employed to shorten the bleeding time in other conditions involving abnormal platelet function (e.g. uraemia, following ingestion of aspirin) and has been used successfully to reduce blood loss following cardiac surgery.

FURTHER READING

Andersen JL, Marshall HW, Askings RW. A randomised trial of intravenous and intracoronary streptokinase in patients with acute myocardial infarction. *Circulation* 1984; **70**: 606–618.

Antiplatelet Trialists Collaboration. Secondary prevention of vascular disease by prolonged antiplatelet treatment. *British Medical Journal* 1988; **296**: 320–331.

Barnett DB. Myocardial ischaemia: progress in drug therapy. *British Journal of Anaesthesia* 1988; **61**: 11–23.

Bentley PG, Kakkar VV, Scully MF *et al.* An objective study of alternative methods of heparin administration. *Thrombosis Research* 1980; **18**: 1977–1987.

Beresford CH. Antithrombin III deficiency. *Blood Reviews* 1988; **2**: 239–250.

British Society of Haematology. *Guidelines on the use and monitoring of heparin therapy: first revision.* 1987: 1–12.

Brown JE, Kitchell BB, Bjornsson TD, Shand DG. The artifactual nature of heparin-induced drug protein-binding alterations. *Clinical Pharmacology and Therapeutics* 1981; **30**: 636–643.

Bull BS, Huse WM, Braven SS, Korpman RA. Heparin therapy during extracorporeal circulation. *Journal of Thoracic and Cardiovascular Surgery* 1975; **69**: 685–689.

Davie EW, Ratnoff OD. Waterfall sequence for intrinsic blood clotting. *Science* 1964; **145**: 1310–1312.

Evarts CM, Feil EJ. Prevention of thromboembolic disease after elective surgery of the hip. *Journal of Bone and Joint Surgery* 1971; **53A**: 1271–1280.

Gallus AS. Antiplatelet drugs: clinical pharmacology and therapeutic use. *Drugs* 1979; **18**: 439–477.

Gallus AS, Goodall KT, Tillet J *et al*. The relative contributions of antithrombin III during heparin treatment and of risk factors, to early recurrence of venous thromboembolism. *Thrombosis Research* 1987, **46**: 539–553.

GISSI. Effectiveness of intravenous thrombolytic therapy in acute myocardial infarction. *Lancet* 1986; **i**: 397–402.

Haagensen R, Steen PA. Perioperative myocardial infarction. *British Journal of Anaesthesia* 1988; **61**: 24–37.

Hambley H, Davidson JF, Walker ID, Menzies T. Prophylactic use of antithrombin concentrate following surgery in congenital antithrombin III deficiency. *Clinical and Laboratory Haematology* 1987; **9**: 27–31.

Hamilton PJ, Stalker AL, Douglas AS. Disseminated intravascular coagulation—a review. *Journal of Clinical Pathology* 1978; **31**: 609–619.

Hammond EC, Garfunkel L. Aspirin and coronary heart disease: findings of a prospective study. *British Medical Journal* 1975; **2**: 269–271.

Harris WH, Saltzman EW, Athanasoulis CA, Waltman AC, Baum S, De Sanctis RW. Comparison of warfarin, low-molecular-weight dextran, aspirin and subcutaneous heparin in prevention of venous thrombo-embolism following total hip replacement. *Journal of Bone and Joint Surgery* 1974; **56A**: 1552–1562.

Harris WH, Saltzman EW, Athanasoulis CA, Waltman AC, de Sanctis RW. Aspirin prophylaxis of venous thrombo-embolism after total hip replacement. *New England Journal of Medicine* 1977; **297**: 1246–1249.

Hennekens CH, Peto R, Hutchinson GB, Doll R. An overview of the British and American aspirin studies. *New England Journal of Medicine* 1988; **318**: 923–924.

Howell WH. Heparin, an anticoagulant. Preliminary communication. *American Journal of Physiology* 1922; **63**: 434–435.

Hull R, Hirsh J, Jay R *et al*. Different intensities of oral anticoagulant therapy in the treatment of proximal vein thrombosis. *New England Journal of Medicine* 1982; **307**: 1676–1681.

Ikram S, Lewis S, Bucknall C, Sram I, Thomas N, Vincent R, Chamberlain D. Treatment of acute myocardial infarction with anisoylated plasminogen streptokinase activator complex. *British Medical Journal* 1986; **93**: 786–789.

Inman WH, Vessey MP, Westerholm B, Engleund A. Thromboembolism and the steroidal content of oral contraceptives: a report to the Committee of Safety of Drug. *British Medical Journal* 1970; **2**: 203–209.

ISIS-2 Collaborative Group. Randomised trial of intravenous streptokinase, oral aspirin, both or neither among 17187 cases of suspected acute myocardial infarction. *Lancet* 1988; **ii**: 349–360.

Kakkar VV, Scully MF. Thrombolytic therapy. *British Medical Bulletin* 1978; **34**: 191–199.

Kitchens CS. Concept of hypercoagulability: a review of its development, clinical application and recent progress. *Seminars in Thrombosis and Haemostasis* 1985; **11**: 293–315.

Kroll MH, Schafer AL. Biochemical mechanisms of platelet activation. *Blood* 1989; **74**: 1181–1195.

Lewis RJ, Trager WF, Chan KK *et al*. Warfarin. Stereochemical aspects of its metabolism and the interaction with phenylbutazone. *Journal of Clinical Investigation* 1974; **53**: 1607–1617.

Link KP. Discovery of dicumarol and its sequels. *Circulation* 1959; **19**: 97–107.

Ljungstrom K-G. Prophylaxis of postoperative thromboembolism with dextran 70: improvements of efficacy and safety. *Acta Chirugae Scandinavia* 1983; **514**(Suppl.): 1–39.

Loeliger EA. The optimal therapeutic range in oral anticoagulation. History and proposal. *Thrombosis and Haemostasis* 1979; **42**: 1141–1152.

Loscalzo J, Braunwald E. Drug therapy: tissue plasminogen activator. *New England Journal of Medicine* 1988; **319**: 925–931.

McCann RL, Sabiston DC. Current management of venous thromboembolic disease. *British Journal of Surgery* 1989; **76**: 113–114.

Macfarlane RG. An enzyme cascade in the blood clotting mechanism and its function as a biochemical amplifier. *Nature* 1964; **202**: 498–499.

Mannucci PM, Tripodi A. Laboratory screening of inherited thrombotic syndromes. *Thrombosis and Haemostasis* 1987; **57**(3): 247–251.

Marciniak E, Gluckerman JP. Heparin-induced decrease in circulating antithrombin III. *Lancet* 1977; **ii**: 581–584.

Mishler JM. Synthetic plasma volume expanders—their pharmacological safety and clinical efficiency. *Clinics in Haematology* 1984; **13**(1): 75–92.

Morris GK, Mitchell JRA. Warfarin sodium in prevention of deep venous thrombosis and pulmonary embolism in patients with fractured neck of femur. *Lancet* 1976; **ii**: 869–872.

Morris GK, Mitchell JRA. The aetiology of pulmonary embolism and the identification of high risk groups. *British Journal of Hospital Medicine* 1977; **18**: 6–12.

Morris GK, Mitchell JRA. Preventing venous thromboembolism in elderly patients with hip fractures: studies of low dose heparin, dipyridamole, aspirin and flurbiprofen. *British Medical Journal* 1977; **1**: 535–537.

Morris GK, Mitchell JRA. Clinical management of venous thromboembolism. *British Medical Bulletin* 1978; **34**: 169–175.

O'Reilly RA. Vitamin K in hereditary resistance to anticoagulant drugs. *American Journal of Physiology* 1971; **221**: 1327–1330.

O'Reilly RA. Vitamin K and the oral anticoagulant drugs. *Annual Review of Medicine* 1976; **27**: 245–261.

Patrono C, Ciabattoni G, Bradrigani P *et al.* Clinical pharmacology of platelet cyclo-oxygenase inhibitors. *Circulation* 1985; **72**: 1177–1184.

Poller L, Taberner DA, Sandilands DG, Galasko CSB. An evaluation of APTT monitoring of low dose heparin dosage in hip surgery. *Thrombosis and Haemostasis* 1982; **47**: 50–53.

PRIMI Trial Study Group Randomised double-blind trial of recombinant pro-urokinase against streptokinase in acute myocardial infarction. *Lancet* 1989; **ii**: 863–867.

Raskob GE, Carter CJ, Hull RD. Heparin therapy for venous thrombosis and pulmonary embolism. *Blood Reviews* 1989; **2**: 251–258.

Rothermel JE, Wessnger JB, Stinchfield FE. Dextran 40 and thromboembolism in total hip replacement surgery. *Archives of Surgery* 1973; **106**: 135–137.

Salzman EW, Weinstein MJ, Weintrub RM *et al.* Treatment with desmopressin acetate to reduce blood loss after cardiac surgery. *New England Journal of Medicine* 1986; **314**: 1402–1406.

Schatt U, Bershus O, Jaremo J. Blood substitution and complement activation. *Acta Anaesthesiologica Scandinavica* 1987; **31**: 559–566.

Scheinberg P. Heparin anticoagulation. *Stroke* 1989; **20**: 173–174.

Sharnoff JG, DeBlasio G. Prevention of fatal postoperative thromboembolism by heparin prophylaxis. *Lancet* 1970; **i**: 1006–1007.

Thomas DP. Current status of low molecular weight heparin. *Thrombosis and Haemostasis* 1986; **56**: 241–242.

Vessey MP, Doll R. Investigation of relation between use of oral contraceptives and thromboembolic disease: a further report. *British Medical Journal* 1969; **2**: 651–657.

Weiss HJ. Drug therapy. Antiplatelet therapy. *New England Journal of Medicine* 1978; **298**: 1344–1347; 1403–1406.

Weston-Smith S, Revell P, Savidge GF. Thrombophilia. *British Journal of Hospital Medicine* 1989; **41**: 368–371.

SIXTEEN

Corticosteroids and Hypoglycaemic Agents

CORTICOSTEROIDS

Corticosteroids ('glucocorticoids') are drugs based on the steroid nucleus that have complex effects on carbohydrate, protein, and fat metabolism. Naturally occurring corticosteroids, e.g. hydrocortisone (cortisol), are secreted by the zona fasciculata of the adrenal cortex. In addition, a wide range of synthetic compounds with similar actions is available (e.g. prednisone, prednisolone, methylprednisolone, triamcinolone, betamethasone and dexamethasone). Both naturally occurring and synthetic compounds have similar effects.

Pharmacological effects

1   Gluconeogenesis (i.e. the deamination of proteins and amino acids, and their conversion to glycogen) is accelerated and enhanced by corticosteroids. Although this action is of little therapeutic importance, it is responsible for many of the side-effects of corticosteroids. Increased protein breakdown causes retardation of growth, reduction in voluntary muscle mass, thinning and ulceration of the skin and mucosae, increased susceptibility to peptic ulceration, appearance of striae, osteoporosis, vertebral collapse, and a liability to pathological fractures. Hypercalciuria may also occur. Decreased carbohydrate uptake and metabolism can cause hyperglycaemia, glycosuria, and the precipitation of diabetes in predisposed individuals.

2   Corticosteroids tend to cause the generalized atrophy of many lymphoid tissues. In particular, there is a marked decrease in weight and cellular activity in the spleen, the thymus, the tonsils, and lymph nodes. There is also a decrease in the number of circulating lymphocytes (particularly T-lymphocytes). Lymphoid atrophy may cause a reduction in antibody formation, and the effects of corticosteroids on immunoglobulin synthesis (particularly IgE synthesis) may account for their use in Type 1 hypersensitivity. Their anti-allergic properties and their use

491

in many types of autoimmune disease may also be partially related to their effects on antibody formation. In addition, corticosteroids may reduce the immunological competence of T-lymphocytes; consequently, they are widely used as immuno-suppressants after organ transplantation. The actions of corticosteroids on lymphoid tissues and antibody production may be responsible for some of their anti-inflammatory effects.

3 Both acute and chronic inflammatory responses are inhibited by corticosteroids, although the pathological processes that lead to inflammation are not affected or modified. In acute inflammation, corticosteroids decrease tissue transudation and oedema, reduce the diapedesis of polymorphs and macrophages, and prevent the access of immunoglobulins to inflamed tissues. Similar changes may occur in chronic inflammatory diseases. Until recently, the pharmacological basis for the anti-inflammatory effects of corticosteroids was obscure. At one time, it was believed that they caused stabilization of lysosomes in inflammatory cells, pre-venting the release of cathepsins and similar enzymes during inflammation. There was also some evidence that corticosteroids modified the function of microtubules in inflammatory cells. Current evidence suggests that the anti-inflammatory effects of corticosteroids (and possibly some of their other actions) are dependent on their combination with intracellular steroid receptors in target cells. Glucocorticoid receptors are cellular proteins that are mainly associated with nuclear chromatin (although some low-affinity binding sites may also be present in the cytoplasm). The highly lipid-soluble corticosteroids readily diffuse across cellular membranes

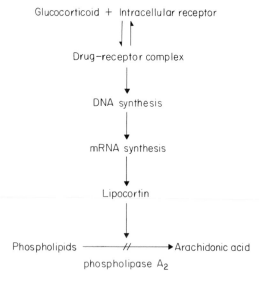

Fig. 16.1 The effects of glucocorticoids on the formation of lipocortin and the synthesis of arachidonic acid by phospholipase A_2. $\nrightarrow$ represents enzyme inhibition.

in inflammatory cells, and are subsequently bound by unoccupied steroid receptors in the nucleus, resulting in the formation of activated steroid–receptor complexes. The activation of these receptors by glucocorticoids modifies DNA and RNA synthesis, and indirectly increases the synthesis of an intracellular glycoprotein (lipocortin). This protein inhibits the enzyme phospholipase A_2, which mediates the conversion of membrane phospholipids to arachidonic acid in inflammatory cells (Fig. 16.1). In this manner, the formation of prostaglandins by target cells is reduced, producing anti-inflammatory effects.

The effects of corticosteroids on inflammatory responses may result in serious side-effects and adverse reactions. The reduction of the inflammatory response modifies resistance to infection, and may lead to the reactivation of latent bacterial infections (e.g. tuberculosis). The symptoms and signs of infection may be suppressed until the condition is advanced. Corticosteroids may also lead to the activation of peptic ulceration, and gastrointestinal haemorrhage or perforation. These effects are probably due to inhibition of prostaglandin synthesis by gastric mucosal cells, leading to decreased mucosal protection.

The anti-inflammatory (and anti-allergic) potency of corticosteroids is extremely variable. Cortisone and hydrocortisone are the least potent steroids in current use. Prednisone and prednisolone are approximately four times more potent than hydrocortisone; methylprednisolone and triamcinolone are slightly more potent than prednisolone. Betamethasone and dexamethasone are the most potent steroids that are currently available; they are approximately 30 times more potent than hydrocortisone (Table 16.1).

4 Corticosteroids also produce indirect or permissive effects, i.e. their presence in the body in physiological concentrations is essential in order for certain

Table 16.1 The relative anti-inflammatory dose and potency of some common corticosteroids. The doses of each drug compared are equivalent to the daily physiological secretion rate of hydrocortisone.

	Equivalent anti-inflammatory dose (mg)	Equivalent anti-inflammatory potency
Cortisone	37.5	0.8
Hydrocortisone	30	1
Prednisone	7.5	4
Prednisolone	7.5	4
Methylprednisolone	6	5
Triamcinolone	6	5
Paramethasone	3	10
Betamethasone	1	30
Dexamethasone	1	30

hormones (e.g. insulin and adrenaline) to produce their actions. Many of the metabolic effects produced by adrenaline are indirectly dependent on the presence of corticosteroids in body fluids. Indeed, the hypotension, vascular collapse, respiratory depression, and delayed recovery associated with general anaesthesia in adrenocortical insufficiency is probably due to the resistance of vascular smooth muscle to adrenaline and other endogenous hormones.

5 Corticosteroids mobilize fats from fat depots and promote their conversion to ketones. In addition, the distribution of fat is altered. Adipose tissue is lost from the limbs, and deposited in the neck, the supraclavicular region, and the trunk. The explanation for these effects is obscure.

6 Finally, some corticosteroids affect electrolyte balance and have actions that are similar to aldosterone. Thus, fludrocortisone (and to a lesser extent, cortisone and hydrocortisone) acts on the distal renal tubule, promoting the retention of sodium and chloride ions (and water) in exchange for the elimination of potassium and hydrogen ions. This type of action ('mineralocorticoid') is present in steroids whose anti-inflammatory potency is weak; the more potent steroids (e.g. prednisone, prednisolone, triamcinolone, betamethasone, and dexamethasone) only have minimal mineralocorticoid activity. They do not cause salt or water retention (except in very large doses). Corticosteroids with significant mineralocorticoid activity may cause oedema and precipitate hypertension or cardiac failure in susceptible patients.

Administration

Corticosteroids may be administered orally, parenterally, or as local therapy (e.g. to the skin, into joints, or to the respiratory tract, ears, or eyes).

Intravenous corticosteroids are most commonly used in emergency situations (e.g. in shock, acute anaphylaxis, and status asthmaticus). High doses can usually be given safely, as the risk of complications is negligible in patients on short-term therapy. Unfortunately, intravenous corticosteroids do not have an immediate action; although they usually begin to act within 1 h, they may take up to 6 h to produce their maximum effects. Intravenous hydrocortisone (100–500 mg) should be given as the sodium succinate salt, which requires reconstitution prior to injection. Although the sodium phosphate salts of hydrocortisone or prednisolone can be given intravenously, they may cause unpleasant side-effects after rapid injection (e.g. generalized vasodilatation and pelvic and perineal discomfort) which may be related to their hydrolysis by phosphatase enzymes.

More commonly, corticosteroids are given orally. Most of these drugs are extensively metabolized by the liver and may be subject to first pass (presystemic) metabolism. Indeed, the effects of both cortisone and prednisone are dependent

Table 16.2 Conditions in which corticosteroids are used systemically in order to suppress pharmacological or pathological processes.

Active chronic hepatitis
Acute anaphylaxis
Bronchial asthma
Bronchospasm
Cerebral oedema
Crohn's disease
Gout
Haemolytic anaemia (acquired)
Malignant conditions (acute leukaemia; non-Hodgkin's lymphoma)
Nephrotic syndrome
Polyarteritis nodosa
Polymyalgia rheumatica
Polymyositis
Rheumatoid arthritis
Rheumatic carditis
Systemic lupus erythematosus
Systemic sclerosis
Temporal arteritis
Thrombocytopenic purpura
Transplantation reactions
Ulcerative colitis

---

on their initial hepatic metabolism (to hydrocortisone and prednisolone respectively). Corticosteroids may be used as replacement therapy (e.g. in Addison's disease, hypopituitarism, or after hypophysectomy or adrenalectomy); in these conditions, oral hydrocortisone, usually supplemented with fludrocortisone, is commonly used. Alternatively, they may be given non-specifically for their anti-inflammatory or antiallergic effects, in order to suppress the manifestations of various diseases. Some of the conditions in which corticosteroids are used are shown in Table 16.2.

Corticosteroids are also given by local application or administration in a wide variety of diseases. For instance, they are widely used in diseases of the skin (e.g. in eczema, lichen planus, discoid lupus erythematosus and neurodermatoses); in diseases of the mouth (oral and perioral ulceration); in ENT diseases (allergic rhinitis and eczematous otitis externa); in ophthalmological conditions (e.g. allergic conjunctivitis, keratitis, and uveitis); in respiratory diseases (e.g. bronchial asthma); and in intestinal conditions (e.g. ulcerative colitis and proctitis). Local preparations of corticosteroids are used whenever possible in order to limit their systemic side-effects. When oral or parenteral preparations are used in the management of rheumatic, inflammatory, or autoimmune diseases, the doses required to control or suppress pathological processes are usually associated with the presence of serious and unavoidable side-effects. Indeed, some of these

Table 16.3 Adverse reactions to systemic corticosteroids.

Causal effects	Reaction
Increased tissue and protein breakdown	Retardation of growth
	Muscle wasting
	Myopathy
	Osteoporosis
	Vertebral collapse
	Fractures
	Thinning of skin, mucosae and hair
	Cutaneous striae
	Ecchymoses and bruising
	Subcutaneous and petechial haemorrhages
	Gastrointestinal bleeding
	Impaired wound healing
Increased carbohydrate turnover	Hyperglycaemia
	Glycosuria
	Diminished carbohydrate tolerance
	Diabetes mellitus
Anti-inflammatory effects	Suppression of normal immunological responses
	Suppression of manifestations of infection
	Diminished resistance to infection
	Reactivation of latent infection
	Peptic ulceration
Salt and water retention	Oedema
	Cardiac failure
	Hypertension
	Hypokalaemia
Abnormal fat deposition	Facial roundness
	Buffalo hump
	Supraclavicular fat deposition
	Truncal obesity
Of uncertain origin	Habituation and dependence
	Euphoria
	Psychoses
	Mental depression
	Acne
	Leucocytosis
	Cataract
	Amenorrhoea
	Peripheral neuropathy

effects may be observed after the use of potent local preparations (particularly when used in the treatment of diseases of the skin). Adverse reactions to systemic corticosteroids are often a limiting factor in their use; although some of these reactions are due to the exaggerated pharmacological effects of steroids, others are obscure in origin (Table 16.3).

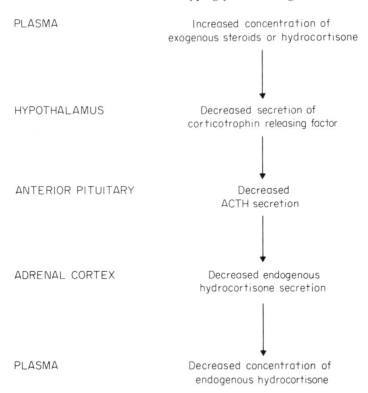

Fig. 16.2   The control of hydrocortisone secretion by the hypothalamic–pituitary–adrenal axis.

Suppression of pituitary–adrenal function

Undoubtedly the most serious long-term complication of corticosteroid therapy is suppression of the hypothalamic–pituitary–adrenal axis. Corticosteroid adminis-tration increases the plasma concentration of hydrocortisone or similar steroids, and suppresses the secretion of corticotrophin-releasing factor by the hypothalamus (Fig. 16.2). This in turn decreases the secretion of ACTH by the anterior pituitary, and reduces the physiological release of hydrocortisone and other corticosteroids by the adrenal gland to negligible levels. Functional suppression of the hypothalamic–pituitary–adrenal axis may be followed by atrophy (particularly of adrenal cortical cells), which persists for a variable time (possibly as long as 3–12 months) after treatment is stopped. In consequence, when patients are stabilized on corticosteroids in doses greater than the normal physiological secretion rate (equivalent to about 30 mg hydrocortisone in 24 h), the abrupt cessation of therapy is dangerous, since pituitary–adrenal function is suppressed and the adrenocortical response to stress may be impaired or defective. It is therefore important to slowly decrease corticosteroid dosage after chronic therapy, so that functional recovery of the hypothalamic–pituitary–adrenal axis may slowly occur. The physiological integrity of the axis can be tested by the morning plasma hydrocortisone concentration or the response to insulin-induced hypo-glycaemia, which normally causes a prompt increase in the physiological secretion of hydrocortisone.

Suppression of the hypothalamic–pituitary–adrenal axis by systemic corti-costeroid therapy can be limited by various methods. These include (1) the use of as low a steroid dose as possible for as short a period as possible; (2) intermittent corticosteroid therapy; (3) the use of a single daily dose, given in the mornings; (4) the use of a double dose on alternate mornings; or (5) the use of ACTH or tetracosactrin.

ACTH (adrenocorticotrophic hormone) is a polypeptide containing 39 amino acids; only part of the molecule (the first 24 amino acids) is identical in all mammalian species and is responsible for the biological effects of the hormone. The remaining amino-acid sequence is not identical in all species (e.g. it is different in man, pigs, and cattle), and is responsible for the immunological specificity of ACTH. The hormone used in man sometimes causes allergic and hypersensitivity reactions. Tetracosactrin only contains the biologically active part of the molecule (i.e. the first 24 amino acids), and hypersensitivity reactions are less likely, although they can occur. Both ACTH and tetracosactrin are available as depot preparations that are complexed with gelatin or zinc, and their action may last for 16–48 h. Although they increase the secretion of hydrocortisone from the adrenal cortex, they suppress the production of corticotrophin-releasing factor and endogenous ACTH. These effects are only occasionally of clinical significance. ACTH and tetracosactrin increase the secretion of endogenous anabolic steroids from the adrenal cortex, and may be less likely to induce muscle atrophy, osteoporosis, and retardation of growth during childhood than corticosteroids. Unfortunately, the adrenocortical response is variable, and the effectiveness of ACTH and tetracosactrin is also variable, since they can only increase the basal secretion of hydrocortisone five to ten times (from 30 mg per day to 150–300 mg per day).

Normal hypothalamic, pituitary, and adrenal function also plays an important role in the metabolic response to surgery. In a normal subject, the response to stress (including surgical operations and dental extraction) is complex; it may be influenced by the extent and nature of the surgical procedure, by drugs used during anaesthesia, and by other factors. One of the important metabolic re-sponses to major surgery is an increase in the endogenous secretion of hydro-cortisone, which may rise from 30 mg per day to 100–300 mg per day in response to operative stress. This response is dependent on the integrity of the hypothalamic–pituitary–adrenal axis. In patients taking the equivalent of 30 mg hydrocortisone (or more) daily, the axis is partially or completely suppressed. Some adrenal suppression may persist for at least 2 months (and possibly for 12 months) after corticosteroid therapy has been slowly reduced and stopped.

The degree of adrenal suppression, and its duration, depends on the dose and the duration of previous steroid therapy. In these conditions, the physiological increase in hydrocortisone secretion normally associated with surgical stress is partially obtunded or absent, and its absence may cause severe hypotension and cardiovascular collapse during surgery. In patients undergoing major surgical procedures, these complications can be prevented by the administration of hydrocortisone (up to 100 mg 8-hourly, by i.m. injection) on the day of surgery. This dose should be given to all patients on corticosteroids (or who have been on corticosteroids during the previous 3 months) on the day of major surgical procedures. Hydrocortisone sodium succinate must also be available during surgery. During the postoperative period, the dosage of steroids can be slowly reduced, and progressively replaced by the normal oral steroid therapy (if any). This process is usually complete by the third to fifth postoperative day. During and after adrenalectomy, a similar regime may be followed, and oral therapy (usually hydrocortisone and fludrocortisone) progressively introduced following surgery.

The use of corticosteroids during minor surgical procedures (or in patients whose steroid therapy has been stopped 3–12 months earlier) is less clearly defined. There is considerable evidence that the use of hydrocortisone on the day of surgery alone (either in three divided doses, or possibly as a single injection) provides ample protection against peripheral vascular collapse. Nevertheless, intravenous steroids should be available during surgery.

HYPOGLYCAEMIC AGENTS

In diabetes mellitus, there is a relative or absolute deficiency of insulin. The disease may be due to the degeneration, destruction, or exhaustion of the β-cells of the islets of Langerhans, to the failure of tissues to respond to circulating insulin, or to the presence or excessive secretion of insulin antagonists (e.g. antibodies, ACTH, hydrocortisone and other corticosteroids, and possibly glucagon and somatostatin). The relative or absolute deficiency of insulin results in defective carbohydrate metabolism, hyperglycaemia, and glycosuria; secondary effects on fat metabolism occur, resulting in the formation of ketone bodies. Protein metabolism is also affected. The aim of the treatment of diabetes mellitus is the correction of the metabolic abnormality and the prevention of complications by the use of hypoglycaemic drugs, which can be divided into three groups:
1 Insulin and its derivatives.
2 Sulphonylureas and related drugs.
3 Biguanides.

Insulin and its derivatives

Insulin is a polypeptide with a molecular weight of approximately 5700. It contains 52 amino-acid residues, in two peptide chains (A and B), which are

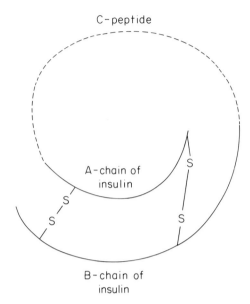

Fig. 16.3 Diagrammatic representation of the structure of pro-insulin. The A-chain and the B-chain of insulin (solid lines) are connected by disulphide bridges; C-peptide (broken line) is released from pro-insulin when it is converted to insulin.

linked by two disulphide bridges (Fig. 16.3). The hormone is synthesized in the form of a larger polypeptide (pro-insulin), in which the A and B chains are linked by a larger fragment (the C-peptide). When insulin is released into the circulation in response to hyperglycaemia, C-peptide is also released and can be measured separately.

Until recently, all the insulin used in the treatment of diabetes was obtained from the pancreas of pigs (porcine insulin) or cattle (bovine insulin), and purified by crystallization. There are minor differences in the amino-acid sequences of these insulins and human insulin; thus, human insulin differs from porcine insulin by one amino acid, and from bovine insulin by three amino acids. In impure preparations of porcine or bovine insulin, both pro-insulin and the C-peptide may be present; subcutaneous injection of these impure crystallized insulins may give rise to localized or generalized insulin allergy, or fat atrophy (lipodystrophy), which can be distressing and disfiguring. These are believed to be immunological reactions, mainly due to species differences between pro-insulins (particularly involving the C-peptide). The occurrence of these complications is minimized by the use of highly purified bovine or porcine insulin; all the pro-insulin and C-peptide in these preparations is removed by gel filtration and ion exchange chromatography. Consequently, almost all insulin preparations of animal origin that are in current clinical use are highly purified, since this minimizes the problems of insulin allergy, lipodystrophy, and insulin resistance (i.e. an insulin requirement of 100–200 units per day).

During the past 10 years, human insulins have been synthesized and used in the treatment of diabetes. These may be prepared semi-synthetically, by the enzymic modification of porcine insulin (enzyme modified porcine or emp insulin); alternatively, they may be made biosynthetically by *Escherichia coli*, using recombinant DNA technology (chain recombinant bacterial or crb insulin). The insulin requirement of diabetic patients is usually reduced (by approximately 10–15%) when bovine insulin is replaced by human insulin; the requirement of patients stabilized on porcine insulin is usually unchanged. Human insulins may be less prone to produce local or general immunological reactions, although all insulins are potentially immunogenic in man. Thus, when insulins are injected subcutaneously, physical changes may occur in solution which enhance their immunogenicity (i.e. dimerization and desamidation).

Insulin lowers blood sugar by activating specific insulin receptors which facilitate the transport of glucose across cellular membranes. Insulin receptors are present in many tissues, and are subject to 'upregulation' and 'down-regulation' by the plasma concentration of insulin. The hormone may also have secondary effects on enzymes concerned with glycogen synthesis. Consequently, the storage of glucose as glycogen in liver and muscle is increased, and glycogenolysis, gluconeogenesis, and ketogenesis are reduced. Insulin also stimulates fat and protein anabolism. Lipogenesis is increased, and lipolysis and the concentration of most plasma lipids is decreased. Protein synthesis from amino acids is enhanced, and there is diminished protein catabolism.

Endogenous insulin secretion is mainly dependent on the concentration of glucose in blood. It is also modified by amino acids, and by drugs that affect α and β-receptors. In the circulation, insulin has a short half-life (4–6 min); it is rapidly broken down by insulinases in the liver and other tissues.

Since insulin is a polypeptide, it is broken down in the gut and must be given by injection (usually subcutaneously, except in the treatment of hyperglycaemic coma and during the perioperative period). Insulin is usually injected into the arms, thighs, or abdomen, and its absorption may be affected by local blood flow; consequently, absorption is increased by physical exercise. It is usually given by needle and syringe, although portable injection devices (pen injectors) which deliver a metered dose are also widely used. Alternatively, soluble insulin can be given by continuous subcutaneous infusion, using a battery operated portable pump. This technique provides a continuous basal infusion of soluble neutral insulin, and also permits supplementary bolus administration before main meals. In spite of its disadvantages, diabetic control and the quality of life may be improved.

Neutral insulin is a buffered solution of soluble insulin (pH = 7.0). It may be prepared from highly purified animal insulins as well as human insulin. After

Table 16.4 Preparations of animal and human insulin in current use. BHP = bovine highly purified insulin; PHP = porcine highly purified insulin; H = human sequence insulin.

Type of preparation	Name of preparation		Subcutaneous injection		
			Onset of action (h)	Maximum activity (h)	Duration of action (h)
Short-acting	Neutral insulin (soluble insulin)	Hypurin neutral (BHP) Velosulin (PHP) Human actrapid (H) Human velosulin (H) Humulin S (H)	0.5	2–4	8
Intermediate-acting	Isophane insulin (NPH)* (isophane protamine insulin injection)	Hypurin isophane (BHP) Insulatard (PHP) Human insulatard (H) Human protaphane (H) Humulin I (H)	3	6–12	18
	Biphasic insulin†	Rapitard MC (BHP) (PHP)	2	5–12	15
	Insulin zinc suspension (amorphous)	Semitard MC (PHP)	2	6–10	15
Long-acting	Insulin zinc suspension (mixed; 30% amorphous + 70% crystalline insulin zinc suspension)	Hypurin lente (BHP) Lentard MC (BHP) (PHP) Human monotard (H) Humulin lente (H)	3	6–15	24
	Insulin zinc suspension (crystalline)	Human ultratard (H)	6	10–24	36
	Protamine zinc insulin	Hypurin protamine zinc (BHP)	5	12–24	36

* Isophane insulin can be combined with neutral (soluble) insulin; two ready mixed preparations of highly purified porcine insulins are available. Similarly, mixed preparations of human insulins may be used.
† Biphasic insulin consists of crystalline bovine in a solution of neutral porcine insulin.

subcutaneous-injection, it usually acts within 30–60 min; its maximum activity is from 2 to 4 h, although it has some activity for 8 h or longer. Human neutral insulin preparations may have a more rapid onset of action, and a shorter duration of action (due to their enhanced aqueous solubility). Neutral insulin may be given intramuscularly and intravenously, as well as subcutaneously, and is the most suitable preparation for diabetic emergencies, and during the perioperative period.

The duration of action of soluble neutral insulin can be prolonged by decreasing the solubility of insulin, and delaying its absorption after subcutaneous injection. This can be achieved by complexing the hormone with various proteins (e.g. protamine), or with zinc alone in specialized conditions (e.g. in insulin zinc suspensions). After subcutaneous injection, the insulin present in these preparations is released and absorbed at varying rates, resulting in preparations with (1) an intermediate onset and long duration of action (maximum activity between 4 and 12 h); or (2) a slower onset and long duration of action (maximum activity between 6 and 24 h). The preparations that are commonly used in the UK are shown in Table 16.4. Preparations with an intermediate duration of action are usually given twice daily; those with a long duration of action are given once daily. In general, they may be mixed with neutral insulin before injection. Protamine zinc insulin should not be mixed with neutral soluble insulin before injection; however, this preparation is only rarely used.

Sulphonylureas

The sulphonylureas lower blood glucose by displacing bound insulin from the β-cells of the islets of Langerhans into the circulation. In experimental conditions, they have been shown to cause degranulation of the β-cells (probably by competing with insulin for intracellular binding sites); they may also increase the number, and cause hyperplasia of functioning β-cells. Some sulphonylureas may also reduce the secretion of glucagon and decrease the activity of hepatic insulinase. Since they mainly act by displacing intracellular insulin, their effects are dependent on the presence of functioning islet cells; they are mainly used in Type 2 (non-insulin-dependent) diabetes. Sulphonylureas are of little value in insulin-dependent diabetes, in patients with ketosis, or in subjects with an insulin requirement of more than 30 u per day.

Many sulphonylureas can cause gastrointestinal side-effects (e.g. nausea, heartburn, anorexia, and diarrhoea), and various hypersensitivity phenomena (skin reactions, cholestatic jaundice, and blood dyscrasias) occasionally occur. The chronic administration of some sulphonylureas (particularly tolbutamide and chlorpropamide) is associated with alcohol intolerance; genetically susceptible patients on these drugs may develop intense facial flushing due to vasodilatation on drinking alcohol. The hypoglycaemic effects of most sulphonylureas may be enhanced by some other drugs (phenylbutazone, salicylates, sulphonamides, probenecid, monoamine oxidase inhibitors, anticoagulants, clofibrate, and β-adrenoceptor antagonists), and antagonized by others (e.g. thiazide diuretics and corticosteroids).

Most sulphonylureas are extensively bound to plasma proteins. They are usually extensively metabolized, with the exception of chlorpropamide; some of their metabolites may possess considerable hypoglycaemic activity (particularly hydroxyhexamide, the main metabolite of acetohexamide). Chlorpropamide is extensively protein-bound, is mainly eliminated unchanged in urine, and has a long half-life. It may produce prolonged hypoglycaemia, particularly in elderly subjects or in patients with renal disease. Drugs that have active metabolites may also have prolonged effects in renal disease.

Some sulphonylureas (e.g. glibenclamide) may produce slight diuresis; others (e.g. chlorpropamide) can have slight antidiuretic effects. Chlorpropamide has been used in the treatment of diabetes insipidus.

Biguanides

Metformin is the only biguanide currently available in the UK; it is a relatively toxic drug, and its use in recent years has declined. It has little effect on blood glucose in normal subjects, although it decreases insulin requirements in diabetes. Metformin is occasionally used in patients with Type 2 (non-insulin-dependent) diabetes who are not adequately controlled by diet and sulphonylurea drugs.

Its mode of action is uncertain. Metformin may decrease carbohydrate absorption from the small intestine, reduce hepatic gluconeogenesis, and increase the peripheral uptake and metabolism of glucose by voluntary muscle. It also affects fat metabolism and lowers the plasma concentration of cholesterol, triglycerides and low-density lipoproteins.

Although metformin frequently produces gastrointestinal side-effects, the most serious hazard associated with its use is the occasional occurrence of lactic acidosis, which often has an insidious onset. Metformin may predispose to this condition by increasing lactate levels in blood, and its use in the elderly, patients with renal or hepatic impairment, or in alcoholic subjects may be particularly dangerous.

The oral hypoglycaemic drugs that are currently available in the UK are shown in Table 16.5.

Hypoglycaemic drugs and general anaesthesia

Surgical procedures in diabetic patients are associated with an increased morbidity and mortality. Diabetic subjects are a high-risk group who are more

Table 16.5 Oral hypoglycaemic drugs in current use.

Drug	Proprietary name	Dose range (mg per day)	Plasma half-life (h)	Elimination
Acetohexamide	Dimelor	250–1500	5	Metabolized to active compounds (hydroxyhexamide)*
Chlorpropamide	Diabinese	100–500	36	Mainly excreted unchanged
Glibenclamide	Daonil	2.5–15	6	Mainly metabolized; some metabolites are active†
	Euglucon			
Glicazide	Diamicron	40–320	11	Extensively metabolized; no active metabolites
Glipizide	Glibenese	2.5–30	3	Extensively metabolized; no active metabolites
	Minodiab			
Gliquidone	Glurenorm	15–120	5	Extensively metabolized; no active metabolites
Tolazanase	Tolanase	100–1000	7	Extensively metabolized
Tolbutamide	Rastinon	250–2000	5	Mainly metabolized to carboxytolbutamide (inactive)
Metformin	Glucophage	500–3000	3	Eliminated unchanged in urine

* Hydroxyhexamide is more active than acetohexamide; its plasma half-life is approximately 6 h.
† Active metabolites are not usually of clinical significance.

likely to develop several postoperative problems, including metabolic and electrolyte abnormalities, cardiovascular sequelae, infection, and delayed wound healing. Management of the disease in the perioperative period is complicated by several factors (e.g. altered calorie intake, the metabolic response to stress, and the effects of procedures and agents that are used during anaesthesia). The metabolic response to stress is particularly difficult to assess, and varies considerably in different patients. Unfortunately, some diabetic patients may not be recognized or detected prior to surgery; the presence of glycosuria should always be excluded (or a fasting blood glucose determined) in all patients before any operative procedure.

In non-diabetic subjects, surgical stress causes a rise in the metabolic rate, changes in carbohydrate, fat and protein metabolism, and the increased urinary elimination of nitrogen, phosphorus, potassium and calcium. The secretion of many pituitary hormones (e.g. ADH, ACTH, GH and prolactin) and adrenal hormones (adrenaline, aldosterone, and hydrocortisone) is increased. Surgical stress also affects the secretion of pancreatic hormones; glucagon levels are increased, and may be raised for several days. By contrast, insulin secretion is normal or decreased during surgery, despite the presence of hyperglycaemia. It is generally accepted that the normal or reduced insulin levels are due to changes in the plasma concentration of endogenous catecholamines (mainly adrenaline). In the postoperative period, insulin secretion rises although hyperglycaemia is sustained (possibly due to enhanced gluconeogenesis). These metabolic changes are related to the extent and duration of surgery. They are slight and unimportant during minor procedures, but are enhanced during major surgery, particularly when complicated by shock or infection.

The management of diabetic patients during anaesthesia and surgery is aimed at the prevention of intraoperative or postoperative hypoglycaemia, and the avoidance of excessive metabolic responses or decompensation. Many regimes have been proposed and used for this purpose, and the management of diabetes during surgery has been a matter of some controversy. Ideally, the use of hypoglycaemic drugs should reflect the physiological changes in insulin secretion that occur during surgical procedures in non-diabetic subjects.

It is generally accepted that patients who are controlled by diet alone, or who are stabilized on low doses of short-acting sulphonylureas, do not require additional therapy during minor surgical procedures. The morning dose of the sulphonylurea should be omitted on the day of surgery, and blood glucose should be frequently measured in order to exclude hypoglycaemia. Small amounts of intravenous glucose may be required preoperatively, depending on the blood glucose concentration. All other patients should be admitted to hospital several days prior to surgery and stabilized on insulin, given two or three times daily. This is particularly important in elderly patients stabilized on chlorpropamide or sulphonylureas with active metabolites (e.g. acetohexamide), when diabetic control is poor, or if major surgery is contemplated. Similarly, metformin should be stopped and changed to insulin before surgery, in order to prevent the possibility of intraoperative hypoglycaemia and lactic acidosis. The aim of these procedures is to ensure that diabetic patients are well controlled, normogly-caemic, non-ketotic, and have adequate glycogen reserves prior to surgery.

In these patients, and in diabetic patients stabilized on insulin who are undergoing surgical procedures, mixed intravenous infusions of glucose, insulin, and potassium salts are widely used during the perioperative period. One common regime is based on the addition of neutral insulin (usually 10 units) and potassium chloride (10 mmol) to 500 ml 10% dextrose, which is then infused at the rate of 100 ml hour^{-1}. This regime can be modified if hyperglycaemia is marked, or if fluid restriction is necessary. Although there is no danger of patients receiving insulin alone, some may be absorbed by glass or by plastic. Alternatively, insulin and dextrose (with potassium chloride) can be separately infused; the rate of insulin infusion (usually 1–3 U hour^{-1}) is controlled by frequent blood glucose determinations. Sufficient potassium is added to maintain its plasma concentration within normal limits (3.5–5.0 mmol litre^{-1}). In the postoperative period, there is commonly an increased insulin requirement (particularly if infection or other complications occur), and a moderate degree of hyperglycaemia is not unusual; frequent monitoring of blood glucose may be needed to prevent the development of decompensation or ketosis. Infusion of intravenous fluids containing glucose, insulin, and potassium salts may be continued for several days, while normal feeding is gradually established. As soon as the patient can take food or fluids orally, normal antidiabetic drug therapy can be resumed.

Emergency surgery (particularly in the uncontrolled or ketotic diabetic patient) presents particular problems; it is generally accepted that ketosis and abnormal fluid balance must be controlled before anaesthesia is induced.

It should be emphasized that the optimum control of diabetic patients during surgery depends on the frequent measurement of blood glucose (and potassium) concentrations. Blood glucose can be rapidly determined on the ward or in theatre by semiquantitative methods (e.g. Dextrostix) which provide a reasonably accurate assessment of the metabolic state. Most authorities consider that the determination of glucose in urine during the perioperative period is an extremely misleading guide, since the blood glucose may be changing rapidly.

Although certain anaesthetics (e.g. ether and cyclopropane) can cause hyperglycaemia, most agents in current use (including nitrous oxide, halothane, enflurane, isoflurane, intravenous barbiturates, opioid analgesics, and all muscle relaxants) have little or no effect on blood glucose. Nevertheless, other drugs that may be used before, during, or after surgery (e.g. β-adrenoceptor antagonists, corticosteroids, adrenaline, diazoxide, ketamine and trimetaphan) may signi-ficantly modify blood glucose levels. β-adrenoceptor antagonists are particularly hazardous, since they may induce hypoglycaemia and obscure all its peripheral clinical signs.

Increased secretion of endogenous adrenaline may cause marked hyperglycaemia in the unpremedicated, nervous, and excitable patient. Similarly, hypoxia and hypercarbia increase adrenaline secretion, and cause a considerable rise in blood glucose concentration.

FURTHER READING

Adams R, Siderius N. Postoperative acute adrenal cortical insufficiency. *Journal of the American Medical Association* 1957; **165**: 41–44.

Alberti KGMM. Diabetic emergencies. *British Medical Bulletin* 1989; **45**: 242–263.

Alberti KGMM, Hockaday TDR. Diabetes mellitus. In: Weatherall DJ, Ledingham JGG, Warrell DA (eds) *Oxford Textbook of Medicine*, 2nd edn. Oxford University Press: Oxford, 1987.

Alberti KGMM, Thomas DJB. The management of diabetes during surgery. *British Journal of Anaesthesia* 1979; **51**: 693–710.

Alieff A. Das Risiko chirurgischer Eingriffe beim Diabetiker. *Zentralblatt für Chirurgie (Leipzig)* 1969; **94**: 857–860.

Allison SP. Changes in insulin secretion during open-heart surgery. *British Journal of Anaesthesia* 1971; **43**: 138–143.

Bayliss RIS. Surgical collapse during and after corticosteroid therapy. *British Medical Journal* 1958; **2**: 935–936.

Beyer HS, Bantle JP, Mariash CN, Steffes MW, Seljeskog EL, Oppenheimer JH. Use of the dexamethasone–adrenocorticotrophin test to assess the requirement for continued glucocorticoid replacement therapy after pituitary surgery. *Journal of Clinical Endocrinology and Metabolism* 1985; **60**: 1012–1018.

Bowen DJ, Daykin AP, Nancekievill ML, Norman J. Insulin-dependent diabetic patients during surgery and labour. *Anaesthesia* 1984; **39**: 407–411.

Bromage PR, Shibata HR, Willoughby HW. Influence of prolonged epidural blockade on blood sugar and cortisol responses to operations on the upper part of the abdomen and thorax. *Surgery, Gynecology and Obstetrics* 1971; **132**: 1051–1056.

Burke CW. Adrenocortical insufficiency. *Clinics in Endocrinology and Metabolism* 1985; **14**: 947–976.

Byyny RL. Management of diabetes during surgery. *Postgraduate Medicine* 1980; **68**: 191–202.

Child CS, Kaufman L. Effect of intrathecal diamorphine on the adrenocortical, hyperglycaemic and cardiovascular responses to major colonic surgery. *British Journal of Anaesthesia* 1985; **57**: 389–393.

Christiansen CL, Schurizek BA, Malling B, Knudsen L, Alberti KGMM, Hermansen K. Insulin treatment of the insulin-dependent diabetic patient undergoing minor surgery — continuous intravenous infusion compared with subcutaneous administration. *Anaesthesia* 1988; **43**: 533–537.

Clarke RSJ. Anaesthesia and carbohydrate metabolism. *British Journal of Anaesthesia* 1973; **45**: 237–243.

Cope CL. The adrenal cortex in internal medicine — Part I. *British Medical Journal* 1966; **2**: 847–853.

Cope CL. *Adrenal Steroids and Disease*. London: Pitman Medical, 1972; 1–883.

Diethelm AG. Surgical management of complications of steroid therapy. *Annals of Surgery* 1977; **185**: 251–263.

Diltoer M, Camu F. Glucose homeostasis and insulin secretion during isoflurane anesthesia in humans. *Anesthesiology* 1988; **68**: 880–886.

Dunnet JM, Holman RR, Turner RC, Sear JW. Diabetes mellitus and anaesthesia — a survey of the peri-operative management of the patient with diabetes mellitus. *Anaesthesia* 1988; **43**: 538–542.

Dunnett SR. Insulin infusion pump. *British Medical Journal* 1985; **291**: 1808–1809.

Dunnett SR. Insulin infusion pump. *British Medical Journal* 1985; **291**: 1808–1809.

Egdahl G. Pituitary–adrenal responses following trauma in the isolated leg. *Surgery* 1959; **46**: 9–21.

Ellenberg M, Rifkin H (eds) *Diabetes Mellitus: Theory and Practice*. New York: Medical Examination Publishing Company, 1983.

Federman DD, Rubenstein E (eds) The adrenal. *Scientific American Medicine* **1**; 1983.

Felig P, Baxter JD, Broadus AE, Frohman LA (eds) *The Adrenal Cortex, Endocrinology and Metabolism*. New York: McGraw-Hill, 1981.

Feiwel M, James VHT, Barnett ES. Effect of potent topical steroids on plasma-cortisol levels of infants and children with eczema. *Lancet* 1969; **1**: 485–487.

Fletcher J, Langman MJS, Kellock TD. Effect of surgery on blood sugar levels in diabetes mellitus. *Lancet* 1965; **2**: 52–54.

Flower RJ. Lipocortin and the mechanism of action of the glucocorticoids. *British Journal of Pharmacology* 1988; **94**: 987–1015.

Fraser CG, Preuss FS, Bigford WD. Adrenal atrophy and irreversible shock associated with cortisone therapy. *Journal of the American Medical Association* 1952; **149**: 1542–1543.

Galloway JA, Shuman CR. Diabetes and surgery. A study of 667 cases. *American Journal of Medicine* 1963; **34**: 177–191.

Gill GV, Alberti KGMM. Surgery and diabetes. *Hospital Update* 1989; **5**: 327–336.

Hall GM. Diabetes and anaesthesia — a promise unfulfilled? *Anaesthesia* 1984; **39**: 627–628.

Hall GM. The anaesthetic modification of the endocrine and metabolic response to surgery. *Annals of the Royal College of Surgeons* 1985; **67**: 25–29.

Hall GM, Desborough JP. Diabetes and anaesthesia — slow progress. *Anaesthesia* 1988; **43**: 531–532.

Halter JB, Pflug AE. Effects of anaesthesia and surgical stress on insulin secretion in man. *Metabolism* 1980; **29**: 1124–1127.

Hertzberg LB, Shulman MS. Acute adrenal insufficiency in a patient with appendicitis during anesthesia. *Anesthesiology* 1985; **62**: 517–519.

Horton JN. Anaesthesia and diabetes. In: WS Nimmo, G Smith (eds) *Anaesthesia*. Oxford: Blackwell Scientific Publications, 1989; 745–758.

James ML. Endocrine disease and anaesthesia: A review of anaesthetic management in pituitary, adrenal and thyroid diseases. *Anaesthesia* 1970; **25**: 232–252.

Jarrett RJ, Keen H. Oral hypoglycaemic drugs. *British Journal of Hospital Medicine* 1974; **11**: 265–267.

Keen H, Jarrett J. Modern management of diabetes. *Medicine* 1978; **11**: 530–536.

Kehlet H. Adrenocortical function and clinical course during and after surgery in unsupplemented glucocorticoid-treated patients. *British Journal of Anaesthesia* 1973; **45**: 1043–1048.

Kehlet H. A rational approach to dosage and preparation of parenteral glucocorticoid substitution therapy during surgical procedures. *Acta Anaesthesiologica Scandinavica* 1975; **19**: 260–264.

Kehlet H, Binder C. Adrenocortical function and clinical course during and after surgery in unsupplemented glucocorticoid-treated patients. *British Journal of Anaesthesia* 1973; **45**: 1043–1048.

King RJB, Mainwaring WIP. *Steroid-Cell Interactions*. London: Butterworths, 1974.

Lacoumenta S, Yeo TH, Burrin JM, Paterson JL, Hall GM. The effects of cortisol supplementation on the metabolic and hormonal response to surgery. *Clinical Physiology* 1987; **7**: 455–464.

Leslie RDG, Mackay JD. Intravenous insulin infusion in diabetic emergencies. *British Medical Journal* 1978; **2**: 1343–1344.

MacKenzie CR, Charlson ME. Assessment of perioperative risk in the patient with diabetes mellitus. *Surgery, Gynecology and Obstetrics* 1988; **167**; 293–299.

Nordenstrom J, Sonnenfeld T, Arner P. Characterization of insulin resistance after surgery. *Surgery* 1989; **105**: 28–35.

Oyama T. Endocrine responses to anaesthetic agents. *British Journal of Anaesthesia* 1973; **45**: 276–281.

Oyama T, Takiguchi M. Prediction of adrenal hypofunction in anaesthesia. *Canadian Anaesthetists*

Society Journal 1972; **19**: 239–249.

Page MMcB, Watkins PJ. Cardiorespiratory arrest and diabetic autonomic neuropathy. *Lancet* 1978; **1**: 14–16.

Plumpton FS, Besser GM, Cole PV. Corticosteroid treatment and surgery. *Anaesthesia* 1969; **24**: 3–18.

Rees GAD, Hayes TM, Pearson JF. Diabetes, pregnancy and anaesthesia. *Clinics in Obstetrics and Gynaecology* 1982; **9**: 311–331.

Ringold GM. Steroid hormone regulation of gene expression. *Annual Review of Pharmacology and Toxicology* 1985; **25**: 529–566.

Salam AA, Davies DM. Acute adrenal insufficiency during surgery. *British Journal of Anaesthesia* 1974; **46**: 619–622.

Salassa RM, Bennett WA, Keating FR, Sprague RG. Postoperative adrenal cortical insufficiency: occurrence in patients previously treated with cortisone. *Journal of the American Medical Association* 1953; **152**: 1509–1515.

Sampson PA, Brooke BN, Winstone NE. Biochemical confirmation of collapse due to adrenal failure. *Lancet* 1961; **1**: 1377.

Sampson PA, Winstone NE, Brooke BN. Adrenal function in surgical patients after steroid therapy. *Lancet* 1962; **2**: 322–325.

Schleimer RP. The mechanisms of anti-inflammatory steroid action in allergic diseases. *Annual Review of Pharmacology and Toxicology* 1985; **25**: 381–412.

Slaney G, Brooke BN. Postoperative collapse due to adrenal insufficiency following cortisone therapy. *Lancet* 1957; **1**: 1167–1170.

Symreng T, Karlberg BE, Kagedal B, Schildt B. Physiological cortisol substitution of long-term steroid-treated patients undergoing major surgery. *British Journal of Anaesthesia* 1981; **53**: 949–959.

Thomas DJB, Platt HS, Alberti KGMM. Insulin-dependent diabetes during the peri-operative period. An assessment of continuous glucose–insulin–potassium infusion, and traditional treatment. *Anaesthesia* 1984; **39**: 629–637.

Uchida I, Asoh T, Shirasaka C, Tsuji H. Effect of epidural analgesia on postoperative insulin resistance as evaluated by insulin clamp technique. *British Journal of Surgery* 1988; **75**: 557–562.

Vandam LD, Moore FD. Adrenocortical mechanisms related to anesthesia. *Anesthesiology* 1960; **21**: 531–552.

Weatherill D. Pituitary and adrenal disease. In: WS Nimmo, G Smith (eds) *Anaesthesia*. Oxford: Blackwell Scientific Publications, 1989; 759–770.

Wright PD, Henderson K, Johnston IDA. Glucose utilisation and insulin secretion during surgery in man. *British Journal of Surgery* 1974; **61**: 5–8.

Glossary

The glossary contains most of the common abbreviations used in the book. The mathematical symbols used in Chapters 2 and 3 are defined separately. Common chemical symbols (e.g. H^+, K^+, Na^+, and Ca^{2+}) have not been included.

Units of length, mass, volume and time

nm	nanometre
m	metre
μm	micrometre (micron)
mm	millimetre
g	gram
kg	kilogram
μg	microgram
mg	milligram
ml	millilitre
h	hour
ms	millisecond
min	minute
s	second

Other abbreviations

AChE	acetylcholinesterase
ACTH	adrenocorticotrophic hormone
ADH	antidiuretic hormone
AMP	adenosine monophosphate
ATP	adenosine triphosphate
AV	atrioventricular
B.P.	British Pharmacopoeia
BP	blood pressure
b.p.m.	beats per minute
ChE	cholinesterase
CNS	central nervous system
COMT	catechol-*O*-methyltransferase

CSF	cerebrospinal fluid
CTZ	chemoreceptor trigger zone
δ-ALA	delta-aminolaevulinic acid
E–C	excitation–contraction
ECG	electrocardiogram
EEG	electroencephalogram
ENT	ear, nose and throat
GABA	γ-aminobutyric acid
GH	growth hormone
GMP	guanosine monophosphate
GTP	guanosine triphosphate
^3H	tritium labelled
Hz	Hertz (a frequency of 1 stimulus per second)
ICP	Intracranial pressure
IgE	immunoglobulin E
IgG	immunoglobulin G
i.m.	intramuscular
iu	international units
i.v.	intravenous
kPa	kilopascals (1 kilopascal = 7.5 mmHg)
LD_{50}	median lethal dose
MAC	minimum alveolar concentration
MHPG	3-methoxy-4-hydroxy-phenylethylene-glycol
MSH	melanocyte stimulating hormone
mV	millivolt

NADPH	reduced nicotinamide adenine dinucleotide phosphate
NSAID	non-steroidal anti-inflammatory drug
$P\text{co}_2$	carbon dioxide tension
$P\text{aco}_2$	carbon dioxide tension in arterial blood
$P\text{ao}_2$	oxygen tension in arterial blood
pH	$-\log_{10}[\text{H}^+]$
pK_a	dissociation constant, negative logarithm of
PAG	periaqueductal grey matter
PG	prostaglandin
PRA	plasma renin activity
RNA	ribonucleic acid
SA	sino-atrial
s.c.	subcutaneous
sp.gr.	specific gravity
$t_{\frac{1}{2}}$	half-life
t.d.s.	thrice daily
u	unit
UDP	uridine diphosphate

V	volume
v/v	volume for volume
VMA	3-methoxy-4-hydroxy-mandelic acid (vanillylmandelic acid)

Greek letters

α	alpha
β	beta
γ	gamma
δ	delta
ε	epsilon
ϰ	kappa
λ	lambda
μ	mu
π	pi
σ	sigma

Symbols

≈	approximately equals
∝	is proportional to
≡	is congruent to

Index

513